Understanding Infection Prevention and Control

Second edition

Shaheen Mehtar

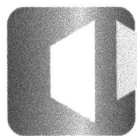

juta

Understanding Infection Prevention and Control

First published 2010
Second impression 2015
Second edition 2023

Juta and Company (Pty) Ltd
First floor, Sunclare building, 21 Dreyer street, Claremont 7708
PO Box 14373, Lansdowne 7779, Cape Town, South Africa
www.juta.co.za

ISBN: 978 1 99896 228 0 (Print)
ISBN: 978 1 48513 076 5 (WebPDF)

Production Specialist: Zainub Gamieldien
Editor: Rod Prodgers
Proofreader and Indexer: Ute Kühlmann
Illustrator: Andre Reinders
Cover designer: Simplicitas Design
Typesetter: Lebone Publishing Services
Typeset in: Chaparral Pro 11.14.3

Contents

Preface xiv

Dedication xv

Author's acknowledgements xv

List of abbreviations xvi

Text acknowledgements xvii

Chapter 1: Infection prevention and control 1

Introduction 1

1.1   Elements of infection prevention and control 3

     1.1.1   Definition 3

     1.1.2   Legislation 3

     1.1.3   Professional bodies 4

1.2   Goals of IPC 5

1.3   The role of IPC programmes 6

1.4   Why the same IPC programme is not universally applicable 6

1.5   IPC and quality improvement 7

     1.5.1   Guidelines 8

     1.5.2   Monitoring and evaluation 8

     1.5.3   Feedback 9

1.6   Types of indicators 9

     1.6.1   Monitoring tools 9

     1.6.2   Effective use of data 10

1.7   Benchmarking 11

     1.7.1   Advantages of benchmarking 11

     1.7.2   Disadvantages of benchmarking 12

1.8   Starting an IPC programme 12

     1.8.1   Aim 12

     1.8.2   Outcome 12

     1.8.3   Structure of IPC programmes 12

     1.8.4   Healthcare facility IPC programme 16

1.9   Community-based IPC programmes 23

1.10   Cost of IPC 23

     1.10.1   Cost of healthcare-associated infections 24

     1.10.2   Cost of setting up an IPC programme 26

1.11 Education in IPC...28
    1.11.1 Introduction...28
    1.11.2 Difference between training and education 29
    1.11.3 Adult teaching methods 30
    1.11.4 Why does adult learning fail?......................................30
    1.11.5 Mentorship...31
    1.11.6 Influences on learning 31
    1.11.7 Teaching methods (IPC) 34
    1.11.8 In-service (on the job) training....................................36
    1.11.9 Practical/demonstration...37
1.12 Know your audience 37
    1.12.1 Healthcare managers 38
    1.12.2 Healthcare workers 39
    1.12.3 Train the Trainers 39
    1.12.4 Link nurses 40
    1.12.5 IPC practitioners...40
    1.12.6 Courses in IPC...41
    1.12.7 Other short courses 43
    1.12.8 Training programmes for community-based structures 44

Chapter 2: Introduction to microbiology 47

Introduction 47
2.1 Micro-organisms...48
2.2 Differences between prokaryotes and eukaryotes............................48
2.3 Bacteria 49
    2.3.1 Classification of bacteria 49
    2.3.2 Staining characteristics 50
    2.3.3 Morphology and growth characteristics..........................50
    2.3.4 Haemolysis 51
    2.3.5 Respiration 51
    2.3.6 Anatomy of a bacterium (Figure 2.1).............................51
    2.3.7 Protection and survival of bacteria................................53
    2.3.8 The growth cycle of bacteria..55
    2.3.9 Other types of bacteria...56
2.4 Viruses..57
    2.4.1 Structure of viruses 57
    2.4.2 Classification of viruses...57
    2.4.3 Transmission of viruses...58
    2.4.4 Replication 59

2.5		Fungi	60
	2.5.1	Morphology of fungi	60
	2.5.2	Reproduction of fungi	61
	2.5.3	Types of fungal infection	61
2.6		Parasites – protozoa and helminths	62
	2.6.1	Classification of parasites	63
2.7		The relationship between pathogen and host	66
	2.7.1	The pathogen	66
2.8		The host	68
	2.8.1	Natural defences	69
	2.8.2	Acquired immunity	70
2.9		Microbes of importance in IPC	71
	2.9.1	Commensal (resident) or normal flora – the microbiome	71
2.10		The microbiome	73
2.11		Healthcare-associated pathogens	74
2.12		Microbiological laboratory and IPC	77
	2.12.1	The laboratory and clinical teams	77
	2.12.2	Taking microbiology samples	78
	2.12.3	The laboratory form	79
	2.12.4	Specimen container	79
	2.12.5	Sampling site	80
	2.12.6	Transportation	81
	2.12.7	Organisms that cannot be cultivated	81
2.13		The laboratory examination process	81
	2.13.1	Registration	81
	2.13.2	The specimen	82
	2.13.3	Interpreting microbiology laboratory results	83
2.14		Antimicrobial tests	84
	2.14.1	Disc sensitivity testing	85
	2.14.2	E-test	85
	2.14.3	Broth microdilution	85
	2.14.4	Automated systems	85
2.15		Laboratory safety	86
	2.15.1	Risk to healthcare workers	86
	2.15.2	Risk-reducing procedures	86
2.16		Antimicrobial agents: Therapy and resistance	86
	2.16.1	Antibacterial agents	87
	2.16.2	Antimicrobial resistance	91
	2.16.3	Mechanisms of antimicrobial resistance	93
	2.16.4	Urinary antiseptics	95

	2.16.5	Anti-tuberculosis drugs	95
	2.16.6	Antifungal drugs	95
	2.16.7	Antiviral drugs	96
2.17	Antimicrobial stewardship		97
	2.17.1	What is One Health?	97
	2.17.2	Combating AMR in animal health	99
	2.17.3	A national plan for AMS	100
	2.17.4	What are the benefits of AMS?	100
	2.17.5	Example of a national AMS programme	103
	2.17.6	An AMS programme at health facility level	104
	2.17.7	Making AMS happen	106

Chapter 3: Decontamination of medical devices — **108**

Introduction			108
3.1	Quality assurance (QA) in sterile services		109
	3.1.1	Essential elements of quality management systems	109
3.2	Legislation and standards		110
3.3	What is validation?		110
3.4	Classification of medical devices		112
3.5	The sterile services department (SSD)		112
	3.5.1	The role of the sterile services department	113
	3.5.2	Staff working in the sterile services department	113
	3.5.3	Calculating the size of the SSD	116
	3.5.4	Layout of a sterile services department	117
	3.5.5	Smaller decontamination units	118
	3.5.6	Infrastructure requirements for an SSD	119
	3.5.7	Reprocessing medical devices outside the sterile services department	126
3.6	Reprocessing of medical devices		127
	3.6.1	Point-of-use care	127
	3.6.2	Cleaning	128
	3.6.3	Cleaning methods	131
	3.6.4	Automated methods for cleaning	133
	3.6.5	Boilers (as disinfectors)	137
	3.6.6	Inspection, assembly and packing	138
	3.6.7	Sterilisation	147
3.7	Tracking and traceability for sterilisation methods		164
	3.7.1	Labelling	164
	3.7.2	Tracking	164
	3.7.3	Traceability	164

3.8	Disinfection	165
	3.8.1	Choosing a disinfection method	165
	3.8.2	Indications for chemical disinfection	166
	3.8.3	Disinfection methods for medical devices	166
	3.8.4	Levels of disinfection	173
3.9	Endoscopy	173
	3.9.1	Decontamination of endoscopes	173
	3.9.2	Sources of infection during endoscopy	174
	3.9.3	Challenges facing endoscopic decontamination	174
	3.9.4	Medical Devices Regulations	175
	3.9.5	Decontamination process	175
	3.9.6	The endoscope	175
	3.9.7	Chemical high-level disinfection/sterilisation	178
	3.9.8	Storage of endoscopes	180

Chapter 4: Risk management in infection prevention and control .. 183

Introduction 183

4.1	What is risk?	184
	4.1.1	What is the difference between hazard and risk?	184
	4.1.2	Carrying out a risk assessment	185
	4.1.3	Planning risk assessment	187
	4.1.4	Review in the risk management process	188
	4.1.5	Analysing risk	188
4.2	Risk-reducing strategies	193
	4.2.1	Multimodal strategy	195
	4.2.2	Hand hygiene	196
	4.2.3	Risk-reducing precautions	210
4.3	Personal protective equipment	225
	4.3.1	General rules about PPE	225
	4.3.2	Gloves	225
	4.3.3	Face covers (medical masks and respirators)	230
	4.3.4	Aprons	235
	4.3.5	Gowns and coveralls	236
	4.3.6	Eye protection	236
	4.3.7	Head coverings	237
	4.3.8	Overshoes	237
4.4	Risk-prone (clinical) procedures in healthcare	237
	4.4.1	Injections	238
	4.4.2	Intravenous (IV) systems	242
	4.4.3	Peripheral intravenous access	247
	4.4.4	Central venous pressure (CVP) catheters	249

	4.4.5	Safe disposal of sharps	253
	4.4.6	Urinary tract infection	254
4.5	Wounds		266
	4.5.1	Pathophysiology	266
4.6	Surgical site infections (SSI)		274
	4.6.1	What is a surgical site?	274
	4.6.2	Surgical wound infection	275
	4.6.3	Classification of surgical wounds and risk of infection	276
	4.6.4	Prevention of SSI	278
	4.6.5	The key elements of an SSI bundle are:	282
	4.6.6	Management of surgical wound infections	282
4.7	Ventilator-associated pneumonia		283
	4.7.1	Prevalence	284
	4.7.2	Pathophysiology	284
	4.7.3	Risk factors	285
	4.7.4	Diagnosis of VAP	285
	4.7.5	Reducing risk for VAP	285
	4.7.6	Key elements of a VAP Bundle	287
4.8	Bundles of clinical risk-prone procedures		287
	4.8.1	What is a bundle?	287
	4.8.2	How are bundles produced?	288
	4.8.3	How can a bundle be used in practice?	288
	4.8.4	Difference between a bundle and a checklist	288
Summary			289
Chapter 5: The built environment			**292**
Introduction			292
5.1	Role of IPC in a project team		293
5.2	Renovations		294
5.3	Designing a new healthcare facility		294
	5.3.1	Population and disease profile	295
	5.3.2	Design elements	295
	5.3.3	Choosing a site	295
	5.3.4	Climatic considerations	296
	5.3.5	Building design	296
	5.3.6	Infrastructure requirements	299
	5.3.7	Water, sanitation and hygiene standards	307
5.4	Workflow and healthcare delivery		308
	5.4.1	Movement of patients	309
	5.4.2	Signage	309

	5.4.3	Movement of staff	310
	5.4.4	Movement of equipment and supplies	310
5.5		Layout of a healthcare facility	310
	5.5.1	Administration (offices) non-clinical areas	310
	5.5.2	Furnishing of clinical areas	311
	5.5.3	Temperature control	312
5.6		Layout of a general ward	312
	5.6.1	Risk of transmission	312
	5.6.2	Bed spacing	313
	5.6.3	Provisions for hand hygiene	313
	5.6.4	Dirty utility (sluice) area	315
	5.6.5	Clean utility area	316
	5.6.6	Treatment room	316
	5.6.7	Disposal room (waste holding room)	316
	5.6.8	Staff areas	317
	5.6.9	Patient waiting areas/day rooms	317
	5.6.10	Play area	317
	5.6.11	Visitors' toilets	317
5.7		Specialised areas of care	318
	5.7.1	Isolation facilities	318
	5.7.2	Operating theatre (OT) complex	319
	5.7.3	Burns unit	328
	5.7.4	Bone marrow transplant unit	331
	5.7.5	Intensive therapy units	333
	5.7.6	Dialysis unit	336
	5.7.7	Neonatal units	339
	5.7.8	Other essential units in the health facility	344
5.8		Mortuaries	345
	5.8.1	Risk of transmission	345
	5.8.2	Design and layout	346
	5.8.3	Personal protective equipment	346
5.9		Healthcare clinics	346
5.10		Community-based clinics	347
	5.10.1	Risk of transmission	347
	5.10.2	Design and layout	348
	5.10.3	Dental clinics	350
5.11		Patient facilities during outbreaks and pandemics	352
	5.11.1	Ebola treatment centres	352
	5.11.2	Transmission risk	352
	5.11.3	Ventilation	353
	5.11.4	The layout of the Ebola unit	353

5.12   Acute respiratory infection treatment centre 355
      5.12.1   Personal protective equipment 355
      5.12.2   Ventilation 356
      5.12.3   Environment 356

Chapter 6: Support services, including environmental cleaning 357

Introduction 357
6.1   Kitchens and food preparation 357
      6.1.1   Layout and workflow 358
      6.1.2   Sourcing raw produce 360
      6.1.3   Storage of raw produce before preparation 360
      6.1.4   Food preparation 361
      6.1.5   IPC measures in catering 361
      6.1.6   Designated preparation areas 362
      6.1.7   Food delivery to wards 364
      6.1.8   The washing of crockery and cutlery 364
      6.1.9   Recommendations on the use of cutlery and crockery 365
      6.1.10   Cleaning of the catering area 365
      6.1.11   Staff health 366
      6.1.12   Education and training 366
      6.1.13   Kitchen waste 366
      6.1.14   Inspection of the premises 366
6.2   Linen and laundry 367
      6.2.1   Types of laundry 367
      6.2.2   The laundry cycle 368
      6.2.3   Laundry collection 368
      6.2.4   Safe handling of linen 369
      6.2.5   Disadvantages of sluicing linen in clinical areas 370
      6.2.6   Storage of used linen 370
      6.2.7   Infested linen 370
      6.2.8   Linen transportation from the wards 370
      6.2.9   Processing of laundry 371
      6.2.10   The cycle 372
      6.2.11   Ozone 373
      6.2.12   Laundry equipment 374
      6.2.13   Returning clean laundry 374
      6.2.14   Storage in the clinical areas 374
      6.2.15   Staff 375
      6.2.16   General 375

6.3		Healthcare waste management	376
	6.3.1	Establish a healthcare waste management plan	378
	6.3.2	Responsibility for healthcare waste management	378
	6.3.3	Types of waste	379
	6.3.4	Source segregation	382
	6.3.5	Clinical areas	383
	6.3.6	Non-infectious waste	384
	6.3.7	Ward storage	384
	6.3.8	Collection of waste	385
	6.3.9	Transportation	385
	6.3.10	Storage	385
	6.3.11	Final (end point) disposal of waste	385
6.4		Environmental cleaning in health facilities	389
	6.4.1	The rationale	389
	6.4.2	The cleaning programme	389
	6.4.3	Education and training	390
	6.4.4	Cleaning protocols	390
	6.4.5	Monitoring the cleaning programme	390
	6.4.6	Staff awareness	391
	6.4.7	Personal protective equipment	392
	6.4.8	Cleaning schedules	393
	6.4.9	Cleaning methods	393
	6.4.10	Procedure for cleaning	394
	6.4.11	Blood spillages	396
	6.4.12	Cleaning equipment	396
	6.4.13	Pest control	397
	6.4.14	The ward environment	398
	6.4.15	Risk assessment for determining environmental cleaning methods and frequency	398
6.5		Patient care articles	398

Chapter 7: Communicable disease and public health **406**

Introduction			406
7.1		Communicable diseases	407
	7.1.1	Control of communicable disease	407
	7.1.2	Notifiable communicable diseases	408
	7.1.3	Factors affecting the spread of communicable diseases	410
	7.1.4	Public health	413
7.2		Applying IPC principles in the community	414
	7.2.1	Mutual trust between health workers and the community	414
	7.2.2	Designated caregiver(s)	414

	7.2.3	Routes of transmission for communicable diseases	415
	7.2.4	Oro-faecal route of transmission	415
	7.2.5	Blood-borne virus transmission	425
	7.2.6	Transmission of infectious agents via the respiratory route	439
	7.2.7	Prions	445
7.3	Occupational health		449
	7.3.1	Legislation governing occupational health	449
	7.3.2	OHS Act	449
	7.3.3	Liability of employer	449
	7.3.4	Compensation	449
	7.3.5	Functions of occupational health	450
	7.3.6	Staff protection	450
	7.3.7	Occupationally acquired HIV	452

Chapter 8: Gathering and applying information in IPC **453**

Introduction			453
8.1	Surveillance		453
	8.1.1	What is surveillance?	454
	8.1.2	Why do surveillance?	454
	8.1.3	Structure of surveillance	455
	8.1.4	The role of surveillance	456
	8.1.5	The plan	456
	8.1.6	Where there are no laboratory services	459
	8.1.7	Levels of surveillance	460
	8.1.8	Who carries out surveillance?	461
8.2	Data collection systems		461
	8.2.1	Storing the data	462
	8.2.2	Paper forms	462
	8.2.3	Computerised systems	462
	8.2.4	Data analysis and interpretation	463
8.3	Audit in IPC		465
	8.3.1	What is audit?	465
	8.3.2	Setting up an audit – what should be in place	466
8.4	Key audit indicators in IPC		468
	8.4.1	Types of indicators	468
	8.4.2	The areas to be audited	470
	8.4.3	Conducting the audit	470
	8.4.4	The audit report	471
	8.4.5	Feedback	471

8.5		Outbreak investigation and management	471
	8.5.1	Definitions of high occurrence of a disease	472
	8.5.2	Alert (warning) system	472
	8.5.3	Types of outbreak	472
	8.5.4	Occurrence	473
	8.5.5	Healthcare facility outbreaks	473
	8.5.6	Investigation of outbreaks	475
8.6		Descriptive and analytical epidemiology	480
	8.6.1	Time	480
	8.6.2	Place	480
	8.6.3	Person	480
	8.6.4	Frequency indicators	480
	8.6.5	Descriptive vs analytical epidemiology	481
	8.6.6	Frequency indicators in analytical epidemiology	485
	8.6.7	Describing time, place and persons in descriptive and analytical epidemiological studies	488
	8.6.8	Person	493
8.7		Important concepts in statistics	493
	8.7.1	Sampling and describing samples	493
	8.7.2	95 % confidence interval	495
	8.7.3	P-values	497
	8.7.4	Chi square	497
8.8		Defining the research question and study objectives	498
	8.8.1	Choosing the right study design	498
	8.8.2	Common qualitative study designs	505
	8.8.3	Study protocol and implementation	507

Glossary 510

Index 514

Preface

The number of excellent evidence-based publications in infection prevention and control (IPC) increases by the day. With the advent of social media, one is constantly bombarded with IPC information and activities all year round. During the COVID-19 pandemic, social media became polarised between those that believed in the evidence of science, such as the protective impact of vaccination, and those that did not. Generally, there was global panic because of the lack of evidence. Over the past years this has effectively improved with sound evidence and effective guidance from the WHO.

Since the last edition, 12 years ago, there has been a substantial increase in publications from low-resource settings, particularly Africa, which allows for the development of regional strategies. The progress in developing robust IPC programmes in low- to middle-income countries is slow but has been greatly enhanced by several pivotal publications including those from the WHO on how to set up national IPC programmes. This very important aspect has been addressed in this, the second edition of *Understanding Infection Control and Prevention*, and it is hoped will lead to the development of robust national IPC programmes.

The Infection Control Africa Network (ICAN) has gone from strength to strength and is recognised as THE organisation delivering a high standard and quality of education and training in IPC for the African region and beyond. This book was initially published as a reference for the various courses offered by ICAN to IPC practitioners – it still holds the same pride of place. This second edition contains updates on various topics, still applying evidence-based principles of IPC that are contextually grounded in the prevailing socio-economic situation.

There is slow progress towards getting IPC recognised in LMICs but, by providing a high standard of evidence-based education, well-trained IPC specialists can apply their knowledge to the workplace and improve patient care and patient safety. They are a great asset to their institution and their country and their contribution cannot be ignored.

Finally, IPC is the most cost-effective health intervention in any country – use this resource wisely!

It is hoped that this book will encourage clarity of thought and decision-making, confidence in clinical practice and safety for oneself and one's patients.

Dedication

This book is dedicated to all the healthcare workers but particularly IPC practitioners who worked tirelessly during the COVID-19 pandemic to provide a safe environment for patients.

A special dedication to the late Ms Christina (Tina) Bradley who, despite her busy schedule, always made time to come and teach on the ICAN Fundamental and International Postgraduate Diploma courses (IPDIC).

Author's acknowledgements

I am grateful to the authors who have given hours of their valuable time and contributed to updating chapters in this second edition with fresh evidence. These are Dr Joost Hopman, Dr Annick Lenglet, Mr Phil de Vries, Ms Buyiswa Lizzie Sithole-Mazibuko and, last but by no means least, Ms Briette du Toit Ludick, who is also the training co-ordinator for the Fundamentals in IPC (FIPC) and the IPDIC, a tireless worker and highly knowledgeable colleague.

I owe particular thanks to Dr Joost Hopman, the co-cordinator for the IPDIC, with whom I enjoy hours of debate on IPC matters, bouncing around new ideas on how to improve IPC teaching and how to break the mould of static knowledge transfer with fresh and innovative ideas. A brilliant mind!

I am most grateful to Lynn Koch for her patience with my timelines for this second edition of *Understanding Infection Control and Prevention*.

Finally, I would like to acknowledge my long-suffering husband of 52 years, Moosa, my son Omar and my two grandchildren Kaya and Louis.

List of abbreviations

AIDS	acquired immune deficiency syndrome
BD	Bowie and Dick Test
BFE	bacterial filtration efficiency
CA-UTI	catheter-associated urinary tract infection
CEN	Comité de Normalisation (European Committee for Standardisation)
CLABSI	central line-associated bloodstream infection
CVP	central venous pressure
DM	deputy manager
EC	European Commission
GMP	good manufacturing practice
GNB	gram-negative bacilli
HACCP	hazard analysis and critical control point
HAI	healthcare-associated infection
HEPA	high-efficiency particulate air
HBV	hepatitis B
HCV	hepatitis C
HCF	healthcare facility
HIV	human immunodeficiency virus
IAP	inspection, assembly and packaging
ICU	intensive care unit
ITU	intensive therapy unit
IHR	international health regulations
IPC	infection prevention and control
IPCP	infection prevention and control practitioner
IPDIC	International Postgraduate Diploma in Infection Control
LMIC	low and middle income countries
MBC	minimum bactericidal concentration
MDR	multidrug-resistant
MBT	mercaptobenzothiazoles
MDV	multi-dose vials
MHC	major histocompatiblity complex
MIC	minimum inhibitory concentration
MPS	mononuclear phagocytic system
MRSA	methicillin-resistant *Staphylococcus aureus*
NHS	National Health Service
NIOSH	National Institute for Occupational Safety and Health
NNIS	The National Nosocomial Infection Surveillance
NNU	neonatal unit
NRL	natural rubber latex
OH	occupational health
OPD	outpatient department
OT	operating theatre
PBP	penicillin binding proteins
PMN	polymorphonuclear
PPE	personal protective equipment
PPM	planned preventative maintenance
PSI	pounds per square inch
RCN	Royal College of Nurses
QA	quality assurance
QM	quality manager
SARS	severe acute respiratory syndrome
SOP	standard operating procedure
SSD	sterile services department
SSI	surgical site infection
TAT	turnaround time
TPN	total parenteral nutrition
TWA	time weighted average
UVGI	ultraviolet germicidal irradiation
VAP	ventilator-associated pneumonia
VHFs	viral haemorrhagic fevers
WHO	World Health Organization

Text acknowledgements

Table 3.5: *Basic Concepts of Infection Control.* Friedman C & Newsom W (eds). 2007. Malta: International Federation of Infection Control.

Figure 3.16: https://www.cdc.gov/infectioncontrol/guidelines/disinfection/tables/figure1.html. CDC. Centres for Disease Control & Prevention. U.S. Department of Health & Human Services. Guideline for Disinfection and Sterilization in Healthcare Facilities (2008)

Figure 3.17: Oh, Tae & Han, Sang & Hong, Kwang & Jeong, Eun & Lee, Hyug & Yun, Jung & Park, Kwang & Lee, Joon & Kim, Young & Chang, Woonki & Park, Chang. (2018). Guidelines of cleaning and disinfection in gastrointestinal endoscope for clinicians. *Journal of the Korean Medical Association.* 61. 130. 10.5124/jkma.2018.61.2.130. License CC BY-NC 4.0

Figure 4.1: Loosely based on *10 Elements to Consider When Conducting an Infection Risk Assessment,* by Marcia Patrick, MSN, RN, CIC June 25, 2016.

Figure 4.2: Australian Commission on Safety and Quality in Health Care. *Guidelines for the Prevention and Control of Infection in Healthcare.* May 2019. The Australian/New Zealand Standard on Risk Management AS/NZS ISO 31000: 2009

Figure 4.3: MCSA. Continuous Improvement. Model 3. 2017. https://asq.org/quality-resources/fishbone; https://www.cms.gov/medicare/provider-enrollment-and-certification/qapi/downloads/fishbonerevised.pdf

Figure 4.9: Adapted from CDC.gov www.cdc.gov/niosh/topics/hierarchy/default.html

Figure 6.1: Workflow in a catering unit. *International Health Facility Guidelines. (iHFG), Part B: Health Facility Briefing & Design Catering Unit.* Figure 1 Functional Relationship Diagram: © TAHPI Version 5 June 2017 Used with permission. www.healthfacilityguidelines.com

Figure 8.6: Helder, O., Kornelisse, R., van der Starre, C. et al. *Implementation of a children's hospital-wide central venous catheter insertion and maintenance bundle.* BMC Health Serv Res 13, 417 (2013). https://doi.org/10.1186/1472-6963-13-417 Open Access

1 Infection prevention and control

Shaheen Mehtar & Briette du Toit Ludick

Learning outcomes

What you should know after reading this chapter:
- Elements of IPC programmes
- Structure of an IPC programme at national and healthcare facility (HCF) level
- Role of IPC team and committee members
- How to set up education and training programmes
- Cost of HAI and IPC programmes

Introduction

Infection prevention and control (IPC) is an evolving process of **developing and implementing safe, evidence-based practice towards improving quality healthcare for all**. It is often part of quality assurance, but preferably should stand alone. The IPC process is constantly evolving, depending on the global disease profile at the time. It encompasses all aspects of prevention and control in healthcare relating to patients and staff, using a quality improvement circle to achieve its goals of reducing healthcare-associated infections (HAI) and antimicrobial resistance (AMR). The IPC elements that influence quality improvement are shown in Figure 1.1.

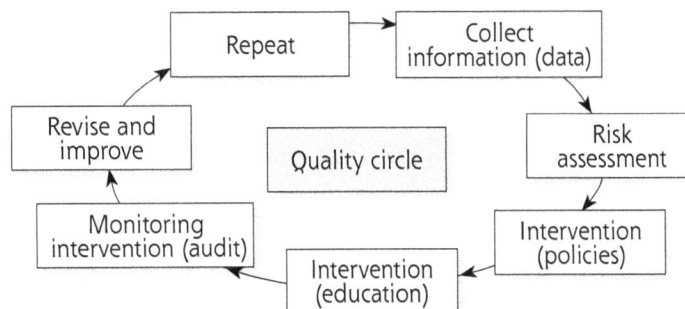

Figure 1.1 Elements that influence IPC programmes in relation to quality of healthcare

IPC covers a wide spectrum from procurement to quality of patient and healthcare worker care. Clearly, this process – understanding the principles and applying them routinely – is inextricably linked with sound knowledge and training for all caregivers, which ideally should embed good IPC practices as second nature. IPC is a specialty in its own right. Application of evidence-based knowledge and regular revision of policies supported by a trained IPC team have significantly improved healthcare delivery and reduced infection rates in hospitals.[1]

IPC programmes should be **proactive** (but are often **reactive**). Systems should be in place to reduce or prevent the risk to patients and staff of acquiring infections during health delivery. Those starting to set up IPC systems should consider stepwise improvements.[2] Healthcare workers (HCW) should be accountable and responsible for their own actions towards protecting themselves and their patients. The ultimate responsibility for IPC lies with the head of the health institution, guided by recommendations from the national departments of health and/or international bodies (WHO). While this duty may be delegated to a deputy, usually the IPC team, accountability to patients is paramount.

In low- to middle-income countries (LMICs) the burden of HAI is fivefold higher than in high-income countries.[3] The impact on healthcare budgets has been catastrophic. Zimlichman et al[4] estimated the burden of the five most common HAIs amounted to $9.8 billion in the USA (2012). The SENIC study[5] clearly demonstrated that the presence of a robust IPC programme reduced HAI (and costs) by approximately 38%, compared with those facilities that did not. This led to the establishment of National Nosocomial Infection Surveillance (NNIS) and benchmarking for HAIs,[6] which is now widely used to compare facilities and drive down the cost of IPC.

There is a misconception that IPC is related to nursing procedures only and therefore is the sole domain of nurses. While professional nursing standards require IPC as part of quality healthcare, there are some notable differences

---

[1]   Haley RW, Quade D, Freeman HE & Bennett JV. 1980. The SENIC Project. Study on the efficacy of nosocomial infection control (SENIC Project). Summary of study design. *American Journal of Epidemiology*, 3(5): 472–485.

[2]   WHO. 2019. Minimum requirements for infection prevention and control. Geneva: World Health Organization. Licence: CC BY-NC-SA 3.0 IGO.

[3]   Allegranzi B, Bagheri Nejad S & Combescure C. 2011. Burden of endemic health-care-associated infection in developing countries: Systematic review and meta-analysis. *Lancet*, 377: 228–241.

[4]   Zimlichman E, Henderson D, Tamir O, Franz C, Song P, Yamin CK, Keohane C, Denham CR & Bates DW. 2013. Health Care-associated Infections: A Meta-analysis of Costs and Financial Impact on the US Health Care System *JAMA Intern Med*, 173(22): 2039–2046. doi:10.1001/jamainternmed.2013.9763.

[5]   Haley RW, Quade D, Freeman HE & Bennett JV. 1980. The SENIC Project. Study on the efficacy of nosocomial infection control (SENIC Project). Summary of study design. *American Journal of Epidemiology*, 3(5): 472–485.

[6]   Jarvis, WR. 2003. Benchmarking for prevention: The Centers for Disease Control and Prevention's National Nosocomial Infections Surveillance (NNIS) system experience. *Infection*. Suppl 2: 44–52.

between IPC and nursing procedures. Nursing procedures are patient-based clinical (and non-clinical) practices, which include IPC measures but do not necessarily take into account evaluation of risk, procurement of products and infection outcome. Procedures are clearly structured acts according to standard operating procedures (SOPs).

IPC, on the other hand, has a wider remit – investigating all areas that influence transmission of microbes – and therefore a sound knowledge of microbiology is necessary. IPC systems evolve continuously, depending on the need, and produce standards of quality care which **underpin** good clinical practice. For example, IPC advice and recommendations when the COVID-19 pandemic struck included a clean environment, procurement of equipment and supplies, particularly face covers, the built healthcare environment and ventilation, workflow and spacing, the application of standards to clinical practice, and training and education of staff. As part of quality improvement, outcomes are measured, such as a reduction in HAI rates and AMR. IPC policies must be evidence-based and should be reviewed frequently following an outcome audit. Thus, a quality cycle is established.

1.1 Elements of infection prevention and control

1.1.1 Definition

The World Health Organization (WHO) defines IPC as 'a practical, evidence-based approach preventing patients and health workers from being harmed by avoidable infections and as a result of antimicrobial resistance. Effective IPC requires constant action at all levels of the health system, including policymakers, facility managers, health workers and those who access health services. IPC is unique in the field of patient safety and quality of care, as it is universally relevant to every health worker and patient, at every healthcare interaction. Defective IPC causes harm and can kill. Without effective IPC it is impossible to achieve quality healthcare delivery.'[7] This is achieved by monitoring infection and implementing IPC measures through education of patients, employees and visitors in the principles and practice of IPC.

1.1.2 Legislation

IPC is legislated for under the International Health Regulations (2005).[8] A wealth of evidence-based information and guidance for setting up a national and healthcare facility IPC programme[9] can be found on the WHO IPC Hub.

---

[7]   WHO IPC Hub. https://www.who.int/teams/integrated-health-services/infection-prevention-control/.
[8]   International Health Regulations (2005), reviewed 2016.
[9]   https://www.who.int/teams/integrated-health-services/infection-prevention-control/.

The National IPC Strategic Framework (2020) outlines the legislation framework for IPC for South Africa[10] and has been adapted from the WHO core components (2016).[11] It is regulated through the Office of Health Standards Compliance (South Africa), IPC (Section 3). Other legislation, including the Health and Safety at Work Act, Occupational Health Act, Public Health Act and constitutional law of the country, support the requirements for an IPC programme.

1.1.3 Professional bodies

A national or regional body of specialists in the field comprises self-appointed groups (society, association or confederation) with common goals (see Figure 1.2). The driving force is its specialist membership that ensures the development and implementation of IPC standards appropriate to its population. There is also a vested interest in protecting jobs and increasing the profile of the specialty. While these organisations do not have legislative powers, *per se*, they often serve as powerful lobby and can influence national legislation by gaining the respect and recognition of legislative authorities, and are often called upon to advise on making of national policies (e.g. COVID-19, TB, HIV). Such organisations may conduct independent local research, review literature from other countries and arrive at evidence-based recommendations for the government to endorse. Their input is invaluable!

Specialist areas of care such as intensive care, operating theatres and dentistry may develop their own IPC programmes, but in consultation with the IPC teams.

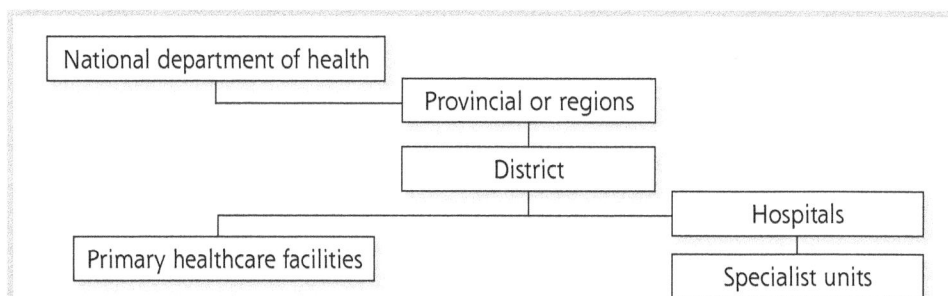

Figure 1.2 (IPC) Cascading system of information and IPC policies

---

[10]   National Infection Prevention and Control Strategic Framework. 2020. Dept of Health South Africa. https://www.nicd.ac.za/wp-content/uploads/2020/04/National-Infection-Prevention-and-Control-Strategic-Framework-March-2020-1.pdf.

[11]   WHO. 2016. Guidelines on core components of infection prevention and control programmes at the national and acute healthcare facility level. Geneva: World Health Organization. https://www.who.int/publications/i/item/9789241549929.

The advantage of such bodies is to provide moral and technical support for their members, assist in setting national standards, network to share and disseminate evidence-based research, develop IPC education programmes and curricula, set uniform audit and outcome measures and publish high-class scientific research.

The disadvantages are that these organisations are not implementing bodies and must work with government structures to achieve their goals and implementation of policy. Funding is usually a challenge and the work is done by volunteers, who as such cannot be regulated or be held accountable.

Where IPC structures do not exist, IPC is sometimes perceived as a 'dumping basket' for clinical and non-clinical-related problems in a health service or a spare pair of hands. IPC is often used as a political tool, particularly during outbreaks, but generally considered a nuisance imposing an extra burden on the finances and infrastructure of the facility, particularly during surveillance, auditing and monitoring clinical practice. In many LMICs it is given low priority since it is not considered directly related to patient care. Finally, under emergency conditions training in IPC is delivered by persons who have little or no specialised knowledge of the subject, thus perpetuating archaic and non-evidence-based practices. Here, professional bodies are invaluable to provide support for IPC personnel.

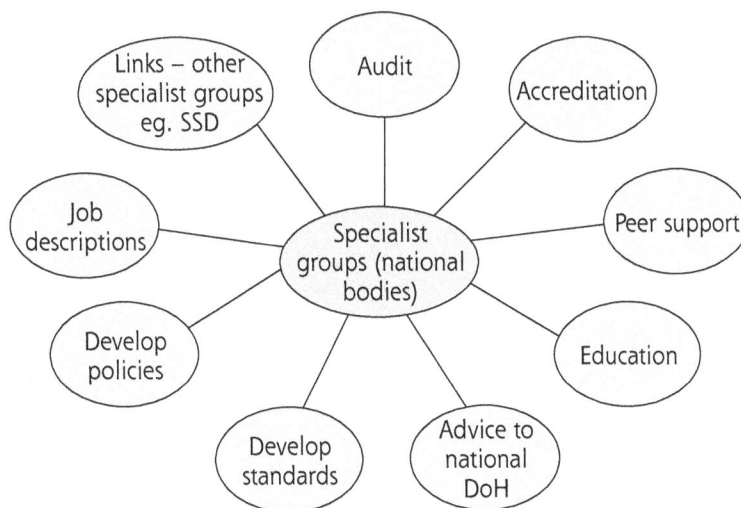

Figure 1.3 (IPC) Activities of national specialist bodies in IPC

1.2 Goals of IPC

The main objective of IPC is to prevent harmful pathogens from reaching anatomical sites where they may cause disease, outbreaks of such disease or mortality among the population, and reducing antimicrobial resistance.

In order to achieve these goals the following bundle of activities is needed:

- to gather evidence (surveillance), from local sources or from further afield, to support sound evidence-based policies
- to develop a set of policies or guidelines which protect patients and healthcare workers while ensuring the best possible standard of care (administration)
- to create awareness of pathogens and their impact on healthcare workers, patients and the environment (education)
- to create barriers that reduce the transmission of infective organisms (interventions)
- to assist healthcare managers to provide cost-effective health without compromising quality (advice).

1.3   The role of IPC programmes[12]

The role of IPC is:

- to provide evidence for best practices nationally and at HCF level
- to prevent and contain the transfer of pathogenic micro-organisms to susceptible hosts
- to contain transfer of pathogens via medical devices and equipment used in providing healthcare services
- to ensure a clean and dry HCF environment
- to apply IPC practices to reduce AMR.

To achieve this, collaboration and buy-in is necessary and the IPC team has to liaise with various departments and units in the facility in which it works as well as related governmental structures (see section 1.8.4.4 on IPC team below).

1.4   Why the same IPC programme is not universally applicable

While the basic principles of IPC remain the same globally, the type of IPC structures will depend upon local conditions – copying blueprints from other countries usually results in unworkable programmes unless these are appropriately modified and adapted.[13]

---

[12]   WHO. 2016. Guidelines on core components of infection prevention and control programmes at the national and acute healthcare facility level. Geneva: World Health Organization. https://www.who.int/publications/i/item/9789241549929.

[13]   Mehtar S. Lowbury Lecture. 2007. Infection prevention and control strategies for tuberculosis in developing countries – lessons learnt from Africa. *Journal of Hospital Infection*, 69: 321–327.

The reasons are as follows:

1.4.1 There are **major differences between countries** and regions based on geography, population distribution and social stratification.

    1.4.1.1 **Geography.** Large countries usually have variance in terrain, which influences differences in populations, manifesting in varied cultures, traditions and disease profiles. In small countries the population is usually homogeneous with a common language and tradition.

    1.4.1.2 **Populations** residing in different parts of the same country vary according to their ability to pay and gain access to healthcare. Some remote areas have no IPC programmes, but may have rudimentary health service delivery.

    1.4.1.3 **Social stratification.** The poor live in crowded conditions with inadequate water, electricity and sanitation and they use the healthcare services provided by the state. The economically better-off reside in areas where the standard of living is high and usually attend private healthcare facilities.

1.4.2 **Differences in healthcare facilities.** Most healthcare systems are tiered to provide primary healthcare in clinics, small inpatient facilities in regional hospitals and tertiary referral hospitals for specialised medicine.

    1.4.2.1 Resources vary by country and within the same country by the type of healthcare facility. In LMICs the private sector has more resources available compared with state-sector hospitals.

    1.4.2.2 Funding of different tiers of hospital varies according to need and government allocation of funds in the state sector; usually priority is given to primary health delivery rather than tertiary hospitals.

    1.4.2.3 Facilities for healthcare delivery depend on the type of patients seen in a particular facility.

    1.4.2.4 Staffing is dependent on the needs of healthcare facilities, distance from cities or urban areas and availability of qualified staff.

1.4.3 **Disease profiles differ between countries.** In LMICs, communicable diseases such as tuberculosis, AIDS and diarrhoeal disease take priority over multiple antimicrobial resistant HAI pathogens.

1.5 IPC and quality improvement

Quality improvement (QI) is a systematic, formal approach to the analysis of practice performance and efforts to improve performance. IPC is a key component of system-wide quality assurance and performance improvement activities – the two are inextricably linked.

Quality assurance (QA) systems are set up to monitor the quality and excellence of goods and services. Their purpose is to:

- ensure best practices guidelines are in place
- ensure each agent is working within quality standards
- monitor, evaluate and redefine parameters and training materials as needed.

1.5.1 Guidelines

A clear set of evidence-based IPC guidelines or polices should be in place which are used to train and evaluate the workforce (National IPC Strategic Framework, South Africa, 2020).[14] These serve to regulate standards in the workplace as well as accountability. These guidelines must be clear, concise, unambiguous and visually acceptable. However, where such policies do not exist, best practices may be used to improve quality of care. Training of the workforce is necessary to ensure that quality standards are understood and maintained (see section 1.11 on Education in IPC).

1.5.2 Monitoring and evaluation

Monitoring and evaluation (M&E) is an integral part of quality improvement. The main purpose of M&E is to review, and modify, processes towards improving the quality of care and practice. The ultimate goal is to achieve behaviour change through feedback towards reducing the risk of HAI and AMR. An excellent example is the COVID-19 Strategic Preparedness and Response (SPRP) Monitoring and Evaluation Framework,[15] which includes definitions and outlines strategies for M&E and is recommended reading.

1.5.2.1 Structure: Regular and/or continuous monitoring and evaluation provides a systematic method to document the progress and impact of pre-established indicators of IPC programmes at national and facility level.

1.5.2.2 Key indicators: These further promote accountability. Sharing results of audits and key indicators with those being audited (individual change), hospital management and senior administration (organisational change) are critical steps to get 'buy-in' and support for the improvement of processes and outcomes.

1.5.2.3 Frequency of evaluation: IPC programmes should be evaluated periodically (preferably annually) to assess the extent to which the objectives have been met and goals accomplished and to identify areas for

---

14   National Infection Prevention and Control Strategic Framework (2020) Dept of Health South Africa. https://www.nicd.ac.za/wp-content/uploads/2020/04/National-Infection-Prevention-and-Control-Strategic-Framework-March-2020-1.pdf.

15   WHO. 2020. COVID-19 Strategic Framework and Response (SFRP), Monitoring and Evaluation Framework.

improvement. Information includes the results of compliance with IPC practices and other process indicators (for example, training activities) and monitoring of outcomes measures (WHO core components, 2016).[16] Carrying out audits too frequently is non-productive because not enough time is allowed to gather data and institute change.

1.5.3 Feedback

Feedback is essential for behavioural change. Engaging stakeholders, creating partnerships and developing working groups and networks strengthens co-operation and compliance. Key indicators further promote accountability. Sharing results of key indicator audits with those being audited (individual change), hospital management and senior administration (organisational change) are critical steps to get 'buy-in' and support for the improvement of processes and outcomes. IPC teams and continuous improvement committees should also be included in the feedback to ensure that improvement initiatives are being developed and implemented.

1.6 Types of indicators

Key Performance Indicators (KPIs) are important decision-making tools that are used to track performance in relation to strategic goals. KPIs monitor whether a facility or organisation is still on track with its strategic goals and objectives. It also serves as an early warning sign, flagging concerns and areas where interventions are required.[17]

Quality improvement tools reflect either outcome (performance) or monitoring of administrative operational function. IPC risk indicators are more useful since these are proactive and identify adverse events and vulnerabilities before problems arise (see 8.1 Surveillance for details of key indicators).

1.6.1 Monitoring tools

Monitoring tools measure standards and compliance to practices. There are various international monitoring tools available for IPC, which could be adapted to local policies and standards for specific clinical areas, but must be validated and tested prior to implementation. Monitoring tools can either measure IPC programmes and adherence to guidelines and standards or individual practices or compliance to practices. Some examples are shown below:

---

[16] WHO. 2016. Guidelines on core components of infection prevention and control programmes at the national and acute healthcare facility level. Geneva: World Health Organization. https://www.who.int/publications/i/item/9789241549929.

[17] Marr, B. The different type of benchmarking – Examples and easy explanations. https://bernardmarr.com/the-different-types-of-benchmarking-examples-and-easy-explanations/ Accessed 2022.01.18.

- WHO instructions for the national infection prevention and control assessment tool 2 (IPCAT2).[18] It provides a general overview of the status of IPC activities according to the guideline recommendations, supports implementation and provides a roadmap to guide IPC interventions (eg WHO core components for IPC Programmes). It does not focus on specific IPC practices or risk factors related to individual patients or practices.
- WHO hand hygiene monitoring and audit tools.[19] These review practices and infrastructure in a systematic way towards a situational analysis of the status of hand hygiene in a facility. This includes infrastructure, training and compliance.
- Water and Sanitation for Health Facility Improvement Tool (WASH FIT).[20] It is directed at improving infrastructure and safe water supply in healthcare facilities and assists in continuous monitoring and improvement of specific high-risk areas.
- An environmental cleaning checklist helps to measure compliance with existing cleaning policies. An international checklist (CDC/ICAN)[21] or a facility environmental cleaning checklist for a neonatal unit in South Africa are excellent examples of effectively using checklists to reduce environmental contamination.[22]
- National monitoring tools, such as Norms and Standards of the South African Office of Healthcare Standards tools,[23] are applied to facilities for accreditation and licensing to ensure safety and high-quality standards.

1.6.2 Effective use of data

Collecting data is time- and resource-consuming and is only of value if utilised correctly to improve IPC practices. Therefore data must be accurate, reliable and presented in a clear and concise manner to ensure that readers understand and interpret it correctly.

---

[18] WHO. 2017. Instructions for the national infection prevention and control assessment tool 2 (IPCAT2). https://apps.who.int/iris/bitstream/handle/10665/330078/WHO-HIS-SDS-2017.13-eng.pdf?sequence=1&isAllowed=y.

[19] WHO. 2010. Hand hygiene self assessment framework. https://cdn.who.int/media/docs/default-source/integrated-health-services-(ihs)/clean-hands-2015/hhsa_framework_october_2010-3.pdf?sfvrsn=98cbf596_3&ua=1.

[20] Water and Sanitation for Health Facility Improvement Tool (WASH FIT). 2018. https://apps.who.int/iris/bitstream/handle/10665/254910/9789241511698-eng.pdf.

[21] CDC and ICAN. Best Practices for Environmental Cleaning in Healthcare Facilities in Resource-Limited Settings. Atlanta, GA: US Department of Health and Human Services, CDC; Cape Town, South Africa: Infection Control Africa Network; 2019. Available at: https://www.cdc.gov/hai/prevent/resource-limited/index.html and http://www.icanetwork.co.za/icanguideline2019.

[22] Dramowski A, Aucamp M, Bekker A, Pillay S, Moloto K, Whitelaw AC, Cotton AF & Coffin S. 2021. NeoCLEAN: A multimodal strategy to enhance environmental cleaning in a resource-limited neonatal unit. *Antimicrob Resist Infect Control* 10: 35 https://doi.org/10.1186/s13756-021-00905-y.

[23] Office of Healthcare Standards Compliance. https://ohsc.org.za/acts-and-regulations/.

Data collected through surveillance, audits and self-assessment are valuable sources to:

- identify trends and risks
- develop benchmarks
- guide IPC strategies and priorities
- monitor and assess the impact and effectiveness of interventions
- assist with outbreak identification and investigation
- assist with the identification of common denominators
- provide feedback to management teams and policy makers
- develop targeted evidence-based policies and standards
- share and publish information about best practices, continuous improvement projects and outbreak resolutions.

Data is a powerful tool to engage stakeholders, motivate for improvement interventions and demonstrate the magnitude of a problem (see section 8.1 Surveillance).

1.7 Benchmarking

The aim of benchmarking is to improve efficiency, quality of care and patient safety, including infection prevention and control and patient satisfaction. Benchmarks are reference points that are used to compare performance against that of others. Benchmarks can compare processes and key indicators. These may be used internally to compare one healthcare facility to another or externally against competitor facilities or organisations.[24] When benchmarking, identify which outcomes or indicators to use, whom to benchmark against and ensure that similar aspects are measured against one another – 'apples are compared with apples'.[25] Benchmarking can be applied to patient characteristics, volume, processes, outcomes or other meaningful categories. It is also a means of measuring strategies and performance against the 'best' internal and external performance.

1.7.1 Advantages of benchmarking

- Gain an independent perspective on how well a facility performs compared to other internal or external facilities
- Identify performance gaps and areas for improvement
- Develop a standardised set of processes and metrics

[24] Marr, B. The different type of benchmarking – Examples and easy explanations. https://bernardmarr.com/the-different-types-of-benchmarking-examples-and-easy-explanations/ Accessed 2022.01.18.

[25] Freytag V & Hollensen S. 2001. The process of benchmarking, benchlearning and bench action. https://www-emerald-com.ru.idm.oclc.org/insight/content/doi/10.1108/09544780 110360624/full/html.

- Establish a culture of continuous improvement
- Establish performance expectations

1.7.2 Disadvantages of benchmarking

- Competitiveness can lead to dishonesty
- Choosing the wrong benchmarks
- It has a narrow perspective of action – it is limited only to a specific organisation
- Facilities that are not comparable are compared, leading to despondency

While benchmarking is a valuable tool, it is not the only answer to improve performance. In order to improve performance one has to set clear strategic goals and objectives, design key performance indicators that assist in monitoring and measuring the goals and objectives and comparing performance.

1.8 Starting an IPC programme

When setting up an IPC programme, countries are advised to refer to the comprehensive WHO core components (2016) and the Minimum Requirements,[26] which provide a step-by-step implementation guide.

1.8.1 Aim

- to establish an IPC programme which conveys the principles of IPC to the healthcare worker irrespective of being in the public or private sector
- to establish skilled and trained person(s) responsible for IPC at each unit level
- to secure a dedicated budget for IPC
- to establish links with management and clinical units
- to implement national or international standards in IPC
- to provide education and training for all healthcare workers in good IPC practices
- to conduct regular audit and revision of IPC policies as required.

1.8.2 Outcome

Cost-effective, improved patient care with a reduction in morbidity and mortality associated with HAI.

1.8.3 Structure of IPC programmes

WHO Guidelines for core component of an IPC programme (2016)[27] are summarised in Table 1.1, which gives clear guidance for a national and healthcare

---

[26]   WHO. 2019. Minimum requirements for infection prevention and control. Geneva: World Health Organization. Licence: CC BY-NC-SA 3.0 IGO.

[27]   WHO. 2016. Guidelines on core components of infection prevention and control programmes at the national and acute healthcare facility level. Geneva: World Health Organization. https://www.who.int/publications/i/item/9789241549929.

facility-level IPC structure; however, there are certain generic aspects that should be taken into account when applying these to local conditions.

Parallel but autonomous structures may develop in individual healthcare units with their own IPC programme, which may or may not be linked to a national programme. The provision of non-standardised IPC services to healthcare facilities may be variable, with no accreditation or continuing education.

Table 1.1 Summary of the core components for national and healthcare facility level IPC programmes

Core component	National	Healthcare facility
1. IPC programme	Active, stand-alone, national IPC programmes with clearly defined objectives, functions and activities should be established for the purpose of preventing HAI, promoting patient safety and combating AMR through IPC good practices.	An IPC programme with a dedicated, trained team should be in place in each acute healthcare facility for the purpose of preventing HAI and combating AMR through IPC good practices.
2. IPC guidelines	Evidence-based, ministry-approved guidelines adapted to the local context and reviewed at least every five years.	Facility-adapted standard operating procedures (SOPs) and their monitoring at primary health level. Expansion to include risk reducing strategies for secondary and tertiary levels.
3. IPC education and training	The national IPC programme should support education and training of the health workforce as one of its core functions.	The panel recommends that IPC education should be in place for all HCWs by using team- and task-based strategies that are participatory and include bedside and simulation training to reduce the risk of HAI and AMR.
4. HAI surveillance	National HAI surveillance programmes and networks that include mechanisms for timely data feedback and with the potential to be used for benchmarking purposes should be established to reduce HAI and AMR.	HAI surveillance should be performed to guide IPC interventions and detect outbreaks, including AMR surveillance, with timely feedback of results to HCWs and stakeholders and through national networks.

Core component	National	Healthcare facility
5. Multimodal strategies	National IPC programmes should co-ordinate and facilitate the implementation of IPC activities through multimodal strategies on a nationwide or subnational level.	IPC activities using multimodal strategies should be implemented to improve practices and reduce HAI and AMR.
6. Monitoring, audit and feedback	A national IPC monitoring and evaluation programme should be established to assess the extent to which standards are being met and activities are being performed according to the programme's goals and objectives.	Regular monitoring/ audit and timely feedback of healthcare practices according to IPC standards should be performed to prevent and control HAI and AMR at the healthcare facility level. Feedback should be provided to all audited persons and relevant staff.
7. Workload, staffing and bed occupancy	Support workload and staffing requirements at a national level in order for the health facilities to function appropriately.	In order to reduce the risk of HAI and the spread of AMR: (1) bed occupancy should not exceed the standard capacity of the facility; (2) HCW staffing levels should be adequately assigned according to patient workload.
8. Built environment, IPC supplies	Budget should be made available to ensure safe patient care through supporting infrastructure and supplies for IPC.	Patient care activities should be undertaken in a clean and hygienic environment that facilitates practices related to the prevention and control of HAI, as well as AMR, including all elements around WASH infrastructure and services and the availability of appropriate IPC materials and equipment. The panel recommends that materials and equipment to perform appropriate hand hygiene should be readily available at each point of care.

1.8.3.1 National IPC programme

A functional national IPC programme should at least consist of an active, stand-alone national unit with a dedicated budget, led by a fully trained IPC practitioner who is capable of managing and supporting an IPC programme at health facility level. National IPC programmes must have clearly defined objectives, functions and activities and be established for the purposes of preventing HAI, promoting patient safety and combating AMR through IPC good practices. National IPC programmes should be linked with other relevant national programmes and professional organisations (Figure 1.4).

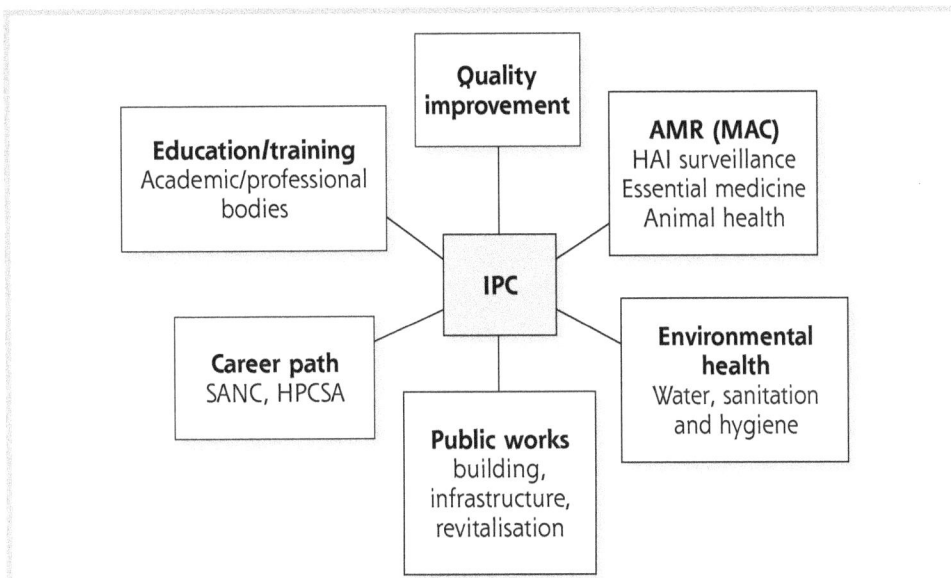

Figure 1.4 The relationship between national IPC and other programmes

1.8.3.2 National IPC committee

An independent national IPC committee consists of the various directorates from within the NDoH that are responsible for specific areas of the national IPC programme. The aim of the national IPC committee is to co-ordinate and support IPC activities of national importance. It should meet at least quarterly to provide advice and information towards formulating or updating policies.

The participating directorates should include Quality Assurance (QA), Affordable Medicines, Communicable Diseases, EMS and Disaster Medicine, Environmental Health, Hospital Management, PHC, District Health Services and Infrastructure.[28]

---

[28] National IPC Strategic Framework (2020) Dept of Health, South Africa.

1.8.4 Healthcare facility IPC programme

The actual implementation of an IPC programme is at health facility level to ensure safety of patients and staff.

1.8.4.1 Responsibility for IPC

The responsibility for IPC lies with the chief executive officer of a hospital or institution, who is accountable to top government management. However, this duty may be delegated to the IPC team. It is also the individual responsibility of each professional healthcare worker to carry out practices which do not harm her- or himself, other members of staff, patients or the environment.

Finally, it must be clearly understood that the IPC team, while more knowledgeable and proactive in implementation of IPC programmes, cannot be held directly responsible for the outcome of such IPC programmes if the necessary support structures are not in place.

1.8.4.2 IPC structure in healthcare facilities

IPC structures in healthcare facilities should consist of at least a functioning IPC committee and an IPC team.

1.8.4.3 IPC committee

There should be an actively functioning IPC committee which meets frequently and regularly with well-kept records and minutes to identify and prioritise IPC matters and make appropriate policies. District-based IPC committees should manage the hospitals within these districts, but each healthcare facility, no matter how small, should have an IPC discussion forum. It is advisable that the IPC committee is independent of the nursing procedures committee (or similar) since it will include non-nursing members.

The IPC committee should be accountable to the management structures of the institution or structure and should report to them.

1.8.4.3.1 Role of IPC committees

These roles may differ from country to country, but generally include the following:
- to implement national IPC policy (where such policies do not exist, local policies should be based on evidence from peer-reviewed publications)
- to establish achievable objectives for improved patient care – few and simple as part of audit and M&E
- to ensure timely and adequate medical supplies to support IPC practices
- to set up and implement an IPC training programme run by trained IPC persons for all hospital staff and conduct continuous in-service training
- to identify areas of risk and prioritise and implement systems to eliminate or reduce them

- to improve patient care and record-keeping with simple yet effective surveillance
- to monitor antibiotic usage and related antibiotic resistance
- to promote the appropriate use of disinfectants
- to respond to surveillance and audit results by instituting improvements
- to produce an infection control manual containing relevant policies and update them regularly.

1.8.4.3.2 Composition of the IPC committee

The list is by no means comprehensive and may vary from one healthcare facility to another, depending on local circumstances.

- chairperson – may be a senior hospital administrator or IPC doctor
- matron or nurse-in-charge of the hospital
- IPC practitioner(s)
- IPC doctor (physician) if not chair
- quality assurance manager
- occupational health representative
- pharmacist
- housekeeping supervisor
- tutors for health services (if present)
- hospital engineer
- representatives from:
    — surgery
    — intensive care unit
    — neonatal ward
    — labour ward
- sterile services department (SSD) manager.

Other members can be co-opted if required, such as catering.

For district IPC committees, the hospital administrators should attend for regular feedback.

Overall, the members are expected to identify and discuss challenges towards implementing IPC programmes. They should discuss policy implementation such as clinical practice and training in IPC, advise on implementation and support audit, monitoring and evaluation. HAI rates and outcomes should be tabled and the findings discussed. Regular feedback to the IPC committee is expected at every meeting. An accurate set of minutes must be kept as a record of activities.

Senior hospital administrator. Ideally the CEO of the hospital should be a member (if not the chairperson) of the IPC committee; however, a deputy senior administrator who has the power to make decisions should be an active member of the IPC committee and might be the chairperson. The role of the administrator is to support IPC activities by providing administrative assistance, endorse IPC policies and provide a budget to implement IPC strategies.

Occupational health (OH). The role of the OH is to report lack of adherence to relevant IPC policies, report IPC-related occupational injuries, support joint IPC/OH audits and report to the committee. The link with OH for prevention strategies such as worker immunisation, personal protective equipment (PPE) and good working conditions is important for IPC and the safety of the staff.

Nurse-in-charge of healthcare facility. The matron or the nurse-in-charge has a major role to play in the IPC committee by ensuring that policies are implemented. The provision for IPC training and education should be supported by establishing a link nurse programme for HAI surveillance and report feedback to the clinical areas. The nurse-in-charge should ensure that any administrative problems encountered are dealt with.

Pharmacist. Recommendations made by the IPC committee regarding antibiotic policies and disinfectants are channelled through the pharmacist to the clinical areas. The pharmacist plays an active role in implementing antibiotic and disinfectant policies by informing individual healthcare units of any changes in antibiotic or disinfectant policy, by supporting implementation of these policies, by keeping records of antibiotic usage, cost and stocks on the ward and by informing the IPC committee of antibiotic or disinfectant audit results and to provide any new relevant information.

Housekeeping supervisor. The housekeeping supervisor implements the recommendations of the IPC committee in best practices in environmental cleaning and appropriate disinfection and reports to the committee any challenges that might occur, including terminal cleaning procedures. Regular training of cleaning staff is essential.

Hospital engineer. The IPC committee works closely with the hospital engineer, who has a pivotal role in ensuring IPC-related equipment functions optimally. This includes maintaining reprocessing equipment such as sterilisers, washer disinfectors and ward washers. The role includes:
- to report any breakdowns or lack of maintenance in the SSD and the wards
- to report on water quality
- to ensure adequate steam supply is provided
- to report changes in ventilation in specialised areas
- to carry out maintenance of non-clinical processing equipment, ventilation systems and infrastructure
- to report on renovations carried out in any part of the hospital or building
- to report on planning of new units which require IPC input.

Clinical team representatives. The acute specialties such as surgery, infectious diseases, paediatrics and neonatology should be represented to discuss training and implementation. They also should have access to the surveillance data and be pivotal in policy development. Often the clinical staff are involved in training.

1.8.4.4 IPC team

The IPC team is the backbone of an IPC programme. The team should be made up of at least an IPC doctor (physician) and nurse practitioner(s) based upon the bed ratio (1 : 250 acute beds, WHO). Additionally, surveillance, data collection and administrative staff should be included. The IPC team should advise on development of IPC policies, procurement of medical devices, appropriate use of PPE, hand hygiene products, disinfectants and other items of clinical and non-clinical equipment used in a healthcare facility. In-depth knowledge of such matters is essential, and regular updates are necessary.

1.8.4.5 IPC team offices

The IPC team (IPC practitioner and IPC doctor) should ideally have its own independent offices close to clinical areas with easy access to the microbiology department.

Requirements are:
- a dedicated budget or allocation for IPC to cover administration, training, surveillance and investigation of potential outbreaks
- an independent area to house the IPC team with access to healthcare facility records and computer access
- continuous internet access and a dedicated computer for IPC
- administrative support.

The IPC team supports staff in ensuring that IPC practice is followed by being available for advice at all times.

A dedicated qualified IPC team:
- is a major resource for the healthcare facility or area
- can implement cost-effective clinical practice
- can prioritise clinical support programmes
- can help with appropriate procurement
- can avert impending outbreaks, morbidity and mortality
- can save a considerable amount of money for the hospital by averting infections.

Working relationships: IPC team

The IPC doctor. The IPC doctor (physician) may be trained in any infection-related specialty. It is useful to have someone who understands the intricacies of the hospital and its functions. The IPC doctor ideally should report to the CEO of the hospital and should hold a salary level of a senior consultant or the head of a unit.

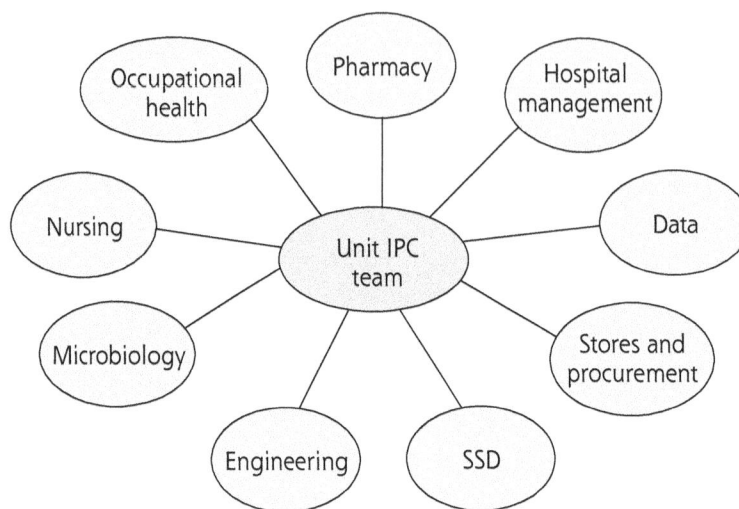

Figure 1.5 Working relationships of the IPC team

The role of the IPC doctor is:
- to report to the CEO regarding pressing IPC matters in the facility
- to liaise between the medical and other staff of the hospital
- to liaise with the microbiology department
- to represent the IPC team at management level
- to establish a close working relationship with the rest of the IPC team
- to be part of policy and decision-making in IPC (with the IPC team)
- to be available for advice on all aspects of IPC
- to promote and support the IPC programme and staff
- to participate in education and training of healthcare staff
- to be an active member of the IPC committee and other committees.

The infection prevention and control professional (IPCP)

The WHO Core Competencies for IPC Professionals[29] define these characteristics as the knowledge, skills and attitudes required for an infection prevention and control (IPC) professional to practise with an in-depth understanding of situations, using reasoning, critical thinking, reflection and analysis to inform assessment and decision-making in the prevention and control of HAI and antimicrobial resistance. The European CDC describes competency as the proven ability to use knowledge, skills and personal, social and/or methodological abilities in work or

---

29   WHO. 2020. Core competencies for infection prevention and control professionals. Geneva: World Health Organization. Licence: CC BY-NC-SA 3.0 IGO.

study situations and in professional and personal development – in other words, what a professional should be able to do (European CDC).[30]

This person should be appropriately qualified and formally trained in IPC in order to function efficiently as a clinical specialist. S/he is pivotal to a sound IPC programme. Since the majority of IPC practitioners are nurses, this section elaborates on aspects of the IPCP work practice. Other IPC practitioners would have similar job descriptions with a different emphasis, depending on training and skills.

The role of the IPCP is:
- to evaluate and improve patient care practices in the hospital or clinical areas by doing daily ward rounds and some night rounds
- to collect appropriate data to support sound IPC policies
- to help with the implementation of IPC policies
- to educate and train all cadres of healthcare staff
- to support the link nurse programme
- to liaise with associated departments/units such as sterile services, engineering and waste management and procurement
- to carry out relevant research
- to attend scientific meetings to update personal knowledge
- to be an active member of the IPC committee and other related committees.

The job description of an IPCP differs from country to country. Where resources are limited, many are designated posts since appointed posts may not exist. This means that the time dedicated to IPC is very limited and the workload is high. S/he may not be supported by an IPC doctor and may have to work single-handed. Some IPCPs may not be formally trained in IPC as they are seconded to a post and have to learn 'on the job'.

The job description of an IPCP should contain the following:
1. Grade of post and salary at the level of a senior clinical nurse manager. This is important for recruitment, retaining staff and respect among peers.

2. **Qualification**
   2.1 **Senior IPCP.** The IPCP should be formally trained in, or in the process of qualifying in, an accredited or structured infection control course. S/he should have and clinical background with at least five years' experience in IPC.

---

[30] Core competencies for infection control and hospital hygiene professionals in the European Union. Stockholm: European Centre for Disease Prevention and Control; 2013 (https://www.ecdc.europa.eu/en/publications-data/core-competencies-infection-control-and-hospital-hygieneprofessionals-european).

    2.2 **Junior IPCP.** This IPCP should have clinical work experience in acute medicine and should work with an experienced IPC team to get good training and experience in IPC. Prior IPC experience (link nurse) is advisable.

3. **Duties**

Duties of an IPCP vary depending on the structure in the healthcare facility, but these are some of the aspects of the job that will support a good IPC programme.

    3.1 **Surveillance.** The IPCP should gather laboratory information regarding alert organisms, especially in high-risk areas, such as the intensive care unit, and keep records of alert organisms. S/he should have computer skills to enter data and maintain the database of HAI.

    3.2 **Investigation of potential outbreaks** and unusual occurrences of alert organisms, monitoring outbreak management and detailed documentation.

    3.3 **Clinical links and advice.** In many countries the IPCP is the sole person responsible for giving clinical advice. Therefore the IPCP should maintain a close working relationship with the clinical staff by regular ward visits, including observation and telephonic discussion. Where necessary s/he should give advice to clinical staff on best practices and improvement of procedures.

    3.4 **Policy development.** The IPCP can help with policy making by using available information to formulate policies, by helping to write policies in conjunction with the IPC team and other relevant stakeholders, by evaluating and monitoring the implementation of policies and by revising policies as required. S/he may assist in the development of an IPC manual with guidelines, policies and standard operating procedures.

    3.5 **Teaching.** The IPCP should provide formal training to healthcare workers as well as short training and discussion regarding IPC matters particularly relating to outbreaks and 'on the job' training while visiting wards.

    3.6 **Research.** The IPCP's operational research activity would include structured investigation into risk factors for IPC and appropriate enhancement of personal development.

    3.7 **Audit** with OH and QA. The IPCP must support a regular (annual) audit of high-risk procedures and policies already in place, the availability of equipment and procurement support and staff response to training and teaching.

    3.8 **Management.** The IPCP must liaise with senior administrative staff in the healthcare facility when the need arises and manage the mentoring, training and support of junior IPC staff.

4. **Skills**

The IPCP must have good personal communication skills, patience, empathy with the staff and the ability to analyse a crisis situation critically and objectively. Computer literacy is essential for writing reports, recording and storing data and recalling information should outbreaks occur.

5. **Self-development**

The IPCP should be encouraged to attend refresher courses, training and scientific meetings and to present scientific papers at national and international seminars.

The number of IPCPs required per healthcare facility is influenced by:
- the number of acute beds (1 : 250 beds, WHO; National IPC Strategic Framework, South Africa, 2020)
- disease profile of the institution or area (predominantly TB/ HIV or HAI)
- number of specialised units such as intensive care units, neonatal units, infectious diseases isolation facilities
- the number of hospital (clinical) staff present.

1.9 Community-based IPC programmes

Community-based structures should be established to support institutions such as care-of-the-elderly homes, primary healthcare facilities and home-based programmes. They should also be involved in public and community education. A district IPC committee could take charge of community health facilities. However, if the community does not have its own structure, the IPC team from the neighbouring facility should provide support in policy development, procurement, design of building and training. IPC training of peer counsellors, community health workers and other support staff will support preparedness in case of outbreaks or pandemics.

By right, all healthcare providers, including families involved in healthcare provision, should be trained in minimum requirements of IPC to maintain and preserve their own health.

1.10 Cost of IPC

There are two considerations for costing IPC programmes – the cost of HAI and the cost of providing an IPC programme. Both of these are complex, but a considerable amount of research has been done which demonstrates that good IPC programmes will save $6 for every $1 spent on IPC!

1.10.1 Cost of healthcare-associated infections

The estimated annual costs of HAI in the UK and USA is estimated to run into billions of pounds sterling and dollars respectively. This has resulted in legislation in these countries to set up IPC programmes which will reduce the number of HAI and cost to the health programme. HAIs in US hospitals have direct medical costs of at least $28.4 billion each year. They also account for an additional $12.4 billion in costs to society from early deaths and lost productivity (CDC).[31]

The SENIC study demonstrated as early as the 1970s that good IPC programmes were associated with lower HAI rates (32%) and healthcare costs.[32] Nyamogoba and Obala estimated that if there is an HAI rate of 8% present in low- to middle-income countries, with an individual cost of between $50 and $500, it is estimated that a 32% reduction would result in a saving of $230 million to $2.3 trillion annually.[33] However, this is dependent on surveillance and analysis of reduction in HAI cost associated with a robust IPC programme. Zimlichman et al[34] estimated the burden of the five most common HAI amounted to $9.8 billion (2012) and reimbursement from medical insurance companies in the USA.[35]

Costing HAI is complex and needs reliable information from several sources, but provides evidence for cost of HAIs and support for IPC. Several parameters are needed to document the cost of HAIs as **direct** and **total** costs and provide standardised methodology towards collecting valuable information.[36] HAIs result in increased length of stay (LOS), resulting in hospital patient treatment and care costs increase. Therefore the LOS used to calculate HAI costs. Device-related infections and surgical site infections costs can be calculated accordingly depending on the increase in LOS. Costs are usually estimated using case control studies and calculating the difference in cost between the two.

The total cost can be extrapolated to a wider group if the HAI incidence is known.[37]

[31] CDC report. https://www.cdc.gov/policy/polaris/healthtopics/hai/index.html#:~:text=HAIs%20in%20U.S.%20hospitals%20have,early%20deaths%20and%20lost%20productivity.

[32] Haley RW, Quade D, Freeman HE. & Bennett JV. 1980. The SENIC Project. Study on the efficacy of nosocomial infection control (SENIC Project). Summary of study design. *American Journal of Epidemiology*, 3(5): 472–485.

[33] Nyamogoba H. & Obala AA. 2002. Nosocomial infections in developing countries: Cost effective control and prevention. *East African Medical Journal*, 79: 435-441.

[34] Zimlichman E, Henderson D, Tamir O et al. 2013. Health Care–Associated Infections A Meta-analysis of Costs and Financial Impact on the US Health Care System. Eyal JAMA Intern Med. 2013; 173(22):2039-2046. doi:10.1001/jamainternmed.2013.9763 Published online September 2, 2013.

[35] Benenson et al. BMC Health Services Research (2020) 20:653 https://doi.org/10.1186/s12913-020-05428-7.

[36] Lee XJ, Stewardson AJ, Worth LJ, Graves N, Wozniak TM, Attributable Length of Stay, Mortality Risk, and Costs of Bacterial Health Care–Associated Infections in Australia: A Retrospective Case-cohort Study, *Clinical Infectious Diseases*, Volume 72, Issue 10, 15 May 2021, Pages e506–e514, https://doi.org/10.1093/cid/ciaa1228.

[37] Manoukian S, Stewart S, Graves Masona NH et al, Bed-days and costs associated with the inpatient burden of healthcare-associated infection in the UK. *Journal of Hospital Infection* 114 (2021) 43e50.

Figure 1.6 Assessing costs for resource allocations[38]

Cost-matrix	Labor costs			Material costs					Infrastructure costs	
Cost category groups / Cost-center groups	Physicians	Nursing	Medical/technical staff	Drugs general	Drugs individual	Implants and grafts	Material	Material individual	Medical	Non-medical
Ward	Care days	Weighted minutes	Care days	Weighted minutes		–	Weighted minutes		Care days	
Intensive care	Weighted hours					Actual usage/unit costs	Weighted hours		Weighted hours	
Dialysis	Weighted dialysis					–	Weighted dialysis		Weighted dialysis	
Operating rooms	Surgery times and setup time		Surgery times and setup time			Actual usage/unit costs	Surgery times and setup time		Surgery times and setup time	
Anesthesia	Anesthesia times		Anesthesia times		Actual usage/unit costs	–	Anesthesia times	Actual usage/unit costs	Anesthesia times	
Delivery ward	Time in delivery ward		Time in delivery ward				Time in delivery ward		Time in delivery ward	
Cardiac diagnostics/therapy	Point system/duration	–	Point system/duration				Point system/duration		Point system/duration	
Endoscopic diagnostics/therapy					Actual usage/unit costs					
Radiology	Point system		Point system				Point system		Point system	
Laboratories										
Further diagnostics/therapy	Point system/duration						Point system/duration		Point system/duration	

A simplified scheme for direct costs is presented below.

Direct costs include

- average length of stay with and without the presence of infection
- additional laboratory costs
- cost of drugs such as antibiotics
- extra sessions in the operating theatre
- cost of dressings and additional nursing support
- additional instrumentation such as intravenous or urinary access
- additional medical consultations.

[38] Vogl M. Assessing DRG cost accounting with respect to resource allocation and tariff calculation: The case of Germany. 2012. *Health Economics Review* 2(1):15. doi:10.1186/2191-1991-2-15.

Table 1.2 A simple costing diagram for IPC. The basic costs are shown in A; additional costs are added from B and C.

Session cost (C)	Surgical or intensive care needs (C)	Basic cost (A)	Individual cases (B)	Additional cost (B)
Extra days – length of stay	• Intensive care • High care • More procedures • More surgical sessions	Bed costs (hotel costs) (What does this cost include?) Cost of acute bed/day	TB cases	• Drugs – antibiotics • Laboratory tests • Personal protective equipment • OPD attendance
Extra staff			HIV	
Extra medication/ pharmacy			H1N1 influenza	
Extra medical devices			HAI	
	Outbreak (HAI) Laboratory tests Extra IPC time Extra staff for isolation rooms			

The information is not readily available in LMICs and therefore the cost cannot be readily estimated, but all attempts should be made to do so. Table 1.2 is an example of how basic costs can be calculated.

Extra costs are incurred during outbreaks of HAI pathogens such as methicillin-resistant *Staphylococcus aureus* (MRSA), multiple antibiotic-resistant gram-negative bacilli, viruses or fungi. Costs associated with the inappropriate overuse of PPE can be calculated and used to document extra costs expense, especially when there are inadequate policies relating to their use. Further costs are incurred when healthcare workers sustain injuries such as needlestick injuries and are given post-exposure prophylaxis and immunisation.

1.10.2 Cost of setting up an IPC programme

It is acknowledged that the cost of setting up an IPC programme from scratch is considerable, but the dividends on such an investment are enormous and the costs can be recuperated quickly. Graves[39] reported that for each dollar spent on IPC a saving of six dollars can be realised, possibly more in LMICs. Vogi published a systematic review evaluating cost of IPC interventions vs HAI reported. The

39 Graves N, Weinhold D, Tong E, Birrell F, Doidge S, Ramritu P, et al. Effect of healthcare-acquired infection on length of hospital stay and cost. Infect Control Hosp Epidemiol 2007;28:280e92. https://doi.org/10.1086/512642.

median savings-to-cost ratio across all studies was US $7.0 (IQR 4.2–30.9), and the median net global saving was US $13 179 (IQR 5 106–65 850) per month.[40]

When setting up a budget, at the very least funding is required for:

Personnel
- staffing – correct bed: IPCP ratios; IPC physicians, administrative staff
- training programmes for IPC staff and healthcare workers
- setting up surveillance
- investigation of infections
- monitoring and evaluation
- regular meetings
- publication of reports.

Benefits
The major contributions of a robust IPC programme are to:
- reduce the number of HAIs
- reduce morbidity and mortality
- improve patient care with early discharge from healthcare facilities
- improve procurement, thereby avoiding costly mistakes
- advise on appropriate facility, building and renovations.

The benefits become apparent when regular surveillance is undertaken.

Case study

The impact of IPC programmes in one intensive care unit (ICU) of a tertiary academic hospital was calculated over a four-year period (Table 1.3). The IPC programme started in 2005 and consisted of one IPC doctor and two IPC nurses. Regular ward rounds, education and lab report communication and feedback with the ICU staff increased. A baseline of number of infections in one ICU was established in 2005–2006 (at the time rates could not be calculated because of lack of access to data). The total (direct and indirect) cost of an ICU patient was determined. The LOS increased five times in HAI patients; the costs varied between R25 000 and R50 000 (US$1 = R15) per day. The decrease in the number of HAI infections from baseline is shown in Table 1.3. In 2007 and 2008 numbers of infections decreased by 31 and 154 respectively. In 2009 the doctor and one IPC practitioner were on leave, leaving only one IPC practitioner to manage 1 300 acute beds! In that year the infections increased by 47. However, in 2010 the IPC doctor returned and the IPC team increased to four IPC practitioners – the HAI infections decreased dramatically by 171 infections! Overall, the saving realised over the four-year period was R8.9 m to R17.8 m. Part of these funds were used to improve IPC training and surveillance and also provide a brand new, state-of-the-art Central Sterile Services Department.

40   Arefian H, Vogel M, Kwetkat A, Hartmann M. 2016. Economic Evaluation of Interventions for Prevention of Hospital Acquired Infections: A Systematic Review. *PLoS ONE* 11(1): e0146381. doi:10.1371/journal. pone.0146381.

Table 1.3   Impact of IPC programme in one tertiary academic hospital ICU

Impact of IPC	Minimum	Maximum	
Feb 11	**R**	**R**	
Cost per infection in ICU	25 000	50 000	
(LOS x 5 times)			
Cost per annum reduction			
Year	**N infections avoided yr on yr**	**Cost**	**Cost**
2006–2007	31 (decreased)	775 000	1 550 000
2007–2008	154 (decreased)	3 850 000	7 700 000
2008–2009	47 (increased)	1 175 000	2 350 000
2009–2010	171 (decreased)	4 275 000	8 550 000
Approx	**Total savings**	**8 900 000**	**17 800 000**

1.11 Education in IPC

1.11.1 Introduction

Evidence-based education and training is the backbone of a robust IPC programme. A well-informed HCW will be confident, carry out safe practice and comply with IPC policy. Core competencies for IPC practitioners (WHO)[41] refer to the knowledge, attitude and skills required to practise, with an in-depth understanding of situations, using reasoning, critical thinking, reflection and analysis to inform assessment and decision-making in the prevention and control of HAIs and AMR. At national and international level, this requires a structured curriculum in IPC encompassing pre-training for undergraduate health trainees, in-service training for the health workforce and post-qualification training for IPC practitioners.

The assumption that anyone who has access to teaching material can train is not true as evidenced by the lack of good IPC practices during large outbreaks such as Ebola and COVID-19. It is best that IPC be taught by a trained, qualified and experienced faculty who understands and has experience in IPC. The question arises, 'When health workers have been trained, why do they not perform well and

---

[41]   WHO. 2020. Core competencies for infection prevention and control practitioners. World Health Organization. https://www.who.int/publications/i/item/9789240011656.

implement policies?' There are several reasons for this, but it is mainly because education and training programmes are not tailor-made to the audience and the essential principles of IPC and understanding these principles are lost because of socio-economic and cultural differences.

- The local conditions of work and staffing levels may differ.
- The cultural norms and language used in training materials adapted from another country may not be clearly understood by the audience.
- The level of teaching needs to be pitched to contextually appropriate local conditions.
- The disease profiles, and therefore emphasis, may differ between countries and this should be taken into account – what is the experience of the audience?
- Tutors are not qualified to train a particular group or level of students.

There are various methods of training, which should be tailored to maximise understanding, depending on the cadre of the audience. The methods could be via lectures, videos, role playing or discussion groups.

1.11.2 Difference between training and education

Tutors should understand the difference between training and education to achieve the correct level of knowledge to be delivered.

1.11.2.1 Training is short term, task orientated and focused on achieving a change of attitude, skills and knowledge in a specific area. It is usually job-related and geared towards increasing proficiency in a skill and helping practitioners feel better about doing it. It answers HOW and WHEN. It is based on practice, rehearsal and repetition. An example would be following a policy or standard operating procedure on the correct insertion method for a peripheral line. It will inform the student about the sequence of steps to be followed in order to carry out the procedure precisely.

1.11.2.2 Education is a lifetime investment. It tends to be initiated by a person in the area of his/her interest. Education answers the WHY questions. It lends weight to various practices and provides evidence, explanation and reason. For example, a clinician can be trained on HOW and WHEN to insert a peripheral cannula correctly, in compliance with an SOP. However, if the risks and hazards arising from a peripheral cannulation are explained, with examples of what can go wrong, then WHY it has to be a careful aseptic procedure is better understood and executed.

Development of an IPC programme including a robust education programme is a long-term investment in IPC human resources which will ultimately pay considerable dividends by reducing healthcare-associated infection.

The aim of training and education is to understand the subject-matter, take ownership of a problem, know what is right and to do it right every time! Further, the aim is to face challenges and deal with them and, ultimately, lead to behavour change.

The tutors must understand their audience and transfer knowledge in a simple and comprehensive way. Factors that influence the students and the tutors' methods will ultimately lead to behaviour change.

1.11.3 Adult teaching methods

Androgogy or adult learning was developed by Knowles,[42] where the students themselves are involved in the learning process. It differs from childhood learning or pedagogy, where the teacher delivers information which must be learnt or memorised in preparation for an examination. Adult learning must always be carried out in a safe environment – no blame or chastising should be allowed since the learning process will be based on both good and bad experiences – lessons learnt!

Knowles (1984)[43] suggested four principles that are applied to adult learning, as shown in Figure 1.7:

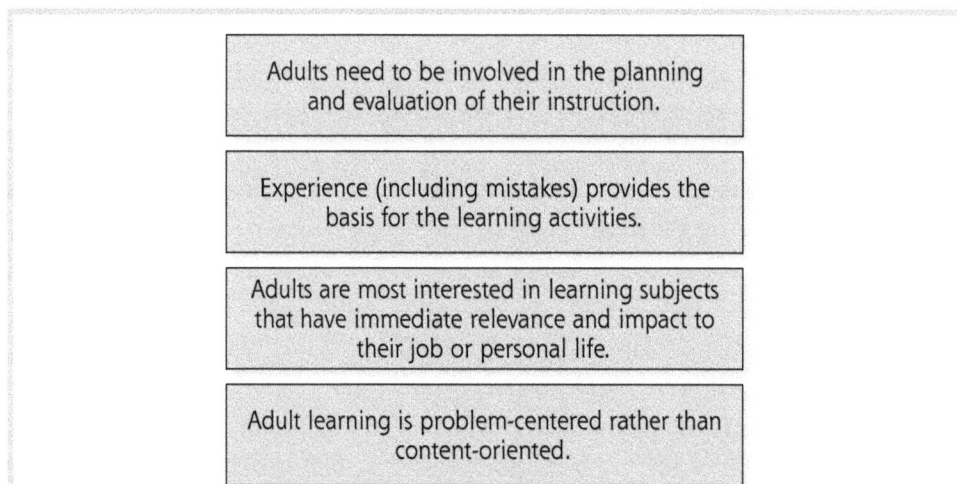

Adults need to be involved in the planning and evaluation of their instruction.

Experience (including mistakes) provides the basis for the learning activities.

Adults are most interested in learning subjects that have immediate relevance and impact to their job or personal life.

Adult learning is problem-centered rather than content-oriented.

Figure 1.7 Four principles of adult learning (Knowles)

1.11.4 Why does adult learning fail?

Despite intensive training, there are often complaints of non-compliance amongst healthcare workers. Some reasons are:

---

[42]   Knowles M. 1984. *Andragogy in Action*. San Francisco: Jossey-Bass.
[43]   Knowles M. 1984. *The Adult Learner: A Neglected Species*. 3rd ed. Houston, TX: Gulf Publishing.

- The teachers or trainers do not understand the subject well enough to allow the adult learners to relate to their own experiences – lack interaction.
- Teaching is carried out by rote learning and facts, sometimes without evidence.
- The material is not contextually appropriate – cut and pasted from another programme without analysing the contents.
- Teaching is done to complete a task rather than provide understanding and knowledge transfer.
- A top-down approach of passing knowledge to the students is used.

1.11.5 Mentorship

Another essential part of adult learning is mentorship. This is when the more experienced colleague or tutor invests in discussing and supporting the student during, and after, the formal teaching has been completed to consolidate and clarify ideas. Again, this must be carried out in a safe space where both the tutor and student are comfortable to discuss matters openly.

1.11.6 Influences on learning

South Africa is a good example of a nation of diverse cultures, each with its own language, traditions and perceptions. Every large organisation such as a hospital will reflect this diversity and employ people from a variety of cultures. This has a profound effect on the teaching of IPC. Educational programmes must take into account and accommodate these differences in understanding of basic concepts, the influence of the individual's set of cultural beliefs and difficulties in fully understanding the language of instruction. All these factors will affect the sustainability of the training programme. In addition, the scarcity of resources will also impinge on the implementation of training.

Even after training, policies are not implemented. There are several reasons for this, including lack of access to robust infrastructure to support IPC practices, lack of understanding and acceptance of new methods, excessive workload or shortage of staff, hierarchical structures, lack of political will and, most importantly, lack of a realistic budget. There are other sociocultural issues that one must be cognisant of when introducing an education programme, which are addressed below.

1.11.6.1 Influence of culture

Despite the diversity of cultures and languages in many countries, there is usually one official language and culture. This influences the way people are taught and what they learn. In South Africa, for example, there are eleven official languages, but English is widely used as the medium of instruction. This does not mean that all teaching is clearly understood; the emphasis may be different and concepts are misunderstood if the teaching method is not attuned to the student's understanding.

The degree of literacy also affects the choice of teaching method. In countries with high literacy, self-teaching using structured modules is acceptable. Where the literacy standard is low, face-to-face oral presentations and practical demonstrations help learners to understand concepts better. In IPC, especially when introducing new programmes, it is more effective to communicate verbally with practical demonstration and then progress to reading, theoretical learning and knowledge tests.

The chat in the corridor between clinical and IPC colleagues usually results in a positive outcome – things get done. Policies may exist but have not been implemented owing to overload or a shortage of staff – the culture of the health facility does not support training.

1.11.6.2 Tradition and perceptions

Usually, HCWs live in the same communities as the general population. The traditions of those communities have been instilled in the psyche of the HCWs and influence the way they conduct themselves in clinical practice. Sometimes IPC policies go against these perceptions and instinctively are rejected. For example, the excessive use of disinfectants in the home environment to reduce germs and disease is a common practice. The impact on antibiotic resistance in the environmental microbiome is neither understood nor contemplated.

Another example is that patients are considered a source of infection or disease and therefore considered 'dirty'. Hospitals are where sick people are admitted, so by definition they are dirty, hence any contact with such a person can only result in harm because of the routes of transmission. This results in the overuse of gloves, aprons, masks and other PPE. To explain the concept of using PPE only for risk-prone procedures is not easy because it goes against traditional perception.

Indigenous knowledge of the local community is frequently overlooked, particularly during large epidemics such as the 2014 outbreak of Ebola in West Africa, when partners from other countries arrive, with preconceived notions, to help and support the local communities and deal with the epidemic. The traditional healers and leaders had considerable knowledge about management of this disease since they had been dealing with Ebola for many years previously, but were not consulted. This resulted in silent hostility and passive resistance, which undermined the efforts to contain the outbreak for a long time.

1.11.6.3 Interpretation of training material

Training and education programmes must be based on most recent evidence, which is constantly evolving and informs good IPC practice; it will require constant review of the curriculum. When curricula or training materials are copied from other countries with different disease profiles, these may not be contextually applicable and the wrong priorities may be emphasised. Therefore, tutors must ensure that the globally recognised evidence-based principles of IPC are taught, irrespective of which country is conducting the training; however, the implementation must be contextually appropriate.

A classical example is hand hygiene. If handwashing is recommended, and the provision of clean running water, soap and hand drying is not available, water tanks with taps (Veronica buckets) can be used. Or alternatively alcohol-based hand rub should be made widely available.

Another challenge is language. Where English is not the first language, teaching must be simple, uncomplicated and unambiguous. Some IPC concepts, such as 'transmission-based precautions', are quite complex to understand and can be misinterpreted if not explained simply. An example is 'standard precautions'. Standard reflects an acceptable level of work performance, hospital design and sterile services, and so on. Standard precautions in IPC takes on a different meaning and means 'routine', or applied in all appropriate situations, such as gloves when accessing the venous system. However, it could be misinterpreted not as 'routine' but 'a goal to strive for' (a standard) and something not yet achieved.

1.11.6.4 Local resources

Training programmes should address the lack of local resources which hinders implementing good IPC practice. There may be a shortage of well-trained IPC tutors, supplies, funds or provisions, which influences training. It is always best to establish what resources exist locally and build on these. When either writing new policies or adapting IPC policies from other countries, local conditions should be a consideration.

1.11.6.5 Sustainability

All or most of the factors previously mentioned affect a sustainable education programme. There has to be ownership of the training and the learners should feel committed, involved and part of the improvement process. Core component 3 (WHO, 2016) is about education in the overall structure and dynamics of a national IPC programme. Education must be funded. The core competencies of an IPC practitioner (WHO) support establishing a career path in IPC with highly competent and dedicated persons in posts at all levels of governance – they must be trained and educated in order to support the IPC programme. Finally, well-run training programmes are part of M&E, and reward for output and excellence should be visible and acknowledged.

To summarise, there are challenges to a sustainable education and training programme.

- Accountability of trained staff to do the correct thing – can be undermined by a lack of consequences.
- Resources – financial constraints mean that budgets for training may not be available.

- Trainers – they themselves may not be well trained and educated in the latest evidence-based information in IPC.
- Relevance of training to work practice – training must be structured to encompass current work practice and must be relevant.
- Refresher courses – once the training is completed, mentorship and refresher courses keep the interest going.

1.11.7 Teaching methods (IPC)

The method of teaching is fundamental to ensure understanding of IPC. Teaching must adapt constantly to the situation and to the needs of the learners. Over the past years, the COVID-19 pandemic has forced trainers to think about innovative ways of transferring knowledge across distance to a wider audience, and necessitated modification of the method of teaching. The teacher must be flexible and creative and use methods that will suit the particular group s/he is teaching. Even the ongoing pressing need for teachers can be solved with some ingenuity, as you will see.

1.11.7.1 Formal

Formal methods are classroom- or web-based, where information is presented in a structured manner. Information is given to the learner, with tasks to complete by self-study, research and testing of knowledge. Tutorials may be held to discuss and debate a particular subject with an exchange of ideas. While tutorials are not structured, they do require an in-depth knowledge of the subject beforehand, moving the student towards education.

1.11.7.2 Contact teaching

For LMICs, contact teaching is most relevant. The students are able to interact closely with the tutors and get personal attention. Bearing in mind that the majority of students have not had learning experience for the past ten years or so, they have to 'relearn to learn'!

There are advantages to this method when:
- English is not the first language. Explanations become essential for understanding and practical demonstrations are necessary.
- Computer and internet access is limited or non-existent.
- Reading skills are not developed to the same level as their peers in other countries, so information has to be visual, simple and, where possible, animated.
- Time can be spent on discussion if a point has not been understood.
- Working conditions can be discussed, and addressed, within the course.
- There are cultural and language differences.

The disadvantages are that this method is very expensive, particularly when the faculty or the students have to travel around the vast continent of Africa. Contact teaching is exhausting for the tutors and marking papers takes a long time. The presentations have to be simple and diagrammatic and sometimes discussions are prolonged.

1.11.7.3 Web-based distance learning

Many excellent IPC courses, especially international courses, are increasingly becoming web-based and available electronically, which is ideal for distance learning, particularly during the COVID-19 pandemic (2020). There are several platforms available such as Zoom, Moodle and Brightspace, which allow virtual classes to be conducted interactively, with practical demonstrations and videos. There is provision for written or verbal interaction between the students and tutors.

The advantages of such a system are:
- A standardised curriculum can reach distant and remote sites so it can reach a wider audience with the same message.
- The students do not have to travel and therefore the cost is lower.
- They can use a computer at their place of work if they do not own one.
- Several colleagues from the same institution can join the class. This can improve communication and peer collaboration.
- Many students can be reached at the same time and taught simultaneously.
- It is less tiring for the tutors and their time can be more structured.

The disadvantages are:
- It is very dependent on a stable internet connection and availability of a computer.
- The tutor has to be very innovative and use several methods of teaching to ensure that the students do not loose track during a teaching session.
- There can be interaction through the chat or white board exercises, but it is not as personalised as contact teaching.
- The quiet students may not get a chance to interact with the tutors.
- A certain basic level of knowledge is expected from the students. Reading material is provided, which should be reviewed beforehand and discussed. Some students cannot manage this type of self-learning.

1.11.7.3.1 Applying web-based learning

Video conferencing has become increasingly popular (particularly during the COVID-19 pandemic), but requires a stable internet connection. It allows access to remote sites to lecture, demonstrate and interact with the audience. Most of the sessions are recorded and the students can return to the lectures and discussions to clarify concepts in their own time.

1.11.7.3.1.1   **Mentorship:** The mentor can have a private discussion with an individual or a general discussion with a group of students at an appointed time. It can be interactive with presentations by the audience, or debates between peers, or indeed quizzes and reminders. It is a non-threatening way to communicate difficult topics. This programme is an excellent way of maintaining interest in IPC and also helping to solve challenges.

1.11.7.3.1.2   **Webinars:** Run for a limited time, webinars can be hosted on such a platform and reach 500 or more persons simultaneously. Webinars are usually one to two hours long and address a single topic of interest to the audience. There is time for interaction and discussion, usually at the end. Webinars have proved to be extremely effective in communicating important messages quickly and succinctly to a wide audience, particularly during the recent COVID-19 pandemic – information was shared widely and quickly across the globe.

1.11.7.4 Informal

Contact with staff on ward rounds, in corridors and tea rooms is used effectively to pass on knowledge and exchange information. It may relate to a particular problem and a non-threatening discussion may be used effectively to clarify matters. Clinical case discussions and other similar occasions are also useful to train informally and sometimes influence IPC policies.

1.11.8 In-service (on the job) training

Regular in-service training should be provided to all HCWs to keep them abreast of the most recent information and advances in IPC. If there is an outbreak or widespread epidemic, in-service training is useful to remind HCWs about IPC policies and practices that will keep their patients and themselves safe. It gives confidence and improves implementation of policies which should be in place already.

In some cases, specific IPC in-service training is provided to specialist areas such as surgery, operating theatres, sterile services, intensive care, neonatology and infectious diseases. Training for non-clinical workers such as cleaners, porters, engineers and environmental health officers can also be arranged to ensure everyone is informed of new or modified policies. It is the role of the IPC practitioner to provide regular in-service training for all categories of staff.

1.11.9 Practical/demonstration

1.11.9.1 Practical teaching: During contact teaching or distance learning, the students visit clinical facilities and apply theory to practice. This has been a most successful method of teaching in LMICs where the students see different clinical settings and can critically evaluate the situation, followed by group discussion. In distance learning a clinical situation can be simulated by asking students to visit clinical facilites, take short videos of their place of work and present these to the class for discussion. This encourages peer-to-peer learning and provides an insight into a variety of environments.

1.11.9.2 Role playing: This is an excellent way of teaching health workers to walk in the shoes of patients with different scenarios relating to infectious disease. This enforces the role of the patient in IPC and helps to improve understanding from the patients' and workers' points of view. It is also interesting to observe the behaviour of the students and their interactions with each other as health worker and patient – ingrained behaviour becomes evident and misconceptions can be corrected.

1.11.9.3 Self-study: Once the contact period is over the students go back to their workplaces, where they complete assignments, usually clinical in nature, and document these in a logbook (portfolio). These assignments usually require the students to apply what was learnt in the classroom to the actual work environment. The students find this most useful since it is the practical application of theoretical learning.

1.12 Know your audience

Before starting a training session, know the level of knowledge amongst the class. This is determined by a pre-assessment test, which gives the tutor an opportunity to address the gaps. The difference between the pre- and post-assessment marks can be evaluated as a percentage of the level of knowledge transfer (Figure 1.8).

An example of pre- and post-test knowledge transfer is shown in Figure 1.8. Group 3 showed the least increase, possibly reflecting the competency of the tutors. Overall a 22% increase in knowledge was documented. The second course was run six months later for the same cohort of students – the knowledge transfer increase was 5%, which probably reflects understanding and retention of information from the first course.

1st IPC training for Ebola, March '15

% Increase in Knowledge

| Class 1 | Pre test average: 11,18 | Post test average: 17,64 | Increase knowledge %: 29,55 |

(Bar chart, Class average 1, 2, 3):
- Class 1: Pre test average 11,18; Post test average 17,64; Increase knowledge % 29,55
- Class 2: Pre test average 13,25; Post test average 18,31; Increase knowledge % 22,99
- Class 3: Pre test average 16,11; Post test average 18,35; Increase knowledge % 10,18

Class average

■ Pre test average ■ Post test average ▨ Increase knowledge %

(Second bar chart — 5% increase):
- Class 1: Pre test 68; Post test exam 74; Median 81
- Class 2: Pre test 69; Post test exam 78; Median 85
- Class 3: Pre test 76.4; Post test exam 77; Median 81
- Total: Pre test 71.1; Post test exam 76; Median 82

■ Pre test ■ Post test exam ▨ Median

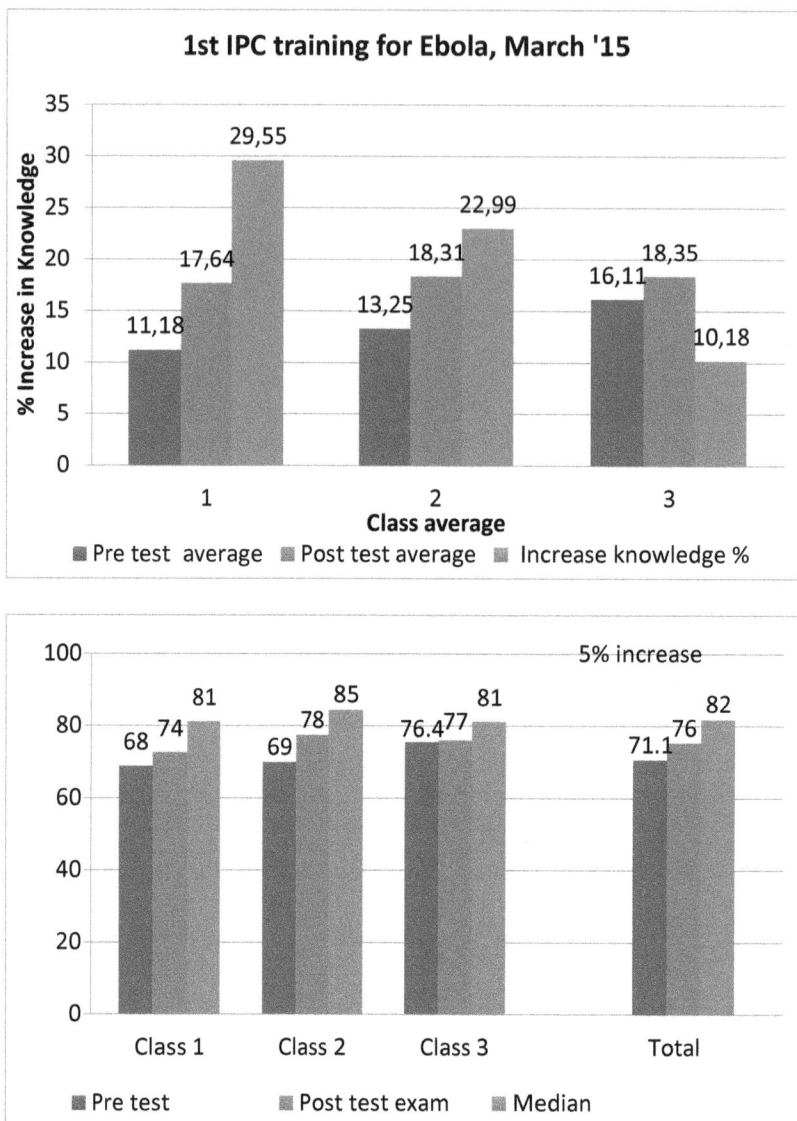

Figure 1.8 A first training programme for three groups

A basic IPC five-day training course should be offered to all HCWs at undergraduate, in-service training and postgraduate level. Specialised IPC courses that feed into a career path should be established at national and healthcare facility level (WHO core component 3).

1.12.1 Healthcare managers

Managers are often too busy or feel they do not need to learn about IPC since there are IPC teams on the ground. Managers should learn the basic principles of

IPC (scope), how it functions (implementation), what it can achieve (cost savings) and what cost benefit can be derived from a good IPC programme. The ultimate responsibility for IPC lies with the managers and so they must know what is happening.

If managers understand IPC, they will be more willing to put resources towards it and ensure HCWs attend training and apply good IPC practice. It is an investment and good marketing tactic for IPC. A course for managers should cover the topics on legislation, cost of IPC, HAI surveillance, disease profiles, hand hygiene, standard and transmission-based precautions, emphasis on high disease prevalence (TB/HIV, HAI and AMR) and policy development. Ward visits should be included.

1.12.2 Healthcare workers

There is little or no IPC training for HCWs at undergraduate level. Where IPC training is provided, the information is obsolete (often 30 years old), poorly taught by non-IPC specialists and even less well understood – in other words, irrelevant to undergraduates, who concentrate on passing examinations.

Formal short courses for HCWs to address particular topics for specific groups should be tailored to their needs. A course in IPC should be considered separately from the disease-based training courses.

It is recommended that all health workers attend at least one IPC training programme in their career. Short refresher courses based on topical matters may be held annually or biannually. Content of such courses should be structured as one hour each of lectures, ward visits and discussion. All relevant topics should be covered, for example risk management in a clinical setting, risk-prone procedures and preventive measures such as hand hygiene, standard and transmission-based precautions and appropriate use of PPE. The emphasis should be on routes of transmission and prevention of common diseases such as TB, HIV or multidrug-resistant organisms (MDROs) as well as the appropriate use of disinfectants and antibiotics.

1.12.3 Train the Trainers

Train the Trainer (TTT) is a way of training a large group of health workers quickly and to pass important messages on to the rest of the workforce. TTT can be chosen from the Basic or Advanced Basic course depending on their interest and understanding of the subject – not everyone can be a trainer so select your group carefully. This group is given additional teaching in adult learning methods and on simplifying complex messages. The trainers could either be a separate group (paid contract workers) or internal staff (part of their job). In order to make this programme sustainable the trainers must be recognised and, where possible, remunerated.

We developed a Train the Trainer curriculum for rapid dissemination of IPC information to select students from the Basic or Advanced Basic course who are interested and committed to teaching IPC. Once they have completed IPC and the Adult Learning Methodology courses (two weeks in total), their 'project' is to train five further people on the information they learnt. They may use any method to teach their students – some are quite innovative. After three months or more, a team of examiners visits the site, either face-to-face or remotely, and tests the knowledge of the five people who were trained. If approximately 75% of the information has been passed on correctly, the trainer will get a Certificate of Competence (TTT) in addition to the IPC course certification. The students get a Certificate of Competence in Basic IPC. If some of the students do not pass, then at least many health workers have been exposed to the basics of IPC.

1.12.4 Link nurses[44]

Trained link nurses in the clinical areas are a great asset to the IPC team and the healthcare programme, particularly where there is a shortage of trained IPC personnel. The link nurse is a person who is ward-based and is involved with day-to-day clinical practice. It can be any clinical person who shows an interest, but it is best if the link nurse is someone who the clinical team has confidence in and will be listened to. The link nurse is trained in Advance IPC (essentials of IPC, surveillance, monitoring and evaluation and guidance for all staff) and acts as the 'eyes and ears' of the IPC team in a positive and constructive way.[45] The advantage of such a programme is that any areas in IPC that require attention are rapidly dealt with. The link nurses are strongly supported by the IPC team with frequent updates and refresher courses. There might be a rapid turnover of link nurses, therefore a continuous training programme for link nurses should be in place where those already trained support each other as well as the ward staff.

1.12.5 IPC professionals

In the core competencies for IPC professionals WHO recommends that an IPC professional (IPCP)[46] should be fully trained, having completed a certified

[44] Williams L, Cooper T, Bradford L, Cooledge B, Elner F, Fisher D, Huws JC, Jones L, Morris S, Rowe N, Sengwe R, Roberts C, Roberts K, Wright J & Griffiths HO. 2019. An evaluation of an infection prevention link nurse programme in community hospitals and development of an implementation model. *J Infect Prev*, 20(1): 37–45. doi: 10.1177/1757177418789480. Epub 2018 Oct 4. PMID: 30719087; PMCID: PMC6346324.

[45] Teare EL & Peacock A. 1996. The development of an infection control link-nurse programme in a district general hospital. *J Hosp Infect*, 34(4): 267–278. doi: 10.1016/s0195-6701(96)90107-3. PMID: 8971616.

[46] WHO. 2020. Core competencies for infection prevention and control professionals. Geneva: World Health Organization. Licence: CC BY-NC-SA 3.0 IGO. https://www.health.gov.za/wp-content/uploads/2020/11/practical-manual-for-implementation-of-the-national-ipc-strategic-framework-march-2020.pdf.

postgraduate IPC training course. Having completed this training, and with more than three years' experience, such a person is a great asset to the healthcare facility.

Formal training in IPC should be provided for all IPC professionals (IPCP) who are in posts or intend to take up a position in IPC, irrespective of their job category. Specialist training in IPC should be based on a single national or international curriculum. By studying together, the skills from different professional groups can be used to effectively build teams, encourage discussion and set up long-lasting networks, working relationships and friendship.

For IPC practitioners the course should be a requirement for a career path in IPC towards becoming an IPC professional (IPCP).[47]

The junior IPCP should attend the Fundamental six-month course in IPC within one year of starting the job.

A senior IPCP should attend the Postgraduate Diploma in IPC after two years of IPC experience.

1.12.6 Courses in IPC

Training and education programmes in IPC are a must for all healthcare workers, including managers. Often managers will require a separate, succinct course which relates more to the advantages of IPC than the actual practical aspects. In some countries doctors and nurses prefer to be trained separately. This is not as effective as training together as teams of doctors and nurses because as a team they can support each other and develop mutual respect for each other's professional ability.

IPC practitioners should be trained to the highest level in IPC so that they can be an asset to the facility. It is always preferable to train IPC practitioners as teams of doctors and nurses.

Different categories of HCW will require the same information on basic principles of IPC, but at different levels, based on their job categories and understanding of the healthcare system. Ideally, one curriculum is developed on the principles of IPC, including the core components, and then it is tailored to the audience. IPC training can be structured as building blocks so that essential information is delivered succinctly and clearly to the group of HCWs to be informed.

All structured training and education must have a pre- and post-assessment. A Certificate of Competence should be issued for all those that satisfy the necessary

---

[47] Infection prevention and control professional (IPCP): Healthcare professional (medical doctor, nurse, or other health-related professional) who has completed a **certified postgraduate IPC training course,** or a nationally or internationally recognised postgraduate course on IPC or another core discipline, including IPC as a core part of the curriculum, as well as **IPC practical and clinical training.** *Source:* Adapted from WHO. 2016. Guidelines on core components of infection prevention and control programmes at the national and acute healthcare facility level. Geneva: World Health Organization. https://www.who.int/publications/i/item/9789241549929.

level of knowledge in IPC. Certificates of Attendance may be offered for in-service training courses, webinars and mentorship classes.

Table 1.4 Categories of staff and the recommended level and duration of training (adapted from National IPC Strategic Framework, South Africa, 2020)

Level of IPC curriculum	Staff category	Duration of teaching
Basic IPC	All HCW	5 days; quarterly refresher 2–3 hours
Intermediate (Advanced) IPC In addition to Basic Course, shorter sessions on specific topics of interest (surgery, ICU, neonatology, outbreaks, COVID-19, antimicrobial stewardship committee members)	Link nurses, clinical teams working with IPC, health managers, emergency medical services, Train the Trainers. Non-clinical teams – cleaners, porters, kitchen, engineers	5-day Basic Course, plus 5–7 additional (1–2 hr) sessions specifically tailored to needs of each group
Fundamentals in IPC (FIPC)	Practitioners starting in IPC, infection-related clinical teams such as ID, microbiology, pharmacists, occupational health, environmental health, policy makers	6 months part time covering 5 modules with didactic teaching, plus homework
Postgraduate Diploma in IPC (PDIC)	IPC practitioners in post for 2 years or more Clinical teams directly involved in IPC	2 years part time; 10 weeks per module plus extra activities

1.12.6.1 Specialist courses in IPC

Training courses for IPC practitioners and specialists are usually based on local or regional needs. No matter how the courses are structured, the basic principles of IPC should be covered (Figure 1.9). National and international courses should be accredited by a recognised body or teaching institution and should be reviewed frequently. Ideally, there should a variety of specialist tutors on the course to improve exposure and confidence among the students.

The course could be designed in many ways, but a modular course helps the learners to complete and understand each section before moving on to the next one. The course may be part time (or full time) to take into consideration that all the students will be employed while on the course.

Basic	Advanced	FIPC	PDIC
			IPC & QI
		ADVANCED IPC PLUS	Multimodal strategies
	BASIC PLUS	Risk-reducing strategies	Operational research
Microbiology	Environmental cleaning and terminal cleaning	Basic epidemiology	Leadership skills and management of IPC structure, budgets, cost of HAI
Transmission	Reprocessing medical devices	Decontamination and sterilisation	
Standard precautions	HAI and AMR	Built environment	
Transmission-based precautions	Audits in IPC practices	WASH	Designing health facilities
Environment	Training adults	Specialised units	Procurement
Disinfectants	IPC legislation	Outbreak response	Ethics
Understanding data		Monitoring and evaluation	Communication
Occupational health	Specialist courses	Mentorship	Advisory role to international organisations
Vaccination		Leadership skills	
		Writing reports and presenting data	

Figure 1.9 The stepwise increment of various levels of IPC training and education (adapted from National IPC Strategic Framework, South Africa, 2020)

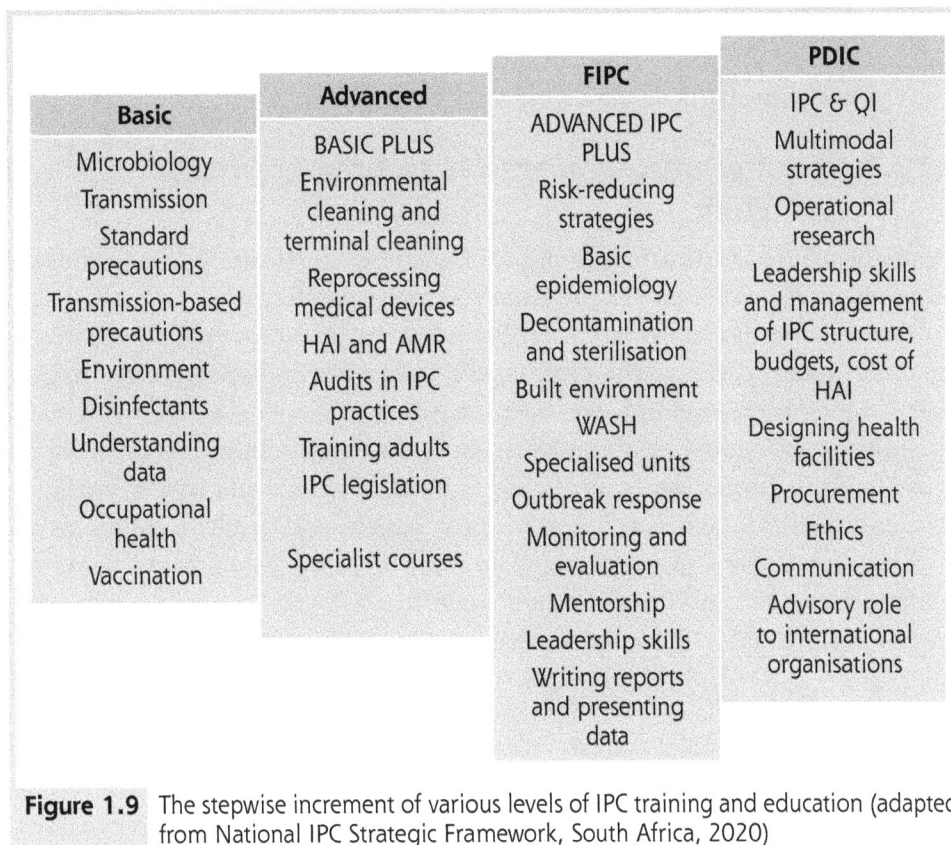

1.12.7 Other short courses

1.12.7.1 Tailor-made courses: Courses on standard and transmission-based precautions for all staff are necessary and should be conducted regularly.

1.12.7.2 Water Sanitation and Hygiene (WASH): WASH and IPC are interdependent. Basic IPC training for environmental health officers, engineers and others working in this field is essential. The course content is set by WASH at WHO, but may be modified to support developing safe IPC practices.

1.12.7.3 Support health staff: Often porters, waste managers and kitchen staff are not included in the training programmes. Short lunchtime courses over several weeks are ideal as they do not interfere with the work plan and the staff is relaxed and feels able to ask questions in a safe environment.

1.12.7.4 Cleaning teams: should have their own in depth training course which explains all aspects of cleaning, materials used for cleaning, and inspection, monitoring and evaluation of cleaning practices.

1.12.7.5 Emergency services: Short courses on reinforcing risk management, hand hygiene and transmission-based precautions are very effective and improve working relationships with IPC. During outbreaks, this forum is most effective in dispelling non-evidence-based policies and clarifying concepts, particularly related to the use of PPE.

1.12.8 Training programmes for community-based structures

Community-based institutions require IPC support, particularly for community HCWs who carry out door-to-door visits and home-based care.

This training should be basic, highlighting transmission of pathogens in the community setting, simple yet effective PPE to be worn and adequate ventilation when attending patients indoors. Understanding where to place the patient (if space allows) to reduce risk of transmission to the household and others must be considered. Healthcare waste, including disposal of sharps and soiled dressings, must be addressed. Communication with the patient and family in simple terms so that good hygiene practices, such as hand hygiene, safe storage of water, sanitation and personal hygiene, are understood. Some essential points are covered in the chapter on communicable diseases.

1.12.8.1 Home-based carers

In countries where families and caregivers play a major role in delivering healthcare the training programmes must be in tune with the level of knowledge and interests of the community. Those caring for loved ones with chronic infectious diseases have to do so over a long period and should be comfortable with the way care is provided safely.

The other aspect is preventive measures. These are different. Here the message has to be given to a large group of mixed age who may or may not have any interest in a healthcare issue at a particular time. An interesting study recently published by Gould et al[48] reflects on the perceptions and knowledge of the community in the United Kingdom – 'they eyed sources of information with suspicion and showed little confidence in the information provided from these sources'.

Community structures will require three things:
- transfer of **accurate knowledge** to patients and their carers
- **support of information** with peer group and lay counsellors, who will sustain the impact of education
- **incentives** to support the health programme.

Transfer of knowledge. There has to be trust between the community and the structures that are giving out information.

[48] Gould DJ, Drey NS, Millar M et al. 2009. Patients and the public: knowledge, sources of information and perceptions about healthcare associated infection. *Journal of Hospital Infection*, 72: 1–8.

The information should be delivered in the simplest format with pictures, pictograms and unambiguous visual information. In countries with low literacy these visual aids, accompanied by verbal communication, seem to be most effective.

Information derived from hearsay or sensational media reports should be clarified with simple yet evidence-based answers. The information leaflets or campaigns must be empathetic and open communication with the Department of Health via telecommunication or other means should be established. The community must be given regular feedback and accurate follow-up to strengthen this partnership.

Peer education and counsellors. There is no one who understands a community better than those who live in it. A group of enthusiastic young people should be recruited and means of teaching should be discussed and followed closely. A mentoring system for these peer-counsellors has to be in place. In a family environment a designated caregiver is an ideal person to be informed and trained.

The training should include basic information on home-based care relating to simple yet effective transmission-based precautions, waste management and patient placing during an epidemic or outbreak.

Regular classes or discussion groups should be held and some of the responsibility of managing the current situation should be given to the community. For example, in a cholera outbreak, appropriate handling of water and food should be delegated.

Incentives. The entire community should have a reason to comply with the procedures put in place. The incentives do not have to be financial – there could be benefit in kind, improvement of child health or family well-being, food or other support. Schools and institutions are a good place to start basic IPC programmes on hand hygiene, safe water and food and sanitation.

Specialist courses in IPC: International Postgraduate Diploma in Infection Control (IPDIC)

The contents of the module are shown in Figure 1.9.

Outcome of the IPDIC

The module marks are distributed equally over a written examination, the logbook and the project. This is to accommodate those who may have difficulty in expressing themselves under the stress of examination but have done well in applying their knowledge during a practical situation. The project reflects what has been learnt and applied, and it provides evaluation of IPC at the place of work.

2 Introduction to microbiology

Joost Hopman & Shaheen Mehtar

Learning outcomes

What you should know after reading this chapter:
- Basic anatomy and physiology of micro-organisms
- Using microbiology laboratory services effectively
- Healthcare-associated infections and how these are transmitted
- The microbiome
- Microbes of IPC importance
- Antimicrobial stewardship

Introduction

Knowledge of basic microbiology is pivotal to understanding IPC programmes. A competent IPC practitioner should understand the role of microbes and their interaction with humans and the surrounding environment. It is not the remit of this chapter to give an in-depth account of microbiology, but more to support IPC knowledge and practices by **understanding transmission of pathogens** and how these can be reduced.

Another area of major global concern is antimicrobial resistance (AMR). Major efforts are under way to curb the increase in AMR – one such vital pillar is IPC. Here, IPC plays a major role in reducing the spread of multidrug-resistant organisms (MDROs) thereby reducing the need to prescribe, and consume, antibiotics.

Micro-organisms are ubiquitous (found everywhere) and play an essential role in our world. The different types of micro-organisms in living hosts, the environment and surrounds are known as microbiomes. Most micro-organisms are harmless and are even considered friendly. They colonise humans, living in harmony with their host, and often prevent the entry of pathogens. Microbes are part of a parallel universe which surrounds us and our environment.

However, microbes can cause disease in humans. This usually follows an event which supports the transfer of microbes via a vehicle to a susceptible host. This either transports microbes to an environment that supports and favours their invasion and multiplication or reduces host defences. Bacteria, viruses and some fungi are of importance in IPC, but in this chapter, parasites (helminths and protozoa) are also addressed. For further information, readers are referred to textbooks or online information on microbiology.

2.1   Micro-organisms

Micro-organisms are living beings classified by genus (groups) and species (subgroups), related by common features such as genetics, metabolism or immunological responses. They are very small (micro) life forms and include bacteria, fungi, microscopic parasites and viruses.

2.1.1   **Bacteria** are unicellular prokaryotes with distinctive biological characteristics and can survive and replicate **independently** of the host.

2.1.2   **Fungi** and moulds are multi-cellular eukaryotes with **independent** survival and replication.

2.1.3   **Parasites** (eukaryotes) include helminths and protozoa and are also capable of **independent** survival and replication.

2.1.4   **Viruses** are not actually considered independently 'alive' since they are only made of genetic material – either DNA and/or RNA – and their survival and replication is **totally dependent** on entering living cells.

2.1.5   **Prions** are not actual micro-organisms because they lack all but nucleic acid; however, they are infectious agents. Prions are minute particles of protein which are infectious in a particular context such as nervous tissue. Most important from an IPC perspective is their resistance to inactivation by routine decontamination and sterilisation means.

2.2   Differences between prokaryotes and eukaryotes

Bacteria are classified as **prokaryotes**, while all the other organisms (except viruses) are classified as **eukaryotes**. There are significant differences between these two groups, which are clinically relevant, particularly when prescribing antimicrobial therapy.[1]

---

[1]   Mims AC, Playfair JHL, Roitt IM et al. 1993. *Medical microbiology.* London: Mosby.

Table 2.1 Comparing prokaryotes and eukaryotes: similarities and differences[2]

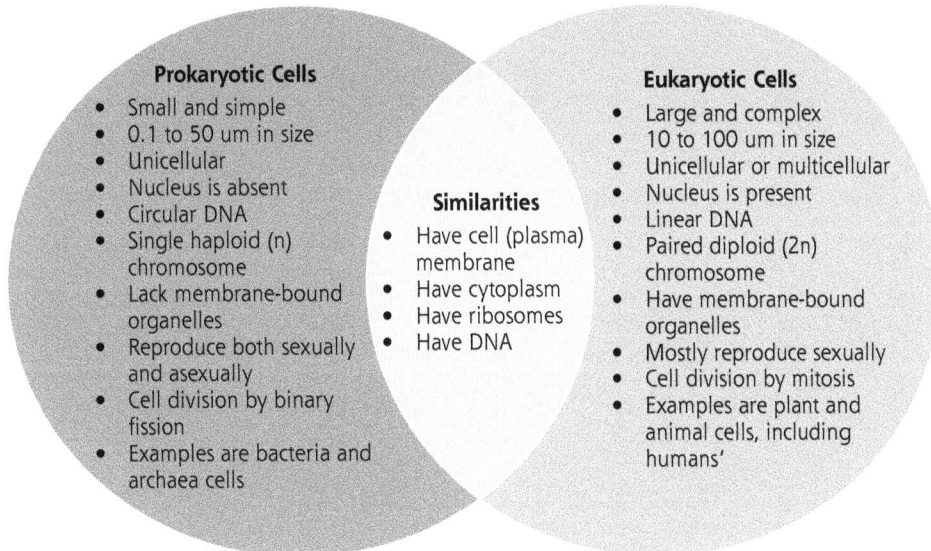

Prokaryotic Cells
- Small and simple
- 0.1 to 50 um in size
- Unicellular
- Nucleus is absent
- Circular DNA
- Single haploid (n) chromosome
- Lack membrane-bound organelles
- Reproduce both sexually and asexually
- Cell division by binary fission
- Examples are bacteria and archaea cells

Similarities
- Have cell (plasma) membrane
- Have cytoplasm
- Have ribosomes
- Have DNA

Eukaryotic Cells
- Large and complex
- 10 to 100 um in size
- Unicellular or multicellular
- Nucleus is present
- Linear DNA
- Paired diploid (2n) chromosome
- Have membrane-bound organelles
- Mostly reproduce sexually
- Cell division by mitosis
- Examples are plant and animal cells, including humans'

2.3 Bacteria

Bacteria have a rigid cell wall (peptidoglycan) and contain both DNA and RNA but no nuclear membrane and therefore no distinct nucleus. It is the rigid cell wall that defines their shapes.

2.3.1 Classification of bacteria

Based on the gram stain, size, morphology and growth characteristics, bacteria can be classified as shown in the abbreviated table, with examples of bacteria of medical importance.

Table 2.2 Examples of common bacteria of medical importance and their identification

Gram stain	Shape	Morphology	Respiration	Examples
Positive	Cocci	Clusters	Aerobic	Staphylococci
		Chains		Streptococci
		Pairs	Microaerophilic	Pneumococci
			Anaerobic	Peptostreptococci

---

[2] https://www.sciencefacts.net/prokaryotes-vs-eukaryotes.html.

Gram stain	Shape	Morphology	Respiration	Examples
	Bacilli (rods)	Sporing	Aerobic	*Bacillus spp*
		Non-sporing	Aerobic	*Listeria spp*
		Sporing	Anaerobic	*Clostridium spp*
		Non-sporing	Anaerobic	*Cutibacterium spp*
Negative	Cocci	Pairs	Microaerophilic	*Neisseria spp*
	Bacilli	Random	Aerobic	*Klebsiella pneumoniae, E coli**
			Anaerobic	*Bacteroides spp*
		Curved, comma shaped	Aerobic Microaerophilic	Vibrios, *Campylobacter spp, Helicobacter spp*
Poorly staining or not at all	Spiral	Corkscrew	Anaerobic Aerobic	Treponemes, *Leptospira spp*
	Bacilli	Beaded on ZN	Microaerophilic	*Mycobacterium spp*

* also known as coliforms

2.3.2 Staining characteristics

Bacteria are classified based on the gram stain, a widely used method to identify the shape of bacteria in the laboratory. Bacteria which retain the blue dye are gram positive, while those that lose the dye (discolouration) and stain pink with the counterstain are known as gram negative. Some are poorly staining, such as spirochetes, vibrios and mycobacteria, and different staining methods are required to visualise them under the microscope.

Mycobacteria have an additional waxy layer outside the cell wall and do not take up the gram stain readily. A modified Ziehl–Neelsen stain uses heat to drive the carbol fuchsin into the cells and withstands decolourisation with acid and alcohol. These are known as acid- and alcohol-fast.

2.3.3 Morphology and growth characteristics

Typically, bacteria range from about 1 μ to about 5 μ – some may be as small as 0,2 μ (mycoplasma) or as large as 15 μ (spiral). They have a characteristic pattern when seen under the microscope and are instantly recognisable. For example, staphylococci appear in grape-like clusters, while streptococci will form chains, albeit short or long, in fluid media. Genus *Klebsiella* and *Escherichia coli* are gram-negative bacilli and follow no particular morphological pattern, while diphtheroids (gram-positive bacilli) appear as 'Chinese lettering'. The reader is referred to a textbook on microbiology for further information.

Bacterial shapes vary depending on the species they belong to:

1. round or ball-shaped (cocci)
2. elongated or bat-shaped (bacilli)
3. spiral or corkscrew-shaped (spirochetes)
4. curve or 'comma'-shaped (vibrios).

2.3.4 Haemolysis

Growth on solid media also differentiates various species of bacteria. Haemolysis of blood agar is a characteristic of some bacteria, notably streptococci, which produce haemolytic enzymes. These are used to classify streptococci growing on blood agar plates.

2.3.4.1 β-**haemolytic.** The area around the growth of the bacteria colony producing this toxin is clear compared with the rest of the blood agar plate. It is characteristic of group A streptococci, but other bacteria can also produce a haemotoxin.

2.3.4.2 α-**haemolytic.** There is partial haemolysis, the surrounding area appearing green. *Streptococcus pneumoniae* is a classical example.

2.3.4.3 **Non-haemolytic.** The area surrounding the bacterial colony does not demonstrate any change compared with the rest of the agar plate, as seen with *Enterococcus spp.*

2.3.5 Respiration

Bacteria can also be divided into **aerobic**, or oxygen-dependent, and **anaerobic** (growing in the absence of oxygen). Some are **microaerophilic** and need oxygen as well as carbon dioxide to survive and multiply.

2.3.6 Anatomy of a bacterium (Figure 2.1)

- **Flagella** are long helical filaments that support motility and allow the bacterium to change its environment. Flagella are built from protein (flagellins) which are strongly antigenic. These (H) antigens are important targets for antibody responses (e.g. *Salmonella spp*).
- **Pili and fimbriae** are external fine hair-like rigid structures (not involved in motion) which allow the bacterium to attach itself to external surfaces – either to a host (common pili) or other bacteria (sex pili); the latter is to transfer genetic information. Common pilus attaches to specific receptors and can change its antigenic configuration to avoid recognition by the host's immune system. If there are numerous pili, the bacterium may escape phagocytosis.

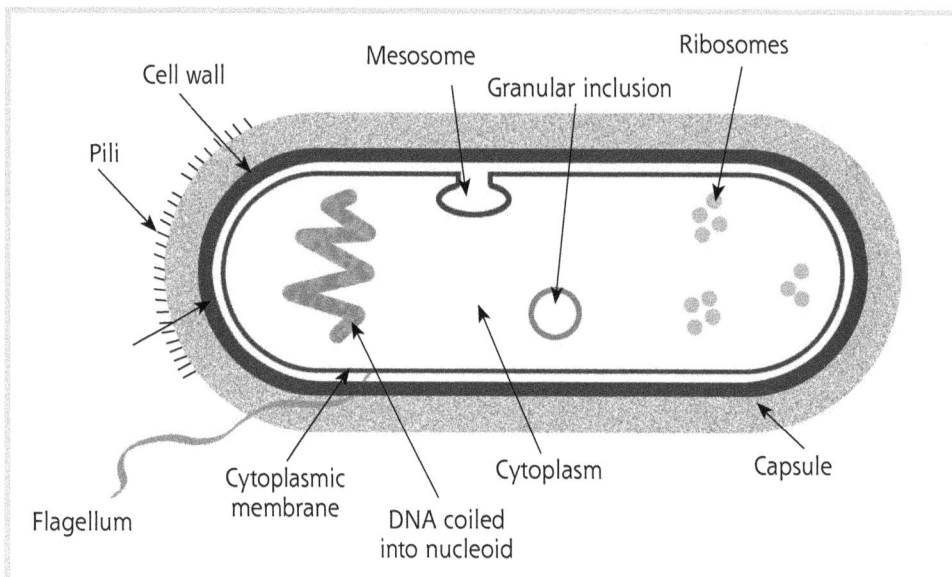

Figure 2.1 A diagrammatic representation of a bacterium illustrating the essential anatomical components

- **Cell membrane** is the lining inside the cell wall which holds the cytoplasm in place. It is semipermeable to essential nutritional elements and removal of waste.
- **Ribosomes** are constantly producing the protein building blocks for rejuvenation of the cell.
- **Deoxyribonuclease (DNA)** is the genetic 'brain' that ensures survival of the cell. It contains important genetic encoded material which defend the cell by various means.
- **Cell wall** (Figure 2.2) is a rigid structure which allows selective absorption and excretion of various substances. In gram-negative bacilli there are inlets or channels called **porins** which allow selective passage into and out of the cell and can be modified, if required, to restrict noxious substances such as antimicrobial agents from entering the cytoplasm. There are clear differences between the cell walls of gram-negative and gram-positive bacteria, as shown in the figure below. The main difference is the peptidoglycan layer in the gram positive cell wall, which is much thicker than the gram negative cell wall. On the other hand, the gram negative cell wall has two lipo-polysaccharide layers, above and below the peptidoglycan layer. The cell wall is a target for several groups of antibiotics, such as β-lactams and glycopeptides.

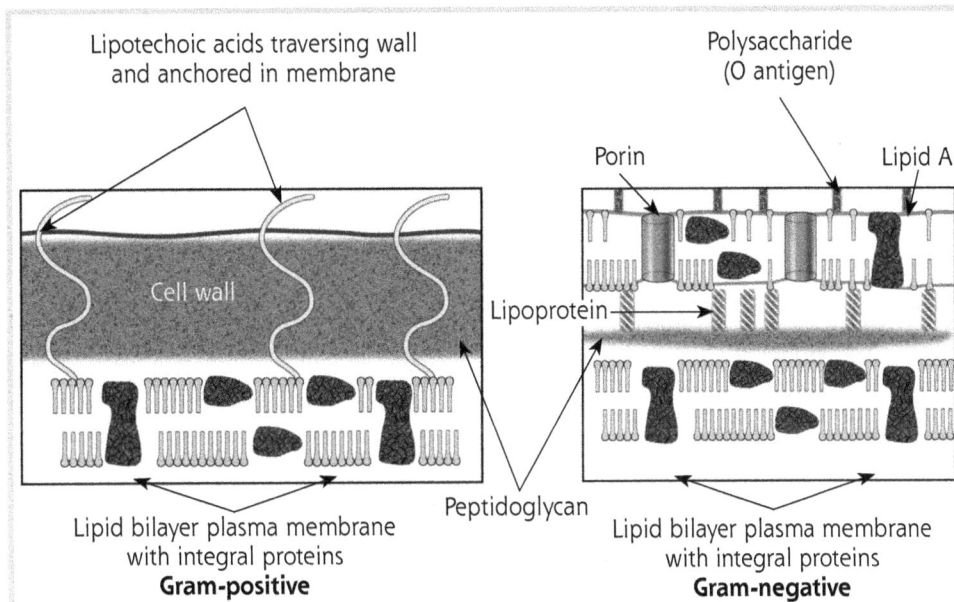

Note: The cell wall in the gram-positive bacteria is much thicker than in the gram-negative bacteria

Figure 2.2 Cell wall of gram-positive and gram-negative bacteria

2.3.7 Protection and survival of bacteria

There are several ways for bacteria to survive: they either move away to a less hostile environment, produce enzymes that destroy the toxic substance (such as β-lactamases) or cover themselves in a protective cover. Despite being unicellular organisms, bacteria are very versatile and ingenious. Their protective mechanisms vary, but at least one mechanism per species exists.

Protective mechanisms by the bacterium are either part of virulence, or a stress response or a combination of both. Various species respond differently by the following means:

Intracellular replication: Some bacterial species can survive and multiply inside neutrophils after being phagocytosed and are capable of causing disease. Examples are *N meningitidis* and *Brucella spp*.

Capsule (made of polysaccharide) **production:** This is usually in response to invasion of the host and is part of the virulence where the bacterium is protected from phagocytosis, as found in *S pneumoniae* and *K pneumoniae*. In some species, such as *K pneumoniae*, capsule production may be induced by plasmids of an outbreak strain as part of its virulence.

Spores: Some species, notably *Clostridioides (clostridium) spp*, respond to hostile conditions by surrounding the DNA, the essential part of the new bacterial cell, with a tough protective coat which can survive long periods of drying and heat. Under favourable conditions, such as temperature and humidity, the bacterium reverts to its original or vegetative form – sporulation. During the process of sporulation, toxins are liberated, which result in clinical diseases.

Toxin production: Determining the clinical significance of a toxin involves many factors, including the toxin's prevalence, virulence and role in disease pathogenesis.[3] Bacteria living in microbial communities or microbiome are highly competitive and part of this competition for nutrition and space is the production of toxins.[4] Many toxins are produced only if the local density is high, using quorum sensing. Bacteria can produce multiple types of toxins and cytotoxins, depending on the virulence. Generally, **endotoxins** are produced and remain inside the bacterial cell. These are released when the bacterium lyses upon its death. This type of toxin is more common in gram-negative bacilli such as *E coli*, *K pneumoniae* and *P aeruginosa*, to name but a few. **Exotoxins** are produced and excreted by the bacterial cell, causing damage to the host tissues and attacking the T cells (usually) as part of virulence. A classical example is *S aureus* producing several different cytotoxins, including TSST1, which causes Toxic Epidermolysis or Toxic Shock Syndrome – Group A streptococci can also produce this type of toxin.

Biofilm (Figure 2.3): Biofilms have attracted considerable interest recently particularly from an IPC perspective. They are made up of a group of different species and micro-organisms that come together as a whole or colony to protect themselves and each other. They secret a slimy substance (glycocalyx), similar to a capsule, which protects them from disinfection and toxic substances. Inside the biofilm, as these colonies grow and expand, they exchange vital survival information via plasmids and chemicals (quorum sensing). The nature of the colony changes. While usually microbes are fiercely competitive for nutrition and space, within the biofilm they live in harmony, protecting each other from harm. They communicate among themselves via quorum sensing. Finally, when the nutrition and essential contents of the biofilm are depleted, the colony bursts and the micro-organisms are released into the surrounding environment.

Biofilm is formed over most inert materials, especially plastic, allowing the bacteria to survive, and indeed thrive, inside it. It is impermeable to most chemotherapeutic agents, including disinfectants. Since most of the medical devices used in modern medicine are made of synthetic substances, the ability to produce biofilms offers the bacteria great advantages and protection from antimicrobial agents- this is a major challenge to IPC.

3   Forbes JD. 2020. Clinically important toxins in bacterial infection: utility of laboratory detection. Clin *Microbiol Newsl*. 42(20): 163–170. doi: 10.1016/j.clinmicnews.2020.09.003.

4   Doekes HM, de Boer RJ & Hermsen R. 2019. Toxin production spontaneously becomes regulated by local cell density in evolving bacterial populations. PLoS Comput Biol.15(8): e1007333. doi: 10.1371/journal.pcbi.1007333.

Environmental biofilms are increasingly being recognised as important reservoirs for multidrug-resistant bacteria. Sinks, showers, toilets and sewerage systems are reported especially in the context of gram-negative bacteria such as *Pseudomonas aeruginosa*, *Acinetobacter baumannii* and *Klebsiella pneumoniae*. Ventilation systems are likely to be involved in the colonisation of high-touch surfaces in patient areas with both gram-positive and gram-negative bacteria. These reservoirs can cause transmission of the same bacteria over extended periods of time (multiple years) and are significant from an IPC perspective.

Finally, it was previously thought that biofilms only formed on moist surfaces, but is now clear that 'dry biofilms' can be detected on surfaces in healthcare facilities – again emphasising the need for thorough cleaning rather than disinfection alone!

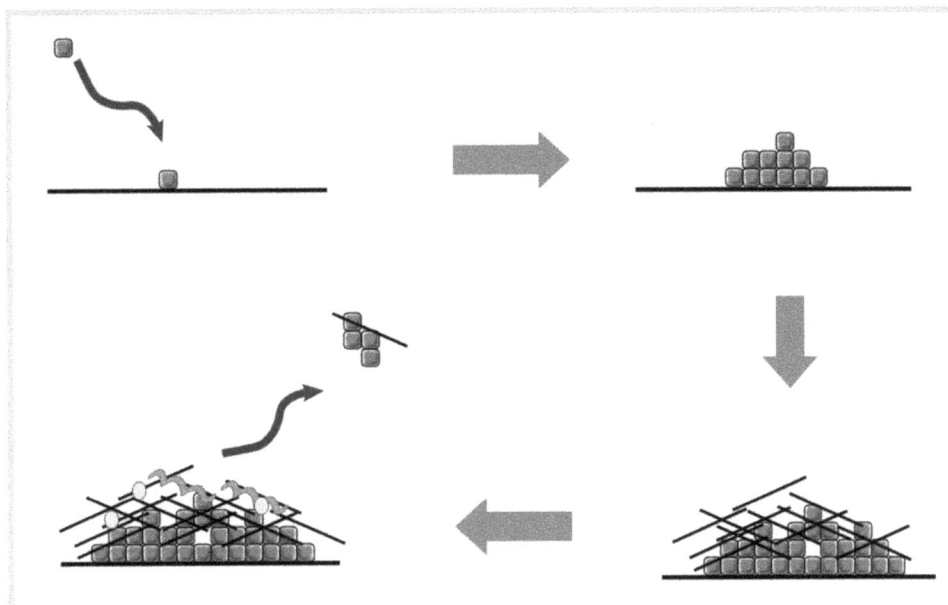

Figure 2.3 Biofilm (glycocalyx) production on foreign body

2.3.8 The growth cycle of bacteria

Bacterial growth occurs when conditions are optimal or sub-optimal. These conditions include temperature, humidity and the presence of nutrients. They replicate by binary fission and generally, under optimal conditions, most bacteria will replicate every 20 minutes, while *Mycobacterium tuberculosis* replicates every 24 hours. There are four distinct phases of growth:

A. **Lag phase.** Nothing happens. There is no increase in cell numbers or size.

B. **Log (exponential) phase.** There is rapid, optimal replication and the bacteria increase rapidly and reach maximum numbers in the appropriate growth medium.

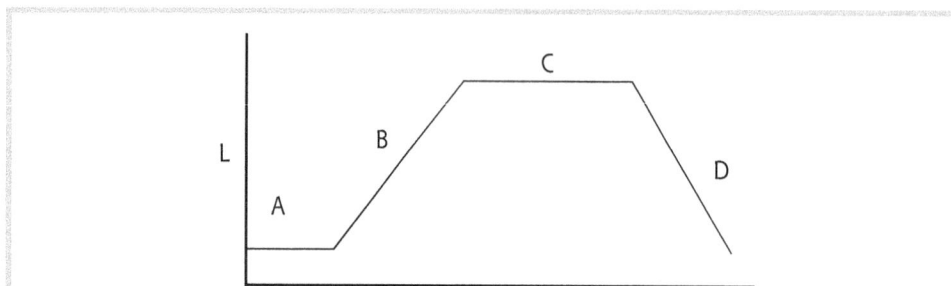

Figure 2.4   Growth cycle of bacteria. A = lag phase; B = log phase; C = stationary phase; D = death.

C. **Stationary phase.** There is no increase in the numbers, possibly due to the nutrients becoming exhausted.

D. **Death.** Lysis occurs and the number of cells starts to decline.

In vitro the log phase is most important because bacteria are metabolising rapidly and are most active and therefore most vulnerable to chemotherapeutic agents.

2.3.9 Other types of bacteria

The diagnosis of other types of bacteria as listed below has to rely on serological methods because routine culture is difficult and often specialised media is required for growth. It takes a long time for these bacteria to grow. The quickest means of diagnosis is via serology, which is accurate and rapid. A point of note is that bacteria that do not have a cell wall cannot be treated with a β-lactam antibiotic.

- **Mycoplasma** are small bacteria that lack a cell wall, but can be grown in the laboratory under special circumstances. These are associated with respiratory infections, particularly atypical pneumonia, and sexually transmitted disease,
- **Chlamydiae.** These are obligatory intracellular bacteria which cannot grow or survive outside a cell and therefore have to be grown in cell culture. Chlamydia is most commonly associated with sexually transmitted infections but can also cause neonatal ophthalmitis, trachoma and respiratory disease.
- **Rickettsiae.** These too are obligatory intracellular bacteria usually transmitted to humans from insect vectors. There are several subtypes of rickettsiae which cause a variety of local and systemic diseases. The common ones affect the skin and lymph nodes, and result in low-grade persistent fevers with lymphadenitis, and/or jaundice.
- **Spirochetes** are long coiled bacteria and can be seen under dark background microscopy. These have a cell wall and can be treated with penicillin. *Treponema pallidum* is the causative organism for syphilis, but other treponemes can cause skin lesions such as yaws. The means of diagnosis is serological, but skin scrapes from open wounds can also be used.

2.4 Viruses

Viruses require the host's systems to survive; therefore viruses infect every life form from bacteria, fungi, plants, to animals and humans.

Intracellular existence offers great advantages to viruses:
- protection against the action of host antibodies and circulating cell mediators
- the use of existing structures within the infected cells to replicate, which reduces the burden of such processes on the virus itself
- the cells infected by viruses are usually those that are part of the host's immune defences, such as macrophages and lymphocytes
- to reach the virus with chemotherapeutic agents without affecting the host cells is a challenge.

2.4.1 Structure of viruses

The structural characteristics of viruses have an impact on the IPC control measures put into place to destroy or remove viruses.
- **Size.** Viruses range from very small (30 nM polio virus) to large (400 nM vaccinia) – the latter being almost as large as bacteria.
- **Shape.** The complete unit of nucleic acid and capsid is called the **nucleocapsid** and is arranged in distinct symmetry. The symmetry can be icosahedral, helical or complex. Often the virus particle (virion) consists only of a nucleocapsid, also known as a 'naked' or an 'envelope-free' virus. In others, the virions are covered with an outer membrane or envelope which is made up of lipid bilayer derived from the host in which the virus protein and glycoprotein are inserted; these are also known as 'enveloped' viruses. *Enveloped viruses (HIV) are more susceptible to disinfectants and anti-viral agents than non-enveloped viruses (polio).*
- **Genetics.** The genetic make-up of various groups of viruses differs considerably, but there are common characteristics. Single-stranded or double-stranded, linear or circular RNA or DNA (but never both) is arranged inside a capsule or capsid and is made up of a number of individual protein molecules known as **capsomeres**. Despite their restricted genetics, viruses have the ability to mutate and adapt to new hosts and to 'jump' between host species – this is commonly found in zoonotic viral infections of which recent examples are Ebola and SARS-CoV-2.

2.4.2 Classification of viruses

Viruses are classified into DNA or RNA viruses depending on the type of nucleic acid they are made up of. They are further classified as single or double stranded.[5]

---

[5] Wikipaedia. Virus classification. Available on www.wikipaedia.com. Accessed on 29 July 2009. 'Virus Taxonomy Portal.' (Website.) *Viral Bioinformatics Resource Center & Viral Bioinformatics – Canada*. Retrieved on 2007-09-27.

Their characteristics of resistance to heat, disinfectants and survival outside the body are relevant to IPC strategies.

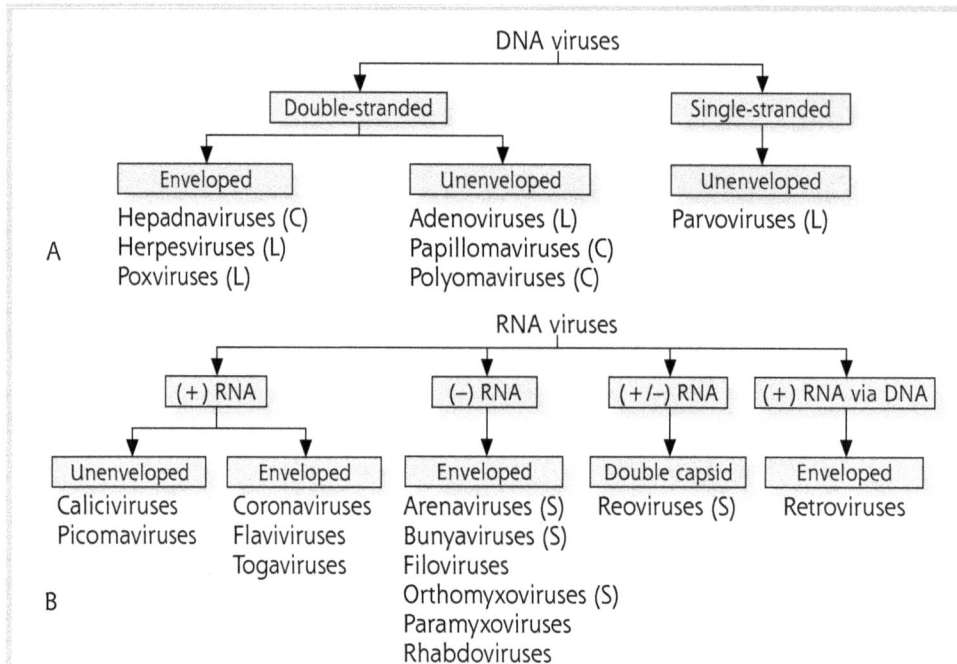

Figure 2.5 Classification of viruses (adapted from https://www.onlinebiologynotes.com/classification-of-virus/)

2.4.3 Transmission of viruses

Transmissibility of viruses is greatly influenced by the differences in susceptibility and survival both in the body and the external environment. Generally, naked or **envelope-free** viruses are more resistant and survive well in the outside world.

Enveloped viruses are more susceptible to environmental drying, gastric acidity and bile. This is important from an IPC strategic point of view since the containment of viruses will depend on their ability to survive in the environment.

Viruses enter the human body by several routes:
- respiratory route via inhaled infectious respiratory particles (rhinovirus, influenza, SARS-CoV-2)
- food and water (hepatitis A, polio)
- direct contact transfer from other infected hosts (HIV, hepatitis B, hepatitis C, Ebola, Marburg virus (VHF))
- bites from vectors such as mosquitoes (yellow fever, dengue)
- sexual transmission (herpes simplex, human papillomavirus (HPV))
- transplacental – mother to child (cytomegalovirus)
- direct skin contact (herpes zoster).

Viruses are host-specific, which restricts them to a single or a small range of host species. The initial basis for specificity is the ability of virus particles to attach to a specific host cell. Therefore, exposure to several viruses does not necessarily result in infection since the specific attachment site may not exist. Viruses can mutate to jump species if circumstances permit, such as Ebola or SARS-CoV-2, resulting in devastating outbreaks and pandemics. Despite this, virus transmission is much faster than bacterial transmission.

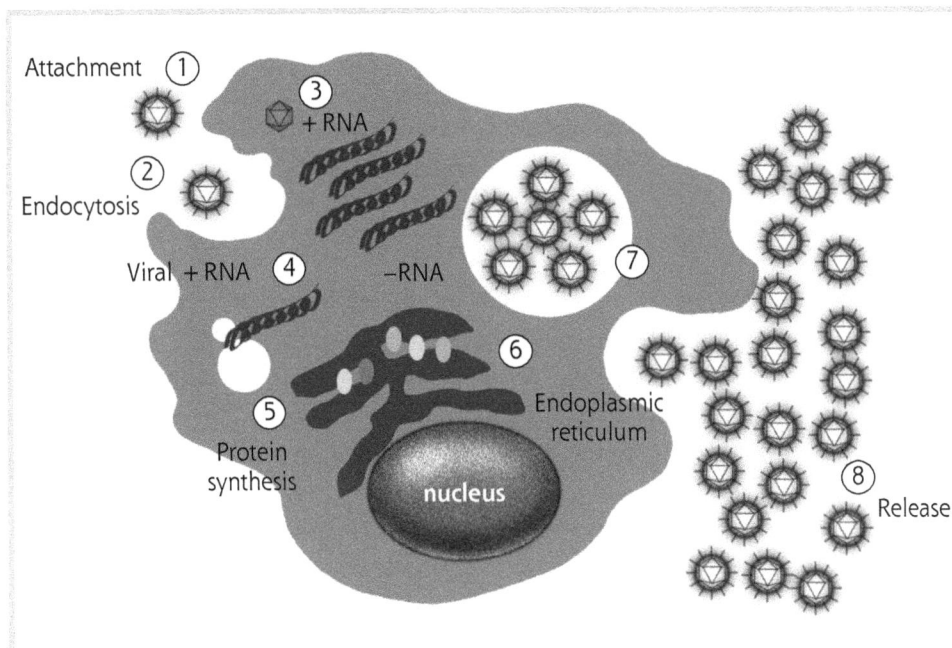

Figure 2.6 Example of replication cycle of a virus

2.4.4 Replication[6]

Step 1. The ability of the virus, naked or enveloped, to attach itself to the host cell is essential. This step is a specific interaction between the virus nucleocapsid or envelope and the molecules on the host cell membrane (receptor). If specific receptors are absent, the virus cannot attach itself.

Step 2. The attachment follows entry into the host cell, and fusion of the nucleocapsid or envelope with the host membrane takes place or phagocytosis occurs.

Step 3. The virus is carried into the cytoplasm across the plasma membrane of the host cell.

---

[6]   Lectures online by Dr Margaret Hunt available at www.pathmicro.med.sc.edu/book/ welcome.html.

Step 4. The envelope and/or capsid is shed, and the viral nucleic acids are released. The virus is now no longer active and this is known as the elipse phase.

Step 5. The viral mRNA starts synthesis of a new viral protein either directly or via the host's genetic machinery.

Step 6. New viral nucleic acids and capsids are produced.

Step 7. The viral replication fills the host cell. **Budding** occurs with enveloped viruses taking on a coat from the host cell. **Cytolysis** (host cell lysis) is seen with naked viruses. Enveloped viruses do not kill the host cells since budding does not require lysis of the cell.

Step 8. The complete new viruses emerge from the host cell, usually following lysis of the latter, and are ready to infect new host cells.

2.5 Fungi

Fungi are eukaryotes and characteristically are multinucleate or multicellular organisms with a thick cell wall (containing sterol) and grow as filaments (hyphae), but other growth forms occur and produce spores. Fungi are ubiquitous in the environment and can be found in decaying matter and growing on organic matter. Healthcare-associated infections (HAI) with *Candida spp* are on the increase, spurred on by aggressive medical interventions, broad-spectrum antibiotic usage and inadequate IPC measures such as hand hygiene, poor environmental cleaning and decontamination of medical equipment. Of particular note is *C auris* as a healthcare-associated pathogen in many ICUs across the globe, with a high mortality.

2.5.1 Morphology of fungi

Those causing disease in humans can be classified either according to growth characteristics or according to the type of infection. Fungi grow as hyphae or mycelia, or as yeasts (forming buds) – some grow both ways and are known as **dimorphic**.

Yeasts are unicellular and reproduce by budding and division. *Cryptococcus neoformans* is a single cell and reproduces by division. Others like histoplasma and *Candida spp* are dimorphic, displaying either filamentous growth or budding, depending on the environmental conditions. Yeast can grow intracellularly, surviving and multiplying within phagocytes.

Filamentous fungi are multicellular filamentous structures made up of tubular cells with cell walls. A mass of hyphae (mycelium) is called **mycelia**. The mycelia form branches; the pattern of branching and the width of the mycelia are aid the morphological identification. If the mycelia do not have septa (divisions), they are called **coenocytic** (non-septate).

The filamentous forms grow extracellularly, invading surrounding host tissue.

2.5.2 Reproduction of fungi

Fungi replicate by asexual reproduction where sporangia are formed, which liberate spores dispersing fungi. The asexual spores may be large (macroconidia, chlamydospores) or small (microconidia, blastospores, arthroconidia).

Yeast-like forms classically replicate by division. Budding may occur and these remain attached to the parent cell and are known as pseudohyphae.

Dimorphic fungi form hyphae at environmental temperatures and can switch to yeast-like forms in the body (temperature induced) – Candida is exceptional in that it forms hyphae in the body.

2.5.3 Types of fungal infection

Infections caused by fungi are known as mycoses. From an IPC perspective fungal infections are mostly seen in either immunocompromised patients, extremely sick patients in intensive care or during the construction and renovation of healthcare facilities. Most severe fungal infections within healthcare facilities are caused by *Aspergillus spp* associated with the built environment or *Candida spp*, which is usually seen in the immunocompromised host. IPC practitioners must be aware of the role yeasts and fungi play in HAI.

There are four types of mycotic diseases specifically caused by fungi:

1. **Hypersensitivity.** An allergic reaction to molds and spores. Indoor air pollution.

2. **Mycotoxicosis.** Poisoning of humans and animals by feeds and food products contaminated by fungi which produce toxins from the grain substrate.

3. **Mycetismus.** The ingestion of pre-formed toxin (mushroom poisoning).

4. **Infection.** See Table 2.3.

Table 2.3 Fungal infections by site, clinical diagnosis and type of fungus

Important fungal infections				
Type	**Site**	**Disease**	**Genus**	**Growth form**
Superficial				
Cutaneous	Hair, skin	Tinea versicolor	*Malassezia*	Yeast
	Epidermis, hair, nails	Dermatophytes (ringworm)	*Microsporum, Trichophyton, Epidermophyton*	Hyphae
Subcutaneous	Subcutis	Sporotrichosis Mycetoma	*Sporothrix —* several genera	Yeast in body Hyphae

Deep				
Systemic	Internal organs	Coccidioidomycosis Histoplasmosis Blastomycosis Paracoccidio-idomycosis	*Coccidioides* *Histoplasma* *Blastomyces* *Paracoccidioides*	Yeast-like spore Yeast Yeast Yeast
Opportunistic	Internal organs	Cryptococcus Candidiasis Aspergillosis	*Cryptococcus* *Candida* *Aspergillus*	Yeast Yeast Hyphae

Superficial mycoses are more common than deep infections. The fungi are transmitted by direct contact with humans or animals with superficial fungal infections. The fungus grows on the body surface in the skin, hair and nails and is usually mild in nature but contagious, especially where the skin integrity is damaged. Secondary bacterial infection may occur.

Deep mycoses are caused by fungi entering the internal organs and causing serious disease, especially in the immunocompromised host. Spores enter either via the respiratory tract or are ingested. Some are part of the normal body flora (Candida) and only cause invasive disease in the immunocompromised host.

Neutrophils are the major defence against invasive fungi. Those species – too large to phagocytose – are killed by extracellular factors released by phagocytes and other components of the immune response.

C neoformans avoids phagocytosis by virtue of its polysaccharide capsule.

2.6 Parasites – protozoa and helminths

Protozoa are free living, single-cell eukaryotes occurring widely in the environment. These are transmitted either via bites of blood-sucking insects or accidental ingestion of infective stages. They are restricted geographically to areas where the vectors live and where the climatic conditions are favourable to the vectors. However, poverty and poor hygiene have a relevant role in transmission. They are considered parasites, deriving all their nutritional and survival needs from another – the host.

Reproduction in humans is usually asexual, by binary or multiple division of growing stages (trophozoites). Cryptosporidium is the exception as it undergoes a sexual cycle in humans. Sexual reproduction either is absent or occurs in the vector. The asexual cycle allows the parasite to rapidly increase in numbers, particularly in the immunocompromised host.

Transmission between hosts depends on reproduction of resistant stages that pass out of the body and are taken up by another host.

Parasites are more relevant to public health than IPC, but in some countries parasitic diseases dominate the health of the population and are a common cause of admissions to healthcare facilities.

2.6.1 Classification of parasites

There are four main divisions based upon the structure and mobility.

- **Sporozoa** contain only intracellular parasites, an example being *Plasmodium* (malaria).
- **Flagellates** move with the beat of one or more flagella.
- **Amoebae** move with pseudopodia and have no fixed shape.
- **Ciliates** move by beating many of their cilia.

Table 2.4 summarises the parasites of medical importance, mode of transmission, clinical presentation and method of diagnosis. Parasites are more of public health than IPC concern.

Table 2.4 Classification of parasites

Organism	Transmission	Symptoms	Diagnosis
Entameba histolytica (amoebae)	Oro-faecal	Dysentery with blood and necrotic tissue Chronic: abscesses	Stool: cysts with 1–4 nuclei and/or trophs Trophs in aspirate
Giardia lamblia (flagellate)	Oro-faecal	Foul-smelling, bulky diarrhoea; blood or necrotic tissue rare	Stool: typical old man giardia troph and/or cyst
Balantidium coli (ciliated)	Oro-faecal; zoonotic	Dysentery with blood and necrotic tissue but no abscesses	Stool: ciliated trophs and/or cysts
Cryptosporidium parvum (sporozoa)	Oro-faecal	Diarrhoea	Oocysts in stool
Isospora belli (sporozoa)	Oro-faecal	Giardiasis-like	Oocysts in stool
Trichomonas vaginalis (flagellate)	Sexual	Vaginitis, occasional urethritis/prostatitis	Flagellate in vaginal (or urethral) smear
Haemoflagellates – vector borne			
Trypanosoma brucei	Tsetse fly	Sleeping sickness, cardiac failure	Haemoflagellate in blood or lymph node
Trypanosoma cruzi	Reduviid (kissing) bug	Chagas disease: megacolon, cardiac failure	Haemoflagellate in blood or tissue

Organism	Transmission	Symptoms	Diagnosis
Leishmania donovani	Sand fly	Visceral leishmaniasis, granulomatous skin lesions	Intracellular (macrophages) leishmanial bodies
Leishmania tropica	Sand fly	Cutaneous lesions	As for *L donovani*
Sporozoan – vector borne			
Plasmodium falciparum P ovale, P malariae and *P vivax*	Female anopheline mosquito	Malarial paroxysm: chills, fever, headache, nausea cycles	Plasmodia in red blood cells, typical of the species involved
Babesia microti	Tick	Haemolytic anemia, jaundice and fever	Typical organism (Maltese cross) in red blood cells
Toxoplasma gondii	Oral from cat faecal material; meat	Adult: flu-like; congenital: abortion, neonatal blindness and neuropathies	Intracellular (in macrophages) tachyzoites
Pneumocystis jiroveci (technically a fungus)	Cough droplets	Pneumonia	Pneumocysts in sputum
Helminths			
Ascaris lumbricoides	Oro-faecal	Abdominal pain, weight loss, distended abdomen	Stool: corticoid oval egg (40–70 × 35–50 μm)
Enterobius vermicularis	Oro-faecal	Peri-anal pruritus, rare abdominal pain, nausea, vomiting	Stool: embryonated eggs (60 × 27 μm), flat on one side
Strongyloides stercoralis	Soil–skin, autoinfection	Itching at infection site, rash due to larval migration, verminous pneumonia, mid-epigastric pain, nausea, vomiting, bloody dysentery, weight loss and anaemia	Stool: rhabditiform larvae (250 × 20–25μm)
Necator americanus, Ancylostoma duodenale (Hookworms)	Oro-faecal (egg), skin penetration (larvae)	Maculopapular erythema (ground itch), broncho-pneumonitis, epigastric pain, GI haemorrhage, anaemia, edema	Stool: oval segmented eggs (30–60 × 20–25 μm)

Organism	Transmission	Symptoms	Diagnosis
Dracunculus medinensis	Oral: cyclops in water	Blistering skin, irritation, inflammation	Physical examination
Trichinella spiralis	Poorly cooked pork	Depends on worm location and burden: gastroenteritis, edema, muscle pain, spasm, eosinophilia, tachycardia, fever, chill, headache, vertigo, delirium, coma etc	Medical history, eosinophilia, muscle biopsy, serology
Trichuris trichiura	Oro-faecal	Abdominal pain, bloody diarrhoea, prolapsed rectum	Stool: lemon-shaped egg (50–55 x 20–25 μm)
Blood and tissue helminths – vector-borne			
Wuchereria bancrofti; W brugia malayi (elephantiasis)	Mosquito bite	Recurrent fever, lymph-adenitis, splenomegaly, lymphedema, elephantiasis	Medical history, physical examination, microfilaria in blood (night sample)
Onchocerca volvulus	Black fly bite	Nodular and erythematous dermal lesions, eosinophilia, urticaria, blindness	Medical history, physical examination, microfilaria in nodular aspirate
Loa loa	Deer fly	As in onchocerciasis	As in onchocerciasis
Organism	**Transmission**	**Symptoms**	**Diagnosis**
Flukes			
Schistosoma mansoni, S japonicum	Skin penetration by cercaria	Dermatitis, abdominal pain, bloody stool, peri-portal fibrosis, hepatosplenomegaly, ascites, CNS	Eggs in stool
Schistosoma haematobium	Skin penetration by cercaria	Dermatitis, urogenital cystitis, urethritis and bladder carcinoma	Eggs in urine
Fasciolopsis buski	Metacercaria on water chestnut	Epigastric pain, nausea, diarrhoea, edema, ascites	Eggs in stool

2.7 The relationship between pathogen and host

Humans are colonised by micro-organisms and usually live in harmony with them; these micro-organisms are known as the human microbiome. Microbiomes vary depending on the part of the body or environment they colonise and this depends on their nutritional, temperature and atmospheric needs. Most colonisation occurs on the skin surface and parts of the body which are open to the outside environment. Areas of the human body which are enclosed, such as tissues, blood, cerebrospinal fluid, vitreous humour in the eye and other internal body fluids, are sterile under normal conditions.

When small numbers of micro-organisms invade parts of the body which are normally not colonised, a host immune response is triggered in an immunocompetent host and this response usually overcomes minor invasions. If the host's immunity is compromised or the invaders are particularly virulent, it results in disease. Thus, a fine balance exists between the host and the pathogen.

2.7.1 The pathogen

Micro-organisms invade the host and cause disease by some or all of the following ways:

- acquisition
- colonisation
- penetration

- spread
- damage
- resolution.

2.7.1.1 Acquisition

That the initial point of contact is with a microbial species is of fundamental importance. Microbes acquired from the host's own flora are known as 'endogenous', while those acquired from external sources are 'exogenous'. Knowledge of both is relevant to containing infection and preventing further spread of the pathogen.

The main routes of transmission are direct and indirect contact, aerosol or droplet and the sharing of non-sterile medical devices. These are of particular relevance to IPC programmes, while others are more relevant to public health but require IPC interventions.

2.7.1.2 Colonisation

After a microbe has been acquired, there is competition between the endogenous flora and the new microbe. Host defences usually reject the intruder. However, if the pathogen has the necessary mechanisms to survive host defences, it can persist in a favourable site on the host. The persistence of a potential pathogen at a site or sites on the host is colonisation.

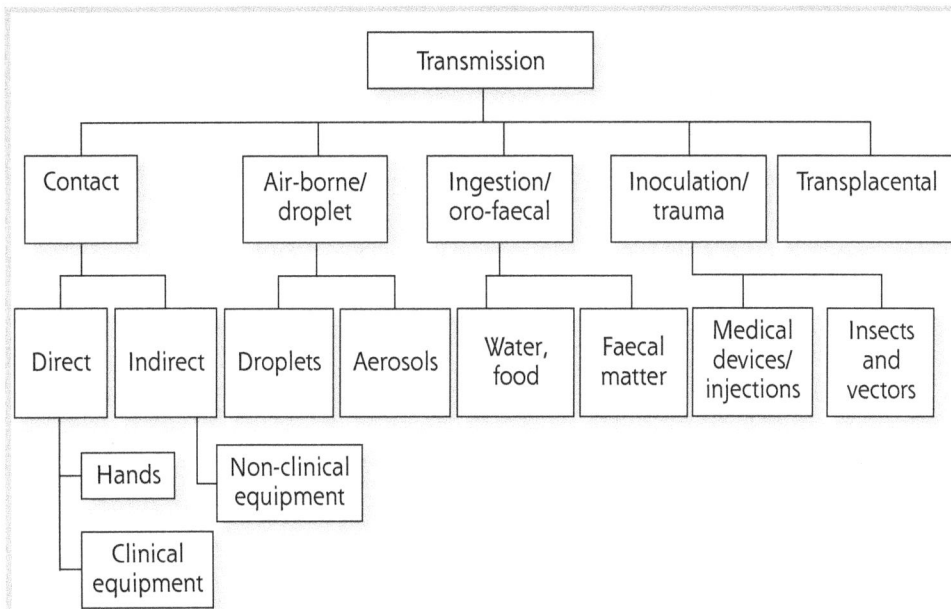

Figure 2.7 Main routes of transmission

These sites are the natural orifices of the body, skin or more commonly broken or damaged skin which has the right conditions of nutrients, temperature and respiratory requirements for the pathogen.

Invasive medical devices such as urinary catheters, intravenous access and endotracheal tubes are classic examples of foreign bodies which support colonisation aided by biofilm formation.

It does not necessarily follow that all colonisation will lead to invasive disease or infection in the initial host. However, the potential to transmit and spread to other humans or hosts is significant.

2.7.1.3 Penetration

In order for the pathogen to invade it has to penetrate several layers of host defences. Microbes have their own mechanisms to increase penetration, known as 'virulence factors', which allow escape from the body's defences (see 2.3.7 Protection and survival). Once they have invaded the host and managed to overcome the host's defences, pathogens find the sites with receptors which will allow them to attach and penetrate. Intracellular organisms will locate the appropriate cell to attach to, penetrate and multiply.

2.7.1.4 Spread

The invader can spread in the host by one or more routes, breaking down barriers in its path:

- direct extension through the surrounding tissues, usually by producing enzymes that break down the tissues and fascia
- along the tissue planes, spreading in the spaces between the tissues
- venous route by entering the bloodstream and spreading along the veins to distant parts of the body
- via the lymphatic system.

2.7.1.5 Damage

Pathogens can damage tissues in several ways:

- **Bulk effect**, where sheer numbers of organisms (for example, helminths) can obstruct an organ.
- **Toxins** which damage surrounding tissues. In bacteria, toxins are either proteins released by the organism or lipopolysaccharides located in the cell wall and liberated during cell growth or lysis. Toxins do not necessarily destroy cells, but can cause sublethal damage or alter cell function.
  - Endotoxins are released during multiplication or lysis.
  - Exotoxins are released during invasion. Many have two components. The B subunit determines tissue specificity, while the A subunit causes cellular damage after binding of B and penetrating the cell membrane.
- **Altering the function** of organs either by the organism or by the host's response to eliminate the pathogen. Examples are diarrhoea due to increased intestinal motility, vomiting to eliminate toxins, or coughing and sneezing.

2.7.1.6 Resolution

The outcome of infection (or invasion) is that the host's defences finally either manage to overcome the infection or succumb. Infections in an immunocompetent host do resolve by themselves over a period of time, but today the duration of bacterial infections is shortened by antibiotics. In the immunocompromised host, disease is more difficult to treat – the lack of body defences increases the risk of overwhelming infection – and the period of infection is often more prolonged.

2.8 The host

The immune system in humans has evolved over many years into 'natural' (innate) defence, which is the first line of defence, and 'acquired' (adaptive), which is a secondary response when the innate immunity is not sufficient to counteract an invading pathogen.

The difference between the two is that the adaptive immune system is a specific memory and improves the response of the innate system.

2.8.1 Natural defences

2.8.1.1 Physical barriers

- **Intact skin** is the first and most important line of defence in humans. It repels multiple possible invasions from microbes each day. In the healthcare environment these microbes can be more aggressive. However, if the skin is damaged, penetration is easier.
- **Mucous membranes** can repel microbial encounters by producing mucus, which encases the invader as well as inhibiting attachment.
- **The respiratory tract** is equipped with ciliated epithelium and mucus-producing cells which attempt to remove microbes. Pathogens of less than 5 μ in size could escape these defences and enter the alveoli. The mucus from the respiratory tract will encase the pathogen and this is then removed by ciliary action, coughing or sneezing.
- **Commensal** bacteria (normal flora or the microbiome) occupy sites along mucous membranes and suppress the growth of potentially pathogenic bacteria and fungi by occupying the available space, competing for nutrients and producing inhibitory substances such as acids or colicins (bacteriocidins).

2.8.1.2 Cellular immunity

- **Mononuclearphagocytic system (MPS).** Macrophages are present throughout the connective tissue, but are concentrated in the liver and lungs and line the lymph nodes. Upon entry into the body the pathogen makes contact with polymorpho (PMN) nuclear cells (neutrophils). It attaches itself to the non-specific receptors on the PMN cells. This stimulates a response within the PMN cell which engulfs the infecting agent into a phagosome. The lysosomes present in the cytoplasm fuse with the phagosome and microbial kill occurs, followed by a release of microbial products.

  A second sequence of events also occurs. Upon entry into the body many bacteria produce chemical substances which attract leucocytes from afar to the site of entry. This triggers a cascade of 'complement', where one reaction acts as an enzymatic catalyst for the next one.

- **Complement.** At the centre of the complement complex is C3, which is abundant and highly complex. Complement is produced in the vicinity of the microbial membrane, binds to its surface and acts as **'opsonins'**. These are molecules which make the organism more susceptible to engulfment by the phagocytes as well as increasing vascular permeability. This stimulates an exudation of fluid and more complement at the site of confrontation. The resulting inflammatory response is when capillary dilation (erythema), exudation of plasma proteins and fluids (edema) and an accumulation of neutrophils occur and these combine in a highly effective way to focus phagocytes onto complement-coated cells. Acute-phase proteins such as interleukin-1 (IL-1), interleukin-6 (IL-6) and tumour necrosis factor (TNF) are released in tissue injury. *During this process C-reactive protein (CRP) is dramatically increased*.

- **IgA.** An antibody produced in response to an infective agent from the cells lining the respiratory tract and gut, it is actively secreted into the lumen and is present in high concentrations. Its function is to coat the infectious agent, thereby greatly reducing its adherence.

2.8.2 Acquired immunity

In *acquired* or **adaptive immunity** cellular response plays a major role since it is based on a specific memory of a previous encounter with the pathogen. **T lymphocytes are pivotal to this process**. During the cycle of microbial invasion, some die within the cells they infect and the proteins derived from the dead organisms are fragmented by intracellular enzymes. These peptides are incorporated into the cytoplasmic vacuoles where they come into contact with molecules of the major histocompatiblity complex (MHC); the latter act as surface markers for infected host cells. Class I MHC is present in virtually every cell in the body; Class II MHC is present on the surfaces of macrophages and B cells.

T-cells have specialised receptors which can recognise (a) foreign antigen and (b) bind the MHC and peptides derived from intracellular organisms. When the T-cell binds to the infected cell indicated by the class of MHC, the former becomes activated and sets up a cascade of mechanisms to deal with the intracellular pathogen. A subset of T-lymphocytes, known as T-helper (Th) cells, deal with *Mycobacterium tuberculosis* and *Listeria monocytogenes* by binding to macrophages with Class II MHC. Thus it is essential for the killing of such organisms that the T-cell function is competent.

In viral infections Class I MHCs are attached by cytotoxic T-cells (Tc), killing the infected cell before the virus has had time to replicate.

Antibodies are synthesised by the host B lymphocytes when the body comes into contact with a foreign agent. The antibodies have a complementary binding site on the microbial surface. The antibody binds with the antigen (microbe) and the complement pathway is activated. The sequence follows the same path as above. Table 2.5 illustrates a comparison.

Table 2.5 Comparison of innate and adaptive immunity

Comparison of natural and acquired immune systems		
	Innate or natural	**Adaptive or acquired**
Soluble (humoural)	Lysozyme, complement, acute phase proteins (CRP), interferon	Antibody
Cells	Phagocytes, natural killer cells	T lymphocytes
Response to microbial infection		
First contact	+	+
Second contact	+	+ + + +
	Non-specific memory	Specific memory
Resistance by repeated contact	Not improved	Improved

2.9 Microbes of importance in IPC

Microbes causing disease in humans are considered either primary or secondary pathogens. HAIs are infections caused by pathogens that are acquired in a healthcare facility or associated with healthcare procedures and are usually secondary invaders. These are of particular relevance to IPC programmes because the differentiation between resident, transient and pathogenic flora will prevent the misuse of antimicrobial agents. Before addressing HAI pathogens, the concept of the microbiome should be understood.

2.9.1 Commensal (resident) or normal flora – the microbiome

There are more microbes colonising the human body than the number of cells it contains. The majority of these are in the large intestine. Normal flora have a protective role and prevent invasion from HAI pathogens. When these are removed by antimicrobial agents, to which they are usually sensitive, a secondary invasion occurs – this should be taken into account when treating patients and staff. The microflora are made up of bacteria, fungi and occasionally viruses. The table below illustrates the distribution of bacteria by sites on the body. These can be reduced, but not completely removed, by cleaning a skin site.

Table 2.6   Examples of distribution of commensals in the human body

Normal flora by site and genus			
Site on body	**Numbers**	**Type of bacteria**	
		Aerobic	**Anaerobic**
Skin (dry)	Few	Coagulase negative staphyloccoci (CNS)	
Skin (moist)	103–107 cfu/cm2	*Staphyloccus epidemidis, Staphylococcus aureus,* coliforms	*Diphtheroids*
Scalp/nails	Few	*Candida spp*	
Nose	1011/gm	Staphylococci, streptococci, coliforms	
Mouth/ gingivae	1011/gm	Streptococci, coliforms, *Candida spp*	(90%) Streptococci, bacteroides, fusiforms
Pharynx/ trachea	Heavy	α & β strep, coliforms *Neisseria spp, Staphylococcus aureus, Gp A streptococci, Streptococcus pneumoniae,* Lactobacilli, *Candida spp, Pneumocystitis jiroveci*	Strep, diphtheroids, gram-negative bacilli, gram-positive cocci
Stomach (acid)	Moderate	Lactobacilli, streptococci	
Upper GI tract	104 per gram	*Streptococci,* gram negative bacilli	
Ileum	108 per gram	*Streptococci, lactobacilli,* Enterobacteria	*Bacteroides spp*
Large bowel	1011 per gram	Many species of gram-positive and gram-negative bacilli	(99%) *Clostridium spp bacteroides sppStreptococcus, spp*
Urogenital tract	108–9 per gram	Streptococci, coliforms, diphtheroids	
Vagina	108 per gram	Changes from Staphylococci/ Streptococci/E coli to lactobacilli, candida and trichomonas (postpuberty)	*Streptococci Bacteroides spp*

2.10 The microbiome

Recently, there has been increasing interest in the existence of microbes in the environment, humans, animals and the built environment. But, what is a microbiome? The microbiome is made up of bacteria, viruses, yeasts and fungi and parasites that make up the microbial flora of almost all surfaces, inside and outside the human body (and all living things).

Each person has his or her microbiome, previously known as commensal flora. Equally, each area of the health facility – the walls, floor, sinks, drains, air and surfaces – has an individual microbiome. In the outside environment, the soil, plants, animals and so on each have a distinct microbiome. So how does this affect IPC?

These independent microbiomes exert a huge influence on each other. Figure 2.8 shows the interaction between people, the built environment and the effect on patient health and safety. The natural microbiome is made up of sensitive microbes, especially bacteria and fungi. If there is extensive use of disinfectants, antibiotics or toxic substances in any of these areas, the microbiome will change, resulting in an increase in antimicrobial resistance and this is leads to the modification of the resistome or antibiotic resistance patterns such as MDROs.

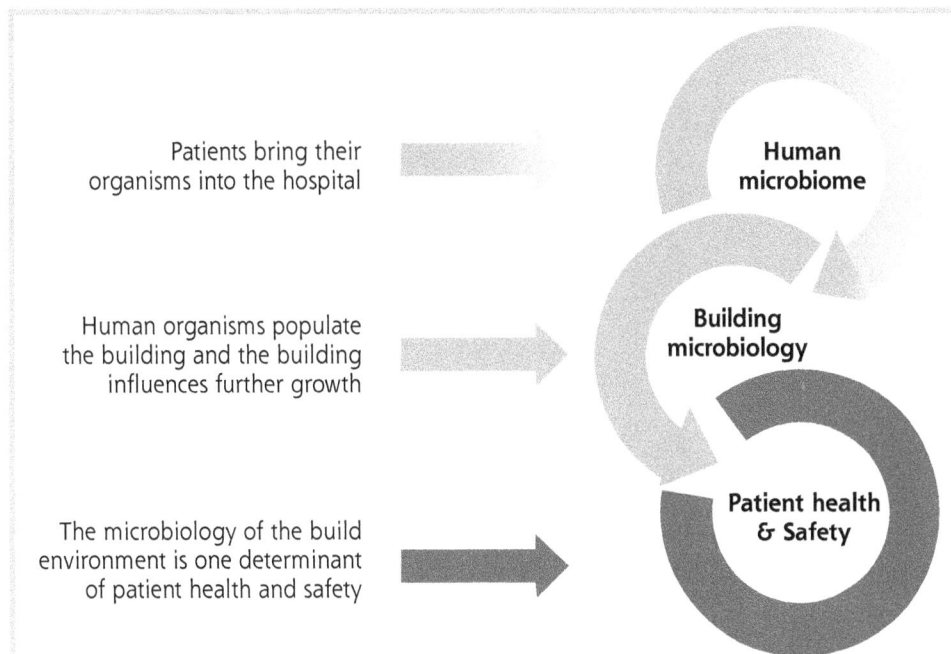

Patients bring their organisms into the hospital

Human microbiome

Human organisms populate the building and the building influences further growth

Building microbiology

The microbiology of the build environment is one determinant of patient health and safety

Patient health & Safety

Figure 2.8 The microbiome and intermingling of organisms in the health environment[7]

---

[7]   Adapted from https://blog.se.com/buildings/building-management/2015/06/09/balance-your-hospital-building-ecosystem-to-improve-patient-safety/.

The microbiome keeps changing and these changes are interdependent on patients coming from different environments, the built environment itself, like the drains, sinks and surface, and the use of antimicrobial agents such as antibiotics and disinfectants.

The role of IPC must be to preserve the sensitive microbiomes which exist in the patients, staff and environment of the healthcare facility. This is done by removing the vehicle of transmission, reducing the level and risk of transmission. One of the ways of doing this is via antimicrobial stewardship, where IPC plays a significant role in the management of patients.

The use of antimicrobial agents such as antibiotics and disinfectant must be judicious and carefully planned with a targeted or focused application which causes minimum modification of the natural sensitive microbiome.

2.11 Healthcare-associated pathogens

Micro-organisms relevant to HAI to are also known as **alert organisms**.[8] The WHO has listed a group of priority pathogens which should be part of research and development. While these priority HAI pathogens are kept under scrutiny in LMICs, there could also be different pathogens of importance in addition the ones listed below.

More recently, the WHO has identified six HAI pathogens that exhibit multidrug resistance and virulence: *Enterococcus faecium, Staphylococcus aureus, Klebsiella pneumoniae, Acinetobacter baumannii, Pseudomonas aeruginosa* and *Enterobacter spp* (ESKAPE). Persistent use of antibiotics has provoked the emergence of multidrug-resistant (MDR) and extensively drug resistant (XDR) bacteria, which render even the most effective drugs ineffective. Extended spectrum β-lactamase (ESBL) and carbapenemase producing gram-negative bacteria have emerged as important therapeutic challenges.[9] Reader, note that these might change from time to time.

Priority 1: CRITICAL
- *Acinetobacter baumannii* – carbapenem-resistant
- *Pseudomonas aeruginosa* – carbapenem-resistant
- *Enterobacteriaceae* – carbapenem-resistant, ESBL-producing

Priority 2: HIGH
- *Enterococcus faecium* – vancomycin-resistant
- *Staphylococcus aureus* – methicillin-resistant, vancomycin-intermediate and -resistant

---

[8] WHO. 2017. WHO publishes list of bacteria for which new antibiotics are urgently needed.
[9] Mulani MS, Kamble EE, Kumkar SN, Tawre MS & Pardesi KR. 2019. Emerging Strategies to Combat ESKAPE Pathogens in the Era of Antimicrobial Resistance: A Review. Front *Microbiol.* 10: 539. doi: 10.3389/fmicb.2019.00539.

- *Helicobacter pylori* – clarithromycin-resistant
- *Campylobacter spp* – fluoroquinolone-resistant
- *Salmonellae* – fluoroquinolone-resistant
- *Neisseria gonorrhoeae* – cephalosporin-resistant, fluoroquinolone-resistant

Priority 3: MEDIUM
- *Streptococcus pneumoniae* – penicillin-non-susceptible
- *Haemophilus influenzae* – ampicillin-resistant
- *Shigella spp* – fluoroquinolone-resistant

The IPC team regard these pathogens as requiring an immediate response when informed by the laboratory or clinical staff since these may be associated with HAI outbreaks. The alert organisms may differ between healthcare facilities, but some are recognised globally as a challenge, such as methicillin-resistant *Staphylococcus aureus* (MRSA). In healthcare facilities the transfer of highly resistant and pathogenic microbes can occur quickly during direct contact with a contaminated surface even with the briefest encounter! These microbes (bacteria, fungi or viruses (transient)) are easily transmitted, but if tackled early enough, can be contained. The longer they persist in the environment or on skin surfaces, the more difficult it is to eliminate them.

The IPC team should investigate every occurrence of HAI to detect and contain any outbreak or potential outbreak as early as possible. This requires constant vigilance and surveillance.

Nosocomial pathogens can occur spontaneously in a healthcare facility (rarely) or may be introduced by staff or patients to the facility. The excessive use of antibiotics has a major impact on flora both from the environment and from the patient, leading to colonisation and spread. It is worth remembering that bacteria never become extinct – only resistant!

Alert organisms. There is a difference between the **acquisition** of antimicrobial resistance resulting from the overuse of antimicrobial agents and **spread** of these pathogens. While it is difficult to prevent acquisition, as will be noted further in this chapter, good IPC practices can reduce the spread by implementing evidence-based appropriate precautions such as hand hygiene and transmission-based precautions. Bear in mind that IPC precautions might be modified depending on the type of pathogen and its route(s) of transmission.

Pathogens not isolated in the healthcare facility previously have the potential to spread and cause outbreaks, but if recognised early, can be contained quite easily with rigorous IPC protocols.

Examples

- *Staphylococcus aureus* introduced by staff (working in other hospitals) or patients previously admitted to other healthcare facilities
- *Salmonella spp* introduced from staff carriers or patients with diarrhoeal disease
- Rotavirus introduced into a neonatal unit by staff or referred patients.

Pathogens in response to changes in medical practice or introduction of new antimicrobial agents. Once these pathogens enter or colonise a unit they are extremely difficult to eradicate because the environment is conducive to their persistence and they thrive in it. Examples of persistent environmental sources for outbreaks with *Acinetobacter baumanni, Pseudomonas aeruginosa* and other priority micro-organisms are numerous in the literature. IPC procedures have to be intense, expensive and continuous. A breach in IPC procedures becomes apparent when these pathogens re-emerge.

Examples

- MRSA introduced by staff who work in several healthcare facilities and carry MRSA from one healthcare facility to another, or patients previously admitted to other healthcare facilities; also, in response to uncontrolled usage of broad-spectrum antibiotics in intensive care units.
- *Acinetobacter spp* in intensive care areas in response to broad-spectrum antibiotics.
- Extended spectrum β-lactamases (ESBL) production among gram-negative bacilli such as *Klebsiella pneumoniae, Enterobacter spp* and *Escherichia coli*.
- *Clostridioides difficile* recognised as a significant nosocomial pathogen in healthcare facilities.

'New' pathogens previously considered commensals or of low pathogenicity. Aggressive medical care and an increased use of antimicrobial agents have resulted in bacteria previously considered commensals or of low pathogenicity emerging with multiple antibiotic resistance and which are difficult to treat. IPC containment measures can be quite drastic and prolonged.

Examples

- Coagulase negative staphylococcus, previously considered a skin coloniser, can cause infection in the presence of foreign bodies such as central lines, intravenous cannulae and urinary catheters.
- *Enterococcus spp* is considered a commensal of the gut, but can cause severe infections in specific patient populations (e.g. ICU).
- *Candida auris* is an emerging fungus that presents a serious global health threat.

Pathogens once considered purely healthcare-facility acquired are now emerging from the community. The reason is simply because healthcare facilities serve a community and the movement between the two is considerable and frequent – the microbiome in all given situations modifies itself to survive in any given environment.

2.12 Microbiological laboratory and IPC

The laboratory plays a key role in IPC programmes and there should be a close working relationship between these two teams. The clinical team directly responsible for clinical care of the patient should be included in all relevant IPC decisions.

In countries with limited resources, laboratories are inadequately funded and are located away from the rest of the hospital and often send out results without any further interaction. In countries where a medically qualified member of staff heads the laboratory services the clinical involvement of the laboratory has extended to clinical management and infection control programmes.

This chapter covers the essentials of microbiological laboratories. Readers are advised to consult other textbooks on the subject for further reading.

2.12.1 The laboratory and clinical teams

The relationship between a well-functioning laboratory, IPC team and the clinical team is close and is based on mutual respect and understanding of each other's knowledge, skills and needs. However, this relationship, as with all relationships, has to be nurtured. Clinicians have a tendency to dismiss microbiology staff as either not being medically qualified or not being clinicians. The laboratory staff may feel intimidated by the clinical staff or may feel it is not within their remit to liaise and discuss management of patients with the clinical team.

In order to work together it is essential that:
- there are regular meetings between the laboratory and the clinical team (including the IPC team if necessary) to discuss important clinical matters and to improve links
- samples are taken as recommended by the laboratory (preferably a written protocol)
- samples are delivered to the laboratory punctually
- samples are processed with the shortest turnaround time as possible (this can be agreed and followed up if delays occur)
- urgent results are reported (by telephone usually) to the relevant member of the clinical team and are not just part of the routine delivery to the ward; this includes an on-call emergency service in some countries

- the clinicians should understand the impact of:
  - antibiotic treatment prior to taking samples for microbiological investigations will distort the results
  - the timing of samples
  - the correct sample (e.g. muco-purulent sputum instead of saliva)
  - appropriate sterile containers
  - clearly written and completed laboratory request forms so that results can be returned
- the laboratory should recognise that:
  - in an emergency samples may be taken after antibiotics have been administered
  - even with a written protocol, samples may be taken at the wrong time, incorrectly or may be contaminated
  - repeat samples, if possible to be taken, can be requested if there is a mishap or breakage
  - the result report should be clear and unambiguous and avoid confusion
- where there are inadequate resources for laboratory services, the diagnosis of infection is usually made clinically:
  - patients with suspected infection are started on antibiotics empirically
  - if treatment fails, laboratory assistance may be sought
- the use of antibiotics has major consequences – it masks and/or hinders accurate laboratory diagnosis:
  - normal flora is replaced by multiple antibiotic-resistant bacteria and this is usually isolated on culture even though it may not be the offending pathogen
  - antibiotic therapy may be changed on the basis of the bacteriology result and this may be both unnecessary and detrimental to the patient's management
  - the infection may be viral in origin and not suspected or diagnosed for some time
  - even if a patient has been treated with an antibiotic to which the bacterium is resistant, the latter may not be isolated on culture because of the inhibitory effect of that antibiotic.

2.12.2 Taking microbiology samples

The outcome of the sample depends on how well the sample was collected and transferred into the appropriate container, how quickly it was transported to the laboratory (or refrigerated if need be) and how rapidly it is processed by the laboratory.

2.12.3 The laboratory form

Ideally an electronic patient system should be in place that connects the microbiological laboratory and the clinical wards. In countries where electronic systems have yet to be established and a paper-based system is used, the following essential elements should be implemented:

- The request form should have the patient's name, hospital number, age, sex and the unit or location (ward or department) **where the results are to be returned to**. Sometimes there is confusion if the patient is admitted from the outpatient department (OPD) or from accident and emergency and the sample is taken there before the patient is transferred to a ward. The unit recorded is stated as OPD; the results are returned there and lost to the patient's records.
- The name of the firm or department (surgery or medicine) and the clinician who ordered the tests and contact details (such as a phone number) should be clearly visible so that the results can be returned.
- The type of tests required should be clearly indicated. Any additional tests should be stated. For example, for a stool specimen from a case of diarrhoea, request for parasites may be additional to culture for salmonella, shigella or campylobacter.
- A brief clinical diagnosis, duration of illness and current or past antibiotic treatment should be recorded. If possible, previous hospital admission, if any, should be stated (this is useful for IPC).
- After the sample has been taken, you should make sure the sample and request form match the patient details.
- It is unwise to leave a stack of signed forms for the ward staff to complete – the clinical information is usually missing or misleading.

2.12.4 Specimen container

- All samples should be taken in a single-use dry sterile container unless otherwise indicated. Re-using or recycling specimen containers is not advisable since cross-contamination can occur.
- A screw-cap, leak-proof plastic container is commonly used in healthcare facilities.
- The container should not come into contact with antiseptic, disinfectant or any other chemical agent as most of these agents are microbicidal.
- All specimen containers must be labelled with the patient's name, hospital number and date and time of sampling.
- At ward or unit level, laboratory containers should be stored in a dry cupboard away from direct contamination – never in the sluice!
- Blood culture bottles are especially prone to contamination because they contain liquid media designed to encourage growth. These must be stored appropriately and used before the expiry date.

2.12.5 Sampling site

Table 2.7 Specimen sites and method of sampling and transportation

Some examples of type of specimen and special precautions required to get the best results		
Type of specimen	**Sample and transportation**	**Reason**
Cerebrospinal fluid	Transported immediately, should be warm and incubated immediately	*Neisseria spp* very susceptible to air and cold
Urine	Taken from sampling port and not the urinary drainage bag or by disconnecting the urinary catheter; can be refrigerated at 4 °C until plated out	Prevent multiplication of bacteria
Faeces	Collect from dry bedpan (warm stools for amoebae)	Reduce contamination
Sputum	Early morning specimen; make sure it is not salivary	Best yield for all pathogens especially *Mycobacterium tuberculosis*
Serous fluid	Sterile sample in a screw-cap container	Possibility of *Mycobacterium tuberculosis* (need much larger sample)
Blood culture (B/C)	Full aseptic technique required; if multiple blood samples taken, inoculate B/C bottle first; may need to take two B/C at different times	Avoid skin contamination; prevent pseudobacteraemia from other containers – false results
Serology	Sterile sample in appropriate container	Contamination leads to haemolysis
Tissue	A large sample in a dry, sterile container; do not add saline or water if possible	Should not be allowed to dry – saline or water can be bactericidal; never add formalin!
Virology	Separate sample of blood for serology; tissue for virology into viral transport media	Contaminants can kill cell lines and give false serological results

The sample is usually taken from the suspected site of infection. Sterile sites, such as blood and cerebrospinal fluid, will require an invasive procedure and therefore require skill to avoid external contamination.

- If the site of infection is not easily accessible or offers difficulty in diagnosis, a sample blood culture may help towards establishing a diagnosis, especially if the patient has a fever (bacteraemia).
- A sample taken from sites (organs or surfaces connected to the outside) which are normally colonised, such as a throat swab or vaginal swab, will require special methods targeted specifically at suspected pathogens.

- Samples from wounds and other infected sites have to be taken with care because colonising organisms are usually prolific and frequently isolated. The sample can thus give false positive results.
- If a device related infection is suspected, a sample from the device, such as a CVP line must always be accompanied by a blood culture from a peripheral site. This is to differentiate between colonisation (biofilm) and pathogen.

2.12.6 Transportation

- Once the sample has been collected it should be placed upright in a clear plastic bag, preferably one with a separate pocket for the request form, and sealed.
- The request form should be facing outwards so that it is clearly visible to the transporter. In the case of accidental breakage, the patient can be identified and another sample requested.
- Non-urgent samples are placed in a marked, robust box at ward level, awaiting collection.
- Once all the laboratory samples have been collected from the healthcare facility they are transported to the laboratory in a robust and safe container.
- The laboratory staff inspect the sample for appropriateness. This means there should be no leakage, it should be clearly labelled and be the correct sample.

2.12.7 Organisms that cannot be cultivated

Some organisms cannot be cultured in routine microbiological laboratory. For such organisms non-culture methods are used. Serological tests can be performed on blood samples or the specimen itself, looking for antigen or antibodies using molecular methods or specialised microscopy. The type of specimen required will be advised by the laboratory. Since many of the non-culture methods are expensive and require automation, specimens are batched and analysed together for cost efficiency. If there is a low turnover of specimens, the results may take some time to come back.

2.13 The laboratory examination process

The aim of the laboratory is to isolate and identify common suspected pathogens from a particular site (such as salmonella from stools), but it also must be vigilant for unusual or less common pathogens. Prohibitive laboratory costs do not allow routine culture for **all** pathogens from **each** specimen and therefore specialised knowledge of microbiology is a great asset when setting standard operating procedures for recovery from each specimen type.

2.13.1 Registration

Samples arriving at the microbiology laboratory are received to an area which registers specimen details. The specimen is then sent to the appropriate area (known as a **bench**) for further processing.

2.13.2 The specimen

Visual macroscopic examination of the sample ensures it is appropriate for processing.

Once the sample has been selected a set protocol is followed to identify relevant pathogens, depending on the laboratory protocol. The steps are briefly described below:

Step 1: Preparation of specimen. Specimens from sterile sites such as cerebrospinal fluid are concentrated, while others such as sputum are inactivated to prevent exposure of the laboratory worker to *Mycobacterium tuberculosis*.

Step 2: Gram stain. Specimens from sterile sites such as cerebrospinal fluid often have an initial gram stain. This helps the clinician with a presumptive diagnosis of meningitis. However, a negative gram stain does not mean there will be no growth on culture.

Step 3: Media. The specimen is carefully plated out onto a set of agar plates made up of non-selective (allowing all bacteria to grow) and selective media (specifically encouraging the growth of certain bacteria). The plates are incubated overnight at 37 °C in an appropriate atmosphere (such as oxygen alone, CO_2 or anaerobic conditions) which will support the growth of potential pathogen.

The following day the plates are examined for growth, characteristics, if any, such as haemolysis, and possible clues to assist with further identification.

Colonies growing on the agar plates are gram-stained and confirmed as either gram-positive or gram-negative.

Step 4: Identification. This step involves the selection of a means of identification:
- **Selective media.** Suspicious colonies are carefully picked and explanted onto a further set of appropriate media and incubated for a further 18–24 hours.
- **Biochemical tests** for gram-negative bacilli help with species classification.
- **Semi-automated systems.** Blood cultures (and other) systems are now available which give an early warning when growth occurs, cutting the time to reporting by more than half compared with previous manual methods.
- **Malditof,** a matrix-assisted laser desorption/ionisation (MALDI) mass spectrometry has evolved into a powerful technology with a diverse range of applications. MALDI coupled to time-of-flight mass spectrometry (MALDI-TOF MS) is used to identify micro-organisms. The sample for analysis

by MALDI-TOF MS is prepared by mixing or coating with a solution of an energy-absorbent matrix which entraps and co-crystallises the sample when dried. The matrix is ionised with a laser beam and transfers the charge to the analytes, generating singly charged ions from analytes in the sample that are then accelerated. Ions are separated from each other on the basis of their mass-to-charge ratio (m/z) before being detected and measured using the TOF mass analyser.

- **Vitek** is another system which gives rapid bacterial identification and antibiotic sensitivity result and is used for the identification of growth in samples, including blood cultures. It picks up growth using an electronic signal system of continuous monitoring of turbidity and, once the growth has reached a certain level of turbidity, an alert signal is activated.

- **Molecular methods.** Recent developments in non-culture methods allow rapid identification of pathogens based on their molecular characteristics. These tests, though extremely useful and becoming more accurate by the day, are expensive. Essentially there are three molecular techniques:
  - genetic
  - biomarker
  - companion diagnostics.

  Genetic and biomarker are sometimes used interchangeably.

For further details consult publications on the subject.

Finally, the **turnaround-time** (TAT) from receiving a specimen to returning results is a priority for the laboratory and recent developments have greatly reduced the TAT. However, it must be said that the skills acquired at the bench through processing specimens manually with care and an in-depth knowledge of bacteria are regretfully fading and being replaced by automated methods.

2.13.3 Interpreting microbiology laboratory results

When empirical antibiotic therapy has been started, and the patient is responding to treatment, there is no need to change antibiotics because the laboratory reports something different. If, however, the patient is not responding after at least 48 hours of appropriate antimicrobial therapy, then a change of management should be considered. Laboratory results are there to assist and guide the clinician. It is a common mistake to change antibiotics based on laboratory findings as this sometimes leads to clinical and IPC problems.

Reporting systems differ from one laboratory to another. The result should be helpful, give good advice and report that which is considered relevant to the clinician.

- Microbiology results from a throat swab, for example, need only state whether recognised pathogens such as Group A Streptococcus are present or not.

- There is no need to mention all the organisms that were grown, especially since most may be commensals. A report like '*Neisseria* species isolated' can confuse the clinician who may interpret it as *N meningitides*, which he or she may consider clinically significant.
- Negative reports are sometimes just as helpful as positive ones. For example, 'Salmonella, shigella and campylobacter not isolated' alerts the clinical staff to look for other possible pathogens.
- A wide range of reported antibiotic sensitivities also can be confusing, especially when the bacterium is reported sensitive to one generation and resistant to another. This is particularly true of cephalosporins. Cross-resistance, where present, should be reported. Inducible β-lactamases should also be reported with a note about its clinical significance.
- An example of inappropriate antibiotic therapy follows:

Example

A 28-year-old man presented with an acute lower respiratory tract infection diagnosed on clinical grounds of a fever, cough with purulent sputum and a chest X-ray showing signs of pneumonia.

He was started on amoxycillin; sputum and blood were sent for culture to the laboratory.
- *H influenzae* was isolated from the sputum and reported as being sensitive to amoxycillin.
- Three days later, although he had improved clinically, he was still pyrexial so a repeat sputum sample was sent. This time the sputum yielded *Klebsiella pneumoniae*.
- The patient was changed to a cephalosporin with an aminoglycoside.
- A few days later the sputum yielded an *Acinetobacter baumannii* and the patient was changed to a carbapenem, with an aminoglycoside and glycopeptide (vancomycin).
- In the next few days *Candida albicans* was isolated from the sputum; the patient now became pyrexial (39,4 °C) and went into respiratory failure.
- He was transferred to the intensive care unit for support ventilation and anti-fungal therapy was added the current regime.
- The sequence of events led to a steady decline of his clinical condition, followed by his demise a few days later.
- On postmortem it was reported that he died of overwhelming nosocomial pneumonia with total organ failure – *H influenzae* was isolated from the lung!

The question is: why was the initial antibiotic changed when the patient was responding to therapy?

2.14 Antimicrobial tests

Once a bacterium has been cultured and isolated in its pure form, antibiotic sensitivity tests may be performed. The most used tests are disc diffusion, Etests, broth microdilution and automated systems.

2.14.1 Disc sensitivity testing

This is a common method for routine testing of bacteria. An array of antibiotics is placed on a non-inhibitory agar plate which has been previously flooded with a pure culture of the bacterium (inoculum of 10^5–10^6 cfu/ml) and dried. The antibiotics are impregnated into a disc of a fixed concentration. Usually, no more than six discs are carefully placed on an agar plate and incubated at 37 °C in the appropriate atmosphere (O_2, 10% CO_2 or AnO_2) overnight. The next morning the plates are examined for inhibition or growth by reading the zone size around the disc. A predetermined zone size indicates sensitivity, intermediate resistance or complete resistance.

Sometimes two antibiotic discs are placed in close proximity to detect β-lactamase production or other synergistic or antagonistic effects.

2.14.2 E-test

This method uses strips of impregnated antibiotics which are marked with zone sizes placed on a solid medium. It gives an indication of the minimum inhibitory concentration (MIC) of the bacterium and is read against a standardised chart of zone sizes.

2.14.3 Broth microdilution

This method requires a range of test tubes or microtitre wells which contain a series of dilutions of an antibiotic. These varying concentrations of the antibiotics and the bacteria to be tested are added to the plate. The plate is then placed into a non-CO_2 incubator and incubated. Following the allotted time, the plate is removed and checked for bacterial growth. If the broth became cloudy or a layer of cells formed at the bottom, then bacterial growth has occurred. The results of the broth microdilution method are reported in Minimum Inhibitory Concentration (MIC), or the lowest concentration of antibiotics that stopped bacterial expansion.

The joint CLSI–EUCAST Polymyxin Breakpoints Working Group has recommended the broth microdilution (BMD) method as the reference method to determine susceptibility to colistin (www.eucast.org).

2.14.4 Automated systems

Automated systems exist that replicate manual processes, for example, by using imaging and software analysis to report the zone of inhibition in diffusion testing, or dispensing samples and determining results in dilutional testing. Automated instruments, such as the VITEK 2, BD Phoenix, and Microscan systems, are the most common methodology for AST.

2.15 Laboratory safety

It is beyond the scope of this book to address details of safety in the laboratories (referred to in current documents as laboratory IPC), but a summary is provided.

2.15.1 Risk to healthcare workers

Laboratory workers are at risk of exposure to pathogens in several ways:
- aerosols generated when opening sputum pots on an open bench
- exposure to blood and body fluids if systems are not in place to carry out these procedures safely
- exposure to splashes during procedures
- exposure to chemicals used in laboratory processing.

2.15.2 Risk-reducing procedures

- A well-planned and organised laboratory with ample space and ventilation; separate specimen reception and administration areas, processing areas and high-risk areas; separate staff rest and eating areas.
- Safety cabinets (with appropriate extraction and filter systems) for processing high-risk samples such as sputum or blood cultures from suspected highly infectious cases.
- Appropriate personal protective equipment for the various areas of work.
- Heat sterilisation of all laboratory equipment and patient samples prior to discard or reprocessing.
- Adequate equipment to carry out safe laboratory practices such as screw-capped centrifuges.
- Hand decontamination facilities.
- All equipment maintained regularly and a record kept with each.
- Protocols for breakages, spillages or accidental exposure.
- Reporting system for all accidents to occupational health, supported by appropriate measures.

2.16 Antimicrobial agents: Therapy and resistance

The use of antimicrobial agents, especially antibiotics, is widespread in medical and veterinary practice. The excessive use of disinfectants and antibiotics has led to the emergence of antimicrobial resistance among bacteria and fungi, leading to major challenges in the management and eradication of pathogens. This is compounded by poor IPC practices in healthcare institutions. The IPC challenges are not only to contain the spread of multiple antimicrobial-resistant pathogens but also to prevent or reduce the emergence of resistance – a problem which preoccupies clinical and IPC teams globally.

This chapter covers the essentials of antimicrobial agents, therapy and resistance. Readers are advised to consult other textbooks on the subject since new antibiotics are being constantly developed and marketed.

2.16.1 Antibacterial agents

These are classified according to
- activity against pathogens: bacteriostatic or bactericidal
- target sites
- chemical structure.

2.16.1.1 Bacteriostatic or bactericidal

Some agents kill (**bactericidal**) while others inhibit (**bacteriostatic**) the growth of bacteria, allowing the body's natural defences to cope with the static population. Bacteriostatic antibiotics are not effective in the immunocompromised host where the body's defences are ineffectual. Equally some antibiotics may act in a bacteriostatic manner for one species of bacteria while being bactericidal for another, but this is a less common consideration these days.

2.16.1.2 Target site for antimicrobials

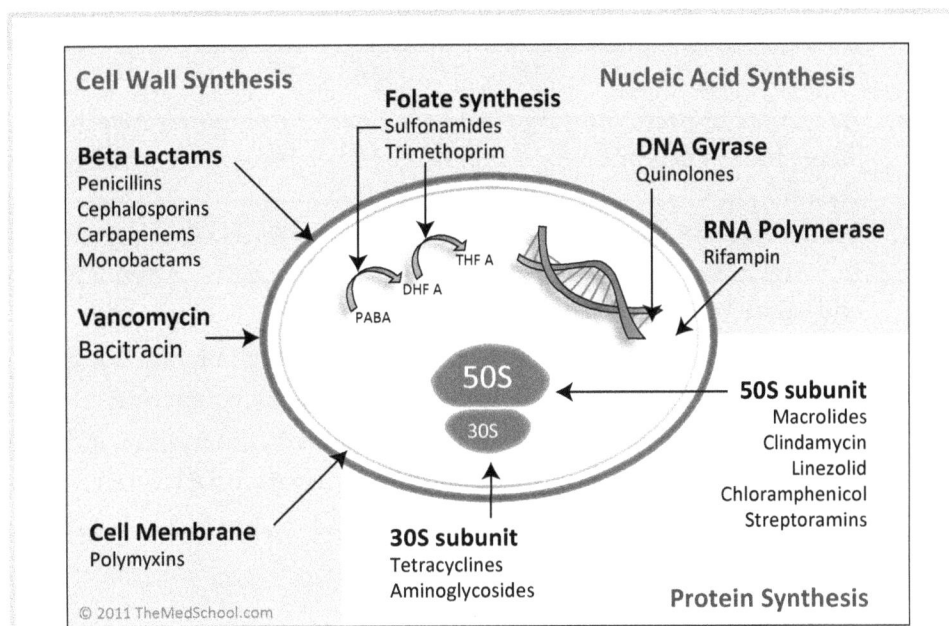

Figure 2.9 The mechanisms of action of common antibiotics[10]

---

[10] Li F, Collins J & Keen R. 2015. Ruthenium complexes as antimicrobial agents. Chemical Society Reviews 44(8) DOI: 10.1039/c4cs00343h.

The antibacterial agents interrupt the growth of bacteria and act at one (or more) stages of growth. The main target sites for antibacterial action are:

- cell wall synthesis
- protein synthesis
- nucleic acid synthesis
- metabolic pathways
- cell membrane function.

2.16.1.2.1 Inhibition of cell wall synthesis (class of antibiotic: β-lactams, glycopeptides, cycloserine, bacitracin)

1. **β-lactams** belong to the same class of antibiotics – the difference between the penicillins and the cephalosporins is a five-membered and six-membered β-lactam ring and the attached structures which give the drug its antibacterial spectrum. It is one of the largest groups of antibiotic used worldwide.

   Mechanism of action: Inhibits cell wall synthesis by binding to the penicillin-binding proteins (PBPs). The result is a weak cell wall which allows the cell membrane to protrude and rupture, resulting in cell lysis.

   Mechanism of resistance
   (a) Alteration of target sites: MRSA synthesises an additional PBP which has a lower affinity to β-lactams than normal PBPs, thus the cell can continue synthesis even when other PBPs are inhibited.
   (b) Alteration in access to target sites is found in gram-negative bacilli, where mutation in the porin genes results in decreased permeability into the cell.
   (c) Production of β-lactamases which hydrolyse the β-lactam ring, resulting in a microbiologically inactive product. The genetic information is widespread on the chromosome and in plasmids

2. **Glycopeptides** (vancomycin and teicoplanin) are active only against gram-positive bacteria.

   Mechanism of action: To inhibit cell wall synthesis by interfering with the cell wall formation during the growing phase of gram-positive bacteria.

   Mechanism of resistance: Plasmid-mediated and transmissible resistance has been reported in *S aureus* and enterococci.

2.16.1.2.2 Inhibition of protein synthesis

These antibiotics interfere with protein synthesis at different levels. (Classes of antibiotic: aminoglycosides, tetracycline, chloramphenicol, macrolides, lincosamides, streptogramines, fucidic acid.)

1. **Aminoglycosides:** These antibiotics are effective against both gram-negative bacilli and staphylococci but not anaerobes or enterococci. They

are actively transported into the cell; both anaerobes and enterococci lack these mechanisms. However, when combined with β-lactams (or any other antibiotic which inhibits the cell wall) they are effective in inhibiting protein synthesis.

Mechanism of action: Aminoglycosides kill by interfering with the binding of transport RNA (tRNA) to the ribosome, thus preventing the initial complex from which protein synthesis proceeds. Streptomycin causes misreading of the mRNA codons.

Mechanisms of resistance
(a) Alteration of the ribosomal target site (especially streptomycin).
(b) Altered permeability.
(c) Altered energy-dependent (active) transport across the cytoplasmic membrane into the cell.
(d) Plasmid-mediated modifying enzymes which are acquired – the enzyme alters the structure of the aminoglycosides which changes the uptake into the cell.

2. **Tetracyclines** are usually bacteriostatic their use is limited to certain infections only.

   Mechanism of action: They inhibit protein synthesis by preventing tRNA from entering acceptor sites on the chromosome. The action is not selective for prokaryotes (bacteria) and bacteria take up tetracycline more than the host cells.

   Mechanism of resistance
   (a) Via a transposon which is expressed in the presence of tetracycline. The synthesis of new cytomembrane protein is induced.
   (b) An efflux pump which reduces accumulation of the drug in the cell.

3. **Chloramphenicol** is bacteriostatic, and is no longer in use.

   Mechanism of action: Blocks peptidyl transferase and thereby prevents protein bond synthesis.

   Mechanism of resistance: Inactivation of drug by producing acetyl transferase (enzyme) which fails to bind to the ribosome and is plasmid-mediated.

4. **Macrolides, lincosamides and streptogramin** These are a group of antibiotics with a similar target site which inhibits protein synthesis and therefore there is cross-resistance between macrolides and lincosamides. The site of action is the rRNA in the 50S subunit.

   Mechanism of resistance: Alteration of the target site which is plasmid mediated and inducible. Erythromycin is the best inducer of resistance.

   Erythromycin-resistant strains will be resistant to lincomycin and clindamycin – known as **MLS resistance**.

2.16.1.2.3 Inhibition of nucleic acid synthesis

2.16.1.2.3.1 Inhibition of precursor synthesis

1. **Sulphonamides**

   These are structural analogues of para-aminobenzoic acid (PABA). It acts by competing with PABA for the essential metabolic pathway of tetrahydrofolic acid (THFA). Bacteria which utilise preformed folic acid are unaffected by sulphonamides.

   Mechanism of resistance: An altered pathway which has a greatly reduced affinity for sulphonamides but not PABA. The cell produces two distinct enzymes- a chromosomally encoded enzyme and a plasmid-mediated enzyme.

2. **Trimethoprim**

   It is a structural analogue to the amino-hydropyrimidine moiety of the folic acid molecule. It acts by preventing the synthesis of THFA. It is often combined with sulphonamides to reduce the emergence of resistant mutants and also for synergy.

   Mechanism of resistance: Plasmid-coded dihydro-reductase with a markedly reduced affinity for trimethoprim. Sulphonamide and trimethoprim-resistant strains are also resistant to co-trimoxazole.

2.16.1.2.3.2 Inhibition of DNA replication

1. **Quinolones** (Class of antibiotics: nalidixic acid; fluoroquinolones: ciprofloxacin, norfloxacin, moxifloxacin, ofloxacin etc) These are a class of antibiotics similar to naladixic acid, but with an improved antibacterial activity.

   Mechanisms of action: Inhibits active DNA gyrase and thereby prevents super-coiling of the bacterial chromosome. This results in the inability of the bacteria to 'pack' DNA into the cell. These drugs inhibit bacterial gyrase but do not affect mammalian cells.

   Mechanism of resistance: Mainly chromosomal, but some reports of plasmid-mediated resistance have been published.
   (a) Changes in the DNA gyrase subunit resulting in a lowered affinity for the drug.
   (b) Changes in the cell wall permeability, thereby reducing uptake.

2.16.1.2.3.3 Inhibition of RNA polymerase

1. **Rifamycins** (rifampicin) This group has activity against gram-positives, but mainly against *Mycobacterium tuberculosis*.

   Mechanism of action: These drugs bind to the RNA polymerase and block synthesis of mRNA.

   Mechanism of resistance: Chromosomally mediated alteration to RNA polymerase target, resulting in lowered affinity for rifampicin.

2.16.1.2.3.4 Other agents affecting DNA

1. **Nitroimidazoles** (Class of antibiotic: metronidazole.) The antimicrobial spectrum includes antiparasitic and anti-anaerobic activity.

   Mechanism of action: Upon entry into the cell the drug is activated by reduction, and it is the reduced intermediate products that have antimicrobial properties, probably by interaction with and the breaking down of DNA. They only act anaerobically.

   Mechanism of resistance: Resistance is unusual, but appears to be due to either an altered uptake or a decrease in cellular reductase activity, thereby slowing activation of the intracellular drug.

2.16.1.2.3.5 Inhibition of cytoplasmic function

1. **Polymyxin:** These are cyclic peptides.

   Mechanism of action: Free amino groups act as cationic agents and disrupt the phospholipid structure of cell membranes.

   Mechanism of resistance: Chromosomally mediated alteration of the membrane structure or reduced uptake of the drug.

2.16.1.3 Selective toxicity

Host cells (eukaryotes) are similar to bacterial cells (prokaryotes) in many ways. Antimicrobial agents are aimed at targets which differ from the host cells, thereby allowing action against the bacterial but not the host cells. This is known as 'selective toxicity'. It is a significant aspect of antimicrobial drug development since toxicity and side effects of therapy in the host should be minimal.

2.16.2 Antimicrobial resistance

Resistance to antimicrobial agents occurs naturally or can be acquired – the latter being highly efficient and evolving over time.

2.16.2.1 Natural resistance

This type of resistance is found in some bacteria. The species is universally resistant to a particular antibiotic and a combination of antibiotics will be required for treatment.

- In the environment, fungi, moulds and bacteria produce **antibacterial substances** (enzymes) that inhibit or kill other bacteria. These are naturally occurring antibacterial agents. This ability gives them the advantage when competing for space and nutrients. Penicillin is a classic example.
- **Lack of target sites.** Some bacteria do not have the required target site for the antibiotic to act.

- **Impermeability of the cell wall.** Some bacteria either have mechanisms to withstand the penetration of antibiotics or the cell structure is impervious to the antibiotic. An example is the difference between the gram-positive and gram-negative cell wall where glycopeptides only act on gram-positive cell walls.
- **Transport mechanisms** to actively carry the antibiotic into the cell do not exist.

2.16.2.2 Acquired resistance

Bacteria which naturally do not have resistance to an antibiotic(s) can easily acquire it from other bacteria of the same species or different species. The gut is heavily colonised with bacteria of varied species; they commonly pass genetic information among themselves, resulting in resistance to antibiotics.

Genetic resistance can be natural or acquired, but the latter is more frequent and most important from a clinical perspective. This type of resistance can be one or more of the following:

2.16.2.2.1   *Chromosome-mediated* (vertical transfer). These are pieces of DNA which are integrated into the bacterial cell's chromosome and can be passed on from mother to daughter during binary fission (cell division). Chromosomally mediated resistance can be either expressed overtly or, more often, expressed only should a relevant antibiotic come into contact with it. For example, resistance to cephalosporins among *Enterobacter spp* and *Citrobacter spp* is carried on the chromosome and will express itself when cephalosporins are administered.

It is noteworthy that exposure to antibiotics, especially broad spectrum, can often express resistance to several antibiotics.

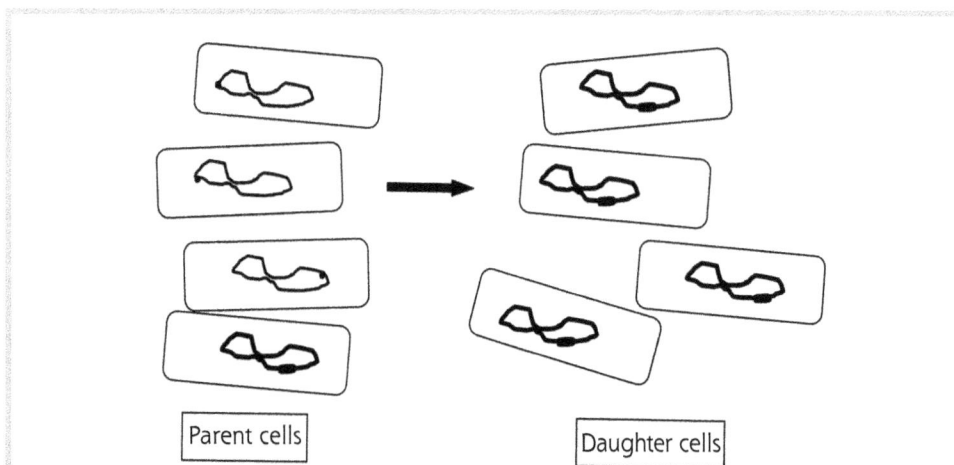

Parent cells   Daughter cells

Figure 2.10   In the parent population only one cell has a resistant chromosome (1). Following cell division particularly in the presence of antibiotics, most of the daughter population have acquired chromosomally mediated resistance.

2.16.2.2.2 *Plasmid-mediated.* This is the commonest type of resistance known to occur. Plasmids are small pieces of **extra-chromosomal DNA** which carry codes for resistance to one or several antimicrobial agents. These are easily transferred between the same species and different species by means of sex pili (known as the F factor). A cell with a sex pilus is known as F+ while one without is F−. Once a plasmid is acquired, the cell changes to F+. A single plasmid can enter a bacterial cell and acquire more antibiotic resistance codes along its journey. Plasmids can influence the metabolism, cell permeability and modification of efflux pumps, in order to protect the bacterium.

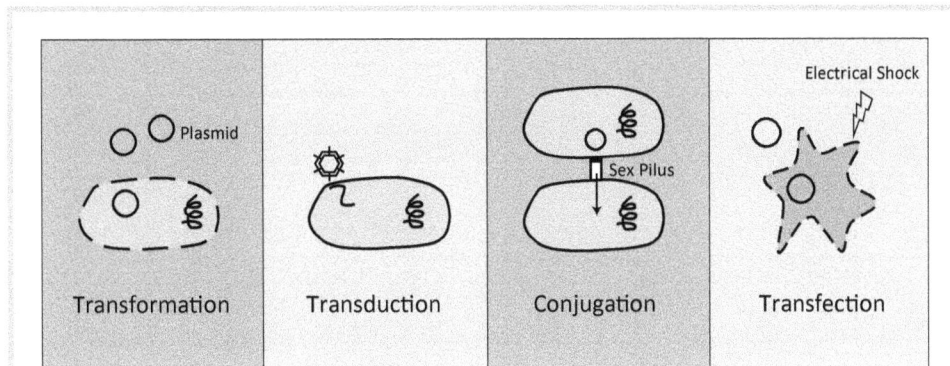

Figure 2.11 Horizontal gene transfer of information between cells[11]

2.16.2.2.3 *Transposons.* These are very small, often single, pieces of extra-chromosomal genetic material that can jump between plasmids (jumping genes) and carry antibiotic and other resistances (see Figure 2.10 above). Some transposons, such as *Tn21*, which confers resistance to trimethoprim, are found worldwide.

2.16.3 Mechanisms of antimicrobial resistance

There are several ways in which bacteria become resistant to antimicrobial agents, including disinfectants, and may employ more than one mechanism of resistance to do so.

1. **Decreased permeability (uptake) of the cell wall.** Some bacteria such as gram-negative bacilli are naturally less susceptible to entry of molecules across the cell wall. They have porins which allow selective entry of substances required

[11]   Adapted from Cecchetelli A . 2019. Plasmids 101: Transformation, Transduction, Bacterial Conjugation, and Transfection https://blog.addgene.org/plasmids-101-transformation-transduction-bacterial-conjugation-and-transfection.

for metabolism. A change in the porin will result in decreased penetration of the cell. This may be general, affecting several antibiotics, or singular, which may affect only one antibiotic.

2. **Alteration of targets.** This is one of the commonest ways of developing resistance where the bacterium modifies or bypasses the target the antimicrobial agent is aimed at. These could be at cell wall, protein synthesis or DNA level.

3. **Alteration of metabolic pathways.** Antibiotics compete for enzymes and sites on the metabolic pathways; bacteria can develop an alternative pathway which bypasses the affected site.

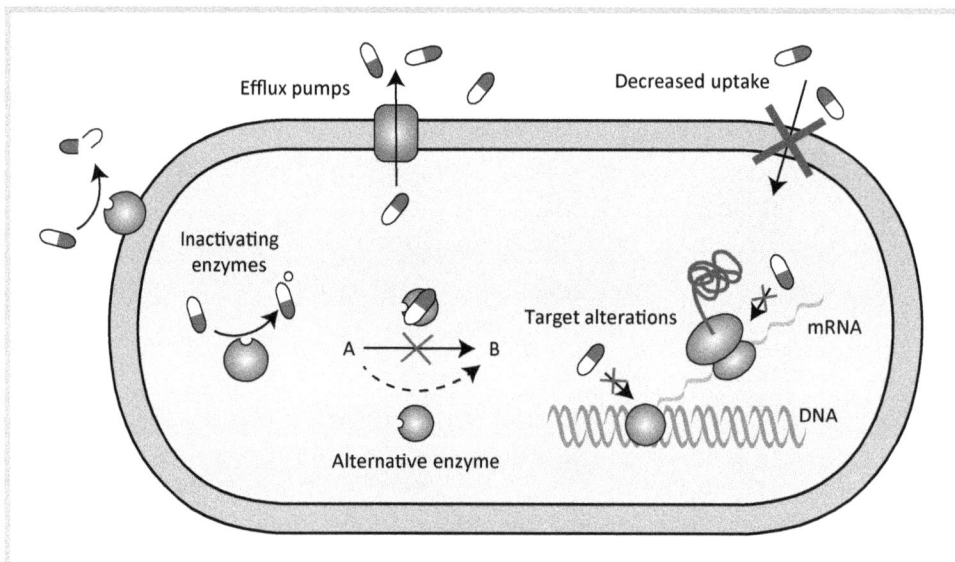

Figure 2.12 Antibiotic resistance strategies in bacteria[12]

4. **Alteration of uptake of the drug.** The bacterial cell modifies the uptake of the drug, thereby eliminating its active carriage into the cell.

5. **Efflux pump.** The bacterium engages mechanisms which 'throw out' the drug once it has entered the cell but before it has had a chance to act.

6. **Enzymatic drug inactivation.** This is perhaps the commonest means whereby the drug is inactivated either before or after it enters the cell.

[12] Courtesy of E. Wistrand-Yuen, from https://www.reactgroup.org/toolbox/understand/antibiotic-resistance/resistance-mechanisms-in-bacteria/.

2.16.4 Urinary antiseptics

Nitrofurantoin and **methenamine** are synthetic compounds which, when taken orally, are absorbed and excreted in the urine. Nitrofurantoin acts only in acid urine. Methenamine is hydrolysed at an acid pH to produce ammonia and formaldehyde. The advantage is that resistance rarely develops.

2.16.5 Anti-tuberculosis drugs

Anti-tuberculosis therapy is a major challenge because *Mycobacterium tuberculosis* has an outer waxy coat and grows intracellularly, which are both impermeable for most antimicrobial agents. Drug delivery and prolonged and uninterrupted treatment regimens can increase the chances of the emergence of resistance and toxicity to the host.

2.16.5.1 First-line therapy

Treatment of tuberculosis is prolonged and difficult. Isoniazid, rifampicin and pyrazinamide are established for primary treatment in uncomplicated tuberculosis. Ethambutol and streptomycin are used as first-line therapy only if there is reason to suspect that the former drugs will not be effective.

Rifampicin and streptomycin have already been addressed.

Isoniazid: The mechanism of action is unclear but may involve inhibition of mycolic acid synthesis and inhibition of the cell wall synthesis. Resistance is plasmid mediated.

Pyrazinamide: The mechanism of action is unknown.

Ethambutol: Inhibits transfer of mycolic acid into the cell wall, thereby inhibiting cell wall synthesis. Emergence of resistance is rapid if used alone.

2.16.5.2 Second-line therapy

When the first-line therapy fails, or a multidrug-resistant strain of *M tuberculosis* has been isolated, additional therapy is indicated following antimicrobial sensitivity testing.

The drugs of choice are clarithromycin or azithromycin (macrolide), ofloxacin, moxifloxacin or gatifloxacin (quinolone) – ciprofloxacin is not recommended. Ethionamide or protionamide is related to isoniazid and inhibits cell wall synthesis. Other drugs are cycloserine, capreomycin and para-aminosalicylic acid (PAS). For further information readers are referred to the WHO and other published guidelines.

2.16.6 Antifungal drugs

Most of the antifungal drugs, such as 5-fluorocytosine and grisofulvin, act on synthesis or function of cell membrane. Table 2.8 outlines the target sites, and mechanisms of action of antifungal drugs.

Table 2.8 Antifungal drugs: Site of action, chemical group and mechanism of action

Target	Chemical group	Examples	Mechanism of action
Cell membrane			
Synthesis	Azoles	Miconazole Ketoconazole Fluconazole Vericonazole	Binds to cytochrome P450, resulting in inhibition of ergosterol synthesis
Cell function	Polyenes	Amphotericin B Nystatin	Binds to sterols in cell membrane; causes leakage of cell components and death
Nucleic acid			
Synthesis	Pyrimidines	Flucytosine (5-fluorocytosine)	Inhibits DNA synthesis and protein synthesis
	Benzofurans	Grisofulvin	Inhibits nucleic acid synthesis; may also interfere with cell wall by inhibiting chitin synthesis

2.16.7 Antiviral drugs

Antiviral agents are few in number and usually have a narrow spectrum of activity. The sites of action of antiviral agents are shown in Figure 2.13. It should be noted that resistance to antiviral drugs can emerge because some viruses can mutate quickly – an example is the human immunodeficiency virus (HIV).

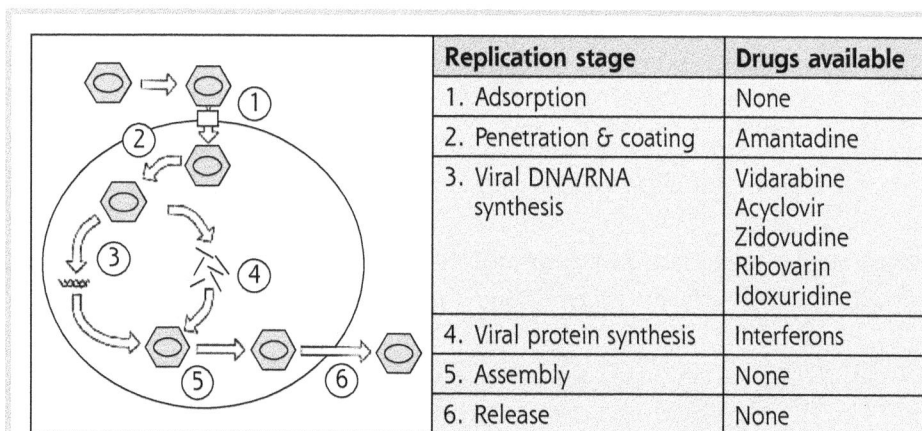

Replication stage	Drugs available
1. Adsorption	None
2. Penetration & coating	Amantadine
3. Viral DNA/RNA synthesis	Vidarabine Acyclovir Zidovudine Ribovarin Idoxuridine
4. Viral protein synthesis	Interferons
5. Assembly	None
6. Release	None

Figure 2.13 Available antiviral therapy and sites of action during replication stage

2.17 Antimicrobial stewardship

International travel and commerce have increased considerably; where humans, animals and food go, there go microbes, carrying their antimicrobial resistance (AMR), or resistome, with them.[13] The microbes are greatly influenced by the wide use of antimicrobials and AMR is becoming more intense. AMR is recognised as a global threat for high- and low- to middle-income countries (LMICs) alike and there are urgent measures called for by the World Health Organisation (WHO) and other similar organisations to reduce the spread of AMR by introducing, and implementing, antimicrobial stewardship (AMS) at national and health facility level. AMS is one of the three pillars of an integrated approach to health systems strengthening – the other two being IPC and patient safety.[14] AMS is very much part of the role of an IPC practitioner as part of the AMS team.

Stewardship is defined as 'the careful and responsible management of something entrusted to one's care'.[15] AMS will require certain administrative structures to be in place, such as AMS guidelines and AMS teams, with a clear yet simple implementation strategy based upon general principles, but specifically aimed at the resources of the health system in question. We are all guardians of antimicrobials and their judicious use. As healthcare workers, we are required to promote AMS not only in healthcare facilities but also in the community through education, extending the role of stewardship beyond the health sector to the health and well-being of the community, guiding health systems at the national and global level.[16] Part of this wider AMS is the recognition of 'One Health'.

2.17.1 What is One Health?

The interaction and close relationship between humans, animals and the environment has been recognised as essential to a concerted effort towards containing anti-microbial resistance. These complex interactions are shown in Figure 2.14. For millennia, humans and domestic animals have had a close relationship. The increasing need for enhanced food production to cater for the needs of an expanding global population has resulted in extensive use of antimicrobials to enhance growth and prophylactically prevent infections in animals and crops. Antibiotics have become part of the normal diet of farmed animals. Antimicrobials are excreted through humans and animals via sewage, and the extensive use of disinfectants, which find their way into the waterways, affects the biodiversity of plants and aquatic life.

---

[13] Report of the Advisory Committee on Animal Uses of Antimicrobials and Impact on Resistance and Human Health Prepared for: Veterinary Drugs Directorate, Health Canada June, 2002.

[14] WHO. 2019. WHO Tool Kit Antimicrobial stewardship programmes in health-care facilities in low- and middle-income countries.

[15] Global framework for development and stewardship to combat antimicrobial resistance: draft roadmap. Geneva: World Health Organization 2017.

[16] Towards better stewardship: concepts and critical issues. Geneva: World Health Organization 2002.

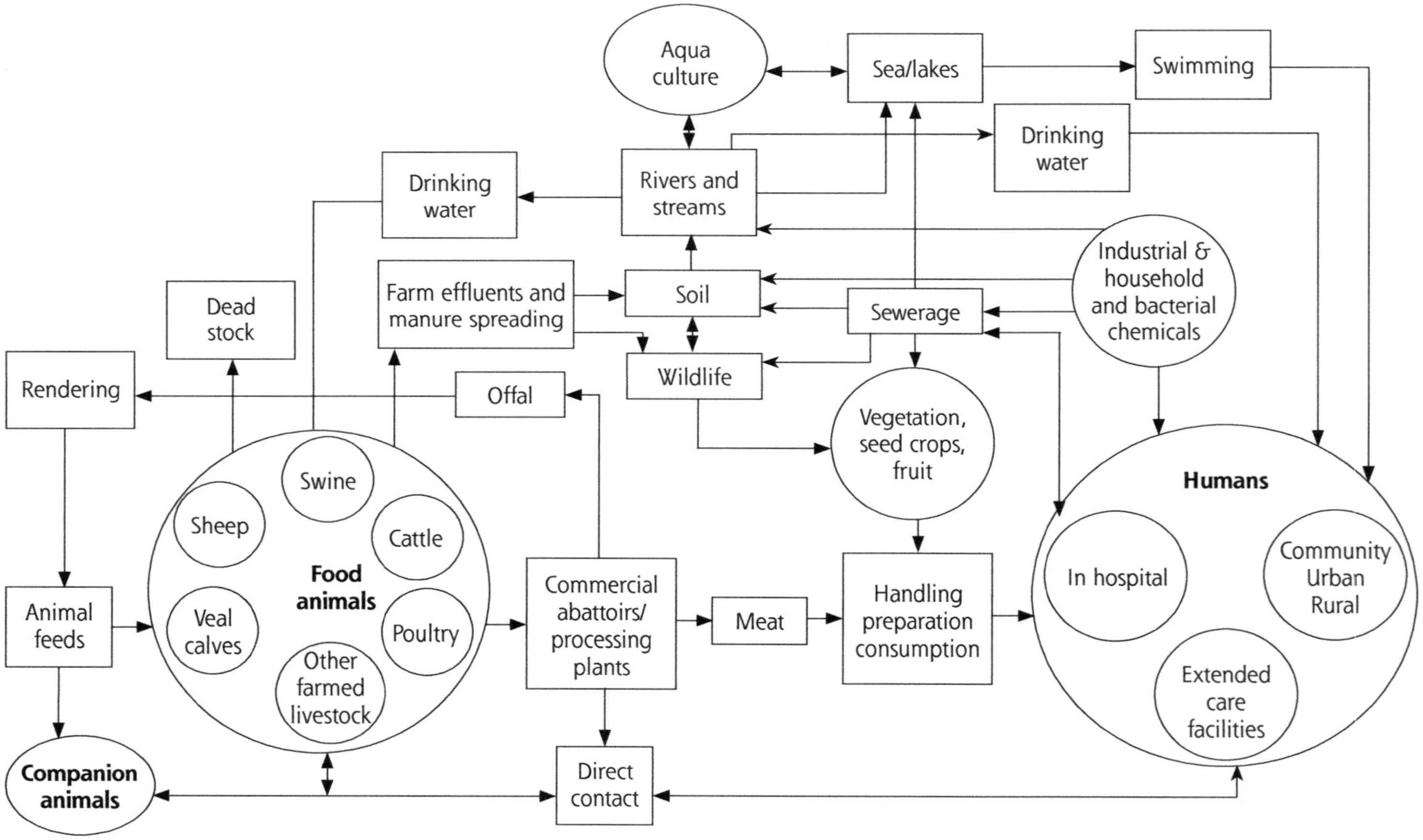

Figure 2.14 Links of AMR through One Health – note the links between humans, animals and farming with the waterways and soil contamination with antimicrobials[17]

17 https://www.canada.ca/en/health-canada/services/drugs-health-products/reports-publications/veterinary-drugs/uses-antimicrobials-food-animals-canada-impact-resistance-human-health-health-canada-2002.html.

Many of these compounds remain in the waterways and soil for extended periods. The emergence of AMR in poultry, animals and vegetables results in outbreaks among humans and animals, particularly in low-resource settings. This has resulted in the banning of unnecessary overuse of antimicrobials. A substantial move globally has been to control antimicrobials in animal husbandry and agriculture, towards reducing the impact on humans, animals and the environment resistome.

In addition to antibiotics, the extensive use of disinfectants has a major impact on the emergence and persistence of AMR in the environment. The mechanisms of resistance for antibiotics and disinfectants are usually the same as previously mentioned.

2.17.2 Combating AMR in animal health

It is beyond the scope of this book to extensively discuss One Health; however, an introduction to the subject is important. There are regulations in some countries to curb the free use of antibiotics in feeds, particularly those groups of antibiotics such as polymyxin (colistin), which are used to treat multidrug-resistant organisms (MDRO) in humans. Feeds which are imported into certain countries are tested regularly for the presence of antibiotics to ensure that the feeds are antibiotic-free.

While antibiotics are being controlled, there is extensive environmental disinfection in animal husbandry and veterinary medicine, often required by environmental health regulations. There is little evidence that random and routine use of disinfectants is useful in preventing infections in animals where good cleaning regimes will suffice. There is a role for disinfectants, but these too must be tightly controlled if AMR is to be combatted.

Finally, it should be noted that in countries where there is poor sanitation, open defaecation and pollution of the waterways, the acquisition of resistant genes (transferrable resistome[18]) by humans is well documented through consumption of contaminated food, particularly uncooked food, and water (Figure 2.15). There are other areas where AMR transmission can take place and these should be considered when setting up a national AMS programme.

---

[18] Blau K, Bettermann A, Jechalke S, Fornefeld E, Vanrobaeys Y, Stalder T, Top EM & Smalla K. 2018. The transferable resistome of produce. *mBio* 9:e01300–18. 156.155.176.94 https://doi.org/10.1128/mBio.01300-18. Downloaded from https://journals.asm.org/journal/mbio on 22 December 2022.

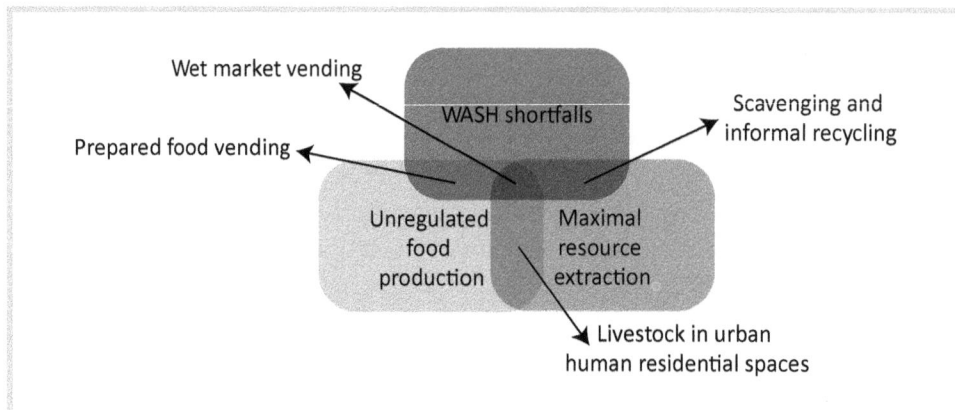

Figure 2.15 Additional potential areas of AMR transmission in low resource settings[19]

2.17.3 A national plan for AMS

The WHO has worked extensively to provide guidance to member states to curb the spread of AMR and MDRO. While it is recognised that low-resource countries will find AMS a challenge, it is always possible to start small and expand, provided there is political support from national departmental structures. AMS is one of the areas where the Department of Health may lead, but animal health, environmental health, sanitation and public works (maintenance) departments must work with it.

2.17.4 What are the benefits of AMS?

The WHO Global Framework[20] outlines the following:
- to improve quality of care and patient outcomes
- to save on unnecessary healthcare costs
- to reduce further emergence, selection and spread of AMR
- to prolong the lifespan of existing antibiotics
- to limit the adverse economic impact of AMR
- to build the best-practices capacity of healthcare professionals regarding the rational use of antibiotics.

19   Adapted from Ikhimiukor, OO, Odih, EE, Donado-Godoy, P et al. 2022. A bottom-up view of antimicrobial resistance transmission in developing countries. *Nat Microbiol* 7: 757–765. https://doi.org/10.1038/s41564-022-01124-w.
20   Global framework for development and stewardship to combat antimicrobial resistance: draft roadmap. Geneva: World Health Organization 2017.

A robust national IPC system to prevent the spread of MDROs, particularly in healthcare facilities, is essential to support the AMS programme at both national and health facility level.

The Global Action Plan on AMR (2015)[21] sets out five strategic objectives as a blueprint for countries for developing national action plans (NAPs) on AMR:

- **Objective 1:** Improve awareness and understanding of AMR through effective communication, education and training.
  - *One of the roles of IPC is to educate and train and communicate to health workers on reducing transmission of pathogens.*
- **Objective 2:** Strengthen the knowledge and evidence base through surveillance and research.
  - *HAI surveillance and data collection is usually under the purview of IPC. This can be reported back to the AMS committee. A point prevalence survey programme is useful (see section 8.1.5.2).*
- **Objective 3:** Reduce the incidence of infection through effective sanitation, hygiene and infection prevention measures.
  - *The role of IPC in ensuring environmental hygiene, clean linen, regular water supply and infection prevention measures. Some of these are achieved through collaboration with the public works and maintenance departments.*
- **Objective 4:** Optimise the use of antimicrobial medicines in human and animal health.
  - *IPC should be an active member of the AMS committee and support AMS.*
- **Objective 5:** Develop the economic case for sustainable investment that takes account of the needs of all countries, and increase investment in new medicines, diagnostic tools, vaccines and other interventions.
  - *While this may not directly relate to IPC, costing of HAIs can help to make a case for improved IPC and AMS measures.*

AMS programmes optimise the use of antimicrobials, improve patient outcomes, reduce AMR and healthcare-associated infections, and save healthcare costs, among others. The Organisation for Economic Co-operation and Development (OECD) report 'Stemming the superbug tide: just a few dollars more', maintained that implementing AMS programmes together with other policies to reduce overuse of antibiotics and promote hospital hygiene could save up to 1.6 million lives by 2050 and US$ 4.8 billion per year in the 33 OECD countries.[22]

[21] Global Action Plan for AMR. Geneva. World Health Organisation 2015.
[22] OECD. 2018. Stemming the superbug tide: just a few dollars more. https://www.oecd-ilibrary.org/social-issues-migration-health/oecd-health-policy-studies_2074319x.

The WHO Toolkit[23] outlines the aim of an AMS programme:

- to optimise the use of antibiotics
- to promote behaviour change in antibiotic prescribing and dispensing practices
- to improve quality of care and patient outcomes
- to save on unnecessary healthcare costs
- to reduce further emergence, selection and spread of AMR
- to prolong the lifespan of existing antibiotics
- to limit the adverse economic impact of AMR
- to build the best-practices capacity of healthcare professionals regarding the rational use of antibiotics.

Key steps in establishing a national AMS programme to enable facility AMS programmes have been adapted from the WHO guidelines on the subject.[24]

1. Establish a governance structure – e.g. a national AMS technical working group (TWG) linked to the national AMR steering committee.
2. Review and prioritise the national core elements:
   2.1 Identify what is already in place and the level of implementation required.
   2.2 Identify the short- and medium-/long-term priority core elements.
   2.3 Identify the resources required.
3. Identify pilot healthcare facilities (public and private) for initial AMS rollout:
   3.1 Tertiary teaching facilities;
   3.2 Regional/state and/or district facilities; and
   3.3 Primary care and/or community (as part of community AMS programmes not covered in this toolkit).
4. Develop a national AMS strategy with national indicators.
5. Dedicate financial and human resources as required.
6. Monitor and evaluate implementation of the national AMS strategy.
7. Facilitate access to and/or support pre- and in-service training on optimised antibiotic prescribing, including community and/or primary care AMS programmes.

Evident from these objectives is the pivotal role IPC plays towards preventing infections, especially HAI, requiring antibiotic treatment and containing the spread of MDROs.

---

23   Antimicrobial stewardship programmes in health-care facilities in low- and middle-income countries. A practical toolkit. Geneva: World Health Organization 2019.
24   National Department of Health, South Africa. 2017. Guidelines on Implementation of the antimicrobial strategy in South Africa: One health approach and Governance.

2.17.5 Example of a national AMS programme

The South African AMR Implementation Plan has also taken into account One Health and the environmental impact of antimicrobial usage. The governance structure has established four pillars:

- diagnostic stewardship
- enhanced surveillance
- antimicrobial stewardship, and
- prevention, including IPC and vaccination.

Each pillar has established a technical working group which addresses areas that are pertinent to its remit. The relationship between IPC and AMS is shown in Figure 2.16, underpinned by a robust training and education programme aimed mainly at health workers and but also the community.

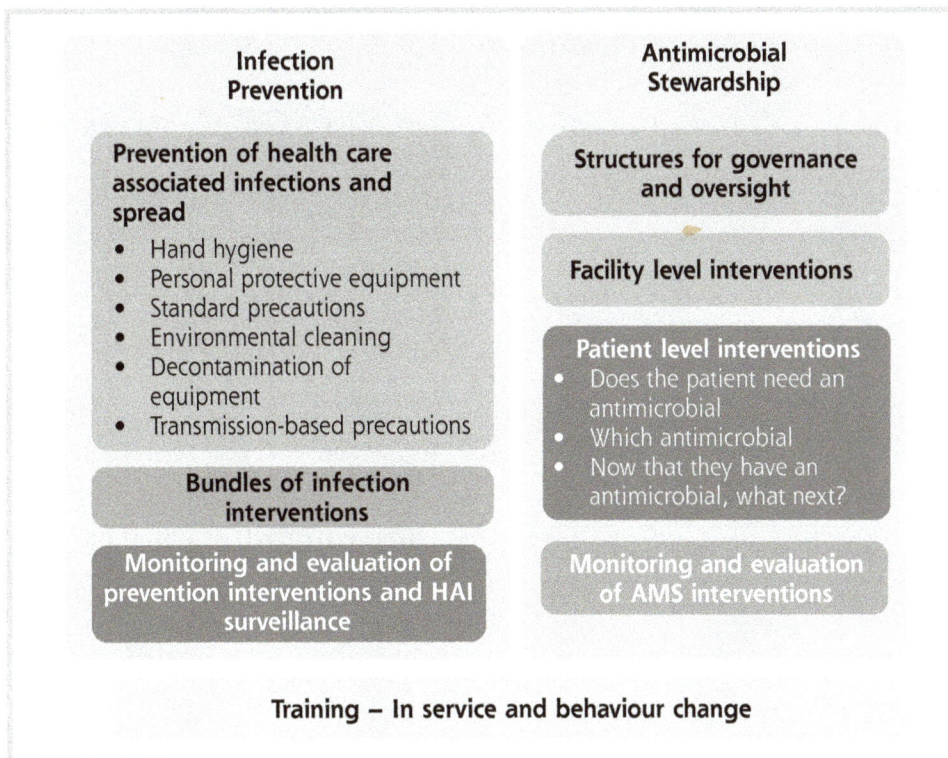

Figure 2.16 Role of IPC in AMS in South Africa. The framework is underpinned by training of health workers and the community.[25]

---

[25] National Department of Health, South Africa. 2017. Guidelines on Implementation of the antimicrobial strategy in South Africa: One health approach and Governance.

2.17.6 An AMS programme at health facility level

Health facility level is where the day-to-day AMS activity resides. The structure is shown in Figure 2.17.

2.17.6.1 The AMS committee

The AMS committee has the advisory role and sets the direction and work programme for the facility. It must have representation from hospital management, preferably the CEO or Deputy CEO. It is a decision-making body. It must have regular meetings, at least every quarter, where the findings from routine HAI surveillance and annual PPS results are reported and discussed. Other matters that affect AMS, such as clean regular water supply, sanitation, hygiene and infrastructure maintenance, should also be considered by the AMS committee. Improvements can start with low-hanging fruit and move up the ladder in a stepwise manner. This information is shared with the AMS team, who are usually part of the AMS Committee.

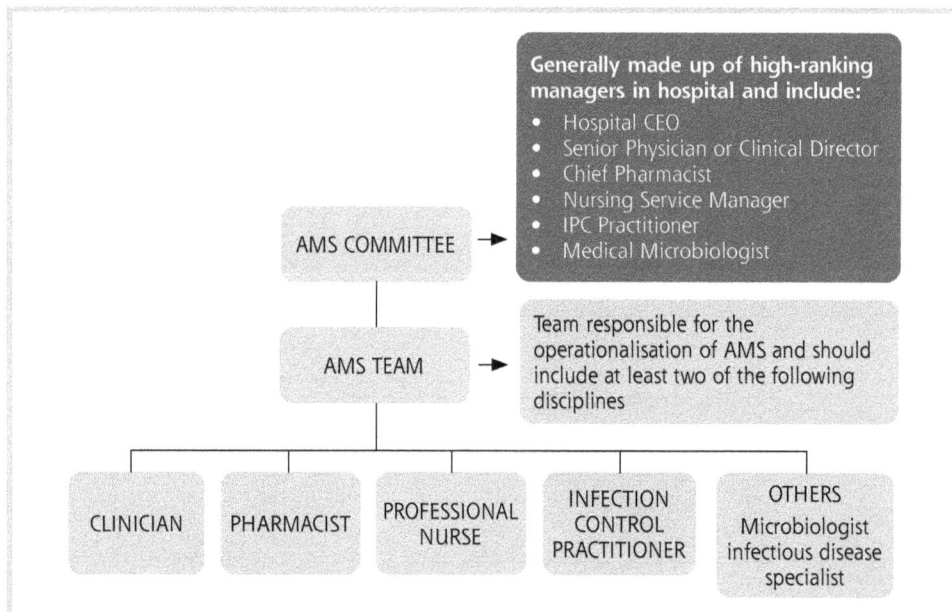

Figure 2.17 AMS structure at HCF level[26]

2.17.6.2 Role of the AMS committee

Figure 2.18 outlines the type of topics the AMS committee should address at health facility level.[27] There may be other issues which concern the AMS committee,

---

26   NDOH Strategic Plan. 2018. https://www.health.gov.za/wp-content/uploads/2020/11/depthealthstrategic planfinal2020-21to2024-25-1.pdf.

27   National Department of Health, South Africa. 2017. Guidelines on Implementation of the antimicrobial strategy in South Africa: One health approach and Governance.

such as maintenance of the infrastructure and constant clean water supply. The AMS committee should be able to advise on improving these and other matters.

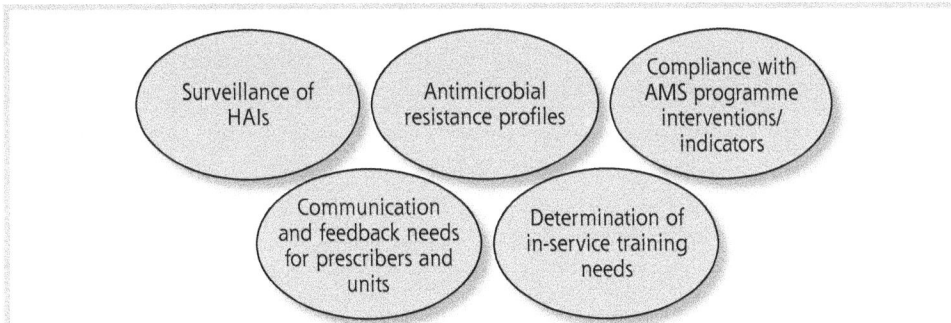

Figure 2.18 Examples of discussion points and IPC matters for AMS committees

2.17.6.3 The AMS team

The AMS team does regular clinical ward rounds, surveillance and monitoring and evaluation. Note that there are several options of who can be part of the AMS team; however, there should be at least two, preferably three, members: clinician, IPC practitioner and pharmacist, particularly in smaller establishments. Irrespective of size, the AMS team must be committed to reducing AMR and support AMS at every opportunity.

Figure 2.19 is an example of a standard approach to conducting AMS on a clinical ward round and helps to follow an algorithm to arrive at a therapeutic conclusion.

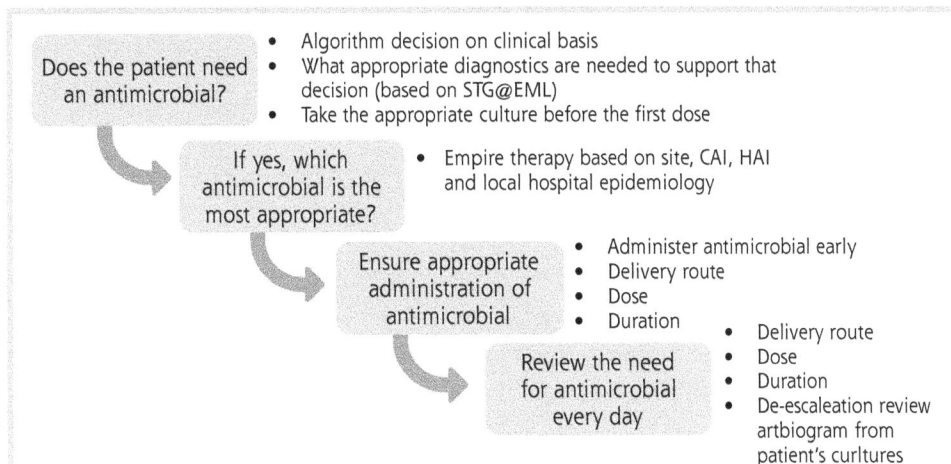

Figure 2.19 A useful example of an approach to AMS when conducting clinical rounds[28]

28   The NDOH Strategic Plan. 2018. https://www.health.gov.za/wp-content/uploads/2020/11/depthealth strategicplanfinal2020-21to2024-25-1.pdf.

2.17.7 Making AMS happen

Once the AMS committee and AMS team structures have been established and responsibilities apportioned, AMS can gradually start happening. Below is an example of an AMS ward round and how reporting, discussion and improvements start with allocated responsibilities.

Step 1: What is our current situation? – *AMS team*
- How many patients are on antibiotics today?
  - Denominator = total number of patients on the ward
  - Numerator – number of patients on antibiotics today

Step 2: Prescription chart – *Pharmacist*
- How long has the patient been on antibiotics?
- Has it been given properly (dose, hang time and route)?

Step 3: Microbiology sample – *Microbiologist*
- Was a microbiology sample taken before starting antibiotics?
- Are the results back?

Step 4: Evaluation – *AMS team clinician(s)*
- Has the patient improved on the current antibiotic regime?
  - Is the patient well enough to come off the antibiotic?
  - Can route change from IV to oral?
- If the patient has not improved,
  - What does the laboratory report say?
  - Does the patient warrant a change of antibiotics?
  - Reassess the cause of not getting better.

Step 5: Are IPC transmission-based precautions required? – *IPC practitioner*
- Type of precautions required.
- Is an isolation or single room needed?
- On the spot teaching of clinical staff – reminder of precautions.
- Contact tracing of other patients if necessary.
- Environmental cleaning (Disinfection).
- Medical device cleaning and disinfection.

AMS is an ongoing process which requires constant vigilance and commitment from all health workers but particularly from management. Figure 2.20 illustrates the relationship between the various components to ensure a successful AMS programme. Leadership commitment is pivotal to a successful AMS programme. There must be accountability from all the members. There should be actions which are regularly evaluated. Education and training at both formal and informal sessions help to maintain interest and the AMS team learns about challenges on the ground. Monitoring and surveillance help with measuring progress made and identifying challenges. Finally, the report and feedback must be not only to the AMS committee but also the clinical areas so that the clinical teams can evaluate themselves.

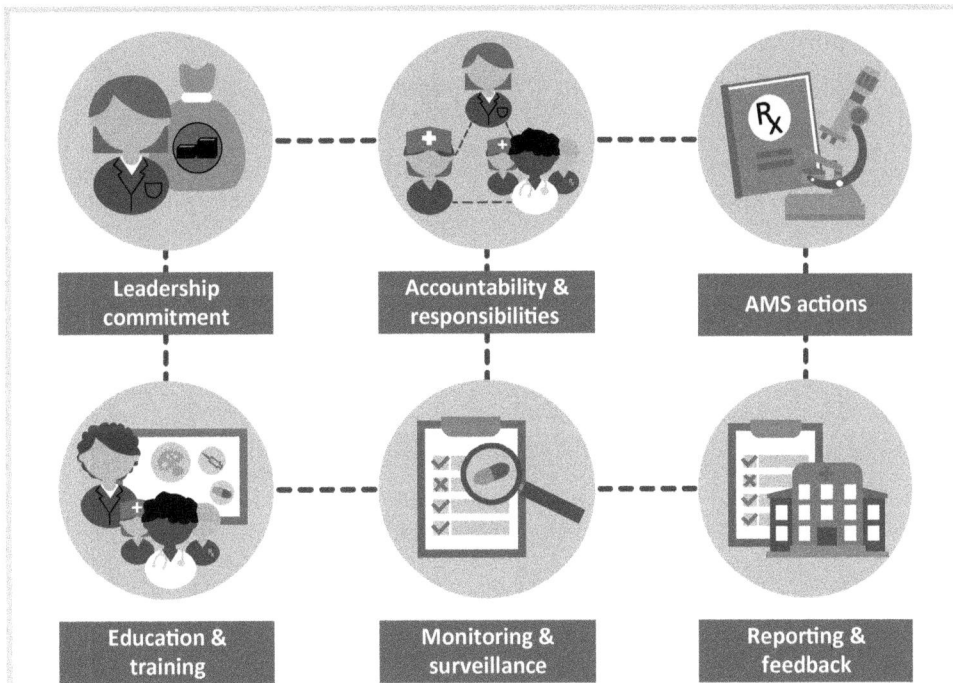

Figure 2.20 The elements required for a successful AMS programme[29]

---

29   Antimicrobial stewardship programmes in health-care facilities in low- and middle-income countries. A WHO practical toolkit. 2019.

3 Decontamination of medical devices

Phil de Vries & Shaheen Mehtar

Learning outcomes

What you should know after reading this chapter:
- Sterile service departments – layout, structure and staffing
  - Functioning of decontamination equipment
  - Processes of decontamination and sterilisation
  - Decontamination of endoscopes
  - Validation of decontamination process
  - IPC interaction with decontamination and sterilisation

Introduction

Decontamination (processing service) is a speciality in its own right and should be housed in an independent stand-alone unit, regulated by extensive legislation and international standards such as ISO and Good Manufacturing Practice (GMP). Specialist knowledge of decontamination and sterilisation lies with the sterile service department (SSD) manager and staff, who are trained in these matters and must remain informed of all recent developments and provide valuable advice and support to the healthcare facility.

The relationship between the IPC team and SSD is a close one, particularly when investigating surgical site infections (SSI). The IPC practitioner must understand the basics of reprocessing of medical devices (MD) and validation of these processes, and, importantly, how the lack of well-documented reprocessing methods can contribute to SSI and HAI. The IPC practitioner should recognise the risks of reprocessing single-use devices, particularly if the processes are not properly controlled. The legal requirements for reprocessing and the production of sterile MD are similar for commercial and healthcare facility units.[1] Each step of the decontamination cycle will require validation as part of the QA programme before a MD is ready for use. The term **'decontamination'** includes both cleaning and disinfection/sterilisation of MD. The final requirement of any of these processes is safe, reusable MDs that will not harm patients.

This chapter has been updated based on the WHO guidelines on Decontamination and reprocessing of medical devices for health-care facilities (2016),[2] which is recommended reading.

3.1 Quality assurance (QA) in sterile services

Documentation and control of process validation at each step of the reprocessing cycle is essential to avoid infections or mishaps from poor reprocessing of medical devices, particularly during surgery. During an investigation of SSI or other related HAIs, the IPC team will require access to all validation and daily testing documentation. Records are usually kept for up to five years, depending on national medico-legal requirements.

3.1.1 Essential elements of quality management systems[3]

The essential elements of quality assurance and management are summarised here. These should be audited regularly to ensure compliance with the regulations.
- Documentation and record-keeping of all stages of the decontamination cycle:
  — steriliser monitoring: use of biological and chemical indicator controls
  — product sterility release criteria: parametric release to ensure that the processed medical device has met the validated process parameters
  — device and process tracking and traceability: manual or computerised system for tracing and tracking to enable tracing from the patient back to the processor and vice versa in the event of a medical device recall
  — storage and transport

---

[1]   The ISO 9001 (general quality) and European norm (EN) ISO 13485 (quality of the installation and maintenance of health products) standards make it possible for a facility to evaluate its system and to guide the steps for its improvement. In the case of sterilisation, the sterilisation assurance level [SAL] 10^{-6} should be ensured so that the sterilisation process generates a product or service according to its predetermined validated specification and in keeping with established quality characteristics.
Note: The European standard EN 46001 1997 stipulates that a medical device determined to be 'sterile' should reach a SAL of 10 colony-forming units (cfu) when it undergoes a validation process. A common requirement of ISO 13485, the European Central Manufacturing Standards (CMS), and the United States (US) GMP and Food and Drug Administration (FDA), is the use of validated processes, as mentioned above.

[2]   WHO. 2016. Decontamination and reprocessing of medical devices for health-care facilities. World Health Organization/Pan American Health Organization. Available at https://www.who.int/publications/i/item/9789241549851.

[3]   Ibid.

- preventive maintenance procedures, schedules and contracts
- procedural or material change standards and policies
- infection prevention and control within the decontamination facility
- Occupational health and safety (OH&S): policies and procedures (including appropriate use of PPE).
- Education and training of all SSD staff: numeracy, literacy and dexterity are essential to perform the duties required.
- Risk management: identification, investigation, evaluation and documentation of all adverse events.
- Knowledge of international standards (for example, ISO 13485:2016 relates to medical devices, quality management systems and requirements for regulatory purposes).

3.2 Legislation and standards

While it is beyond the scope of this chapter to discuss all the necessary legal requirements, the essential norms and standards are mentioned here. Each step of the decontamination cycle requires validation and is regulated by standards established by European Council (CEN) and/or International Organization for Standardization (ISO) and national regulations; while these laws may not apply directly to all countries, the principles remain the same.

3.3 What is validation?

All those using sterile services, including the IPC practitioner, must understand what validation means and how it is applied to each part of the decontamination cycle so that sterility of the product is ensured.

The validation process consists of verifying in a certified and clearly documented manner that a process meets the requirements for which it was designed. For example, for sterilisation, labelling a health product with the word 'sterile' is only permissible when a validated sterilisation process has been used. While it is beyond the scope of this book to provide details of validation for automated reprocessing equipment, readers should be familiar with the terms.

Validation for automated equipment should consist of the following:
- Installation qualification (IQ)[4]
- Operational qualification (OQ)[5]

---

[4]   IQ: A process of obtaining and documenting evidence that equipment has been provided and installed in accordance with its specification.

[5]   OQ: A process of obtaining and documenting evidence that the installed equipment operates within predetermined limits when used in accordance with its operational procedures.

- Performance or process qualification (PQ)[6] documentation
- Microbiological performance qualification (MPQ)
- Validation report and certificates.

A summary of each part of the decontamination cycle and measurements for validation are shown in Table 3.1. IPC practitioners should be aware of these methods and frequency when reviewing SSD documents during any investigation into HAI.

Table 3.1 Validation of decontamination processes should happen for each process on a per item, per process or daily basis (adapted from WHO guidelines on decontamination and reprocessing of medical devices for health-care facilities (2016)

Process	Daily	Per item	Per load	Per process
Cleaning – manual	Use of detergent and disinfectant	Visual inspection	NA	NA
Cleaning – automated washer disinfector	Inspection of chambers, jets and function	Visual inspection	Physical indicators – AWD	Soil test Residual soil tests
Disinfection	Concentration, temperature and pH	NA	Exposure time	NA
Chemical sterilisers	Inspection of equipment	External indicators		Indicators – Biological Chemical Physical
Dry heat (hot air oven)	Biological indicators	External indicators		Physical
Moist heat (steam steriliser)	Bowie-Dick (pre-vacuum) leak test	External indicators		Biological Chemical Physical

Assessing and managing risk. Consider how a device is to be used and whether it can be safely reprocessed with adequate facilities available on site (point of use) or whether it has to be sent away? But, most importantly can the processes on site be validated? This is particularly relevant to low-resource settings.

Depending on the level of risk of infection, based on the Spaulding classification (Table 3.2), one can assess whether or not the local facilities have the means to reprocess such devices.

---

[6]   PQ: A process of obtaining and documenting evidence that the equipment as installed and operated in accordance with operational procedures consistently performs in accordance with predetermined criteria and thereby yields a product meeting its specification.

3.4   Classification of medical devices

Spaulding (Table 3.2) classified the application of devices based upon the level of risk of infection from their use. This classification has become a standard for evaluating process requirements. The MD must be fit for purpose and safe for the patient.

Table 3.2   Spaulding classification for reprocessing medical devices to reduce risk

Classification	Area of use	Requirement	Examples
Critical items	Sterile tissues and cavities, vascular system (bloodstream)	**No** microbes, including spores **Cleaned and sterilised before patient use**	Surgical instruments
Semi-critical	Contact with intact mucous membranes (usually sites which are previously colonised) or broken skin	No vegetative forms of bacteria – a few spores acceptable **Cleaned and high-level disinfection**	Respiratory equipment, non-invasive endoscopes, vaginal speculae
Non-critical items	Coming into contact with intact skin such as common-use objects	No nosocomial or transmissible pathogens **Thorough cleaning with possible low-level disinfection**	Patient care articles, thermometers

It follows, therefore, that items that cannot be thoroughly cleaned and retain organic matter, such as hypodermic needles and syringes, should be 'single use' devices only and discarded after each use. Narrow lumen medical devices, for example endoscopes, must go through a rigorous cleaning and decontamination process before being considered safe for use.

3.5   The sterile services department (SSD)

The SSD plays a pivotal role in the hospital.[7] It is responsible, as an equal partner, in the prevention of SSIs.

The design of the SSD must ensure that the principles of safe practice are observed:

- Workflow moves from dirty to clean areas.
- Staff cannot physically cross over between workstations without changing PPE.

---

[7]   NHS Estates. 2004. HBN 13 Sterile Services Department. Available at https://www.england.nhs.uk/publication/planning-and-design-of-sterile-services-departments-hbn-13/.

- The ventilation moves from clean (positive pressure) to dirty (negative pressure).

3.5.1 The role of the sterile services department

The SSD has a responsibility to reprocess (all) medical devices according to recommended national and international standards so that no harm comes to patients, staff working in the SSD and the clinical areas or the environment.

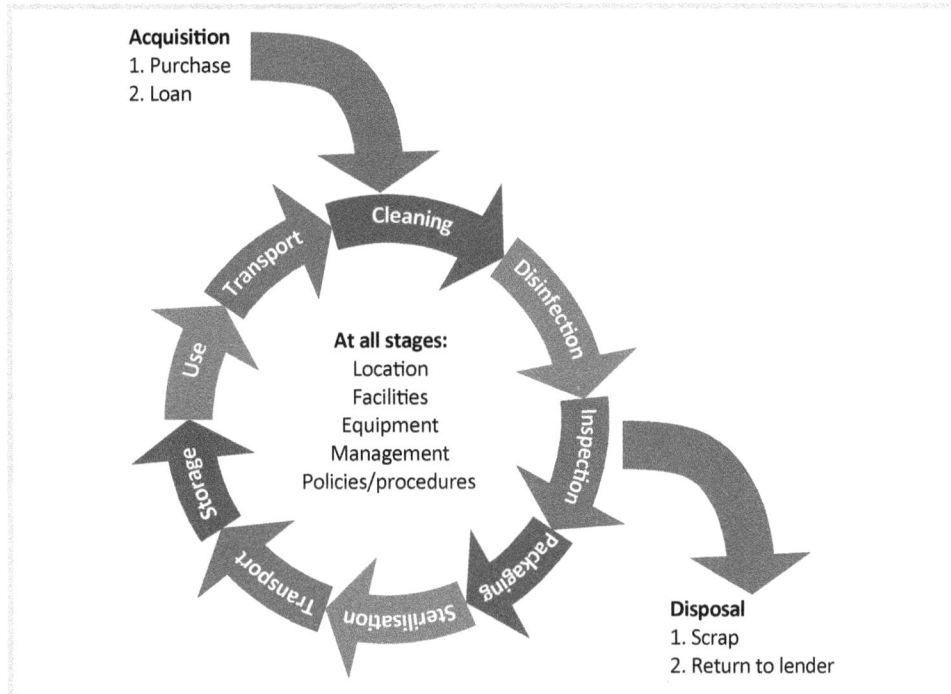

Acquisition
1. Purchase
2. Loan

Cleaning

Transport

Disinfection

Use

At all stages:
Location
Facilities
Equipment
Management
Policies/procedures

Inspection

Storage

Transport

Packaging

Sterilisation

Disposal
1. Scrap
2. Return to lender

Figure 3.1 The process of decontamination of medical devices (adapted from the World Federation of Hospital Sterile Supplies)

The reprocessing cycle of used medical devices is illustrated in Figure 3.1 and will be expanded on in each section.

3.5.2 Staff working in the sterile services department

3.5.2.1 **Staff conduct**. The staff should feel part of quality healthcare delivery. All staff working in the SSD are responsible for good personal hygiene and cleanliness of the working areas. Preferably, staff should work in uniforms or scrubs and close-toed shoes, and if possible a laundry service should be provided at the place of work. The work environment should be comfortable with adequate ventilation, light and uncluttered space; all surfaces and floors should be cleaned regularly. Eating and drinking are not allowed in the working area. Jewellery should be kept to a minimum, for example a wedding band may be allowed.

3.5.2.2   **Staff qualification.** There are no clearly defined qualifications for SSD staff in many countries; however, the entry level operator qualification should be a high-school-leaving certificate. Nonetheless, job descriptions should be clear and well defined with roles and responsibilities to which the staff can be held accountable. Structured competency training programmes (see WHO Decontamination Manual (2016) for recommended training curriculum) for all levels of staff are recommended. Basic IPC training should include standard precautions including hand hygiene, use of PPE, routes of transmission of pathogens and the impact of poor sterilisation techniques on SSI. Furthermore, all staff should be aware of workflow, demarcation of dirty and clean areas and the significance of non-compliance to the areas of demarcation.

In-service training should be provided regularly to update the staff of any changes in procedure, for example the introduction of a new chemical washer/disinfector, steriliser or medical device.

3.5.2.3   **Staff support** (also see 7.3 Occupational health). All operators and management working in the SSD should be offered:
- appropriate use of PPE in the areas of the SSD
- immunisation against hepatitis B, tetanus
- pre-employment medical check up
- access to occupational health in case of accidental injury
- occupational health and safety training in safe practices in an SSD
  - exposure to biological hazards
  - exposure to chemical hazards
  - exposure to high temperatures and pressure equipment such as sterilisers
  - carrying heavy loads and proper lifting practices
- health monitoring on a regular basis.

An accident record book should be kept by the SSD manager.

3.5.2.4   **Staffing structure in sterile services department**

The staffing structure will depend on the national SSD programme, but there are some essential posts that should be considered and these are usually based on the staff–workload ratios.

3.5.2.4.1 Staffing ratios

Calculating the number of staff required in an SSD varies greatly from country to country and the roles the staff plays. There are two methods recommended as a rough guide.

1. The number of operations or consultation episodes, calculated as 3 000 per year per member of staff. This calculates the staff contingent as a whole.

2. A time and motion study of each area, type of devices reprocessed and numbers of trays by surgical specialty over a specific time period (usually six months to cover all variations in practice). This considers the job category and hours of work in each area or station.

3.5.2.4.2 Staffing levels

Depending upon the size of the SSD, there should be at least one administrative person, and one each of supervisors and operators for the clean and dirty areas.

The manager. A fully qualified manager should be in charge of sterile services, be knowledgeable of recent developments, understand management and function independently. S/he must take full responsibility for safe processing of devices and understand the processes involved in the SSD, including what can go wrong, and provide support for staff. The IPC team works closely with the manager during investigations of SSI and outbreaks. In larger SSDs, a deputy manager may be appointed to support the manager.

Quality manager (QM). This post is usually missing in low-resource settings, but is pivotal to the smooth running of the SSD and ensures both staff and the processes are satisfactorily maintained. If not appointed, a person can be delegated to this position.

The responsibility of the QM is to ensure that all the processes are validated and comply with the regulations. All policies and SOPs should be up to date and the staff trained in processes. There should be availability of PPE, stock of raw materials, recorded validation of all processes and quality checks of the finished products. The QM is responsible for validation and the ultimate safe reprocessing of medical devices.

Supervisor. Ideally there should be a supervisor for each section in the SSD, **but the minimum would be one each for the dirty and clean areas**. Some larger SSDs have more than one supervisor per section. This person works 'hands-on' at the floor level and should be well trained in all aspects of SSD procedures. S/he should be able to stand in if a member of the team is absent.

Operatives. The operative is the technical person working at the bench or processing area. There are usually several operatives in each section and their function should ideally be sufficient to meet the workload in each area. Most operatives start directly after school and are trained as apprentices. However, they should be literate and numerate and have formal training in sterile services. They can be taught practical skills as they rotate through the SSD. S/he reports to the supervisor.

The **responsibility** of the operative is to understand the role s/he plays in maintaining the high quality and standards of the SSD as a vital part of the team.

Additional support staffing is required to work with or in the SSD. They are:

- **Storekeeper.** This may be a dedicated or rotational post in the SSD.
- **Delivery personnel.** SSDs may have their own staff to deliver and receive SSD items or use the hospital staff. Either way, the delivery personnel should be trained and be aware of the role they play in the SSD programme, including health and safety aspects of SSD.
- **Cleaning services** should preferably be dedicated to work only in the SSD. If other cleaning services are used, clear SOPs should be drawn up and regular training provided.
- **Office administration.** There should be administrative staff to deal with the receiving and dispatch of packs, stocktaking and ordering and making appointments for the managers.
- **Engineers/technicians.** In larger SSDs there are dedicated engineers or technicians. Their role is to ensure the processing equipment is fully functional and that all equipment is regularly maintained and tested. A report (logbook) should be available with each item of reprocessing equipment, such as a steriliser or washer-disinfector. Some sections of the logbook are completed every day and others less frequently, depending on the frequency of maintenance processes in place. There should be planned preventive maintenance (PPM) that is carefully adhered to and monitored by the SSD manager.
- A quarterly engineering report on the state of the equipment should be presented by the SSD manager to the IPC committee.

3.5.3 Calculating the size of the SSD

When calculating the size of the SSD, it is not only the reprocessing area (wash room, IAP, sterilisation) but also storage of raw materials, including chemicals, trolley parking and cleaners' facilities, that should be taken into account.

There are several ways of calculating the size of the SSD, related to the workload and the number of sterilisers in use.[8]

1. To **calculate the number of beds** in a hospital and the use of the SSD by specialty such as surgery, maternity and so on. This considers the case mix in the hospital and works on a department gross square metre (DGSM) per bed depending on the number of sterilisers required to carry the workload.

---

[8]   Australasian Health Facility Guidelines, Part B Health Facility Briefing and Planning, Rev 5, 2016; see website https://healthfacilityguidelines.com.au/aushfg-parts.

2. To determine **the workload and how this is performed**, particularly applicable to LMICs. For example:

   2.1 Is all the washing done manually or is there an automated washer-disinfector? Manually cleaning will require more space.

   2.2 Is there adequate space for inspection, assembly and packaging (IAP)?

   2.3 Are there enough sterilisers to manage the workload safely?

   2.4 Is there adequate space for storage of sterile packs and devices?

   2.5 Is there adequate space to accommodate healthcare waste, storage of raw materials, offices and dispatch areas with the necessary equipment?

3. The **number of surgical trays** reprocessed daily. This method works well when there is expansion or variation in the number of trays reprocessed every day or week.

4. The number of shifts per day and the number of staff per shift.

5. Quality and size of the equipment used to reprocess medical devices, e.g. whether these are front-loading or the pass-through type with double doors.

6. Central supply of high-quality water, medical quality of air and pre-generated steam. These are essential elements and the space to house or produce these must be included in the calculation for space.

Whichever method for planning the space for the SSD is used, the SSD should be housed in a separate building, with an efficient transportation system, with adequate space and with future expansion of services in mind.

3.5.4 Layout of a sterile services department

The workflow in an SSD consists of movement of (a) staff, (b) contaminated items including unprocessed raw material coming in and (c) sterile items leaving from the dispatch area.

There should be strict access control with no unauthorised person coming into the work area of the SSD. The engineers should have access to the sterilisers from a separate outside entrance, but if they need access to the front of the sterilisers, the engineers will be required to gown up.

> **Irrespective of the size of the SSD, the workflow is always unidirectional from dirty to clean!**

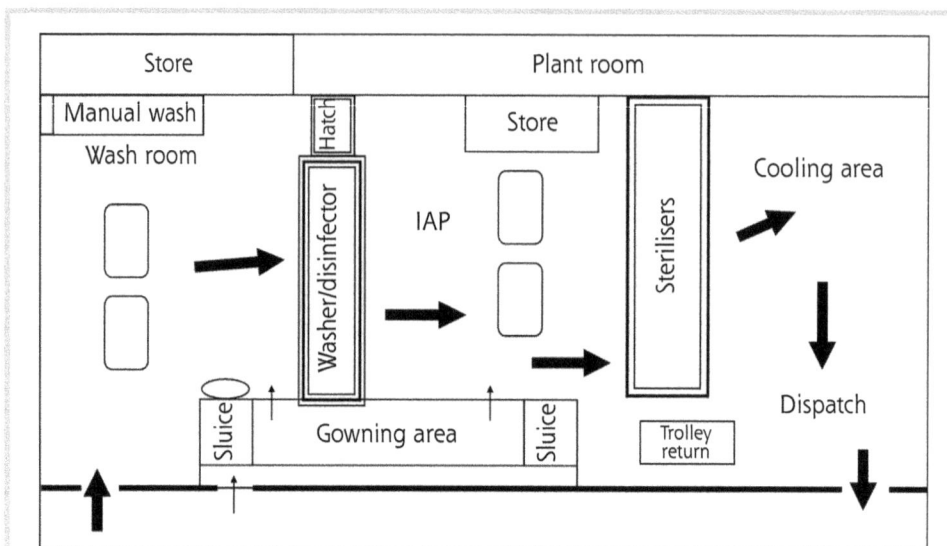

Figure 3.2 An example of an SSD layout showing the distinct areas. The bold arrows show the route for medical devices. The thin arrows show the movement of personnel.

The SSD is clearly demarcated into the following work stations:

- a '**dirty**' or **wash room** or decontamination area which receives used instruments which may have been pre-cleaned but not safe to handle
- a '**clean**' or **inspection, assembly and packaging** (IAP) area where medical devices are inspected, sorted and packed after having been washed and cleaned – from this point onwards the medical devices are clean and can be handled safely
- **sterilisation (clean)** area where packed items are processed in sterilisers
- **cooling (clean)** area where sterile packs are placed prior to dispatch
- **dispatch (clean)** area or sterile store.

> The wash (dirty) area must be physically separated from the clean area in even the smallest decontamination unit.

3.5.5 Smaller decontamination units

In smaller clinics such as dental, outpatients or community centres, decontamination of medical devices often takes place in the clinic. A designated separate area should be made available which allows the principles of SSD workflow and practice to be followed. These units usually have only one room, but a trained person can learn to work from dirty to clean without crossing over and to maintain safe practice.

3.5.6 Infrastructure requirements for an SSD

The essential requirements for a properly functioning SSD are summarised below.

Air is required for drying lumen of medical devices. Air should be medical-grade quality (free from bacteria, dirt or large particles).[9] ISO 8573 on air quality standards and ISO12500 on compressed air filter recommend a 1.0 micron particulate filter, which will help to prolong the service life of the pressure gun.

Water quality in the SSD is critical to the functioning of the reprocessing equipment and must be soft water, which means it has a low mineral and salt content.[10] Modern machines are highly sensitive to impurities in water and soft water is essential to ensure there is no adverse reaction with the devices or reprocessing equipment. Water is needed for cleaning of devices and producing high-quality steam for the sterilisers. Routine testing of water is essential to maintain a low content of mineral and salt in the water. Water softening methods are as follows:
- **Filtration** of the water supply selectively removes minerals and salts.
- **Reverse osmosis (RO)** removes chlorides and is recommended by most manufacturers for the more modern and sophisticated machines.
- **Water softening** systems are installed to add chemicals that soften water.
- **Ion exchange** selectively removes ions and softens the water.

If water-softening systems are not readily available, an effort should be made to install some sort of system to protect the SSD equipment and will prove cost-effective in the long term. The cost of processing water is expensive, therefore soft water can be used for the final rinse to reduce cost. Modern sterilisers are more economical and use much less water compared to the older ones, but do demand a high quality.

Steam[11] used in sterilisers, especially the modern, sophisticated ones, must be of high quality. If the steam source is far from the steriliser, the piping serving the steam must be robust and maintained regularly to avoid leaks and contamination. Modern sterilisers with independent integral steam generation systems cater to the requirements of the machines and are recommended if affordable.

The quality of steam must not interfere with the sterilisation process or damage the MD being sterilised. The quality of steam must be checked regularly and documented. This is addressed later in the chapter under steam sterilisation.

---

[9] ISO 8573-1:2010. Compressed Air Contaminants and Purity Classes 2010; ISO 12500-1:2007. Filters for compressed air — Test methods — Part 1: Oil aerosols.
[10] Huys J. 2010. Water quality. In Sterilisation of Medical Supplies by Steam. 3 edition. MHP-Verlag.
[11] ISO 17665-1:2006 Sterilisation of health care products – Moist heat – Part 1: Requirements for the development, validation and routine control of a sterilisation process for medical devices.

Ventilation in the SSD flows from clean to dirty and should be provided by an independent air-handling unit (AHU). Wall-mounted air conditioners are not recommended because the air is not filtered. Generally, 20 air changes per hour (ACH) are recommended. In the absence of an AHU, direct introduction from outdoors is possible, with 10–20 ACH in the dirty area and 12–24 ACH in the clean areas. The wash area is under negative pressure compared to the IAP room and clean areas, which are under positive pressure. To provide negative pressure in the dirty area an extraction fan is installed to expel the air to the outside atmosphere.

> **In the SSD, air direction must flow from clean to dirty.**

Relative humidity in the SSD is recommended to be 40–50%, but may be higher in hot countries, up to 70%, which can affect the sterile barrier.

Ambient temperature in the SSD should be well controlled because the processing equipment generates heat.

The recommended temperatures are
- dirty (decontamination) area 18–20 °C
- clean areas 18–23 °C
- sterile storage 15–25 °C

In warm countries it might be difficult to maintain the required temperatures and there is a tendency to open the windows, particularly in sterilisation rooms – this is not recommended because the trays can become contaminated. If pedestal or other fans are used, these should be directed away from the trays, particularly during packaging.

Surface coverings must be smooth, without cracks, leveled and easy to clean and should withstand regular cleaning and disinfection chemicals. The surfaces and sinks should be waterproof and easy to clean, for example stainless steel. Wood or laminates are not recommended because they absorb chemicals.

Ceilings must be smooth, straight and without cracks and should be moisture-proof. Panel ceilings are not recommended.

Walls should be continuous, smooth and covered in washable paint or material. The corners should be protected with metal ridging or similar to prevent damage from carts and trolleys.

Floors should be level, smooth and able to withstand the load of heavy carts and constant traffic. Preferably the floors should have a continuous non-slip finish, with coved corners up to 4 cm up the wall, to ensure good cleaning.

Lighting in the SSD must be of high quality. Natural light is preferred, but if that is not possible, then a mixture of natural and artificial light should be provided.

3.5.6.1 Staff changing rooms

Staff and visitors should enter the SSD only through the changing area. Constant traffic in and out of the SSD or decontamination unit is not recommended. Changing facilities for male and female staff should be equipped with lockers, changing areas and toilet facilities with a clinical handwash basin and showers.

After changing into work clothes staff should be allocated to either the wash (dirty) or the clean area. They enter their work station via the dedicated gowning area for the section and stay in that area until they leave.

> If there is need for staff to move from one station to another, the person must take off his/her PPE, wash hands and wear a fresh set of PPE before entering the other area. This applies equally to single-space units such as dental clinics.

3.5.6.2 Wash (dirty) area gowning-up area

The wash area receives used and contaminated medical devices and is considered a dirty area. Therefore the PPE should offer protection to eyes, mucous membranes and hands.

- The gowning-up area should be located just outside the wash area close to the changing rooms.
- PPE: Those entering in the wash area must wear a plastic apron, non-sterile gloves, visor or masks and goggles. Headgear and overshoes are not necessary.
- Adequate supplies of PPE (apron, mask, gloves, face shield) in various sizes should be available and laid out neatly.
- There should be hand hygiene facilities available.
- Entry and exit to the wash room should be controlled.

3.5.6.3 Wash room (decontamination area)

Ideally, there should be a physically separate area for receiving and holding used surgical devices with controlled access to the wash area. If this is not possible, used items sent to the SSD for reprocessing may be received in the wash area – space should be set aside for this purpose. The received items should be registered (logged in) and forwarded to the sorting area.

There should be sufficient space to accommodate the workload of the SSD, particularly for sorting used devices.

Functions of the wash room are:
- checking contaminated returns
- disassembly and preparation of re-usable instruments prior to cleaning, disinfection and drying

- sorting and loading of instruments into washer-disinfectors
- selecting devices for manual cleaning
- transfering items to the inspection, assembly and packaging area (IAP).

Requirements for the wash room are:
- direct access to used devices from the wards and operating theatres, waste removal and laundry returns
- located adjacent to the IAP
- no direct movement of staff from the wash room to the IAP other than via the gowning area
- automated washer-disinfectors (preferably double-door) installed between the decontamination and IAP to allow a one-way flow of processed items
- an area for manual cleaning available and fully equipped
- a separate pass-through hatch to IAP for manually cleaned or rejected items
- handwashing facilities.

Distribution of space in the wash room should make provision for:
- receiving area large enough to take the trolleys and the return workload
- an area to keep registers/logs, computer and records
- a clinical handwash basin with liquid soap and paper towels near the entrance
- a flat inspection table used for a quick inspection prior to washing to remove paper, linen and plastic
- trolleys or containers to carry used instruments to the washing stations
- an area to wash down trolleys if no other site is available
- a healthcare waste station for clinical waste
- a designated area for manual cleaning including appropriate-sized sinks
- adequate space for location of and access to washer-disinfectors for use and engineering requirements.

3.5.6.4 Inspection, assembly and packing (IAP) gowning-up area

The IAP and sterile areas are considered clean areas; MD have been cleaned thoroughly and are safe to handle.
- The IAP area should be accessible only from the IAP gowning room, which should be close to the changing facilities.
- The recommended PPE is a plastic apron and head cover. Gloves, masks and visors are not necessary. Closed-toes shoes should be worn.
- Powder make-up is not permitted as it can contaminate the devices during IAP.
- Men with facial hair should wear a beard cover to prevent hair from falling onto devices.

- Hand-washing facilities should be provided in the gowning area.
- There should be access to the IAP and the doors should have vision panels and interlocking devices.

3.5.6.5 Inspection, assembly and packing area

The IAP room receives clean instruments from the wash room and flows into the sterilisation area.

Functions of the IAP room are:
- for staff to inspect, carry out function testing, assemble and package clean medical devices
- to carry a supply of raw materials such as instrument replacements, packaging and indicators which are used to prepare the devices for sterilisation.

Requirements of the IAP room are:
- access to IAP via gowning area only with controlled entry and exit
- access to sterilisation area wide enough to accommodate loading trolleys
- hatch between wash room and IAP for manually washed or returned equipment
- stores for raw material supplies used in preparing surgical trays
- storage area for replacement equipment
- register for log of discarded items or those sent for repair
- inspection table for processed items prior to packaging
- a bright light and magnifying glass to inspect the devices
- adequate number of work stations with storage area (if indicated) for SSD workload
- staff access to the steriliser area
- no handwash basin or washing up in this area.

Factors in the **distribution of space** are:
- adequate space for work stations to ensure running and flexibility of workflow
    - receiving area for the washed and disinfected items
    - adequate space for inspection of instruments prior to replacement, condemning and packaging
- easy passage of trolleys from packing stations to sterilisers
    - loading area for trolleys
    - parking area for trolleys not in use
- equipment store for replacement items in surgical trays
- shelving with slats/wire mesh, free-standing, mobile and easily cleaned
- raw material stores; used within 24 hours
- display boards with documentation on SOPs etc.

3.5.6.6 Sterilisation area

In an SSD with an open-plan layout the sterilisers are either placed along one side of a large IAP room or installed as pass-through (double-door) sterilisers between the IAP and cooling room, which allows loading at one end and unloading into the cooling room.

Functions of the sterilisation room are as follows:
- The sterilisation room receives trolleys with packaged items prior to sterilisation.
- The packs are loaded on trolleys and placed in the sterilisers.
- Once the packs are sterilised they may be held in a cooling area prior to dispatch.
- The sterile packs are taken for storage to the sterile store and/or dispatch area.
- A double-door steriliser allows the sterile packs to arrive directly into the sterile store.
- Single-door sterilisers should have adequate space in front of them to load and unload trolleys easily.
- There should be means to record the load and attribute it to a particular steriliser.

Requirements[12] of the sterilisation area are as follows:
- sterilisation area adjacent to the IAP with easy access
- easy passage for trolleys from the IAP to the sterilisation area
- appropriate PPE including heat-resistant gloves
- means to reduce heat gain from steriliser
- easy access to steriliser for testing and maintenance
- separate area for items undergoing an alternative sterilisation process.

Distribution of space
- There should be adequate space to allow free access to and from the steriliser.
- Trolleys used to unload the sterilisers should have a storage area.
- There should be a separate section where items are quarantined following failure of sterilisation cycle.
- There should be a designated area for keeping records for each of the sterilisers and quality and traceability records.
- Each steriliser should have space for documents such as its own logbook, which contains information on its quality records, maintenance and repairs.

---

[12] ISO 14664-1:2015 – Cleanrooms and associated controlled environments – Part 1: Classification of air cleanliness by particle concentration stipulates that a SSD clean room (IAP) must achieve compliance with ISO 13485:2003 – Quality management – Requirements for regulatory purposes.

3.5.6.7 Cooling area (sterile store)

Functions of the cooling area are as follows:

- Once the packs have been processed they are moved to a designated area, ready for dispatch to the clinical areas.
- Surplus surgical packs and equipment should be stored in an area separate from the processing sites.
- After being logged in a register, equipment is dispatched from here in closed containers or trolleys to the designated clinical area.

Requirements of the cooling area (sterile store):

- The storage area should be cool and dry. Any moisture or excessive heat may jeopardise the integrity of the protective cover of sterile packs.
- Storage racks should be robust, with open shelving for air circulation (solid shelves are not recommended).
- There should be ample space for ease of movement between the shelves with a trolley or other containers.
- The shelves should have clips or holders to keep documentation – these should be clearly visible.
- Sterile packs should be dry when placed on the racks. **Wet packs are not sterile**.
- Sterile packs should be placed next to each other and not stacked high. Stacks can trap moisture between the packs.
- If sterile packs have to be stacked, the method of stacking should allow air circulation between the packs and minimise damage to the packs and contents.
- Each rack should be clearly labelled with the type of pack or item and a list of how many of each are currently stored. This list is updated each time a pack is removed or added.
- Each pack should be placed in such a way that the name of the surgical pack (for example, major abdominal pack), date of processing (for example, 01/01/2009) and all relevant information is clearly visible.
- A daily check of all stores should be carried out and any discrepancy with the dispatch log or register should be recorded.
- Stock should be rotated on a 'first in/first out' basis.

The distribution of space must make provision for:

- adequate space to allow storage of sterile items with easy movement of trolleys between them
- an area for documentation tracking and traceability, registration and stocktaking.

3.5.6.8 Dispatch area

Ideally, there should be only one dispatch station so that stock movement can be controlled.
- All items that leave the storage area must be logged and signed for by the person receiving the goods.
- A simple yet robust tracking system should be in place.

3.5.6.9 Other areas

- separate cleaner's room with dedicated sluice for cleaning equipment
- raw materials storage for packaging, replacement devices and spares holding enough supplies for four weeks and be replaced regularly
- store room for chemicals and volatile products
- dispatch/holding area
- IT system and good traceability and tracking of surgical trays and packs
- staff facilities such as tea room, seminar or conference room
- office space for management.

3.5.7 Reprocessing medical devices outside the sterile services department

Although not recommended, lack of sterile services or shortage of MD drives the need for point-of-use reprocessing, particularly ventilator and other tubing. If any processing of medical devices takes place outside the SSD, the appropriate rules and regulations must apply and be strictly adhered to.
- There should be a dedicated space for cleaning and reprocessing MD.
- The person carrying out the cleaning and decontamination must be well trained.
- Each item that is reprocessed must be logged for medico-legal reasons.
- Stations must be fully equipped to carry out manual cleaning to a satisfactory standard.
- Separate handwashing facilities and gowning area should be provided.
- The packaging should be of good quality.
- Usually, non-wrapped items are reprocessed off site, such as in the operating theatre.
- The Immediate Use Steam Steriliser (IUSS) or flash steriliser must go through the same validation systems, be tested regularly and maintained.
- Accurate record-keeping is essential.

3.5.7.1   **Dedicated cleaning area.** A separate room should be allocated away from the clinical areas with:
- appropriate PPE for staff
- a wide sink dedicated to cleaning devices, with proper fittings
- running hot and cold water

- surface to allow items to dry
- correct detergents and chemicals – clearly labelled with contents and expiry dates
- good ventilation
- storage area.

The door to the cleaning area must be clearly labelled and a biohazard sign should be displayed. The room should be secure with a lockable door.

3.6 Reprocessing of medical devices

All devices requiring re-processing should be sent to the SSD or a decontamination unit (such as a dental clinic). Soiled instruments are wiped or rinsed at point of use to remove gross contamination, and transported to the point of reprocessing. Once the devices are cleaned these are safe to handle. The devices are inspected, packaged and marked before sterilisation (or disinfection). After sterilisation the items are stored ready for dispatch to the appropriate clinical areas. Each of these steps must be validated and audited regularly (see Figure 3.1).

3.6.1 Point-of-use care

After use the soiled devices are taken to an area in the operating theatre where they are wiped down to remove coarse debris or rinsed under running water to prepare them for safe transport and to reduce risk to SSD staff.

Wear appropriate PPE such as gloves, apron and face mask or shield. Remove all disposable items. Open all hinged devices. Remove all visible organic matter. Spray with an enzymatic cleaner. Place the devices in a solid container with a damp cloth over them and send to the SSD. This is to ensure that the organic matter does not dry on the devices, making them difficult to clean and disinfect. The details can be found in the WHO decontamination and reprocessing guidelines.[13]

Preparing devices at the point of use does not replace the cleaning process. DO NOT soak in a disinfectant before cleaning.

The principles for reprocessing are:
- Ideally, devices should be cleaned and decontaminated using automated and validated processes.
- Monitoring of critical variables for each cycle, e.g. time and temperature, should take place.

---

[13] WHO. 2016. Decontamination and reprocessing of medical devices for health-care facilities. World Health Organization/Pan American Health Organization. Available at https://www.who.int/publications/i/item/9789241549851.

- Decontamination equipment should be fit for intended use, well maintained, validated and tested.
- Decontamination processes should be validated to prevent adventitious contamination.
- Conditions should be controlled.
- Tracking systems should be in place.
- Reprocessing requirements should be reviewed before purchase of new equipment.
- Single-use instruments must not be reprocessed.
- Appropriate dedicated facilities should be used.
- A management system should be in place for stock control.
- There should be sufficient staff to ensure the smooth running of the department.
- There should be no health and safety risk to patients, staff or visitors.
- Planned preventive maintenance and testing programmes should be in place.

3.6.2 Cleaning

Cleaning is the first essential step in the reprocessing of medical devices before any process of disinfection or sterilisation can be carried out.

Once devices have been received in the SSD and 'logged in' (registered), they must be thoroughly cleaned. Point-of-use wiping before dispatch to the SSD reduces heavy soiling. Modern automated systems remove soil effectively and are much safer than manual cleaning for patients and staff.

3.6.2.1 Reasons for cleaning

MD must be cleaned before processing:
- Organic matter and chemicals can damage the reprocessing equipment and the devices.
- Organic material, particularly biofilm, allows micro-organisms to thrive and protects microbes during the process of disinfection and sterilisation.
- Organic matter may inactivate certain disinfectants.
- Any cleaning method, manual or automated, must use the correct detergents and chemicals, at the right temperature with the correct contact time to remove all visible organic matter.
- All devices must be dismantled and cleaned thoroughly. They should be rendered safe to handle for inspection before further processing.

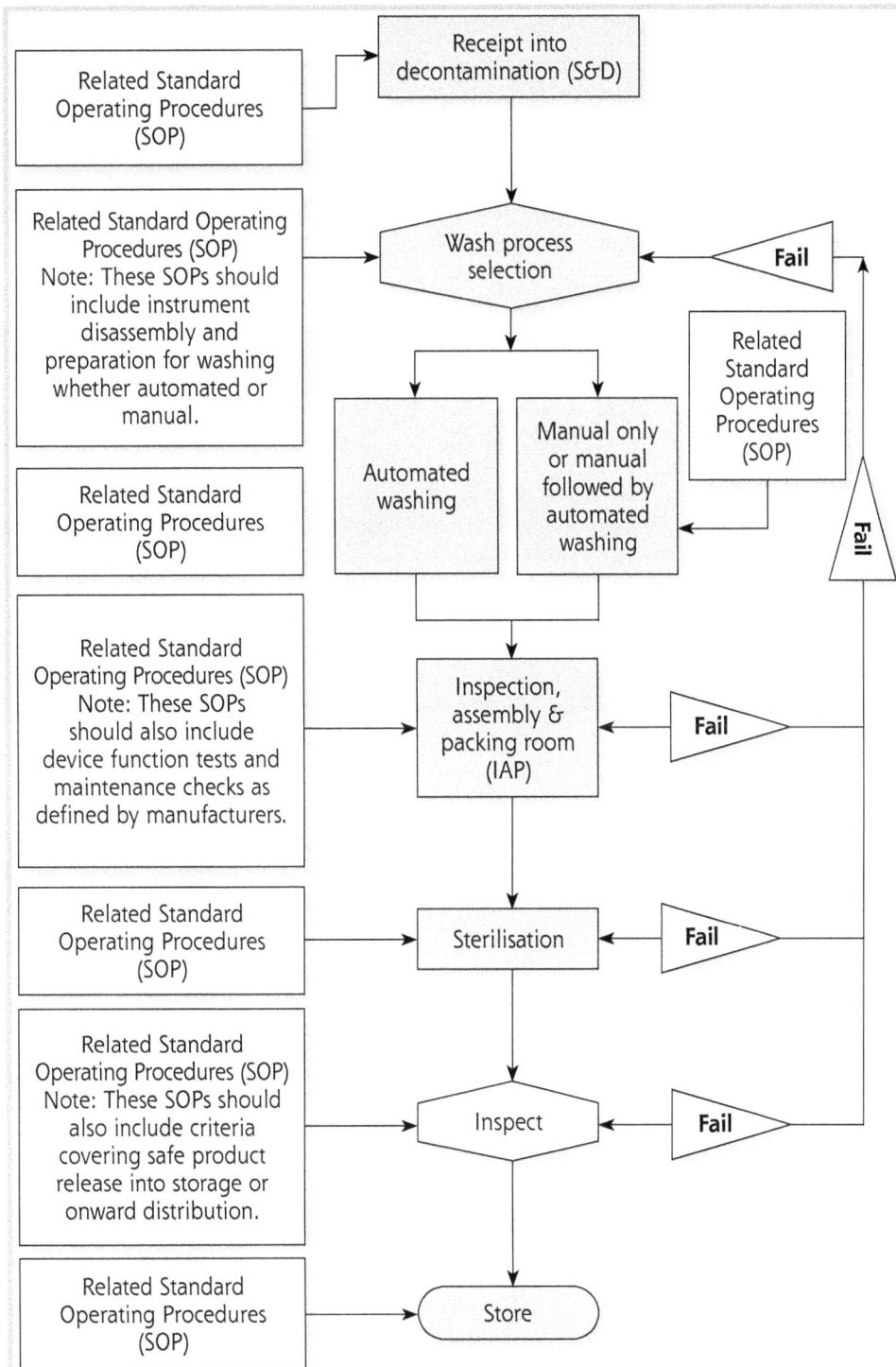

Figure 3.3 Decontamination process showing the flow of work and SOPs (The Global Decontamination Discussion Group)

3.6.2.2 Factors that affect cleaning

- The amount and type of soil present – the presence of organic matter will inactivate certain cleaning chemicals.
- Water quality and temperature. Certain chemicals are designed for specific temperatures.
- Hard water contains high levels of calcium and other salts, which will interfere with cleaning and deposit scales on the equipment.
- High level of chlorides in the water will cause damage to the devices.
- Staff training in manual and automated methods is as important as knowing the devices being processed.

3.6.2.3 Cleaning Circle

Cleaning (Sinner's Circle, 1959) requires the combination of three forms of energy: **mechanical** (brushing/flushing), **thermal** (temperature) and **chemical** (detergents, enzymes) plus contact time with the chemicals. All of these are of equal importance and greatly affect the outcome of any cleaning method.

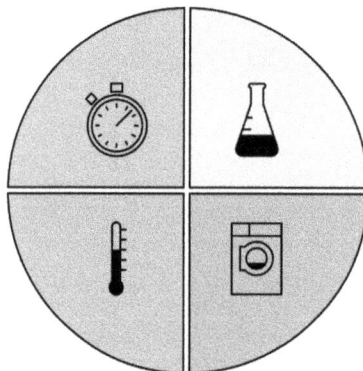

Figure 3.4 Sinner's Circle cleaning, showing the relationship between time, temperature, chemical and contact time (Wikimedia commons. Free media repository. https://upload.wikimedia.org/wikipedia/commons/7/78/Sinner%27s_Circle. svg)

3.6.2.4 Chemicals used in the cleaning process

For the total cleaning process one or more chemicals is used, especially in automated washer-disinfectors (AWD). In manual cleaning a single detergent at the correct dilution and temperature is usually sufficient.

AWDs are equipped with dosing systems which can be programmed to inject the required amount of each individual chemical at the right moment in the process.

3.6.2.4.1 **Detergents.** In order for water to clean, it has to come into contact with all surfaces of the device, which is prevented by surface tension. Detergents and soap are **surfactants** and improve the contact between water and the device by lowering the surface tension. A hospital-quality detergent should be pH neutral.

> Detergents must be prepared to the optimal dilution (manufacturer's recommendation) for the best function – increasing the strength will not improve effectivity.

3.6.2.4.2 **Alkali detergents (pH 8–10.8)** are substances that improve the activity of surfactants, help to emulsify and remove fats and oils and break down water-insoluble proteins. Some bind to hardness ions, such as calcium and magnesium, and soften the water.

3.6.2.4.3 **Corrosion inhibitors.** Stainless steel is hardly affected by the detergent solutions. However, aluminum is corroded by alkaline detergents. The addition of corrosion inhibitors such as aluminum silicates forms a protective oxide layer on the device.

3.6.2.4.4 **Enzymes (proteolytic).** They are biological catalysts that break down large molecules such as proteins, fats and starch, which can then be removed by washing. Enzymes are integrated into cleaning agents for increased activity.

3.6.2.4.5 **Lubricants.** Surgical instruments are prone to corrosion, especially in the hinges. Stainless steel has a protective layer of chromium oxide, which becomes thicker with time and damaged during friction. Mineral residues in the hinges stimulate corrosion. Lubricants (usually paraffin oils), which form a protective layer on the steel, are added to the rinsing water. However, these can introduce contamination and should be considered only where non-purified water is used.

3.6.2.4.6 **Rinse aids.** Their routine use is not recommended.

3.6.3 Cleaning methods

3.6.3.1 Manual cleaning

Cleaning by hand may be necessary when:
- mechanical methods are not available
- delicate or difficult instruments have to be cleaned
- complex instruments have components which may be destroyed by heat or chemicals
- narrow-hollow lumen need special cleaning methods.

When cleaning manually, put on appropriate PPE such as a pair of domestic gloves, a plastic apron and visor/goggles to protect the eyes and mucous membranes from splashes. Do not use metal brushes and ensure the detergent is compatible with the devices being cleaned. Always hold the device below the level of the water to avoid splashing. Manual cleaning requires a neutral detergent and friction to remove soil. Commercially available products offer cleaning and disinfection in one. The correct procedure is described in **Appendix A**.

For cleaning long hollow lumen tubing, high pressure jet nozzles at 5 bar or 75 psi should be used by fixing one end of the tube to the water tap and allowing the water to run through while holding the tube underwater. It is important to ensure that the detergent is used in accordance with the manufacturer's instructions regarding concentration, temperature and contact time.

Validation

Manual cleaning cannot be validated. A clear SOP is required.

3.6.3.2 Rinsing after cleaning

After the cleaning process, chemicals must not remain on the devices that could cause adverse reactions with the equipment, user or patient. Proper rinsing is essential as the chemical residue can damage the mucous membranes of humans and affect the devices during drying or during steam sterilisation.

The final rinse should be carried out with high-quality water, for example water prepared by de-ionisation or reverse osmosis.

3.6.3.3 Good cleaning practice

- Where possible clean instruments immediately after use.
- Automated methods of cleaning are preferred and should be used as frequently as possible.
- Manual cleaning should be reserved for delicate devices.
- Follow the manufacturer's instructions and recommendations for detergents – **do not use household detergents**.
- Open hinged/jointed instruments to ensure access.
- Disassemble instruments before cleaning.
- Use only suitable cleaning tools and accessories – do not use wire brushes or abrasives.
- Rinse thoroughly after cleaning and dry.
- Do not overload trays – it prevents proper access and cleaning.
- Inspect instruments thoroughly after cleaning.

3.6.4 Automated methods for cleaning

Automated methods have major advantages of minimising handling of contaminated medical devices, save time, can reprocess a larger load than manual cleaning and are controlled by validated processes that reliably clean devices provided they are properly used. They have built-in controls and computerised processes which are self-validating, producing reports which can be kept in the SSD records.

3.6.4.1 Ultrasonicators

Ultrasonicators are baths with lids containing water plus a detergent. Dirt is removed by high-power output of 0.44 W/cm², which vibrates at a high frequency and dislodges organic matter. They are recommended for delicate devices which cannot withstand vigorous processing of an AWD. These work by cavitation, a process of creating minuscule bubbles or cavities in the water which dislodge the dirt. Ultrasonic cleaning units are available as freestanding units or may be integrated into modern automatic washer-disinfectors.

3.6.4.1.1   **Application of ultrasonicators.** Ultrasonic treatment can be used for stainless steel instruments, especially for instruments sensitive to mechanical impact: microsurgical instruments and dental instruments.

3.6.4.1.2   **Method of using an ultrasonicator**

Fill the bath and use a non-foaming cleaning agent in concentrations and temperature recommended by the manufacturer. De-gas the bath with warm water (no more than 40 °C). Any gases present in water reduces cavitation and the cleaning effect. Do not allow the water temperature to go above 55 °C. Renew the water frequently, preferably after each use. Make sure the items are fully immersed. Trays should not be overloaded; hinged instruments must be opened and laid side by side.

3.6.4.1.3   **Ultrasonicators** are <u>not</u> recommended for:
- Flexible endoscopes or optical lenses. They should never be treated in an ultrasonic bath.
- Elastic or silicone materials. These absorb the ultrasonic waves and weaken cleaning action.
- Minimal invasive surgery (MIS) instruments or rigid endoscopes. These may only be cleaned in an ultrasonicator if the manufacturer recommends it. Optical systems should not be cleaned in an ultrasonic bath.

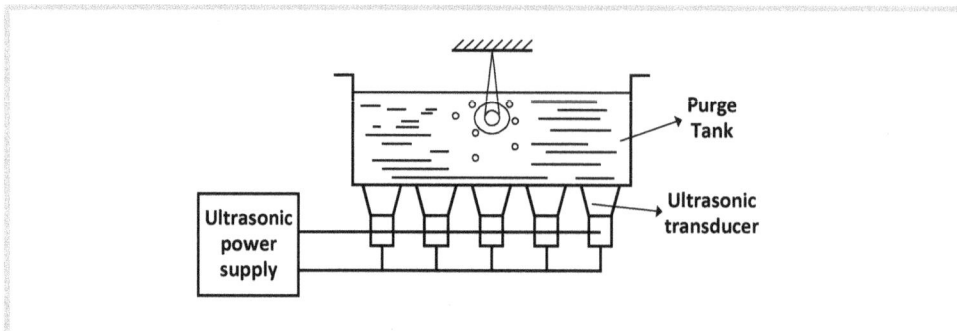

Figure 3.5 Components of an ultrasonicator[14]

3.6.4.1.4   Testing of ultrasonicators Daily testing is required and the results should be documented.

Testing performance of ultrasonic cleaners. There are two simple tests for checking the performance of your ultrasonic cleaner:

1. **Aluminium foil test** requires the placing of small pieces (usually nine strips) of aluminium foil suspended in the ultrasonicator and running the cycle for 10 minutes. Visually inspect the foil pieces and look for an even distribution of perforation and wrinkling.

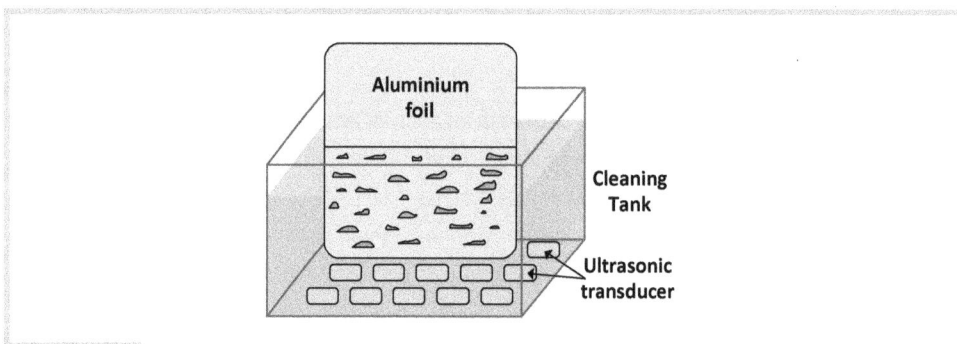

Figure 3.6 Aluminium foil test showing the perforations caused by the ultrasonicator[15]

2. **Chemical indicators for checking cavitation (annual).** The test device is a closed vial/capsule containing a chemical indicator containing glass beads. The vial is placed in the ultrasonic bath, which is switched on to a specified frequency, time and temperature. With effective cavitation, the colour in the vial changes from green to yellow. The advantage of this system is that it can be placed in with the load during the cleaning cycle, but is expensive.

---

[14]   From Xin Cheng. 2020. Research and application of ultrasonic cleaning technology in medical equipment cleaning under computer control system. *J Phys: Conf Ser* 1574 012042.

[15]   Adapted from Fuchs FJ. 2015. *Ultrasonic cleaning and washing of surfaces.* Power Ultrasonics.

3.6.4.2 Automatic washer-disinfectors (AWD)

AWDs have widely replaced manual and ultrasonic cleaning. Modern machines are sophisticated and economical to run, and have reduced the physical workload. They use pressurised water to physically remove the bioburden, followed by rinsing, heat disinfection, a final rinse and drying. There are several designs of washer-disinfectors including multi-chamber, batch and tunnel types, each designed for a specific size of SSD and the number of trays required to be processed per cycle.

Figure 3.7 illustrates the various phases of the AWD cycle, which are briefly described here:

1. **Pre-rinse.** Initial rinsing of the load with cold water. A major part of the soils is flushed away. The temperature should not exceed 35 °C.

2. **(Enzymatic) Cleaning.** The detergent is added and the water is heated up to approximately 45–55 °C. The major cleaning takes place during this phase.

3. **Neutralisation.** When an alkaline cleaning agent is used, the water is chemically neutralised with a weak acid to prevent corrosion.

4. **Intermediate rinse.** All remaining soils are carefully washed away with fresh cold water.

5. **Heat disinfection.** This occurs with hot water, at temperatures of 90 °C for 6 seconds, 80 °C for 1 minute (60 seconds), or 70 °C for 10 minutes (600 seconds) (ISO 15833). A lubricant is added which will reduce the drying time. Time and temperature will depend on the load.

6. **Drying.** In order to prevent recontamination it is essential that the load is dry by the time it is removed.

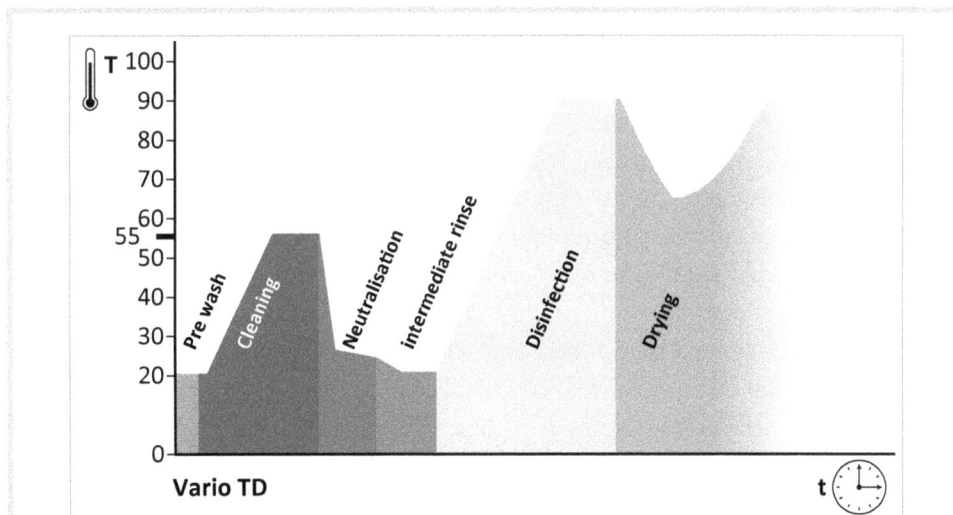

Figure 3.7 Phases of the automatic washer disinfector cycle

The **advantages** of AWDs are:
- fully automated cycles, which reduce subjective evaluation by the operators
- cleaning and disinfection is a part of the cycle
- minimised device handling
- performance can be monitored and validated
- no toxic residues.

The **disadvantages** are:
- unsuitable for complex hollow lumen devices without dedicated load carriers
- unsuitable for some heat-sensitive and delicate items
- expensive to run and maintain
- need expertise to maintain
- at the end of the cycle the devices are not sterile.

3.6.4.3 Validation for AWD

According to the new standard for WD (ISO 15883), the cleaning performance must be validated for each type of load (see WHO decontamination and reprocessing manual). There are complex standard test soils and process challenge devices for cleaning processes. Once the process of cleaning (and disinfection) has been completed the devices should be tested for cleanliness – in this case detecting the presence of residual soil or organic matter. See Table 3.1 for a summary of validation.

- **Inspection of the AWD.** Each morning the AWD must be checked to ensure the chamber, jets and chemicals are in working condition – any faults should be logged.
- **Visual inspection.** Close inspection of each item should be carried out to ensure there is no visible soiling after the cycle is over. While SSD staff are trained to inspect quickly and thoroughly, occasionally there may be a residue, which will require the device to go through the cleaning process again.
- **Soil removal.** A standardised test soil (commercially available) is applied to a batch of devices and run through a normal cycle of the AWD. Once completed the residual amount can be assessed by visual or chemical means. The test soil being processed should be compatible with the chemicals and detergents in the washing process.
- **Residual soil tests.** Once a washing cycle has been completed the detection of residual soil is possible with chemicals which react with protein and other organic matter such as ninhydrin, biuret, ortho-phthalaldehyde (OPA) and hydrogen peroxide. There are also commercial kits available which are more expensive.

The IPC team should be informed of any failure of validation of the AWD.

Washer-disinfector cycles fail because of:
- delays before processing – equipment with dried protein, blood and fats
- too high initial wash temperature (above 55 °C, which coagulates the protein)
- blocked or misdirected jets
- failure to irrigate hollow devices
- badly placed instruments
- shading effects – one device covers another
- overloading the trays
- insufficient or incorrect detergent
- too short cycle
- jammed motor arms.

3.6.5 Boilers (as disinfectors)

Before automated methods were available, boilers were used to heat-disinfect equipment. Some were used for sterilising devices, especially in community-based facilities or for field ambulances. These are no longer recommended for routine use because the process cannot be validated. However, they are still used in some countries and readers should familiarise themselves with its use.

Method. Devices are disassembled, cleaned manually and placed in the chamber of the boiler (unwrapped). Electric boilers are thermostatically controlled, and the cycle is run for 10 minutes once steam appears. They are fitted with a pressure and temperature gauge. At the end of the cycle, the boiler is turned off and allowed to cool before removing the devices.

Validation. There is no recognised method of validation for a boiling steriliser. A clear SOP is recommended.

The **advantages** are:
- cheap
- portable – can be carried to the site of use
- effective for small devices
- no toxic residues.

The **disadvantages** are:
- unsuitable for heat-sensitive items
- no process controls, i.e. time/temperature interlock
- scald risk to staff
- items must be cleaned before immersion
- forceps required for instrument removal
- devices come out wet and therefore sterility cannot be guaranteed.

3.6.6 Inspection, assembly and packing

This is an important step in ensuring that the devices are clean and ready for end-stage reprocessing – sterilisation – and that the packs are complete, safely packaged and will maintain sterility during storage.

3.6.6.1 Inspection

Once the devices are rendered safe following cleaning, they are visually inspected carefully by trained staff to ensure the devices function properly. Devices such as forceps and other hinged instruments should be scrutinised to make sure they are fully functional, for example that the tips or points are sharp and the hinges and clips work properly. The devices should not show pitting, loss of metal or wear at the hinges. Instruments should be carefully inspected to ensure there is an absence of organic matter in the hinges and teeth – areas which are difficult to clean. Instruments which do not satisfy these criteria should be replaced immediately or condemned and a replacement ordered.

3.6.6.1.1 Reason for inspection

- The devices are fit for purpose.
- Damaged devices are either replaced or sent for repair.
- Contents of packs, major and supplementary, are available.

3.6.6.1.2 Function of inspection

In order to ensure inspection is carried out optimally, the minimum requirement in the inspection area is a bright light and a magnifying glass to carry out inspection.

For details, see the WHO Decontamination and Reprocessing of Medical Devices for Healthcare Facilities (2016) guidelines section on Inspection.

3.6.6.1.3 Requirements for inspection area

The area where inspection is carried out must be airy and well lit, and have adequate surfaces to allow for inspection, including of narrow-bore hollow lumen devices.

3.6.6.2 Assembly

Challenges in assembly and packaging

- In some countries all surgical devices are first soaked in hypochlorite, which destroys metal. The instruments become pitted, rusted and brittle – they break when exposed to steam sterilisation.
- Replacement instrument stocks may be low or non-existent. Because replacement devices are not readily available, substandard devices continue in use. These are harmful to both the staff and the patients.

- Some surgeons will only work with a particular set and will not accept replacements if these vary from the original set – damaged devices remain in use. Instruments are controlled by the operating theatre, which should not be the case.
- The control of ordering medical devices lies with the operating theatre and often they are not replaced because of lack of resources.

3.6.6.2.1 Reason for assembly

- After inspection the devices are re-assembled individually according to the manufacturer's recommendations.
- Surgical and other packs are assembled according to the standard lists provided.
- A traceability (labelling) system (computerised or manual) for each tray has to be put in place.
- A record must be kept of all devices which have been inspected and tested.

3.6.6.2.2 Requirements for assembly area

- All the raw material needed for assembly must be available.
- There must be adequate surfaces to assemble packs or individual packages.
- Internal and external indicators should be put in place.
- Trays should be assembled according to the checklist.

A summary of points to remember is outlined below:[16]

- All devices are present in accordance with the surgical tray, are re-assembled according to the manufacturer's instruction and placed in the correct manner to ensure ease of use by the user.
- When packaging for sterilisation, it is essential that all surfaces are presented to the sterilisation media – the devices must be disassembled and presented in this state; rachet devices should be loosely closed to first rachet.
- Keep similar devices together; place devices in a single layer on the tray.
- Line the base of the surgical tray with a tray liner.
- Spread the weight of the devices evenly; spread plastic devices evenly across the tray.
- Protect sharp devices with protectors that allow steam penetration.
- Ensure protection of delicate devices.
- Report any missing or extra devices to the supervisor.

16   WHO. 2016. Decontamination and reprocessing of medical devices for health-care facilities. World Health Organization/Pan American Health Organization. Available at https://www.who.int/publications/i/item/9789241549851.

3.6.6.3 Packaging

Knowledge about the application and use of packaging is essential for the IPC practitioner to ensure the devices have been exposed to the method of sterilisation and the packaging is intact, safely stored and the microbial barrier is maintained until opened. Devices for sterilisation require packaging and are covered in depth in the WHO decontamination guidance. There are international standards for various types of packaging for different sterilisation methods.[17]

Reason for packaging
Packaging is required to:
- keep the contents of the packs intact
- allow safe transport and storage
- allow sterility to be maintained when the pack is opened for use.

Function of packaging
In order to fulfil these requirements, there should be at least two – but preferably three – layers of packaging as follows:
- **Primary packaging** with the purpose to prevent recontamination with dust and/or microbes and maintain sterility during transport and storage, e.g. two layers of paper or fabric, or a combination.
- **Secondary packaging** to facilitate transport and storage, e.g. extra layer.
- **Transport packaging**, which allows the delivery of sterile packages and is removed after delivery of the sterile packs.

3.6.6.3.1 Requirements of packaging

Materials used for packaging must be appropriate to the devices being sterilised and should:
- Enable sterilisation: allow movement of steam and gases in and out of the packaging.
- Be compatible with the sterilisation process including chemicals, temperature, pressure, and humidity changes.

---

[17]   EN-ISO 11607:2017 Packaging for terminally sterilised medical devices. The EN 868 series provides requirements and test methods for a range of specific materials and configurations of sterile barrier systems. The series now comprises:
Part 1:2018 Requirements for materials, sterile barrier systems and packaging systems
Part 2:2017 Sterilisation wrap
Part 3:2017 Paper for use in the manufacture of paper bags and pouches and reels
Part 4:2017 Paper bags
Part 5:2018 Sealable pouches and reels of porous materials and plastic film construction
Part 6:2017 Paper for low temperature sterilisation
Part 7:2017 Adhesive coated paper for low temperature sterilisation processes
Part 8:2018 Re-usable sterilisation containers for steam sterilisers
Part 9:2018 Uncoated nonwoven materials of polyolefins
Part 10:2018 Adhesive coated nonwoven materials of polyolefins.

- Maintain sterility and do not allow recontamination.
- Be strong, withstand tearing and impact.
- Ensure product integrity and patient safety: there should be no release of chemicals or particles onto the devices and they should be lint-free.
- Have external indicator which shows whether the pack has been processed.
- Make it clearly visible if damage occurs (use of coloured wraps).
- Facilitate aseptic opening without recontamination of devices.

It should be evident if the package has been opened. It should not re-seal itself.

3.6.6.3.2 Types of packaging material

There are several types of packaging commonly used. The application, uses, advantages and disadvantages are shown in Table 3.3, but are summarised below. The application of packaging material is shown in Appendix B.

- **Sterilisation wraps** are made up of a combination of bleached crepe paper, cellulose and synthetic fibres. These are widely used for steam, dry heat and ethylene oxide (ETO).
- **Rigid containers** are reusable and are made of aluminium, high-density polymer or a combination. Their use is for steam sterilisation and can be re-used several times provided they are not damaged during sterilisation or transportation.

> **Cardboard boxes are known to carry spores and are not recommended.**

- **Fabrics**, such as cotton (woven) and some non-woven sheets, are re-used. These are usually used for primary packaging for pre-vacuum or gravity sterilisers. *Fabric*[18] packaging is of four types:
  - **Cotton or linen** (textile) has been widely used in LMICs as an inner wrapping for instrument sets and/or outer dust protection. **Textile alone is not suitable as primary packaging!** There are some major disadvantages in using textiles (Table 3.3) and they are no longer recommended. 'Linting' from woven fabrics occurs, which results in fibres contaminating the devices, which are transferred to surgical wounds and cause 'sterile' wound infections.
  - **Paper sheets** have largely replaced textiles and are used as primary packaging for wrapping of textile packs and instrument sets in trays. They are also used as inner packaging in containers. Paper sheets are for single use only.

---

[18] ISO 11607-1:2019. Packaging for terminally sterilised medical devices. Part 1. Requirement for materials, sterile barrier systems and packaging systems.

- **Paper sterilisation bags** are used for packaging of individual instruments or small sets used in nursing stations and wards. The bag has a chemical indicator visible on the outside. It is sealed with a device. Sterilisation bags are for single use only.
- **Non-woven sheets** are used as primary packaging for wrapping of textile packs and instrument sets in trays. These are also used as inner packaging in containers. Non-woven sheets contain a certain amount of synthetic fibre. The combination of these fibres creates a tortuous path to prevent migration of micro-organisms. Non-woven sheets are for single use only.

- **Glass or metal** (non-perforated) is used for dry heat sterilisation.
- **Glass bottles**, vials and ampoules are also used for dry heat sterilisation.
- **Aluminium foil** – thicker grade is used for dry heat sterilisation.
- **Laminated film pouches** are used for primary packaging of individual instruments or small instrument sets and have largely replaced paper sterilisation bags. The pouches consist of a sheet of paper or non-woven material and a sheet of laminated transparent plastic, which are sealed together to form a pouch. The pouches must be loaded correctly in the steriliser to ensure the sterilant penetrates inside. The open end of the pouch is closed with a sealing device The pouch is opened by peeling back the laminated sheet from the paper sheets. Pouches are available in many sizes.
  - **Transparent pouches** are recommended for steam and ETO. Some are specifically made for hydrogen peroxide plasma and dry heat.
  - **Bonded polyethylene** (superior) is similar to non-woven and can be used for steam, ETO, low-temperature steam formaldehyde and hydrogen peroxide plasma.

Table 3.3 Types of packaging with their advantages and disadvantages (WHO decontamination manual)

Type of packaging	Method of sterilisation	Advantage	Disadvantage	Comment
Paper (medical grade) Bleached crepe paper Cellulose and synthetic fibres	Steam Dry heat ETO	Penetration of steam, air, chemicals Effective barrier in dry, clean conditions Free from loose particles Single use only	Fibres and loose particles if torn or shredded Not to be used for hydrogen peroxide plasma – absorbs hydrogen peroxide Does not facilitate aseptic opening	Double wrap may reduce steam penetration Paper bags are not very strong Unable to see inside

Type of packaging	Method of sterilisation	Advantage	Disadvantage	Comment
Reusable rigid containers – metals, aluminium	Steam sterilisation for large sets of surgical devices	Keeps the devices safe after sterilisation and during transportation	Containers must be loaded properly to avoid problems of moisture and increasing drying times	Training on loading and unloading metal containers is essential. Not all types of packaging material can be used.
Woven fabrics Two layers of cloth or one each of cloth and paper Primary packaging	Steam pre-vacuum or downward displacement (gravity)	Heavy pack Stronger – resistant to tearing Reusable	Poor bacterial barrier Holes in the fabric render them ineffective Impede air penetration and air removal if thick or tight Cannot be used alone If too dry, will cause overheating of steam and failure of sterilisation 'Sterile' wound infections from lint	Store clean and dry Need to be inspected carefully and quality assessed during use and re-use Not recommended for primary packaging alone, must have another (secondary or layered) cover with it
Synthetic woven fabric	Steam sterilisation	Durable and good to use	Needs to be validated for sterilisation and reliable drying in the facility	Validation required for sterilisation
Transparent (laminated film) pouches Paper and polymers e.g.: polyethylene PVC polypropylene polycarbonates nylon	Steam ETO Hydrogen peroxide plasma Dry heat only	Good antimicrobial and dust barrier Single items (one medical device per pouch) Maintain sterility	Can tear or perforate Need to be properly heat-sealed without leaks to maintain sterility	Use for single devices or light materials Some polyethylene pouches do not tolerate vacuum

Type of packaging	Method of sterilisation	Advantage	Disadvantage	Comment
		Contents easily visible Can be heat-sealed Has an incorporated chemical indicator	Some impede steam removal and increase air removal time	PVC and nylon pouches are not recommended
Tyvek bonded polyethylene Superior bonded, paper-like non-woven	Steam ETO Low-temperature steam formaldehyde Hydrogen peroxide plasma	Robust Good barrier properties Low absorption of chemical sterilants Can be heat sealed Has an incorporated chemical indicator	None, but expensive Not widely available	Good non-woven substitute for linen
Non-perforated containers of glass or metal	Dry heat	Sterilisation of needles	Poor conductor of heat – increases drying time	Not recommended
Glass bottles, vials and ampoules for liquids	Dry heat sterilisation of liquids and oils	Sterilisation of liquids and oils	Limited use, if any	Rarely used

3.6.6.4 Wrapping

During opening, the contents of a pack containing sterile devices must not get contaminated. Wrapping techniques for packs and sets have been developed to assure aseptic opening. The most common wrapping techniques applied for packaging of textile packs and surgical sets are the **envelope fold** (Figure 3.8) and the **parcel fold** (Figure 3.9). The unfolded outer wrapper covers the instrument table and provides a sterile field. The techniques can be used with sheets of textile, paper and non-wovens.

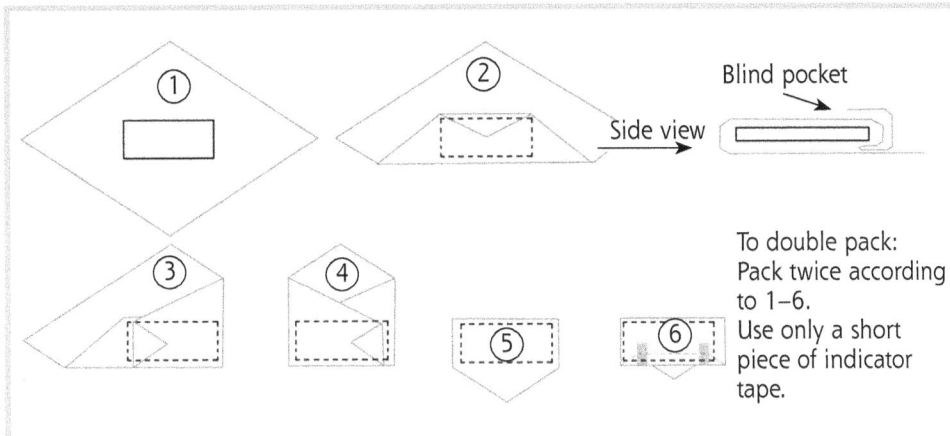

Figure 3.8 Small-item wrapping technique

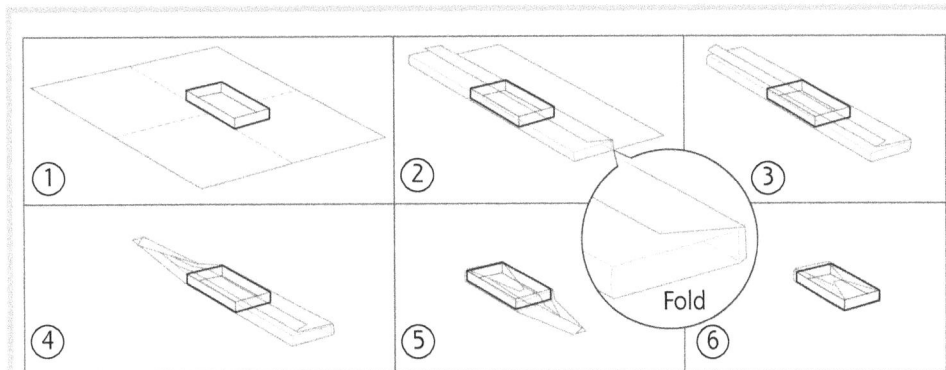

Figure 3.9 Larger packs wrapping technique

3.6.6.5 Sealing, indicators and labelling[19]

Heat sealing of flexible packaging materials is the best method for these materials. Seal the laminate to the paper with a continuous adhesive seal of 3–15 mm. In the event of breakdown of the heat sealer, a seal may be formed by first folding the corners of the open end inwards, then making two or three width-wise folds of the entire open end of the pack, followed by securing of the folds with adhesive tape (autoclave indicator tape).

The heat-sealing process should be undertaken with care. Creases in the packaging material can result in an inadequate or uneven seal. When double-wrapping using heat seal pouches, the packages should be used in such a way

---

[19] WHO. 2016. Decontamination and reprocessing of medical devices for health-care facilities. World Health Organization/Pan American Health Organization. Available at https://www.who.int/publications/i/item/9789241549851.

so as to avoid folding the inner package to fit into the outer package. Edges of inner heat seal pouches should not be folded as air may be entrapped in the folds and inhibit sterilisation. When double-wrapping using paper/plastic heat seal pouches, the paper portion should be placed together to ensure penetration and removal of the sterilant, air and moisture. This also enables the device to be viewed. It is important to wrap the device securely to avoid contamination, which could compromise sterility. Use an adhesive device identification label – *do not write on the paper side of the pouch*. The device identification label is placed on the outside packaging.

> **When loading paper/plastic pouches into the steriliser, the packages should be placed in the same direction (i.e. paper/plastic, paper/plastic). If one heat seal pouch is placed inside another, care should be taken to select the appropriate sequential sizing.**

Self-sealing packages are to be used in accordance with the manufacturers' instructions. Staples must never be used because they perforate the packaging material.

Accessories for packaging include:
- **Adhesive tape** is autoclave/indicator tape. This keeps the package together and has an external chemical indicator.
- **External chemical indicator.** All device trays or packages must have an external indicator which the user should take note of before opening the package. A colour change (choice of colour varies with the manufacturer) will occur when the package has been exposed to the sterilisation method.
- **Trays** for arranging instruments (stainless steel) should be of a standard size so that they can fit into all the processing equipment such as washer-disinfectors and sterilisers easily. They should be able to fit into rigid containers of standard dimensions.
- **Baskets** are used for small items to assist with loading of sterilisers and provide extra protection. They keep smaller packs upright to allow optimal access of the sterilising agent to the packs.
- **Protection materials** such as tip covers for sharp devices are to protect the tips and prevent them from damaging the primary packaging. They should not be too tight and allow the sterilising agent to reach the surfaces of the instrument.
- **Dust covers** over the primary package provide extra protection and may extend the expiry period.

3.6.6.6 Labelling

Packages to be sterilised should be labelled before sterilisation. The information on the label should include the following:

- name of product
- name of wrapper
- expiry date and/or sterilisation date
- where appropriate, the word 'sterile'
- load number.

A piggyback batch control label system or computer-generated system is to be used on all items that are to be used as a sterile product.[20]

This label is to be placed in the patient's procedural record by operating theatre staff to assist with the ability to recall items.

3.6.6.7 Validation of the packaging system

It is essential that a packaging system with its contents meets the requirements for sterility maintenance and protection of its contents. Packaging should be validated in combination with the actual load and the sterilisation process used. When testing a packaging system, handling transport and storage conditions should be included.[21]

3.6.7 Sterilisation

An IPC practitioner should know the various methods of sterilisation (heat and chemical) and how these systems are monitored and validated. During investigation of SSI, HAI or outbreaks, this information is invaluable.

3.6.7.1 Types of sterilisation

Heat is the most common type of sterilisation method used in healthcare. More recently chemical methods for sterilising heat-sensitive equipment have been introduced. This section will concentrate mainly on steam sterilisation, but will summarise the other methods (Figure 3.10).

There are two types of heat:
- dry heat
- steam.

---

[20] Recommendations for manual batch labelling and manual tracking of instruments trays for operating suite. Available at https://www.health.qld.gov.au/chrisp/.
[21] ISO 11607-2:2019.

Chemical sterilisation can be carried out with ethylene oxide (ETO), hydrogen peroxide in gaseous or plasma form, ozone (not used very often) or low-temperature steam formaldehyde, which has limited use in certain countries. Chemical disinfectants are often called sterilants, but these are not true sterilants – they can only provide high-level disinfection and are not suitable for critical devices.

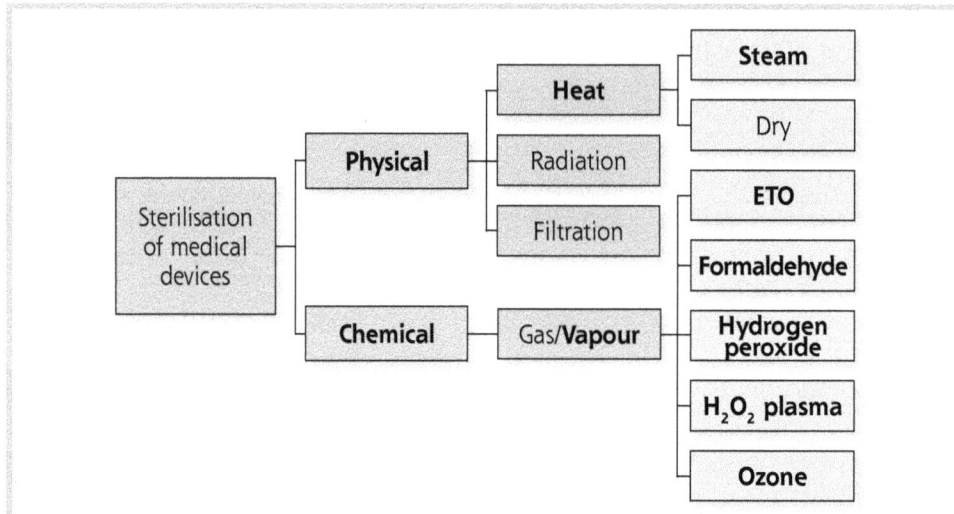

Figure 3.10   Types of sterilisation methods used in healthcare facilities (those in bold are more often used)

3.6.7.1.1 Dry heat[22]

Dry heat or hot air ovens are based upon gravity or mechanical convection (similar to kitchen ovens). The element heats the air within the chamber, which is circulated by a fan. This method of sterilisation is erratic and often has cold spots inside the chamber unless well regulated.

Temperature: The exposure time and temperature vary according to the item to be sterilised, typically two hours at 160 °C, one hour at 170 °C or 30 minutes at 180 °C.

Indications: This method of sterilisation is rarely used, but there are a few indications:

- for critical devices that will be damaged by moisture, pressure and/or vacuum
- rarely used clinically for the sterilisation of restricted types of material, such as glassware, oils, powders and instruments that are moisture-sensitive materials/devices.

---

[22]   ISO 20857:2010 Sterilisation of health care products – Dry heat – Requirements for the development, validation and routine control of a sterilisation process for medical devices

Monitoring and validation:

- each cycle – physical indicator
- each package – chemical indicators
- daily – biological indicators.

While hot air ovens (dry heat) are non-corrosive and can reach internal parts (by heat conduction) if the device has not been disassembled and is relatively inexpensive, it is not recommended for widespread use. The length of exposure time because of slow heat conduction can be up to 180 minutes, depending on the temperature, and cooling the load post-sterilisation also takes a long time. Some types of materials can get damaged and this is a limitation. It penetrates poorly and like all heat sterilisation methods, heat-labile items are destroyed; it cannot sterilise liquids and is not suitable for dental hand pieces.

3.6.7.1.2 Steam sterilisation

Steam sterilisation is the most common and widely used method for processing re-usable heat-stable medical devices. It also has the most developed methods of validation prior to allowing medical devices to be released from the sterilisation area (parametric release) after having been monitored and validated according to the required standard.

3.6.7.1.2.1 *Principles of steam sterilisation*

Heat is a major and the cheapest form of energy used for sterilisation. Water (liquid) is heated to boiling point to produce steam (gaseous).

The essential components of steam sterilisation are shown below. In principle, water is heated and at boiling point it converts from its liquid form to an expanded gaseous state of steam. When the steam comes into contact with a cooler surface, such as the packs in the chamber, it starts to convert back to its liquid state, and during this process releases latent energy (heat), which is transferred to the load, enabling it to reach sterilisation temperature. The contact time between the items and the steam has to be for a prescribed duration and this sterilises the items it comes into contact with. Additionally, when steam condenses into water it occupies a much smaller space so steam condensation within a sealed vessel – a chamber – will create a vacuum.

Pressure

When water is heated in a closed container it expands as it changes from a liquid to a gaseous state. If there is no escape for the steam, the chamber will explode because of the immense pressure built up inside the chamber. That is why sterilisers have safety valves to let off excess steam. If the lid is left open, there is no pressure build-up and the steam escapes as it is produced. Pressure inside the chamber can be used to control the temperature. There is a fixed relation between the temperature and pressure of saturated steam, making the process easy to control and validate.

3.6.7.1.2.1.1 *Quality of steam*

The quality of steam can be described in many ways including:

- the amount of water trapped in it
- the amount of impurities contained in it
- its temperature relative to its boiling point.

Definitions of steam include:

- **Saturated steam.** This is steam at a particular set of saturation conditions – boiling temperature and pressure. Saturated steam may, or may not, contain water droplets, but does contain latent energy. **Penetration of the load is good – it reaches inside the packs and kills organisms**.
- **Superheated steam.** This is steam that has been further heated above its saturation temperature. Superheated steam is dry. **The packs are over-dried and medical devices, linen and other items in the load can be damaged.** It does not penetrate the packs very well and kills organisms much more slowly.
- **Wet-saturated steam.** This is steam at saturation conditions that contains too much water; the wetness in the steam clogs the pores of packed loads and prevents the steam from properly penetrating wrapped loads or sealed pouches. The wetness prevents the steam from penetrating the load. **The packs come out wet and are not considered sterile.**

3.6.7.1.2.1.2 *Vacuum and air removal*

If the air is removed from a closed chamber by means of a vacuum, the steam will penetrate the packs inside the chamber better because there is no air to block its movement. This is the principle of vacuum sterilisers. Figure 3.11 demonstrates these principles.

> **To summarise, steam is produced, or introduced, into a closed chamber, and it carries a large amount of latent heat. As the steam builds up pressure, in the absence of air, it penetrates the contents of the chamber. A drop in temperature when in contact with the objects, allows the steam to release the latent heat. This heat has excellent sterilisation properties. Once a designated contact (or sterilisation) time has been achieved, the steam is removed.**

Why is steam such a good sterilising agent?

- Humidity of steam facilitates the killing of micro-organisms, including spores.
- As soon as it cools down slightly, it will condense to water, releasing its heat.
- It can penetrate packages in the steriliser well because of the change of volume when it condenses.

- It is clean and non-toxic.

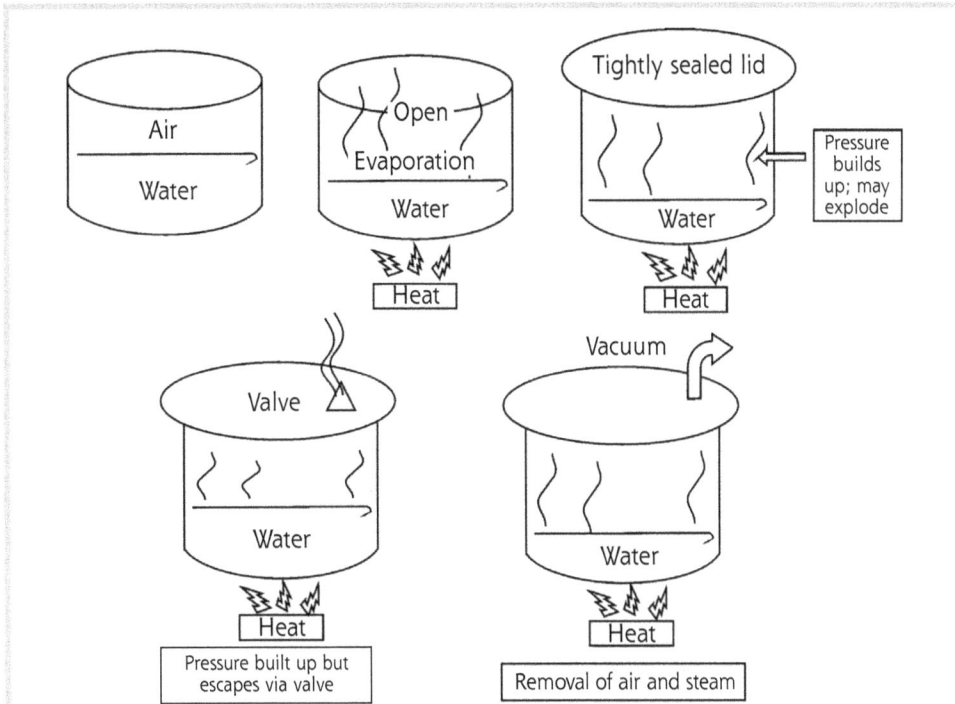

Figure 3.11 Applying heat to open vessels of water results in evaporation. However, if the container is tightly sealed, the pressure builds up.[23]

3.6.7.1.2.2 *The process of sterilisation*

There are some essential considerations when undertaking steam sterilisation:

- Blood and organic matter reduce steam penetration and therefore all devices must be clean before packing for autoclaving.
- The steam supply to the jacket and the chamber should come from a common source, which makes it easier to control. It also makes the validation of each stage of the process easier. Steam from different sources may not be effectively controlled and the difference in temperature and pressure can result in non-removal of air, leaving 'cold spots' where steam cannot penetrate owing to the presence of air.

Other important points are:

- Steam is lighter than air and forms a layer above air. The removal of air is done either by displacing it (downward displacement) or by extraction (vacuum).
- Steam cannot penetrate in the presence of air and thus the sterilisation will fail.

23   Huys J. 2010. Water quality. *In Sterilisation of Medical Supplies by Steam*. 3 edition. MHP-Verlag.

3.6.7.1.2.3 Components of a steam steriliser

- pressure vessel, with lid and gasket
- temperature/pressure control
- valves for air removal, steam release
- safety device
- steam supply
- electricity or an energy source
- water or steam source.

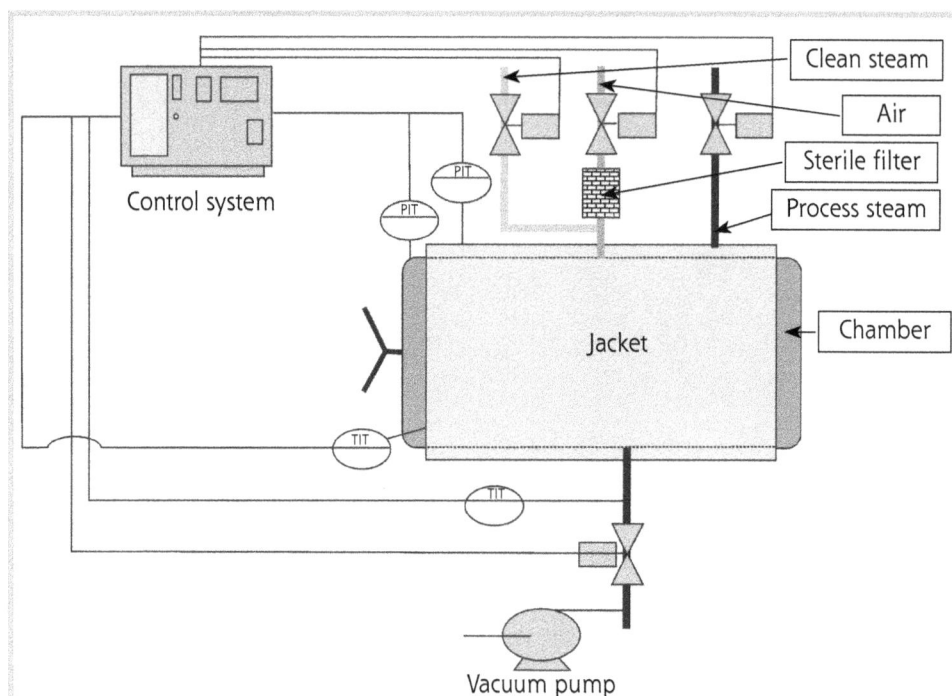

Figure 3.12 Elementary diagram of a steam steriliser

These basic components can be developed to build small portable sterilisers as well as large fixed ones.

3.6.7.1.2.4 Types of sterilisers

There are several types of steriliser available depending on the types of devices to be reprocessed and the validation methods applicable to the process. **All moist heat (steam) sterilisers are based on the same principles of sterilisation.**

3.6.7.1.2.4.1 Immediate-use steam sterilisers (IUSS) – 'flash' sterilisers

This type of steriliser is used where there is an urgent need to re-sterilise a device quickly, often during a surgical procedure, such as dropped instruments. This sterilisation method should be avoided as the material is sterilised *without packaging* and the cycle eliminates *drying*. As a result, the possibility of recontamination of the material increases. Validation of such sterilisers is by physical indicators.

3.6.7.1.2.4.2 *Tabletop sterilisers*

The tabletop model is the most frequently used steam steriliser in smaller decontamination units such as dental and rural clinics. It has a small chamber volume and generates its own steam when distilled or deionised water is added by the user. These sterilisers are designed for small instruments, such as dental instruments, and not recommended for any lumen instruments. The chamber must be packed methodically to allow steam to penetrate the packs and trays and must be visibly dry at the end of the cycle as wet packs are not considered sterile. Unwrapped items are vulnerable to contamination. These sterilisers are monitored and validated by mechanical, chemical and biological indicators (see section 3.6.7.1.2.9).

3.6.7.1.2.4.3 *Downward-displacement (gravity) steriliser*

These sterilisers are less commonly used for general purposes. The steam is introduced from the top of the chamber and the air is driven downwards by the pressure of the steam. Validation is by physical, chemical and biological indicators.

Downward-displacement sterilisers have several disadvantages:
- Are not effective for wrapped load and hollow instrument sterilisation because air removal may be incomplete.
- Can only be used for unwrapped, non-hollow instruments and fluids.
- The sterilisation cycle is longer because it takes time for the steam to penetrate the load.
- Packing of the load has to be done carefully and methodically to allow the movement of steam and air in the chamber.
- Wet loads are common because of condensation of steam.

3.6.7.1.2.4.4 *Pre-vacuum sterilisers*

The process for pre-vacuum sterilisers is complex because the total removal of air has to be ensured for sterilisation to occur. The quality of steam must be optimal. Temperature regulation has been improved by an outer jacket that covers the sterilising chamber. A vacuum system is attached to the chamber to ensure air removal at the beginning of the cycle and removal of steam and drying at the end of the cycle.

Challenges with pre-vacuum sterilisers

There are several **challenges** to producing a sterile load, most of which are related to the efficient removal of air from the packs in the chamber. This is because a mixed load of a variety of packaging material will affect air removal and steam penetration.

- Narrow-bore devices may not allow complete air removal. This means that steam cannot penetrate inside the lumen and the device will not be sterile.
- Packing the steriliser correctly is essential to ensure complete air removal.

Improving the sterilisation process

There are several ways in which the sterilisation process can be improved. These are the correct loading of the steriliser, improving quality of steam and improving steam penetration.

3.6.7.1.2.5 Loading the steriliser

The steriliser chamber must be loaded correctly to ensure maximum circulation of steam in and around the packs. The chamber must not be overloaded. Packaging material which does not allow steam or chemicals to penetrate must not be used.

Method of loading steriliser[24]

Steam sterilisers shall be loaded in the following manner to ensure sterilant contact and penetration:
- package placement to avoid overloading
- non-perforated tray and container placed on their edges
- packages away from chamber walls
- concave devices on an angle to avoid condensate pooling
- textile packs perpendicular to the steriliser cart shelf
- laminated pouches on their edges with multiple packages being placed *paper to plastic*
- rigid containers not stacked unless advised by the manufacturer and validated for that configuration.

The operator responsible for loading and initiating the cycle should be documented.

Method of unloading a steriliser

Upon completion of the cycle, the operator responsible for unloading the steriliser must review the steriliser printout for the following:
- correct sterilisation parameters
- cycle time and date
- verification that the cycle number matches the lot control label for the load
- verification and initialing that the correct cycle parameters have been met
- examining the load items for:
  - any visible signs of moisture
  - any signs of compromised packaging integrity.

---

24   Huys J. 2010. Water quality. *In Sterilisation of Medical Supplies by Steam*. 3 edition. MHP-Verlag.

Printed records of each cycle parameter (i.e. pressure, temperature, time) shall be retained in accordance with the healthcare setting's requirements.

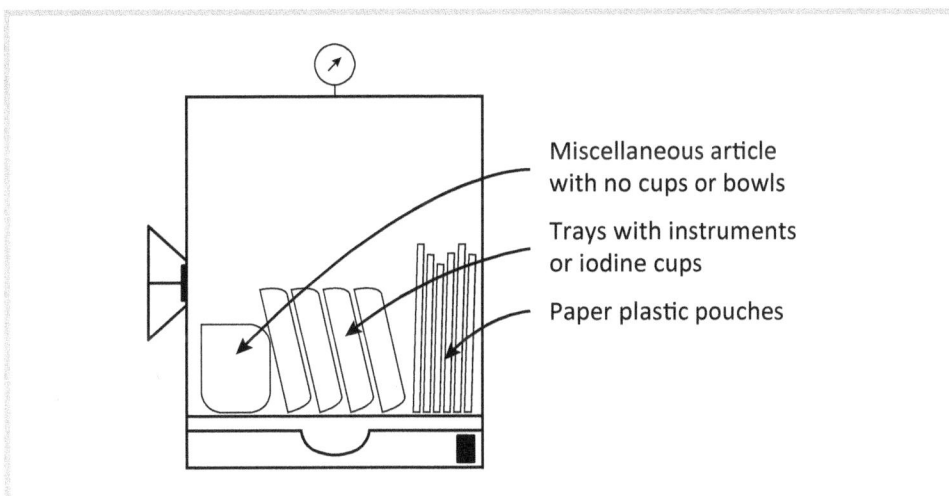

Miscellaneous article with no cups or bowls

Trays with instruments or iodine cups

Paper plastic pouches

Figure 3.13 Loading a table top steriliser allowing room for removal of air, circulation and penetration of steam into the packs

3.6.7.1.2.6 Steam

Steam is the essence of moist heat sterilisation. Steam can either be produced at a distant plant and piped to the SSD or each steriliser can have a self-generating steam component. Either method is acceptable as long as the quality of the steam is optimal and there are no leaks in the pipes carrying the steam to the SSD.

3.6.7.1.2.6.1 Air removal and steam penetration

In order for the steam to penetrate the packs effectively, air must be removed to avoid cold spots forming (in the presence of air) which prevent steam penetration. There are several ways to remove air from inside the chamber, allowing steam to enter and sterilise the contents of the steriliser.

3.6.7.1.2.6.2 Introducing steam into the chamber

The introduction of steam into the chamber can happen by the following methods:

Bleeding. During the pre-vacuum cycle, small amounts of steam are injected into the chamber. First a vacuum is drawn and at a particular stage of the air removal, small amounts of steam are introduced into the chamber above atmospheric pressure while the vacuum pump is running. The air is gradually flushed out of the packs assisted by the vacuum and small amounts of steam.

Pulses of steam are admitted above atmospheric pressure into the chamber, followed by the release of pressure. Steam penetrates deep into the packs, displacing and removing air within the packs. The process is carried out several times and ensures complete air removal, especially from textile packs. Temperature measurements show that after the second pulse the temperature inside the pack is the same as that of the chamber.

Fractionated pre-vacuum. A vacuum is drawn first and steam admitted under pressure below or just above atmospheric pressure. At the end of the first pulse both air and steam will remain in the chamber. With the second vacuum both air and steam will be withdrawn and a new jet of steam will be admitted. Subsequent pulses will reduce the amount of air and increase steam in the chamber and the packs. With this method the pressure of pulses is low, requiring less steam and the rapid changes in pressure increase the amount of steam into the packs, resulting in rapid air removal.

If steam pulses remain below atmospheric pressure, there is a likelihood of air being sucked into the chamber and is subject to leakages, which can be easily detected.

3.6.7.1.2.7 *Steam steriliser cycle*

Steam sterilisation cycle with its temperature components at the various stages (Huys, 2010).

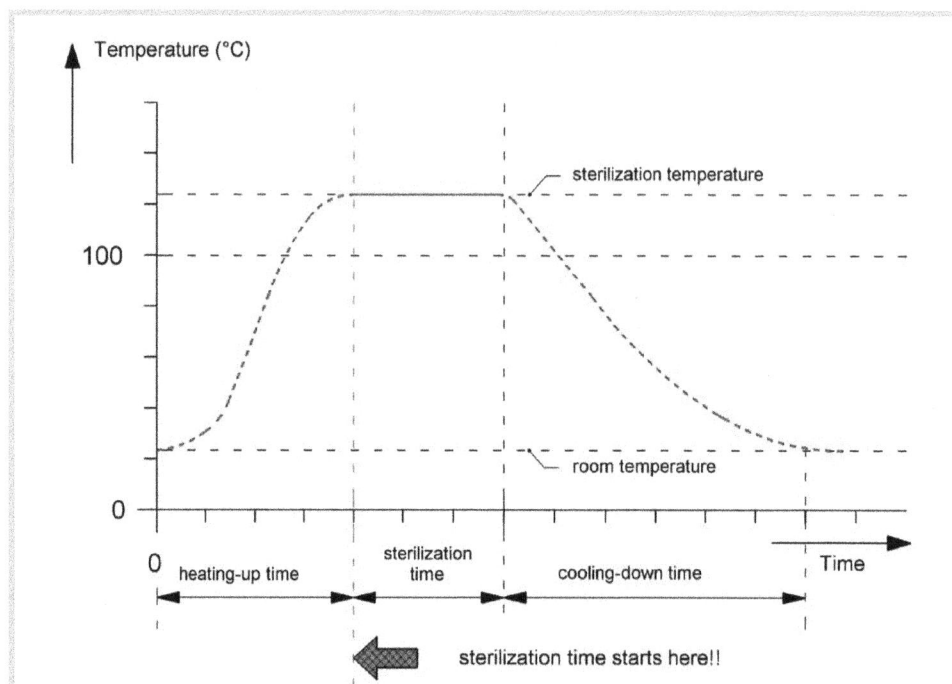

Figure 3.14 An example of a pre-vacuum steam sterilisation cycle[25]

---

[25] Huijs J. 2010. Water quality. *In Sterilisation of Medical Supplies by Steam.*

The sequence of steps occurring in the chamber are shown in Figure 3.14 and are summarised as follows:

1. Warming up of the chamber
2. Vacuum extraction
3. Pre-steam penetration time
4. Steam penetration time
5. Holding time
6. Cooling time.

3.6.7.1.2.7.1 *Cycle time.* A full sterilising cycle takes about 45 minutes with a holding time of 3 minutes at 134 °C (this is essentially the contact time). For complete sterilisation to take place, air removal from the load must be complete and therefore a vacuum system is essential.

3.6.7.1.2.7.2 *Condensate removal.* Sterilisation requires that, to evaporate all condensate in the load, the amount of water should be as low as possible to ensure that the packs are dry when the cycle is completed. Water condenses, especially at the beginning of the cycle, and falls to the bottom of the chamber. The condensate is removed by a drain at the lowest point of the chamber, which opens when the autoclave is under pressure and until steam is discharged. The drain pipe is fitted with a steam trap which has sensors to detect the difference between water and steam and opens when condensate is present. A strainer is placed before the steam trap to prevent dirt or debris from entering it. Regular maintenance of the steam trap is essential for the functioning of a steriliser.

3.6.7.1.2.8 Testing of steam sterilisers

A trained IPC practitioner should know about validation methods and parametric release. The reader is referred to Table 3.1 on the methods of validation for all sterilisation methods. Those for steam sterilisation are mentioned here.

3.6.7.1.2.8.1 *Physical – charts and gauges.* Visual observations of temperature and pressure printouts should be recorded for each sterilisation cycle.

All records of each cycle should be kept for at least one year and should be available for inspection by the engineers and the IPC team in the event of a mishap or outbreak.

3.6.7.1.2.8.2 *Leak test.* This test is performed when the steriliser is hot. The chamber is evacuated to 7 kPa by using a vacuum. The valves are closed and two readings are taken 10 minutes apart. There should not be an increase of more than 0.13 kPa (1.3 mbar) per minute. Ideally the test should be carried out weekly by the manager or engineer.

3.6.7.1.2.8.3   *Bowie-Dick (BD) test.* The Bowie-Dick test is the most widely used and should be carried out daily before the first sterilisation cycle of the day. In Europe the BD test indicates for air removal from a standard pack used in large sterilisers (EN 285:2016), while in the United States the same test is used for assessing steam penetration.

3.6.7.1.2.8.4   *Alternative BD tests (EN11140-4:2007)* requires that 'alternative' Bowie-Dick products have 'equivalent' performance to the towel pack. Reference pack (towel pack) and 'alternative' are tested alternately in both good 'pass' cycles and corrupted 'fail' cycles. The criteria are strict and these should comply.

3.6.7.1.2.8.5   *Thermocouple testing.* Several leads are introduced into the chamber, drains and packs via sampling ports by the engineers. Any variations in temperature at these sites are recorded – the usual reason is inadequate air removal. The chamber should be airtight during the tests. Thermocouple testing is carried out when commissioning a new steriliser and three-monthly thereafter for a year and should be done regularly as part of maintenance, and is carried out by the engineers. Thermocouple tests are an important part of the performance qualification and periodical performance requalification of the steriliser.

3.6.7.1.2.9 Indicators

Biological indicators. These indicators use spores that should be killed when placed in a sterilisation cycle. The modern indicators reflect this with a colour change, which can be recorded within a short space of time.

Chemical indicators. Chemical indicators are dyes or chemicals which change colour when exposed to a particular level of temperature of steam, but do not necessarily indicate length of exposure. They are produced as tubes, strips of paper or steriliser packs which are impregnated with chemicals that respond to a particular requirement. For proper validations, other tests such as BD and the charts and gauges should be used in conjunction with chemical indicators in **each cycle**.

Classification of indicators (ISO 11140:2014) is summarised below:
Class 1: Process indicators

Class 2: Indicators for use in specific tests
Class 3: Single-variable indicator
Class 4: Multi-variable indicators
Class 5: Integrating indicators
Class 6: Emulating indicators

Table 3.4 Types of chemical indicators (from WHO decontamination manual)

Types	Purpose
Type 1 Process indicators	These indicators are intended for use with packs or containers to indicate that they have been directly exposed to the sterilisation process and to distinguish between processed and unprocessed units
Type 2 Indicators for use in specific tests	These indicators are intended for use in specific test procedures, such as, the Bowie-Dick test for air removal
Type 3 Single variable indicators	These indicators are designed to react to one of the critical sterilisation variables, e.g. time and temperature, and are intended to indicate exposure to a predetermined sterilisation process variable, e.g. 134°C
Type 4 Multivariable indicators	These indicators are designed to react to two or more of the critical sterilisation variables, e.g. time and temperature, and are intended to indicate exposure to a predetermined sterilisation process variable, e.g. 134°C, 3 minutes
Type 5 Integrating indicators	These indicators are designed to react to one of all critical variables of the sterilisation process, e.g. time, temperature and presence of moisture, and are intended to be equivalent to or exceed the performance requirements given in the ISO 11138 series for biological indicators
Type 6 Emulating indicators	These indicators are designed to react to all critical variables of the sterilisation process, e.g. time, temperature and presence of moisture, and are intended to match the critical variables of specified sterilisation cycles

3.6.7.1.2.10 *Cycle monitoring*

3.6.7.1.2.10.1 *Parametric release.* The physical parameters that can be measured without opening the pack such as temperature, pressure and sometimes steam quality.

3.6.7.1.2.10.2 *Load control.* Both chemical and biological types of indicators are used. Load control provides the assurance that the correct parameters for effective sterilisation were present in the load. Physical evidence is retained and stored with the cycle, physical printout providing proof for inspection.

3.6.7.1.2.10.3 In-pack monitoring. Generally, a Class 4, 5 or 6 chemical indicator is placed in the tray or wrapped item. The classification of the indicator would determine the level of assurance offered by this indicator.

It provides the assurance that effective sterilisation conditions were present within each tray and is physical evidence for the end-user to record.

Chemical indicators may fail because of inaccurate loading of the steriliser, wrong packaging or wrong packaging material; in-pack monitoring allows the operator to review these practices.

3.6.7.2 Chemical (low-temperature) sterilisation methods

Chemical gas (low-temperature) sterilisation is used to sterilise heat- and moisture-sensitive medical devices. With medical advances in developing delicate and intricate surgery such as minimally invasive surgery, some very expensive but heat-sensitive devices have been developed which cannot be processed by heat or steam.

In the past, liquid chemicals provided high-level disinfection at best, however recent developments have vastly improved the sterilant effect of chemicals and these are widely used for highly delicate medical devices that cannot be processed via other means. The process must be carefully structured and monitored with clear written policies. Be aware that not everything can be processed with every chemical and each medical device must have specific clearance from the manufacturer, to carry out a particular chemical sterilisation method. Chemical sterilisation will require the same steps of thorough cleaning, IAP and labelling. The packaging material may differ from system to system to allow adequate penetration of the chemical and removal after the process has been completed.

Process monitoring and product validation is paramount.

Written policies and procedures for chemical sterilisation should include:
- staff qualification, education/training and competency assessment
- preparation and packaging of medical devices
- steriliser operating procedures
- monitoring and documenting of chemical or cycle parameters
- workplace health and safety protocols specific to the chemical sterilant
- handling, storage and disposal of the sterilant (consult sterilant manufacturer's instructions for use and local regulations).

Chemical sterilisation methods are mainly based on converting chemicals into a gaseous state (Figure 3.15) to improve penetration and contact time under controlled conditions.

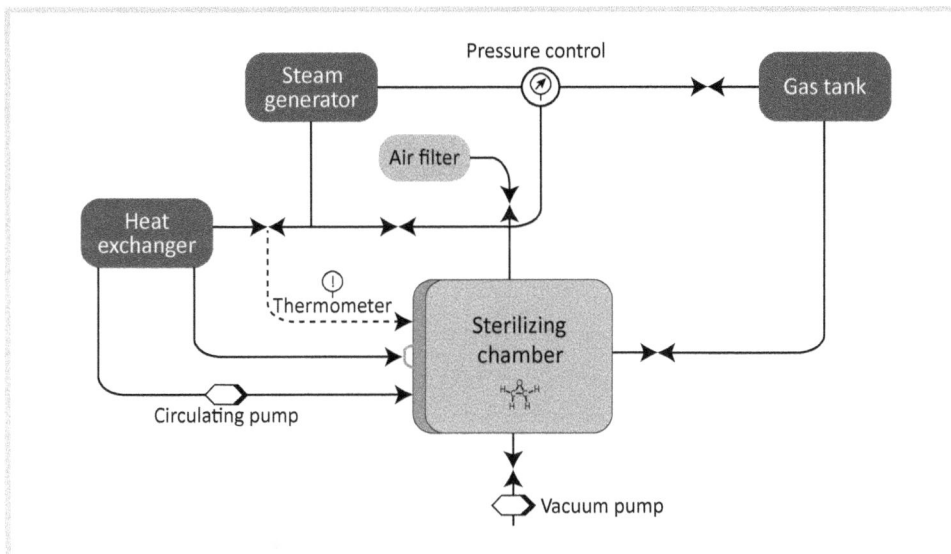

Figure 3.15 Generic gas sterilisation process diagram[26]

The process efficiency depends on the concentration of the gas, humidity, time of exposure, temperature and the bioburden. The mechanism of action will depend upon the sterilising agent, such as oxidation or alkylation that damage protein and DNA. After the process has been completed, complete removal of all agents and residues must be secured.

The essential steps are
- vacuum to remove air
- humidification to improve conditions within the chamber
- introduction of the gas
- sterilisation
- post-vacuum aeration, dependent upon the type of chemical gas used.

Chemical sterilisation has limited and specific use. It must be borne in mind that most of the present chemical sterilisation systems cannot sterilise liquids, textiles and cellulose-based materials (including paper packaging systems).

3.6.7.2.1 Validation for chemical sterilisation

Physical, chemical and biological indicators for specific chemicals should be used such as *B subtilis* for ETO and *G stearothermophilus* for hydrogen peroxide.

[26]   Adapted from Galante R, Pinto TJA, Colac OR & Serro, AP. 2017. Sterilisation of hydrogels for biomedical applications: A review. J *Biomed Mater Res* Part B 2015.

3.6.7.3 Types of chemical sterilisation

Some commonly used chemical sterilisation methods are summarised below.

3.6.7.3.1 Ethylene oxide (ETO)

ETO has been used to sterilise heat-sensitive equipment for many years. It is a colourless gas that is toxic, flammable and explosive and must be used in controlled conditions. The essential aspects which influence the effectiveness of ETO are:

- gas concentration
- temperature
- relative humidity
- exposure time.

These must be meticulously controlled.

Advantages of ETO

- can be used for heat-sensitive equipment
- good penetration into short lumen devices
- can reprocess unwrapped medical devices (instruments) or packs.

Disadvantages of ETO

- ETO is potentially toxic to humans and must be used only in controlled conditions – complete removal of ETO is essential prior to use of items.
- ETO is absorbed by many materials such as rubber and some plastics. For this reason items must be thoroughly aerated prior to handling or use following sterilisation, according to the device manufacturer's recommendations.
- The aeration cycle must not to be interrupted for any reason. Do not open the chamber to retrieve devices for use.
- Similar to all sterilisation processes, the effectiveness of ETO sterilisation can be altered by lumen length, lumen diameter, inorganic salts and organic materials.

3.6.7.3.2 Hydrogen peroxide gas (plasma)

Hydrogen peroxide (H_2O_2) has been used as a disinfectant for a long time. The conversion of hydrogen peroxide to gas and plasma state has greatly expanded its use in sterilisation of heat-sensitive equipment. Hydrogen peroxide gas sterilisation activity is primarily dependent on the gas concentration, exposure time and the process temperature. Materials and devices that cannot tolerate high temperatures and humidity, such as some plastics, electrical devices and corrosion-susceptible metal alloys, can be sterilised by hydrogen peroxide gas.

Advantages of hydrogen peroxide gas
- Depending on the concentration and contact time, hydrogen peroxide gas is considered an effective antimicrobial, including rapid bactericidal, fungicidal, virucidal and sporicidal activity.
- The gas is safe for use on most device and material types, including electrical components and electronics.

Disadvantages of hydrogen peroxide gas
- The equipment is expensive.
- Hydrogen peroxide is absorbed by paper and needs therefore expensive special packaging.

3.6.7.3 Ozone with or without hydrogen peroxide gas

Ozone is a potent antimicrobial chemical, but requires high levels of humidity. The steriliser creates its own sterilant internally from oxygen, steam-quality water and electricity. The sterilant is converted back to oxygen and water vapour at the end of the cycle by passing through a catalyst before being exhausted into the room. Duration of the sterilisation cycle is approximately 4 hours 15 minutes. The hydrogen peroxide and ozone gas combination versus only ozone has the benefit of a shorter cycle time and greater lumen penetration capability.

Advantages of ozone
- Ozone is compatible with a wide range of commonly used materials, including stainless steel, titanium, aluminium, ceramic, glass, silica, PVC, teflon, silicone, polypropylene, polyethylene and acrylic.
- This process is safe for use by the operator as there is no handling of the sterilant, no toxic emissions, no residue to aerate.
- A low operating temperature means that there is no danger of an accidental burn.

Disadvantages of ozone
- Incompatible with some materials (e.g. aluminum, brass and polyurethane).

3.6.7.4 Formaldehyde gas or low-temperature steam formaldehyde

Formaldehyde gas is biodegradable over approximately two hours in the environment. However, it is known to be a toxic, irritating and allergenic chemical; it is also referenced as a suspected carcinogen. Low-temperature steam formaldehyde is indicated for all materials used for haemodialysis. It is not widely used.

3.7 Tracking and traceability for sterilisation methods

Keeping good records of equipment and its movement is essential to the functioning of an efficient SSD. If possible, all equipment should be labelled and tracked so that any mishap can be followed up and, if necessary, a batch recalled. Devices should also be traceable so that a record of stock can be kept.

3.7.1 Labelling

All items which are processed through the IAP should be clearly labelled. The contents of each pack are clearly laid out on a sheet and are used during packaging. This sheet also acts as a worksheet and a checklist before the items are dispatched.

Labelling each pack or item gives an indication of the workload, assists with batch recall in the case of infections or problems with surgery, and can link the patient with a particular batch of processed equipment. Labelling also ensures that the load placed in a particular autoclave can be traced back to that autoclave in case of process failure. A register or log is kept of all receipts and dispatches each day.

The minimum information required is:
- cycle number/steriliser number
- date of processing
- expiry date
- contents
- sterilisation indicator.

3.7.2 Tracking

All items processed in an SSD should be logged so that there is:
- stock control
- stock rotation
- scheme for identifying the location of items, e.g. in storage, SSD etc
- a record of returned items after use
- record of arrival and dispatch of items into/out of the department.

3.7.3 Traceability

A workable system, either manual or computerised, should be in place to identify all stages of the decontamination process and use of equipment. This identifies the movement of items from the patient through the SSD processes and back to patient areas. The system could be manual or computerised. It should contain the following:

- Patient
  - Name
  - Unique ID
  - Location
  - Date
  - Instruments used
  - User/operator
- Process
  - Sterilisation cycle number
  - Date of process
  - Proof of successful process
  - Proof of validation of washer-disinfector/steriliser

3.8 Disinfection

Disinfection is a process which reduces the numbers of pathogenic microbes (except spores) to a level that is not harmful to human health. It is not recommended for sterilisation of a medical device, only high level disinfection, such as for endoscopes.

Disinfection of reprocessed medical devices can be achieved by heat or chemicals, although heat is preferred. Most automatic washer-disinfectors (AWD) combine cleaning and heat disinfection in one cycle (see section 3.6.4.2 on AWD).

In this section only the disinfection of medical devices will be addressed.

3.8.1 Choosing a disinfection method

Choice of disinfection method will depend on:

Patient susceptibility to infection: Immuno-compromised patients will need high-level disinfection or sterilisation for the devices used in their treatment.

Tolerance of device to heat, chemicals, pressure, moisture: Some devices such as endoscopes and other fibre-optic equipment are unable to withstand the temperatures required to achieve sterilisation and therefore chemicals are used.

Nature of the contamination/micro-organisms present: More resistant micro-organisms will require sterilisation in preference to chemical disinfection.

Time available for processing. Chemical disinfection is generally quicker than thermal cycles since the latter requires time to heat and cool down before use. With chemical disinfection, the process may be quicker but should be effective.

Risks to staff. Some chemicals are highly toxic and, in the absence of appropriate personal protection, can adversely affect staff working in the area.

Cost of processing. Some facilities may not be able to afford, or have available, newer more efficient, disinfectants which are usually expensive.

Availability of processing equipment. In low-resource countries disinfection is determined by the availability and regular supply of products and maintenance of equipment.

3.8.2 Indications for chemical disinfection

The use of disinfectants in clinical practice is limited to a few indications:

- Heat-sensitive devices and equipment that cannot be sterilised by heat, such as endoscopes and electrical items.
- The environment such as floors, ceiling and other surfaces do not require routine disinfection. However, occasionally there is an indication to disinfect with a chemical, such as body fluid spills, worktops in infectious isolation areas, mattress covers (rarely) and baths (occasionally).

3.8.3 Disinfection methods for medical devices

3.8.3.1 Thermal disinfection

This has already been covered under washer-disinfectors (see section 3.6.4.2). Temperatures of 80 °C for 10 minutes' holding time are recommended.

3.8.3.2 Pasteurisation[27]

This is a method usually used for milk and food products, but has also been used for respiratory and anaesthetic equipment. The device or fluid is exposed to 70–75 °C for 30 minutes. The higher the temperature, the shorter the exposure time – for flash pasteurisation the fluids may be exposed to 90 °C for less than one minute. Pasteurisation has been superseded by other more reliable methods in sterile services, but is still used in the food and beverage industry particularly for milk products.

3.8.3.3 Chemical disinfection

> **Before disinfection, devices must be thoroughly cleaned. This reduces the bioburden, removes biofilm and prepares the device for disinfecton. By cleaning, maximum exposure of all surfaces of the device to the disinfectant is facilitated.**

---

[27]   Gardner JF & Peel MM (eds). 1998. *Sterilisation, disinfection & infection control.* 3rd ed. Edinburgh: Churchill Livingstone.

In many countries chemicals are widely used to 'sterilise' items. The reasons for this are:
- lack of proper heat-processing equipment in the SSD
- turnaround times on devices too long and processing occuring in clinical areas
- the belief that 'disinfection' and 'sterilisation' are the same thing
- the belief that all chemicals are sterilants
- considered to be cheaper than investing in an SSD
- clinical staff wanting to be in control of processing.

It should be made clear that, **by definition, a disinfectant is not a sterilant** and should not be expected to replace sterilisation unless specifically proven to do so. Chemical disinfectants can be used alone or in combination.

Before embarking on purchasing and using disinfectant, consider the following:
- Make sure it is the correct disinfectant for the purpose for which it is intended to be used.
- Disinfectants harm living cells and therefore may harm humans.
- There is cross-resistance between antibiotics and disinfectants since the mechanisms of action are similar for both.
- Disinfectants may harm the environment (some are not biodegradable).
- They cost money – some are more expensive than others.
- They have specific indications for use and have limited value in healthcare settings.

3.8.3.3.1 Choice of disinfectant

The following should be considered in the choice of disinfectant:[28]
- Range or spectrum of antimicrobicidal activity – some devices will need a wider range.
- Rate of kill at use which refers to the log reduction[29] – a >6 log reduction is the standard used for quantifying disinfection by the EPA.
- Toxicity, irritancy, sensitisation of staff should comply with safety regulations.
- Compatibility with other agents and chemicals used – can irreparably damage expensive instruments.
- Inactivation by organic matter – will not be effective for surgical devices.
- Stability at use, dilution, room temperature and in the work environment.

---

[28]   Hoffman P, Bradley C & Ayliffe G (eds). 2007. Disinfection policy. In *Disinfection in Healthcare*. 3rd ed. Oxford: Blackwell, p 17.

[29]   EPA Product Performance Test Guidelines (2012). OCSPP 810.2200: Disinfectants for Use on Hard Surfaces – Efficacy Data Recommendations. Available at https://www.regulations.gov/document?D=EPA-HQ-OPPT-2009-0150-0021.

Further considerations are:

- **Efficacy.** Destroys pathogenic spores, mycobacteria, non-sporing bacteria, viruses and fungi.
- **Compatibility.** Non-damaging to instruments and processors.
- **Safety.** Non-irritating to patients and staff
- **Environmentally friendly.**
- **Cost.** Consider use concentration, stability and associated costs, e.g. processors, personal protective equipment.

3.8.3.3.2 Categories of disinfectants

Disinfectants are categorised according to the spectrum of activity based on standardised testing methods. The list of disinfectants is shown in Table 3.5 with their range of activities and their advantages and disadvantages.[30]

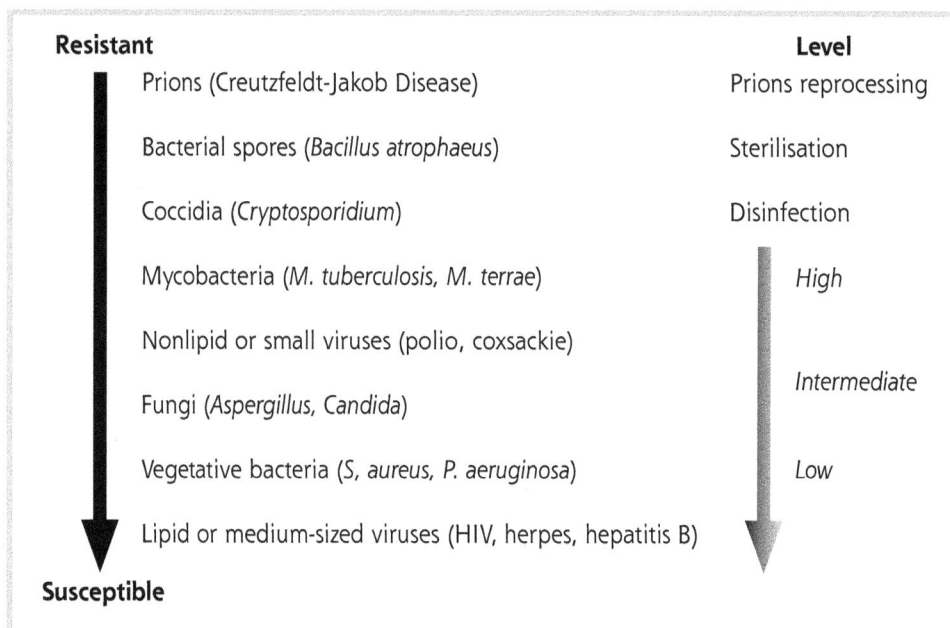

Figure 3.16 Level of antimicrobial resistance and level of disinfection required (https://www.cdc.gov/infectioncontrol/guidelines/disinfection/tables/figure1.html)

---

30   Friedman C & Newsom W (eds). 2007. *Basic Concepts of Infection Control.* Malta: International Federation of Infection Control.

Table 3.5 Disinfectants: spectrum, uses, advantages and disadvantages

Disinfecting agents	Spectrum (level)	Uses	Advantages	Disadvantages
Alcohols (60–90%) including ethanol, isopropanol	Low to intermediate	• Semi-critical and non-critical • Thermometers, stethoscopes • Rubber stoppers on multi-dose vials • Spot cleaning on surfaces	• Fast-acting • No residue • No staining • Low cost • Widely available	• Volatile, flammable • Irritant to mucous membranes • Inactivated by organic matter • May harden rubber, cause glue detoriation or crack acrylic
Chlorine and related compounds Sodium hypochlorite (3–8%) house bleach at a concentration of 100–5000 ppm free chlorine	Low to high	• Tonometers • Spot disinfection of surfaces • Dental appliances • Hydrotherapy tanks	• Low cost • Fast-acting • Readily available • Liquid, tablets, powder	• Corrosive to metal in high concentrations (>500 ppm) • Inactivated by organic matter
		• Water system in haemodialysis (high concentrations or chlorine gas)		• Discolouration/bleaching of fabric • Releases toxic chlorine gas when mixed with acids[31] • Skin and mucous membrane irritant • Unstable if left uncovered, exposed to light or diluted

31   https://en.wikipedia.org/wiki/Sodium_hypochlorite#Packaging_and_sale.

Disinfecting agents	Spectrum (level)	Uses	Advantages	Disadvantages
Aldehydes Glutaraldehyde: >2% aqueous solution buffered to pH 7,5–8,5 with sodium bicarbonate	High level to sterilant	• Endoscopes • (20 min at 20 °C)	• Good material compatibility	• Allergenic, irritant to skin and respiratory tract • Direct contact causes skin injury • Relatively slow activity against *M tuberculosis*
Other formulations available				• Requires monitoring for continuing efficacy levels • UK maximum exposure levels: 0,05 ppm (0,2–3mg/m3) • Short-term exposure (15 min) • Long-term exposure (8 h Time Weighted Averages)
Peracetic acid 0,2–0,35% and other stabilised organic acids	High level to sterilant	• Automated endoscopic systems • Sterilisation of heat-sensitive items, e.g. haemodialysers • Suitable for manual instrument processing	• Rapid sterilisation cycle time at low temperature (30–45 min at 50–55 °C) • Active in the presence of organic matter • Environmentally friendly by-products (water, oxygen, acetic acid)	• Corrosive to some metals • Unstable when activated • May irritate skin, conjunctivae, mucous membranes

Disinfecting agents	Spectrum (level)	Uses	Advantages	Disadvantages
Orthophthalaldehyde 0,55%	High level to sterilant	• Endoscopes	• Excellent stability over wide pH range • No need for activation • Superior mycobactericidal activity compared with glutaraldehyde	• More expensive • Stains skin and mucous membranes • Stains items not thoroughly cleaned • Eye irritation on contact • Hypersensitivity reactions • Slow sporocidal activity • Monitoring for continuing efficacy levels
Hydrogen peroxide 7,5%	High level to sterilant	• Cold sterilisation for heat-sensitive items 30 min at 20 °C	• No activation • No odour • Ecofriendly	• Material compatibility concerns with metals such as brass, copper, zinc etc
Hydrogen peroxide 7,5% plus peracetic acid 0,23%	High level to sterilant	• Haemodialysis disinfection	• Fast-acting (high-level disinfection in 15 min) • No odour • No activation required	• Material compatibility concerns with metals such as brass, copper, zinc etc • Damage to eyes, skin
Glucoprotamin	High level	• Manual endoscope processing, 15 min at 20 °C	• Good mycobactericidal activity • High cleansing performance • No odour	• Lack of activity against some spores and enteroviruses

Disinfecting agents	Spectrum (level)	Uses	Advantages	Disadvantages
Phenolics	Low to intermediate	• Environmental decontamination and non-critical items • To be avoided	• Not inactivated by organic matter	• Leaves a residual film on surfaces • Harmful to the environment • No antiviral activity • Reported hyperbilirubinaemia in infants (avoid in nurseries)
Iodophores (30–50 ppm free iodine)	Low level	• Disinfection of non-critical items, hydrotherapy tanks • Main use is as an antiseptic (2–3 ppm iodine)	• Relatively non-irritating and non-toxic	• Inactivated by organic matter • Adverse reaction with silicone tubing • May stain fabric • Not commonly in use as a disinfectant
Quaternary ammonium compounds	Low level Narrow spectrum	• Environmental surfaces • Skin antiseptic	• Stable • Non-irritating • Good cationic detergent	• Not recommended unless combined with other disinfectants

Adapted from Basic Concepts in Infection Control (International Federation of Infection Control, 2011)

3.8.4 Levels of disinfection

There are three levels of disinfection. Figure 3.16 illustrates the type of microbes and where disinfection can be applied. The recently discovered SARS-CoV-2 is an enveloped (also known as lipid) virus and can be added to hepatitis B and HIV.

- **High-level disinfection.** Disinfectants that kill all vegetative forms of bacteria, including mycobacteria and viruses, but require prolonged exposure time to kill spores. They are used for heat-sensitive critical items such as endoscopes and dialysis systems.

    Exposure for high-level disinfection as a general rule is 10–45 minutes at 20–26 °C, but longer exposure times are required for sterilisation. All items should be rinsed after exposure to remove any soil residue. High-level disinfection is commonly used in healthcare facilities. Good-quality water should be used to remove disinfectant residues (final rinse) to avoid recontamination of processed items with water-associated contamination. Sterile water is advised if sporicidal activity is required.

- **Intermediate level.** These disinfectants destroy all vegetative bacteria, fungi and most, but not all, viruses. They do not affect spores.

- **Low level.** These disinfectants destroy only fungi, vegetative bacteria (except mycobacteria) and enveloped viruses.

3.9   Endoscopy

Endoscopes are widely used for the following reasons:
- It is minimally invasive for the patient.
- Patient recovery is quick following an endoscopy.
- More patients can be investigated in a shorter period of time, eliminating the need for overnight hospital stay.
- Endoscopies can be conducted in designated clean areas outside the operating theatre.
- The cost per procedure is minimal.
- Complications are minimal.
- The infection rates are low.
- Technical skills among both clinical staff and those processing endoscopes have improved over the years.

3.9.1 Decontamination of endoscopes

Thorough cleaning and decontamination of an endoscope is a regulated process and is essential to ensure safety of the patient, care and prolonging the life of the instrument and, most importantly, reducing cross-infection. Blood-borne viruses such as hepatitis B and C, enteric pathogens (*Salmonella typhi*) and mycobacteria have been reported following endoscopy with inadequate cleaning and disinfection.

Flexible endoscopes probably pose the greatest challenge as they are heat-sensitive and the structure is complex, with some endoscopes containing numerous lengthy channels. Newer rigid endoscopes will withstand the temperatures required to achieve thermal disinfection and sterilisation. The manufacturer's instructions for reprocessing should be followed at all times. Failure to do this may invalidate any warranties associated with the equipment.

Most endoscopic procedures are carried out on the alimentary tract and the bronchial tree, which are normally colonised with endogenous flora. In this situation there is **intermediate risk** to the patient (Spaulding classification) and **high-level disinfection** is usually adequate. However, if sterile cavities, such as articulated joints, are entered, there is **high risk** and **sterilisation** is indicated.

3.9.2 Sources of infection during endoscopy

- Previous patient with an infection which is transmitted to the next patients owing to inadequate decontamination of endoscope before re-use.
- Contamination of the endoscope during reprocessing and storage.
- Endogenous skin, bowel or mucosal flora.
- Contaminated lubricants, dyes, irrigation fluids, rinse water.
- Inadequate decontamination of processing equipment – inadequate control of the process.
- Hands, air and the environment contaminating the instrument after it has been processed.

3.9.3 Challenges facing endoscopic decontamination

- Instruments and accessories are expensive – technical knowledge of the structure/channel configuration of the endoscope and the decontamination procedure is essential.
- Fibre optics are damaged by heat and pressure so careful processing is essential.
- They are complex instruments with multiple channels which are difficult to clean and dry.
- Penetration of channels by chemicals and detergents is uncertain.
- Disinfectants used for endoscopes are often toxic, damaging or ineffective so good knowledge of the types of available disinfectants is essential.
- Only short periods available for decontamination – a rapid turnover of patients with inadequate number of instruments can lead to:
  — exposure to toxic chemicals
  — inadequately cleaned and processed instruments
  — transmission of pathogens.

- Automated systems and environmental controls are expensive; sometimes funding is inadequate – the number of endoscopes is usually limited and often shared between institutions.
- Rapidly advancing technology – it is difficult to keep up with all the latest developments unless regular training is provided.

3.9.4 Medical Devices Regulations

The Medical Devices Regulations stipulate that manufacturers are required to provide information on the appropriate methods of cleaning, disinfection, packaging and, where appropriate, sterilisation to allow re-use of the device they supply (ISO 17664:2018).[32]

This should include compatibility with heat, pressure, moisture, processing chemicals (e.g. detergents, disinfectants) and ultrasonics. The provisions of this document are applicable to medical devices that are intended for invasive or other direct or indirect patient contact. Processing instructions are not defined in this document. These regulations do not apply to most developing countries but should be considered as part of the quality assurance.

3.9.5 Decontamination process

The processing of an endoscope is a specialised procedure and must be carried out by trained and dedicated staff in a dedicated room which is fully equipped with appropriate processing items. In order for proper decontamination to take place, the staff should understand the components of an endoscope. A brief description of the parts follows.

3.9.6 The endoscope

There are two types of flexible endoscopes available:

1. **Fibrescope** (fibre-optic endoscope). The flexible endoscope has an eyepiece for the operator to visualise the target site. A camera (video converter) is attached to the eyepiece which allows transmission of images to a monitor for better viewing of the anatomical site.

2. **Videoscopes** were popular in the past. These do not have an eyepiece and the image is directly transmitted to the monitor. However, these have been superseded by endoscopes.

---

[32]   ISO 17664:2018. Processing of health care products – information is provided by the manufacturer for the correct processing of medical devices intended for invasive or other direct or indirect patient contact. Processing instructions are not defined in this document.

3.9.6.1 Components of an endoscope

The flexible endoscope is highly complex, made up of channels with multiple accessories passing to the target site via a single insertion tube.

There are three functions (or systems) operating in an endoscope:

1. **Mechanical system**, which allows the distal tip to rotate for maximum visual clarity of the anatomical site.

2. **Plumbing system** through which water for irrigation is introduced and body materials, water, air or surgical smoke is removed.

3. **Optical system** transmits images back to the eyepiece or monitor so that appropriate therapeutic or investigative management can be provided.

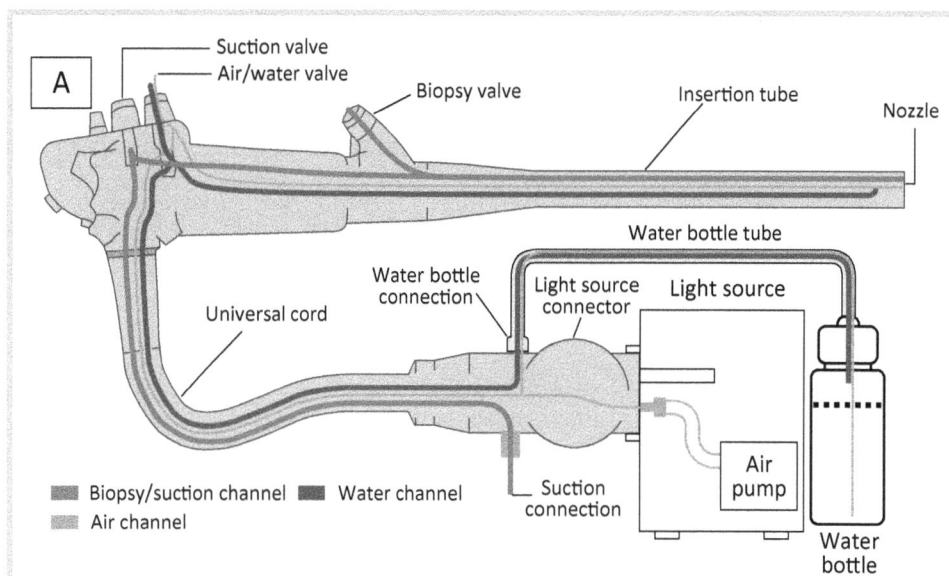

Figure 3.17 Anatomy of a flexible endoscope (courtesy of Olympus)

The main components are briefly described:

1. **Control body (A in Figure 3.17)**. This is the major junction where all the facilities of the endoscope come together
   (a) The control body houses the plumbing system for controlling instillation of air and water entry and providing suction.
   (b) Biopsy instruments are introduced via the biopsy channel for taking samples or undertaking minor cutting operations.
   (c) The control knobs for a complex angulated system are housed in the control body, which work either with a chain drive or a pulley wire design.

Precautions

- A dry lubricant is used to allow free movement of the components in the control body. If fluids enter the internal structure of the endoscope, the lubricant converts into a gritty sludge which damages the internal components.
- The junction between the control body and the insertion tube is stressed through repeated external bending and flexing. Although a reinforcement sleeve may be applied to reduce stress, over-extension and poor handling can damage the scope.

2. **Insertion tube.** This is the long, flexible part of the endoscope that contains the various channels and visual components of the endoscope. These internal components are made up of wires, glass fibre bundles and channels which transmit the essential components of an endoscope. A light is situated at the distal end via a guide light connector. The light is transmitted through thousands of fine glass fibres. If these are damaged, the light at the target site is reduced.

Precautions

- Insertion tubes can be damaged during a procedure if the patient bites and pierces it, allowing fluid to enter during processing.
- Damage can also be caused by the transportation box lid if handled carelessly.
- Ultrasonic cleaners must not be used on fibre-optic endoscopes because the tiny glass fibres become damaged by the vibratory motion.
- The biopsy channels are easily damaged by sharp or rough cleaning instruments.
- If a flexible endoscope is even slightly angulated during the passage of an instrument, the inner lining can get punctured or ripped.

3. **Bending/distal tip.** This is made up of metal coils reinforced by braided wires over the coils. It houses the biopsy port, air/water port, lens covering the image system and the lens covering the light.

Precautions

- The distal part is subject to the most manipulation and requires the most repairs. Most fluid invasion damage also occurs at the distal tip.
- Damage to the lens at the distal tip can be caused by mishandling, banging or knocking the distal tip.

4. **Light-guide connector.** The light-guide connector is attached to the light source. Other ports may also be connected to the light-guide connector so when removing parts or manipulating the light-guide connector during cleaning it may become loose and fluid can penetrate it. You should always ensure

the connector is tight. The channels are also present in this part of the endoscope and are attached at the light-guide connector for suction, air and water.

It is important that staff carrying out the decontamination process understand the structure of the endoscope and handle it very carefully.

3.9.7 Chemical high-level disinfection/sterilisation

Always follow the manufacturer's instructions.

1. **Pre-cleaning.** The first step in processing an endoscope is pre-cleaning and should be performed each time the endoscope has been used. Once the endoscope has been removed from the patient, the insertion tube is wiped with a damp cloth soaked in a detergent and the suction channel flushed. Using an adaptor valve, the air and water channels are flushed with water from the water bottle. This is an essential step in processing and usually takes place in the procedure room.

   The subsequent stages should take place in a dedicated decontamination room with facilities suitable for cleaning and disinfection. Access to a hand washbasin is essential.

2. **Leak testing.** After it has been wiped down, the endoscope must be tested for leaks to avoid fluid penetration into the various components of the endoscope and costly repair.

   The endoscope is disassembled and inspected carefully. The leak tester is attached and the endoscope pressurised. The entire endoscope is held under water and any air bubbles are noted. The distal end should be bent and moved in all directions to ensure no leakage occurs.

   If there is no leak, cleaning can take place; however, if there is a major leak, cleaning should not be attempted and the endoscope should be sent away for repair.

3. **Cleaning.** Each channel should be cleaned with the entire endoscope submerged under water to avoid splashing. Use only detergents and chemical agents that are recommended by the manufacturer. Brush all accessible channels (suction/biopsy) with a brush of the correct length and diameter. After brushing, irrigate all channels using the flushing adaptor with freshly prepared detergent solution, ensuring it is at the recommended temperature and concentration. An enzymatic detergent solution is preferred. Ensure that even channels which have not been used during the procedure are thoroughly cleaned. This prevents bacterial contamination

4. **Rinse** all channels to remove all detergent residues. If left behind, these can affect the disinfection/sterilisation process and may damage the endoscope.

5. The channels of the endoscope should be **flushed with air** before proceeding to chemical disinfection or sterilisation.

6. **Chemical disinfection.** Whichever method of disinfection is preferred, it is essential that the manufacturer's guidelines are followed when making up the solution to ensure its efficacy. Prolonged use of disinfectants does not enhance killing and may damage the instrument. Equally, overuse of a solution will reduce its efficacy over time. **It is important to ensure that the disinfectant accesses all internal and external surfaces of the endoscope for the required contact time.**

7. After the required **contact time** the disinfectant residues must be removed by thorough rinsing with water of a quality that will not recontaminate the endoscope. The rinse water should be used once and discarded to avoid the build-up of disinfectant that could remain in the endoscope. There have been reports of irritation of the patient mucosa by disinfectant residues.

8. **The final stage** is to blow air down the channels and to dry the external surfaces.

   Remember: (a) Documentation should be in place to record that the endoscope has been processed and is ready for patient use. (b) Sterilisation may be achieved with ethylene oxide and sporicidal activity with peracetic acid.

   When choosing a chemical disinfection system, consider the following:
   - It should be suitable for heat-sensitive instruments such as endoscopes.
   - Items cannot be packaged to prevent recontamination so it should be effective in providing high-level disinfection.
   - Disinfectants are often toxic and sensitising.
   - Thorough rinsing is necessary to remove toxic residues.
   - Often inadequate process controls/validation are noted with disinfectants.
   - Traceability is essential.

9. Once the disinfection cycle is completed, the instrument must be **rinsed thoroughly** and dried.

   There are no short cuts to the processing cycle and premature removal of an instrument can lead to serious consequences such as transmission of pathogens and inadequate removal of chemicals.

10. **Maintenance and repair** of all endoscopes is essential to ensure safe and effective usage of the instrument.

3.9.7.1 Automated washer-disinfectors for endoscope

Automatic washer-disinfectors are preferred to manual decontamination; however, there are some shortcomings:
- The processing machine might become contaminated because of inadequate cleaning, disinfection or regular maintenance.

- There may be static water in the tanks and pipeworks, which is highly colonised with pathogens.
- The quality of water may be poor and inadequate to allow good cleaning and thus residue may be left behind or interact with the recommended chemicals.
- There may be biofilm formation within the machine, which will act as a source of contamination.

The water used for rinsing endoscopes should be bacteria-free. This is achieved by various means (see section 3.5.6, Water quality).

3.9.7.2 Validation of decontamination

There are numerous tests described in HTM 2030, but the minimum is for the user to ensure:
- All channel irrigation occurs.
- Disinfectant is within the minimum effective concentration.
- Quality of water is adequate:
  — total viable count – weekly
  — environmental mycobacteria – annually
  — bacterial endotoxins – annually.

3.9.7.3 Traceability

Endoscopes, like other medical devices, should be traceable in case of an adverse event such as an outbreak or chemical contamination; in the UK Variant Creutzfeldt-Jakob disease (vCJD) is a major cause for concern and the relevant legislation requires traceability by law. All endoscopes should have a unique identifier and, when used on patients, this should be recorded in the notes.

3.9.8 Storage of endoscopes

Endoscopes that have been processed by high-level disinfection and have been left for longer than three hours should be reprocessed (MDA DB2002(05)).

Failures occur usually owing to human error. The staff are not adequately trained to understand the significance of their role in patient safety, especially when processing items. The causes usually are:
- inadequate cleaning
- unsuitable disinfectant
- damaged instrument
- contaminated rinse water
- contaminated washer-disinfector.

Occupational health and exposure

It is the responsibility of the manager of the SSD to ensure that all workers are well trained in health and safety and IPC, are fully immunosterilised and are clear about their responsibilities towards preserving their own health.

Appendix A

Manual cleaning

There should be a dedicated sink or basin for manual cleaning.

- Hot and cold running water taps.
- Drainage area for washed items.
- Mark the sink or basin with a level to which water will be filled.
- Plug the sink.
- Add a measured amount of detergent.
- Fill tepid water to the marked level.
- Wear rubber gloves, plastic apron, mask/visor or goggles.
- Carefully place the instruments into the water ensuring full visibility to avoid accidents.
- Using a soft brush, clean the surfaces with the device held below the water level to avoid splashing.
- Lift and inspect for complete removal of organic matter, especially at the hinges and teeth of the instrument.
- Once clean, rinse and allow to dry.

Hollow instruments (ideally cleaned in a washer-disinfector) should be cleaned with a high-pressure nozzle water jet (5 bar or 72 psi) which is attached to the tap. In the absence of a water jet, a large syringe (50 ml) may be used to flush the lumen through several times. Inspect and ensure it is clean.

To prevent spreading a possible contamination, keep the hollow instrument under water while spraying.

Appendix B

Choice of materials and methods for packaging of sterile supplies (primary packaging)

Depending on what is to be packaged, a choice is made for the materials and method of packaging. Often the manufacturer of instruments and other medical supplies may give specific instructions for packaging and sterilisation that must be adhered to. Any combination of load, its packaging and sterilisation process should be validated. The number of layers for primary packaging will depend upon local practice, but it is usually one for clinical areas and two for operating theatres. The following serves as a guideline for steam sterilisation:

Item	Recommendation
Textile packs	• Two sheets of packaging material: parcel-fold or envelope-fold • Container, laminated film pouch
Small quantities of textile and/or bandages/swabs	• One laminated film pouch or two • Container
Instrument sets in trays/baskets	• Two sheets of packaging material: parcel-fold or envelope-fold • Container, laminated film pouch
Individual instruments	• Laminated pouch • Container
Bowls and trays (small)	• Laminated film pouches • Container
Catheters, tubing, hoses	• Laminated film pouch • Two sheets of packaging material • Paper bag • Container
Scopes	• Special container • Laminated film pouch • Two sheets of packaging material, paper bag
Fine surgical instruments	• Laminated film pouches • Special container • Two sheets of packaging material in combination with a support system/rack

4 Risk management in infection prevention and control

Briette du Toit Ludick, Buyiswa Lizzie Sithole-Mazibuko
& Shaheen Mehtar

Learning outcomes

What you should know after reading this chapter:
- Carrying out risk evaluation in IPC
- Interruption of transmission of infectious agents
- Transmission-based precautions
- Appropriate use of personal protective equipment
- Reducing risk from aseptic procedures
- Application of bundles

Introduction

Identification and analysis of risks associated with healthcare delivery is pivotal to an infection prevention and control programme.[1]

Risk management provides a systematic approach towards identifying and managing infection risks. Millar describes infection prevention and control (IPC) risk as 'the probability of exposure to a potentially harmful infective agent, the severity (potential seriousness) of the consequences of the exposure or a product of the probability and severity of harm'.[2]

The European Commission (EC2000B) defines risk as 'the probability of and severity of an adverse effect/event occurring to man or the environment following exposure under defined conditions to a risk source'.[3] A systematic application of risk management improves clinical practice and safety

---

[1]   Australian Government National Health and Medical Research Council. 2019. Australian Guidelines for the Prevention and Control of Infection in Healthcare. https://www.nhmrc.gov.au/about-us/publications/australian-guidelines-prevention-and-control-infection-healthcare-2019#block-views-block-file-attachments-content-block-1.

[2]   Millar M. 2009. Infection control risks. Journal of Hospital Infection 71(2): 103–7.

[3]   European Commission. 2000. First report of harmonisation of risk assessment procedures – part 2. Brussels: European Commission.

for both patients and staff. This concept has recently been extended to 'bundling', which will be addressed later in this chapter.

IPC risk management is important to:
- proactively reduce the risk
- identify unsafe and hazardous practices
- improve clinical practices
- improve clinical outcomes and reduce healthcare-associated infections
- ensure safety of patients, visitors and healthcare workers
- recommend cost effective preventive measures.[4]

The elements of risk management are:[5]
- **leadership** with insight and an understanding of the importance of IPC, demonstrating accountability and leading by example
- **a functional IPC committee** that has the mandate to assist with risk assessments and implementation of corrective actions
- **clear and concise policies and procedures** outlining the IPC programme and guiding practices
- **ownership by and accountability** of healthcare workers
- **strong culture of training and education**[6]
- **trust** between the various teams involved in risk management.

4.1   What is risk?

In order to understand risk we should consider the difference between a hazard and a risk. IPC is based on risk assessment and the outcome or interventions will depend on the type and extent of risk a particular situation poses.

4.1.1 What is the difference between hazard and risk?

4.1.1.1 Hazard

A hazard is anything with the potential to cause harm to
- a person (e.g. injury or illness)
- property (e.g. financial losses)
- the environment (e.g. contamination).

---

[4]   International Federation of Infection Control. Risk Management. December 2013.
[5]   Australian Government National Health and Medical Research Council. Australian Guidelines for the Prevention and Control of Infection in Healthcare. 2019 https://www.nhmrc.gov.au/about-us/publications/australian-guidelines-prevention-and-control-infection-healthcare-2019#block-views-block-file-attachments-content-block-1.
[6]   Dramowski A & Mehtar S. 2014. *Infection Prevention and Control*. Bettercare.

4.1.1.2 Risk

Risk is a combination of the following:

- frequency of exposure to the hazard – how often does exposure to a hazard occur?
- probability of an outcome (given the exposure) – what will happen when exposure to a hazard has occurred?
- severity of the outcome – how serious is the outcome of this exposure?

Risk = Exposure x Probability x Severity

Risk is determined by the interaction of an individual with a hazard.

Example:
A freshly cleaned floor is usually slippery (hazard). Several people might walk carefully across it without any problem. There is a risk of slipping, but it is low. An elderly patient, who is less steady on his or her feet, might slip and fracture his or her hip (high risk). This has serious consequences for both the patient and the hospital management (outcome).

4.1.2 Carrying out a risk assessment

Managing risk requires understanding, confidence and constant application of good practice to ensure risk is reduced.

4.1.2.1 What is IPC risk assessment?

Risk assessment **is the process** where hazards and **risks** that have the potential to cause harm (**hazard** identification) are identified. These are analysed and evaluated as to the level of risk associated with each hazard (risk analysis and evaluation) (Figure 4.1).

An IPC risk assessment should include the elements[7] discussed next.

4.1.2.1.1 Identify hazards

- by area – divide the facility into specific areas, e.g. ICU, wards, theatre etc
- by task – identify hazards associated with each task, e.g. urinary catheterisation, central line placement
- by process – identify hazards at each step of a process, e.g. 'delivering surgery in the hospital'

---

[7]   Canadian Centre for Occupational Health and Safety. https://www.ccohs.ca/oshanswers/hsprograms/risk_assessment.html.

- by group – identify hazards related to a specific group of persons, e.g. employees, nurses, doctors, specific groups of patients

  Other hazards particularly relevant to IPC include:
  — source of the pathogen
    — patients
    — visitors
    — healthcare workers (MRSA carriers)
    — the patient's environment
  — identification of the pathogen
    — bacteria, virus, fungus
    — anything special such as antimicrobial resistance
  — routes of transmission
    — liquid (blood/body fluids)
    — aerosol (airborne)

4.1.2.1.2 Analyse and evaluate risks associated with the hazard

Determine how likely it is that the identified risk will cause harm and how serious the harm will be.

4.1.2.1.3 Determine appropriate measures to prevent, reduce or control the hazard

What preventive measures can be implemented to prevent or control the harm.

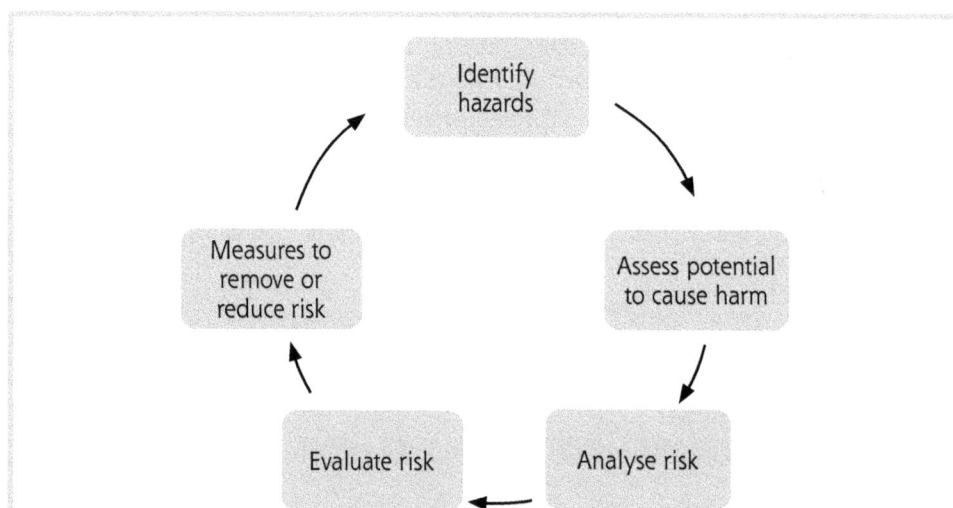

Figure 4.1 Risk assessment and management flow for IPC (https://www.infectioncontroltoday. com/view/10-elements-consider-when-conducting-infection-risk-assessment)

4.1.3 Planning risk assessment

You need to develop a structured plan of action based on the evidence gathered from assessing the risk. The plan should include other departments such as occupational health, clinical, nursing and engineering.

The advantages of such an approach are to assess how well an intervention has worked, re-assessment of the situation and organisational learning as a continuous process or audit cycle.

4.1.3.1 Steps in planning a risk assessment

- **Perform an assessment** of the service to establish the context within which it operates (e.g. population demographics, services offered, size, complexity, stakeholders etc).
- **Identify infection risks** using a structured approach in identifying relevant areas of risk in a facility.
- **Analyse identified risks in relation to the consequences and likelihood of occurrence** and determine what controls are in existence.
- **Evaluate the identified risks to determine management priorities**, review treatment options (control measures) and develop and implement plans to mitigate risk.
- **Continually monitor and review risks** and control measures to ensure effective management and to reduce or prevent risk.

Risk assessment should be carried out with the knowledge and co-operation of stakeholders, and it requires justification to both staff and patients.

4.1.3.2 Evaluating (assessing) risk

While perception of risk differs, standardised tools should be developed to evaluate risk against a set standard to eliminate subjective assessment (Figure 4.1). Evidence-based tools are developed but influenced by local conditions such as disease profile, resources and existing structures. The results should yield maximum information with minimum effort and should be simple to carry out.

For example:
- How much is this risk? **Measure extent**
- How often does it happen? **Surveillance**
- Why does it happen? **Provision or lack of knowledge**
- Can this risk be eliminated? **Education, training, provision**
- If not, then can it be reduced to a minimum? **Audit, monitoring and evaluation**

The same principles apply to IPC; therefore a risk assessment must be carried out when dealing with any opportunity which requires an IPC intervention no matter how big or small (Figure 4.1).

4.1.4 Review in the risk management process

The following areas are for review in the risk management process in relation to the core elements of an infection control programme.

4.1.4.1 Effective management of the core elements of infection control practice[8] include:

- standard precautions
- additional (transmission-based) precautions
- employee health (immunisation)
- HAI surveillance
- environmental cleaning
- reprocessing of reusable medical and surgical equipment
- equipment/product purchases
- waste management
- building and refurbishment
- food safety
- laundry management.

4.1.5 Analysing risk

Identification and analysis of risk requires a systematic and comprehensive approach. Analysis is based on information, both previous and current, to provide a complete picture of occurrences. There could be several reasons such as the absence of policies, lack of training or lack of provisions, but most important is accountability. If such data is not available, a surveillance should be established and, once the information is available, it should be channelled towards appropriate interventions to minimise risk.

A risk analysis matrix may assist with risk analysis and evaluation and decision-making on whether the risks need action, and what the most appropriate risk mitigation strategies and methods may be.

---

[8]   Queensland Health. *Infection Control Guidelines*. Available at http://www.health.qld.gov. au/chrisp/ic_guidelines/sect2_elements.pdf.

Likelihood	Consequences				
	Insignificant	Minor	Moderate	Major	Catastrophic
Almost certain	Medium	High	High	Extreme	Extreme
Likely	Medium	Medium	High	High	Extreme
Possible	Low	Medium	Medium	High	High
Unlikely	Low	Low	Medium	Medium	High
Rare	Low	Low	Low	Medium	Medium
Low risk	Manage by routine procedures.				
Medium risk	Manage by specific monitoring or audit procedures.				
High risk	This is serious and must be addressed immediately.				
Extreme risk	The magnitude of the consequences of an event, should it occur, and the likelihood of that event occurring, are assessed in the context of the efectiveness of existing strategies and controls.				

Figure 4.2 Risk analysis matrix[9]

4.1.5.1 Methods of analysing risk

There are several methods that can be used to identify risks, the commonest being a fishbone diagram or the 5 Whys.

4.1.5.1.1 Fishbone diagram

The fishbone diagram[10] – also called the Ishikawa diagram or 'cause and effect' diagram – (Figure 4.3) is used to identify and analyse all the potential causes or contributing factors of a specific problem or event.

Causes are usually grouped into different categories and the following can be included:

- People: Anyone involved with the process
- Method: How the process is performed and the specific requirements for doing it, such as policies, procedures, rules, regulations and laws
- Equipment: Any equipment, tools, instruments etc required to accomplish the task
- Material: Raw materials, medication, parts, pens, paper, information and so on used in the process

9   The Australian/New Zealand Standard on Risk Management AS/NZS ISO 31000: 2009 outlines a stepwise approach to risk management: Australian Government National Health and Medical Research Council. Australian Commission on Safety and Quality in Health Care. Australian Guidelines for the Prevention and Control of Infection in Heathcare. May 2019.

10   MCSA. Continuous Improvement. Model 3. 2017. https://asq.org/quality-resources/fishbone; https://www.cms.gov/medicare/ provider-enrollment-and certification/qapi/downloads/fish bonerevised.pdf.

- Measurement: Data generated from the process that is used to evaluate its performance
- Environment: The conditions, such as location, time, temperature and culture in which the process operates

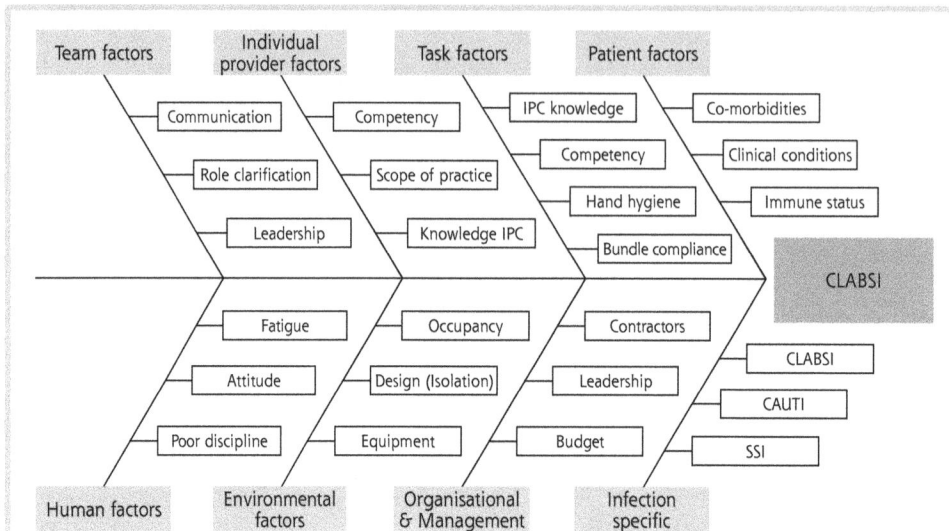

Figure 4.3 Practical example of using a fishbone diagram

4.1.5.1.2 The 5 Whys'

Another method that can be used to analyse risk is the '**5 Whys**', where you keep on asking 'why' until you have the answer. By repeatedly asking the question 'Why?' you can peel away layers of symptoms, which can lead to the root cause of a problem. For example:[11]

- **Why did the patient develop a CLABSI?**
  Because he had a central line inserted.
- **Why is the central line insertion site a risk in this case?**
  Because the femoral artery site was used.
- **Why is the femoral area a problem?**
  Because the risk of infection is much higher.
- **Why is the risk higher?**
  The area is potentially colonised with gram-negative pathogens, moist, skin folds, higher risk of contamination with body fluids etc.

---

[11]   American Society for Quality (ASQ). Five Whys and Five Hows Model 3. 2017. https://asq.org/quality-resources/five-whys.

- **Why is catheter type and duration important?**
  Multiple lumens provide multiple access sites and a possible risk of contamination. The longer the line is in situ, the higher the possibility of an infection occurring.
- **Why, why, why . . .**

4.1.5.2 Minimising or reducing risk

Risk is reduced when specific interventions are put into place (if these do not already exist) and the outcome is assessed. Risks should be prioritised and the highest risk should be attended to first. The priorities should be set for the entire healthcare facility, including management, and be reviewed regularly.

The following administrative structures are for risk reduction in IPC:

- **Establishing an effective IPC committee** plays an important role in facilitating the introduction and reinforcement of appropriate infection control practices. This must be done with input from other departments and result in the desired behaviour in the organisational culture.
- **Policies and procedures** for infection control established and adopted throughout a healthcare organisation provide the foundation for a safe healthcare environment for staff and patients. Standard operating procedures (SOP) for each unit should be established.
- **Behavioural change** is required to implement clinical governance and facilitate the continuous improvement of quality in healthcare.

Key areas influencing behaviour include effective leadership, clinician ownership, education and training, and research and development.

Effective leadership brings about:
- political commitment, resulting in responsibility and accountability
- involvement of senior management of the organisation on the IPC committee to increase top-level commitment and support for an organisation-wide approach towards improvement
- provision of resources to enable behavioural change
- promotion of an organisational culture that facilitates identification, discussion and response to incidents and complaints
- rewarding of achievements to reinforce desirable behaviour.

Clinician ownership has the following effects:
- encourages clinician-driven change through empowering staff to identify problem areas and solutions and to contribute to policy decisions
- nominates opinion leaders to advocate for and demonstrate desired behaviour

- engages clinicians in the risk management process when developing the policies to improve risk identification and ownership of risk minimisation interventions
- promotes local accountability through use of infection control liaison representatives to facilitate communication between clinical staff and infection control personnel
- facilitates compliance with infection control policies and procedures by including this in the annual staff performance review.

Education and training accomplishes the following:
- provides consistent information regarding infection control principles to all staff
- ensures infection control information is provided in the facility orientation programme, including students and undergraduates
- ensures easy access to the infection control manual and IPC policies.

Research and development accomplishes the following:
- involves clinicians in review of clinical data (surveillance results) and engages them in the development of appropriate interventions
- forms collaborative links with clinicians to improve quality in areas posing infection risks (e.g. collaborating on research projects).

An example of applying risk management
The situation shown below is complex and involves several departments or units, such as management, occupational health, procurement of medical supplies, engineering and several clinical units.

A surgical patient is admitted to the ward for a surgical condition and is incidentally found to have had a persistent cough for the past four weeks. On investigation he is diagnosed with pulmonary tuberculosis.

The IPC and occupational health teams are called in to carry out a risk assessment. The plan is put into action after an initial meeting to discuss and approve the plan.

Risk factors	Yes	No
Patient diagnosed with TB within 48 hours of admission – early diagnosis (smear positive)		
Anti-TB therapy started immediately – within 24 hours		
TB IPC policies are in place		
Patient placed in isolation or separated from other patients		

Risk factors	Yes	No
Ventilation and airflows on the ward satisfactory		
Immuno-compromised patients on the ward separated from source		
Immuno-compromised staff not nursing patient		
Staff understand airborne precautions and fully implement them		
Personal protective equipment (PPE) – gloves, masks/ respirators readily available		
PPE used by all staff		
TB notification within one week to provincial structures		

4.1.5.3 Applying the plan

1. **Risk assessment.** Where is the patient located? Who else may be exposed? Where has the patient been in the hospital? What is the immune status of healthcare workers and other patients, availability of PPE, ventilation and policies?

2. **Identify the risk.** Applying the questionnaire above, the following can be established: If the answer to all the questions is 'yes'– the risk (or probability) of transmission is low. If the answers are 'no' to the majority of the questions, the risk of transmission is medium to high.

3. **Analyse the risk.** How many people could become infected? Who is most at risk of infection?

4. **Evaluate the risk.** What is available currently? What can be implemented quickly? What will take time to establish? Establish priorities.

5. **Monitor and evaluate risk reduction.** Have the current interventions such as providing PPE, stricter policies, introducing IPC measures worked? What else needs to be done?

4.2 Risk-reducing strategies

In the healthcare environment risk can be reduced by appropriate interventions and behavioural change.

High risk	Risk assessment	Low risk
Poor	Immune status	Good
No	Appropriate PPE	Yes
No	Well-trained staff	Yes
No	Adequate resources	Yes
No	Good management	Yes

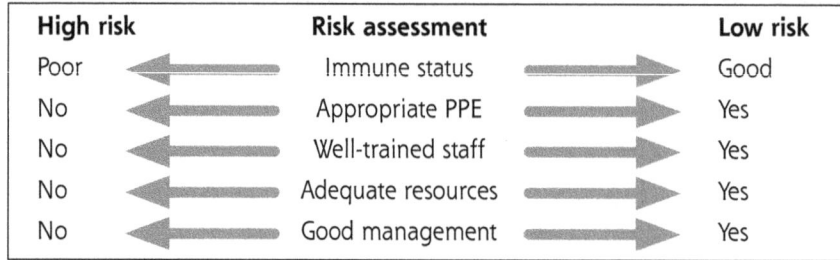

Figure 4.4 Risk can be changed from high to low with appropriate IPC interventions and behavioural change

Table 4.1 Transmission routes and levels of risk which can be reduced by effective interventions

Transmission route	High risk	Medium risk	Low risk
Hands	• No hand hygiene prior to aseptic procedure	• Touching an insertion site with unclean hands	• Bathing a patient with intact skin, bed-making
Airborne droplet Airborne (aerosol)	• Bronchoscopy • Induced sputum • Not wearing a face cover • Poor ventilation	• Crowded patient area • Standing in front of a coughing patient without a mask	• Proper PPE • Ventilation • Well trained in procedure and IPC
Clinical/non-clinical equipment	• No washing or cleaning facilities for equipment • Poor disinfection methods by unskilled staff	• Manual cleaning by untrained staff • Lack of PPE	• Good cleaning • Heat disinfection • Dry storage of clean items
Blood and body fluids (intravenous therapy) Sharps disposal	• Lack of PPE • Lack of skill • Absence of robust sharps boxes	• Bare hands: no gloves or other PPE • Rushed procedures • Sharps box far from procedure	• Appropriate PPE • Well-executed procedure • Safe sharps disposal

Risk can be reduced by understanding and consistently applying the following:
- knowing the modes of transmission
- appropriate and timely IPC intervention
- proper application of aseptic or safe technique
- use of appropriate PPE

- improving environmental factors such as cleaning and ventilation
- advising on procurement of appropriate medical devices and protective clothing
- producing simple yet effective guidelines or policies, for example antibiotics, disinfectants and use of PPE
- monitoring the implementation of such policies.

There should be routine practices in place which reduce the risk of transmission and these should be:
- simple and easy to follow
- for every indication where the risk is potential or real
- for every time it is indicated
- procedures carried out safely on patients.

4.2.1 Multimodal strategy

The WHO promotes a multimodal strategy (MMS)[12] as part of the core components for all IPC interventions which efficiently brings together five elements and requires commitment and involvement of the healthcare facility management team plus all the other teams.

These five elements are summarised as follows:

4.2.1.1 **System change** (Build it). To support and enable IPC practices such as infrastructure, supplies, equipment and other resources.

4.2.1.2 **Training and education** (Teach it). Increase and improve healthcare worker knowledge. This is crucial for IPC to be accepted by the other teams.

4.2.1.3 **Monitoring and feedback** (Check it). To assess the problem, drive appropriate change and document practice improvement.

4.2.1.4 **Reminders and communication** (Sell it). Promote the desired outcomes and constant reminders for IPC. Annual campaigns are also part of this.

4.2.1.5 **Culture of safety** (Live it). This provides a safe, blame free environment to facilitate an organisational climate that values the intervention, with a focus on involvement of senior managers, champions or role models.

The MMS is not easy to establish and takes a lot of hard work and dedication to ensure it comes to fruition and can be sustained. It requires a persistent team effort from management, IPC teams, clinical teams, procurement and engineering departments.

---

[12]   WHO multimodal improvement strategy. Geneva: World Health Organization; 2017. https://cdn.who. int/media/docs/default-source/integrated-health-services-(ihs)/infection-prevention-and-control/core-components/ipc-cc-mis.pdf?sfvrsn=5e06c3d5_10&download=true.

4.2.2 Hand hygiene[13]

4.2.2.1 Introduction

Eighty per cent of pathogen transmission both inside and outside healthcare facilities occurs via hands. Hand hygiene is a general term referring to any action of hand cleansing and has proven to be an effective risk reduction procedure. It has become the primary measure for reducing such transmission in healthcare facilities. In-depth information is available from the WHO website; here hand hygiene is summarised as a significant risk-reducing measure.

Hand hygiene is one of the most important ways to reduce the transmission of infections in healthcare settings. Included in the term 'hand hygiene' is any activity that reduces the level of contamination with micro-organisms, for example handwashing, alcohol-based handrub and surgical hand scrub. Hand hygiene should be part of one's behaviour and culture both at home and, more importantly, in the healthcare setting.

The most common micro-organisms transmitted to patients from the hands of healthcare workers are bacteria and fungi but viruses such as influenza, rotavirus and chickenpox can also be transmitted via hands (following transfer from contaminated surfaces). Parasites may occasionally be transmitted via contaminated hands (e.g. eggs from intestinal worms and scabies mites). Indirect contact with healthcare equipment and the patient environment may result in transmission. Respiratory particles (droplets) settle on surfaces after being expelled from the source. These land on surfaces surrounding the patient and can be transmitted through physical contact from these surfaces to humans.

> **The essential aspect of hand hygiene is not HOW, but WHEN, to carry out hand hygiene in order to protect the patient and the healthcare worker.**

Transient flora are usually carried on the skin for a short time only and is easily removed by hand hygiene and the action of rubbing. Resident flora live in the deeper skin layers (dermis) and are more difficult to remove.

Damaged skin is associated with changes in microbial flora of the damaged surface and increased colonisation with more species of microbes. Some are from the patient's own flora and others from external sources. In hospitals, colonisation of damaged skin with MDROs is common.

---

[13]   World Health Organisation. 2009. *WHO guidelines on hand hygiene in healthcare: First global patient safety challenge* Available at: http://whqlibdoc.who.int/ publications/2009/9789241597906_eng.pdf.

4.2.2.2 Transmission of pathogens via hands

Transmission of HAI pathogens from one patient to another via a healthcare worker's hands requires **five sequential elements**:

1. Organisms must be present on the patient's skin or have been shed onto inanimate objects immediately surrounding the patient.

2. Organisms must be transferred to the hands of the healthcare worker (during care activity).

3. Organisms must be capable of surviving for at least several minutes on the healthcare worker's hands.

4. Hand hygiene must be inadequate or entirely omitted, or the agent used for hand hygiene is inappropriate.

5. The contaminated hand/hands of the caregiver must come into direct contact with another patient or inanimate object that will come into direct contact with the patient.

> The main vehicle for transmitting infectious pathogens in healthcare settings is the contaminated hands of healthcare workers.

4.2.2.3 Reducing risk of transmission via hands

Handwashing action, i.e. friction, rinsing and drying, removes and kills transient flora from the superficial layers of skin; alcohol-based handrub (ABHR) results in further killing by reducing the micro-organism load on HCWs' hands and thus reduces transmission to the patient.

4.2.2.4 Barriers to effective hand hygiene

4.2.2.4.1 **Jewellery:** Skin under these items is heavily colonised with micro-organisms that are difficult to remove

4.2.2.4.2 **Nails:** Nail polish, long nails and artificial nails make hand hygiene difficult. Artificial nails and nail extenders increase the bacterial load up to nine times compared with bacteria found on hands. Nails should be a maximum of 6 mm long and should not extend past the end of the finger

> Long nails, nail polish, artificial nails and the wearing of jewellery prevent the healthcare worker from performing proper hand hygiene and carry microbes under the nails and around the nail bed.

4.2.2.4.3 **Skin:** Skin cracks, dermatitis or cuts can trap bacteria and may place patients at an increased risk.

4.2.2.5 Water temperature and products

- Warm water removes less protective oils than hot water, whereas hot water increases the likelihood of skin damage.
- To prevent contamination, products must be dispensed in a disposable pump container that is not topped up.
- An adequate amount of soap is required to dissolve fatty materials and oils from hands as water alone is not sufficient to clean soiled hands.

4.2.2.6 Effect of inadequate hand hygiene measures

- transferring microbes between patients
- increased morbidity and mortality among patients – septic shock and death
- outbreaks of HAI such as methicillin-resistant *Staph aureus* (MRSA), *Acinetobacter spp* and other multiple antibiotic-resistant gram-negative bacteria and rotavirus
- transmission of viruses from a contaminated environment, such as SARS-CoV-2
- self-colonisation of nose, throat and gut by HAI pathogens
- transferring bacterial and viral pathogens to yourself, your family and social circle
- medico-legal impact.

4.2.2.7 Principles of hand hygiene

The WHO has identified five times when hand hygiene should be performed by healthcare workers. These times have been named the 'WHO 5 Moments for Hand Hygiene' and form part of a global hand hygiene awareness initiative for healthcare workers. The five moments are:

- before patient contact
- before a clean or aseptic task/procedure
- after body fluids exposure risk
- after patient contact
- after contact with the patient's surroundings.

> **The WHO 5 Moments for Hand Hygiene serve as a reminder of when hand hygiene should be performed by healthcare workers.**

4.2.2.7.1 Hand hygiene and glove use

Some healthcare workers use gloves to avoid performing hand hygiene. Micro-organisms can be transferred through microscopic perforations (holes) in the gloves onto the healthcare worker's hands. If hand hygiene is not performed after glove removal, the healthcare worker's contaminated hands can then transfer micro-organisms to the next patient or patient environment.

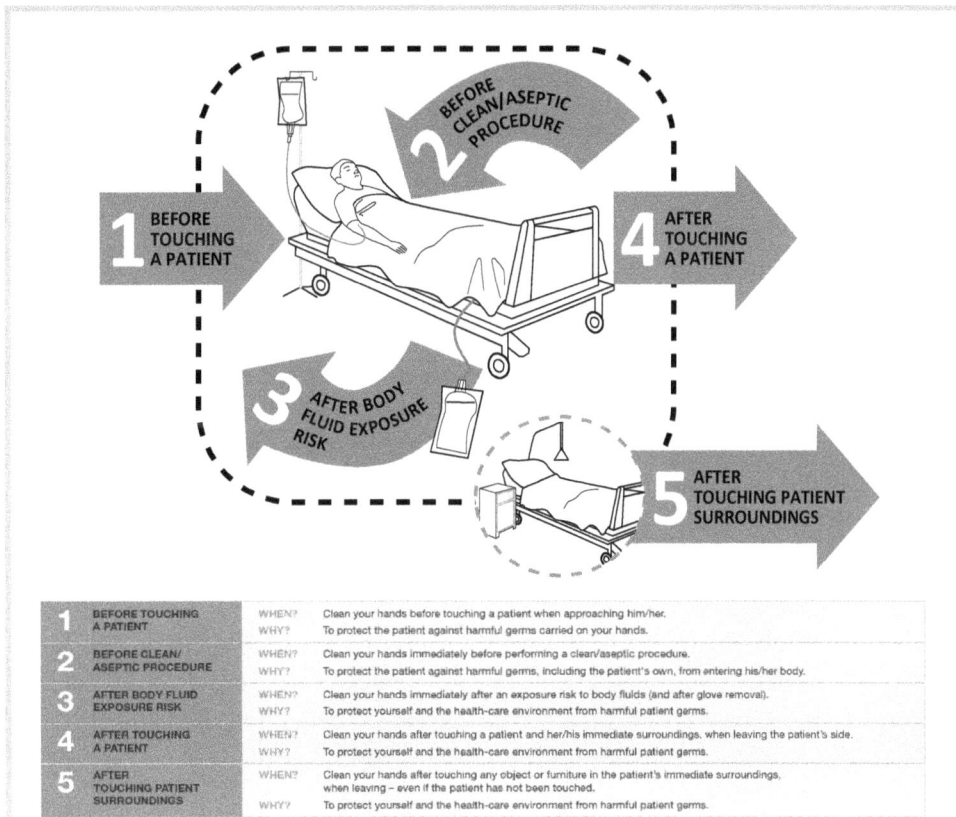

Figure 4.5 WHO 5 Moments of Hand Hygiene

Healthcare workers should use ordinary, clean gloves when direct contact with blood, body fluids, respiratory secretions, mucous membranes and non-intact skin is anticipated. Sterile gloves should be worn for any aseptic task, e.g. inserting a urinary catheter or performing a lumbar puncture. There is no need to wear gloves for routine patient care, e.g. turning, feeding or bathing a patient. All gloves are single-use only and should never be washed or used while caring for multiple patients. Gloves should be changed between each patient, when dirty or contaminated and when moving from a contaminated body area to a 'clean' area of the same patient.

NEVER USE GLOVES TO SUBSTITUTE THE NEED FOR HAND HYGIENE!
Micro-organisms can still be transferred through pores in the gloves.

For healthcare workers to understand the WHO 5 Moments of Hand Hygiene properly, they need to understand the patient zone, the healthcare area and point of care.

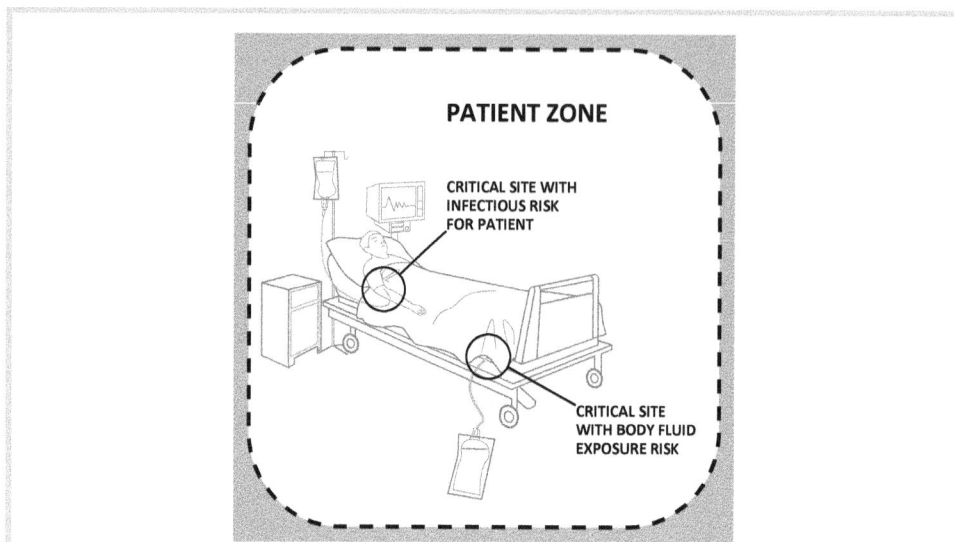

Figure 4.6   Healthcare area and patient zone are clearly illustrated

The **patient zone** (Figure 4.6) includes the patient and some surfaces and items that are exclusively dedicated to him or her, such as all inanimate surfaces that are touched by or in direct physical contact with the patient (e.g. bed rails, bedside table, bed linen, chairs, infusion tubing, monitors, knobs and buttons and other medical equipment).

The **patient zone** has two critical sites: clean site and body fluid site. Patient flora rapidly contaminates the entire patient zone and must be cleaned after each patient has been discharged.

The **healthcare area** contains all surfaces in the healthcare setting outside the patient zone (Figure 4.6). It includes other patients and their patient zones and the wider healthcare facility environment. The healthcare area is characterised by the presence of various and numerous microbial species, **including multi-resistant pathogens** and make up the microbiome.

Table 4.2 Summary of WHEN: WHO Five Moments for Hand Hygiene

Indication	From	Hand transition and micro-organism transmission risk	To	Major negative outcome	Examples
1. Before touching a patient	Surface outside the patient zone	From the healthcare environment to the patient	Patient's intact skin and other surfaces inside the patient zone	Colonisation of the patient by hospital pathogens	Opening the curtains and then shaking hands with the patient
2. Before aseptic/clean procedure	Any surface	From any surface (including the patient's skin) to a site that would facilitate invasion and infection	Critical site for infection in the patient	Endogenous or exogenous infection of the patient	Preparing the equipment and then giving an injection
3. After exposure to body fluid	Critical site for body fluid exposure	Exposure to patient's body fluids potentially containing blood-borne or other pathogens	Any surface	Potential HCW infection by patient blood-borne pathogens	Drawing blood and then adjusting the cannula
4. After touching a patient	Patient's intact skin and other surfaces inside the patient zone	From the patient flora to other surfaces	Surface outside the patient zone	Spreading patient flora to the rest of the healthcare environment and potential infection risk to HCW	Shaking hands with the patient, moving the bedside table, and then touching the door handle
5. After touching patient surroundings (without touching the patient)	Surface inside the patient zone if the patient was not touched	From the patient flora to other surfaces	Surface outside the patient zone	Spreading patient flora to the rest of the healthcare environment and colonisation of HCW	Touching the bed rail (without touching the patient) and then touching the door handle

The **point-of-care** refers to the place where three elements occur together: *the patient, the healthcare worker, and care or treatment involving patient contact* (within the patient zone). The concept embraces the need to perform hand hygiene at recommended moments exactly where care delivery takes place. This requires that a hand hygiene product (e.g. ABHR if available) be easily accessible and as close as possible (e.g. within arm's reach) to where patient care or treatment is taking place. Point-of-care products should be accessible without having to leave the patient zone. This enables healthcare workers to quickly and easily fulfil the five indications (moments) for hand hygiene. Availability of ABHR in point-of-care is best achieved through HCW carrying personal handrubs (pocket bottles), wall-mounted dispensers or handrubs affixed to the patient's bed or bedside table or to dressing or medicine trolleys that are taken into the point-of-care. In Table 4.2 on the previous page, Sax et al[14] clarified the WHO 5 Moments of Hand Hygiene and when and how to apply them.

4.2.2.8 Hand hygiene methods available for healthcare workers

1. Handwashing
2. Handrub with alcohol-based handrub
3. Surgical hand scrub.

4.2.2.8.1 Washing hands

Washing hands with plain soap and water is recommended when hands are visibly soiled. Hands must be dried thoroughly after washing as wet hands serve as a medium for micro-organisms to multiply. Medicated soaps are not recommended for routine handwashing because there is no added value, and some promote antimicrobial resistance.

4.2.2.8.1.1 Hand drying

Wet hands have higher bacterial counts and lead to dryness and cracked skin and increased latex allergies. Hands should be dried on disposable paper towels.

> **Air dryers are not appropriate in healthcare settings. They carry a risk of air dispersal from the hands to the surrounding environment.**

---

[14]   Sax, H, Allegranzi, B, Chraïti, MN, Boyce, J, Larson, E & Pittet, D. 2009. The World Health Organization Hand Hygiene Observation Method. *American Journal of Infection Control* 37: 827–34. https://doi.org/10.1016/j.ajic.2009.07.003.

0 Wet hands with water;	1 Apply enough soap to cover all hand surfaces;	2 Rub hands palm to palm;
3 Right palm over left dorsum with interlaced fingers and vice versa;	4 Palm to palm wit fingers interlaced;	5 Backs of fingers to opposing palms with fingers interlocked;
6 Rotational rubbing of left thumb clasped in right palm and vice versa;	7 Rotational rubbing, backwards and forwards with clasped fingers of right hand in left palm and vice versa;	8 Rinse hands with water;
9 Dry hands thoroughly with a single use towel;	10 Use towel to turn off faucet;	11 Your hands are now safe.

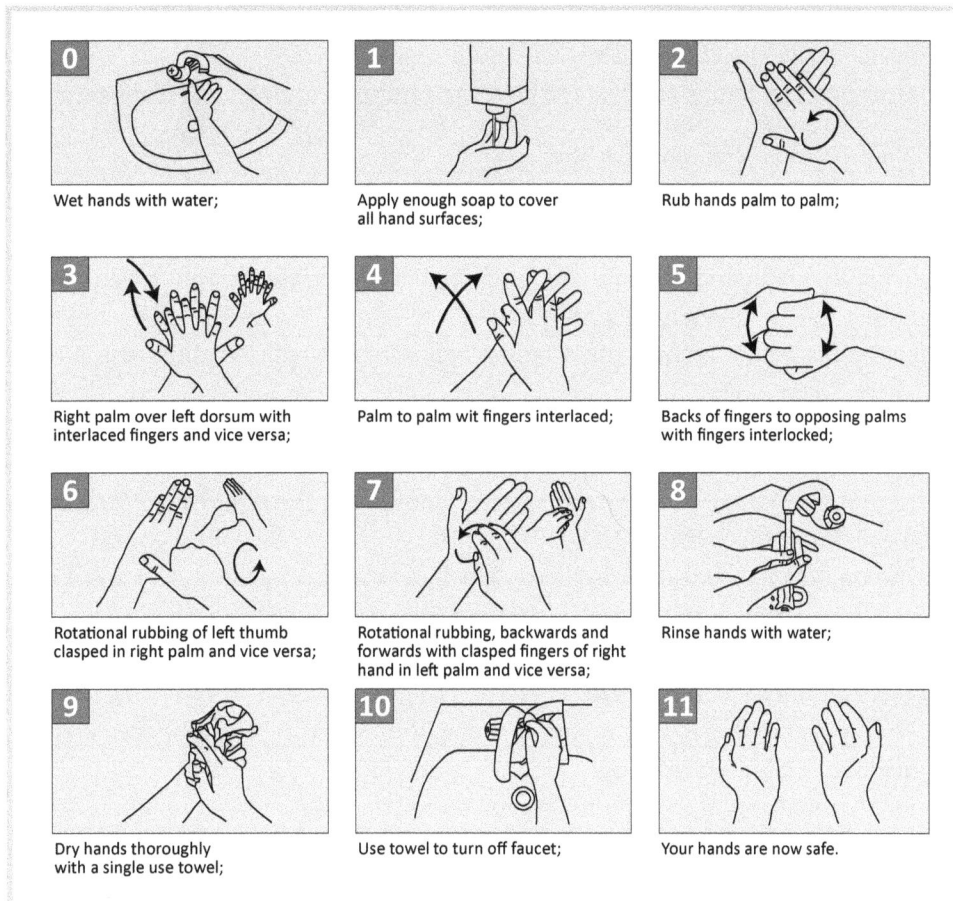

Figure 4.7 Illustration of the WHO technique on handwashing. Note: palm-to-palm rubbing to start.

4.2.2.8.1.2 *Placement of handwash facilities*

The location of handwash facilities is also critically important to encourage hand hygiene compliance **Handwash basins should be placed away from direct clinical areas to avoid splash contamination of the patient zone**. Ideally these should be placed just outside or just inside the entrance.

Some examples are shown below at the entrance of all wards and clinical areas
- inside treatment rooms and physical examination rooms
- inside or close to each nursing station
- inside each dirty utility room (in addition to sinks)
- inside all isolation rooms
- at the entrance of the medication room
- inside any room where food is handled/prepared (hospital kitchen, ward kitchen, breast milk and baby formula handling areas)

- close to each laboratory workstation
- inside each clinical laboratory and morgue
- in areas where hands are likely to be contaminated – storage and disposal areas.

4.2.2.8.1.3 An ideal handwash station

The ideal handwash station should be located at the exit of the clinical area (see Chapter 5 on the Built Environment) and are dedicated for handwashing only. Liquid soap and paper towels are preferred. Pedal-operated 'no touch' waste bins are ideal to prevent recontamination of hands. A laminated poster with instructions on how to wash hands effectively should be placed above the sink.

4.2.2.8.1.4 Liquid soap

Wall mounted holders for liquid soap which are either supplied as single use sachets (500 ml) or closed containers with plungers. If the liquid soap containers are re-used, ensure that:
- The liquid soap container is clearly labelled with its contents, an expiry date and 'For Handwashing Only'.
- The nozzle is clean and working properly.
- The container should not leak.
- The empty containers are replaced and sent for cleaning and (if possible) heat disinfection before refilling.
- There is no topping up of liquid soap at ward level.

4.2.2.8.1.5 Bar or tablet soap

These are used in some hospitals. They are acceptable only if the soap is stored dry either on a stand or suspended (soap-on-a-rope) and kept dry.

4.2.2.8.1.6 Hand drying

Paper towels are usually used to dry hands and are the best option. They should be of good absorbent quality, otherwise several sheets are used at a time, which is wasteful and expensive. Cloth towels are not recommended for aseptic hand hygiene since the cotton absorbs moisture and may harbour potentially pathogenic microbes. Single cotton towels (squares) placed in a pile, used once only and then discarded into a laundry basket, are acceptable; however, there is a problem of theft. Another option is cotton roller towels that are pulled down for each use and laundered when the roll is used up, and then replaced with a fresh one. The disadvantage is cross-infection with healthcare-associated infection (HAI) pathogens.

Air dryers are commonly found in public places, but are inappropriate for health facilities. They carry a risk of air dispersal from the hands to the surrounding environment and are not recommended.

4.2.2.8.2 Alcohol-based handrub (ABHR)

In almost all instances it is preferable to use ABHR, rather than soap and water. The entire handrub procedure is much faster than handwashing, less drying to the skin and alcohol achieves better and faster bacterial killing. ABHR should not be used if hands are visibly soiled with dirt, blood or body fluids, or after potential exposure to spore-forming pathogens (e.g. *C difficile*). **If one has washed hands with soap and water, it is unnecessary to use ABHR in addition.**

4.2.2.8.2.1 *How does ABHR work?*

Alcohol penetrates the cell membrane of bacteria and fungi or the viral envelope, causing damage (denaturing) of the micro-organism's genetic material and thereby killing the micro-organism. It is important to note, though, that to achieve maximal killing the alcohol must be in contact with the skin at sufficient concentrations and must be allowed to dry.

> **WHO recommends alcohol formulations with at least 60–80% alcohol content, as this concentration is most effective at killing micro-organisms. See WHO ABHR Formulations https://www.who.int/publications/i/item/WHO-IER-PSP-2010.5.**

DO NOT USE ALCOHOL HANDRUB!
- If hands are visibly soiled with dirt, blood or body fluids, use soap and water to clean.
- Alcohol is not effective at killing bacterial spores and less effective at killing certain types of viruses (non-enveloped viruses, e.g. noro- and rotavirus).
- In patients with *C. difficile* infection (a spore-forming bacterium that causes severe gastrointestinal disease), healthcare staff should wash hands with soap and water.

> **There is evidence that alcohol-based handrubs (with concentrations above 60% alcohol) are still better than soap and water for killing gastrointestinal, non-enveloped viruses.**

4.2.2.8.2.2 *Handrub technique (for ABHR)*

New evidence has come to light that required revision of the handrub technique from the palm-to-palm method to **dipping fingertips in the alcohol rub first**. The latter gave the best results in reducing bacterial counts. The palm of one hand is filled with alcohol rub and the fingertips of the opposite hand are dipped into the alcohol, and then the alcohol rub is poured into the other palm and the **opposite hand's finger tips are dipped into the alcohol contained in the palm**. The rest of the sequence is to be followed as previously described.

Rub hands for hand hygiene! Wash hands instead when visibly soiled.
Duration of the entire procedure: 20 - 30 seconds.

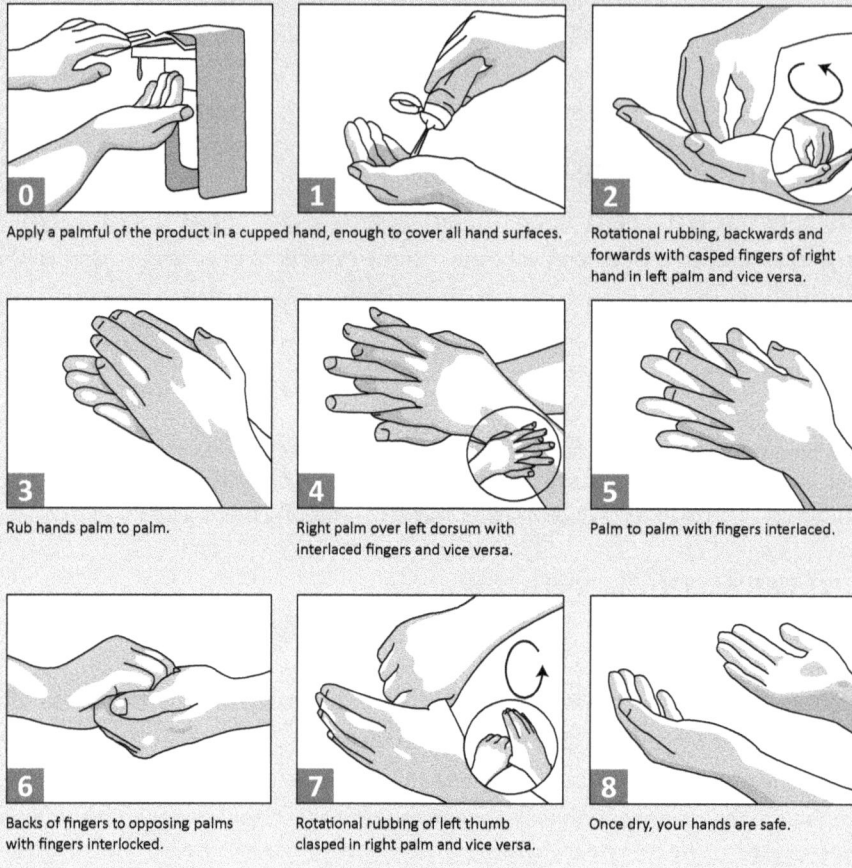

0 Apply a palmful of the product in a cupped hand, enough to cover all hand surfaces.

1

2 Rotational rubbing, backwards and forwards with casped fingers of right hand in left palm and vice versa.

3 Rub hands palm to palm.

4 Right palm over left dorsum with interlaced fingers and vice versa.

5 Palm to palm with fingers interlaced.

6 Backs of fingers to opposing palms with fingers interlocked.

7 Rotational rubbing of left thumb clasped in right palm and vice versa.

8 Once dry, your hands are safe.

Figure 4.8   Illustration of handrub technique. Note: dipping of finger tips in alcohol first.

4.2.2.9 Hand hygiene compliance

Staff and patient education, making ABHR available, reminders in the workplace (posters, campaigns), administrative sanctions and rewards, routine observation and feedback, and maintaining an institutional patient safety climate (where all healthcare workers are individually accountable for adverse events like healthcare-associated infections) are some of the factors associated with an increase in hand hygiene compliance.

4.2.2.9.1 Monitoring hand hygiene compliance

The best way to establish your healthcare facility's overall hand hygiene compliance rates is to directly observe healthcare workers during routine clinical care. There are many tools and forms available for monitoring and scoring hand hygiene compliance, such as WHO Observation tool available at https://www.who.int/gpsc/5may/tools/en/.

> **Education, compliance monitoring and provision of acceptable hand hygiene products are the most effective ways to improve hand hygiene compliance rates.**

4.2.2.9.2 Monitoring a facility-based hand hygiene programme (WHO MMS)[15]

The hand hygiene self-assessment form allows a healthcare facility to evaluate its hand hygiene practices towards behavioural change. It is a gradual process, but shows sustainable change. **It is recommended for all healthcare facilities and has the following steps:**

Step 1: Facility preparedness – readiness for action
Step 2: Baseline evaluation – establishing the current situation
Step 3: Implementation – introducing the improvement activities
Step 4: Follow-up evaluation – evaluating the implementation impact
Step 5: Action planning and review cycle – developing a plan for the next five years (minimum)

Ideally, hand hygiene audits must be done six-monthly, with results available to staff and managers. Other facilities promote hand hygiene programmes through campaigns, which include awards and incentives for areas with the highest compliance.

4.2.2.10 Components of hand hygiene

4.2.2.10.1 Antiseptics. Antiseptics are used on living tissue and are a major component of hand hygiene. The two commonly used ones are chlorhexidine gluconate and povidone iodine, both of which have a sustained effect on reducing bacteria although are not used as often.

4.2.2.10.2 Alcohol-based handrub. Alcohol is also an effective antiseptic and is widely used as a handrub (with emollient). It has several advantages and is becoming increasingly popular, especially in situations where quick hand hygiene is needed. The advantages of ABHR are that it:
- is a waterless antiseptic agent
- dries rapidly

---

[15] https://www.who.int/publications/i/item/a-guide-to-the-implementation-of-the-who-multimodal-hand-hygiene-improvement-strategy.

- contains the right concentration of emollients and thus it is not harmful to hands
- is accepted by most healthcare workers
- can be portable (on treatment trolley) or carried by staff in smaller containers
- can be placed close to patients as required
- does not need a handwash basin, towels and water
- can be supplied to the community during outbreaks.

Alcohol rub can be produced inexpensively by following the WHO in-house formulations (see Appendix A) and contains isopropyl alcohol (60–70%) with chlorhexidine (4%) and an emollient.

4.2.2.11 Poor adherence to hand hygiene

Although it is widely preached and recognised by healthcare workers and the public that hand hygiene is paramount in preventing transmission of pathogens, adherence to the practice is difficult. Several studies have reported adherence rates of up to 67% at best. Most of the studies reveal that healthcare workers do not wash hands willingly. Some reasons are:

- Hand hygiene agents cause irritation and dryness, especially if used inappropriately.
- Cheaper products tend to be purchased, which cause irritation (60–70% isopropyl alcohol vs methylated spirits or raw alcohol (90%)).
- Sinks are inconveniently located or absent – staff too busy to walk more than 10 m away from patient's bed.
- Lack of soap and paper towels at handwash basin – inadequate provision.
- Staff feel they are too busy or have insufficient time or may be called away in the middle of a procedure.
- Patient needs take priority and therefore the need for giving urgent attention often precludes proper hand hygiene.
- Perceptions that the risk of infecting patients is low, so staff are unconcerned.

4.2.2.12 Strategies for improving hand hygiene compliance

The main strategy should be to take hand hygiene to the healthcare worker. This can be achieved by wide use of ABHR, which is portable.

Another way is to provide emollients and creams to the healthcare workers, but this is not always affordable. Communal-use emollients have been known to harbour and transfer bacteria from one healthcare worker to another. Healthcare workers may carry their own personal hand creams provided the container is small and discarded when empty.

Other strategies to overcome challenges to hand hygiene are shown in Table 4.3.

Table 4.3 Challenges to hand hygiene and strategic solutions to overcome them

Obstacle	Strategy to improve hand hygiene
Lack of knowledge	Educate, instruct, revisit; feedback on behaviour and infection rates
Lack of motivation	Direct observation and regular feedback; role models; studies on hand disinfection; hand hygiene programmes for patients and families
Hand hygiene facilities	Convenient location of handwash basin, outside or just inside every room, including procedure rooms and offices; adequate supplies of hand disinfection and drying material; taps – elbow operated; ABHR readily available
Hand products	Need high level of acceptability by the staff; cost and supply; need mobile containers for ABHR
Allergies and dermatitis	Lotions to prevent dryness; testing products before purchase, compatibility between products and gloves; approved by ICU team
Traditional behaviour	Evidence-based teaching; discussion with staff on compliance

(WHO Hand Hygiene Guidelines, 2009)

4.2.2.13 *Care of hands*

All healthcare staff working in clinical areas should ensure the following:
- The hands are in good condition with intact skin. If the skin is broken or cut, it should be covered with a waterproof dressing.
- Finger nails are short and clean.
- Synthetic nail extensions or similar are unacceptable because:
  - They harbour micro-organisms.
  - The nails cannot be properly cleaned.
  - Antiseptics cannot reach the nail bed and surfaces.
  - Antiseptic may interact with the synthetic nails and cause a reaction.
  - Fungal infections of the nail bed may occur.
  - Staff with nail extensions often avoid hand hygiene.
- Jewellery, except a wedding band, should be removed. Several studies have shown the persistence of gram-negative bacteria beneath rings.
- Sleeves are loose enough so that these can be rolled up to the elbows.

All allergies (especially to latex, nuts or resins), dry skin or chronic dermatitis should be reported to the manager. The occupational health department should keep a record of all incidents of allergies.

4.2.2.14 Damage to hands and skin

Hands can get very dry and develop cracks from excessive washing, vigorous scrubbing, using alcohol agents without emollients or because of allergies to the antiseptic. Dryness can also occur if the hands are not dried thoroughly after washing. Skin damage ranges from mild to severe and may jeopardise clinical activity. The consequences of damaged (dry, cracked) skin are:

- increased colonisation with transient pathogens
- increase in latex and other allergies
- increase in chronic dermatitis
- restricted work practice.

4.2.3 Risk-reducing precautions

Clinical procedures require physical contact between HCW, patients and equipment and have the potential to transmit infection. The use of personal protective equipment (PPE) is only one aspect of reducing transmission and is not effective as a sole measure of IPC. The hierarchy of IPC interventions should be applied as a bundle and include administrative, engineering controls and PPE provision. Analysis of the route(s) of transmission is an important factor in determining IPC interventions to reduce risk to both patients and staff (see 4.2.3.6 Transmission-based precautions).

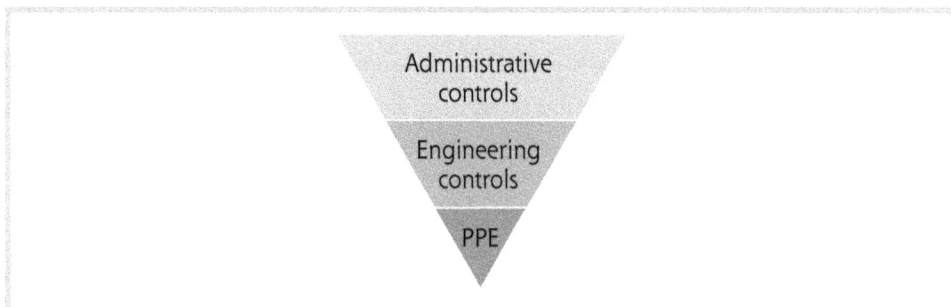

Administrative
controls

Engineering
controls

PPE

Figure 4.9 Hierarchy of controls for IPC risk management (adapted from CDC.gov www.cdc.gov/niosh/topics/hierarchy/default.html)

4.2.3.1 Administrative controls

These are the first requirement and provide the structure for sound and safe IPC practices where evidence-based policies and procedures are in place. These inform healthcare workers and teams on what to do, how and when to do it. Ideally, reporting systems are in place.

4.2.3.2 Engineering controls

These provide the infrastructure for safe IPC practices and address the layout and workflow in a healthcare facility. Ventilation, clean water supply, power supply, placing of IPC essential equipment and maintenance of essential healthcare equipment are addressed.

4.2.3.3 Personal protective equipment (PPE)

PPE is the least effective in the hierarchy of interventions and provides limited safety without the previous two controls being in place. The use of PPE is based upon preventing the transmission of microbes to and from the patient and therefore should be applied appropriately, based on evidence of the routes of transmission. Not all patient–healthcare worker interactions will require PPE.

It is the responsibility of the IPC team, in conjunction with the clinical teams and management, to ensure all precautions are understood and carried out optimally. The IPC team should also be involved in support, education and monitoring of the situation.

> **PPE is the least effective of the hierarchy of IPC measures and should be reserved for risk-prone procedures.**

4.2.3.4 No PPE required

PPE is not indicated when the healthcare worker attends to routine needs of patients who have no known infectious disease, such as bathing, feeding, handing out oral medication or helping a patient out of bed. Equally, making beds or general cleaning does not require PPE unless indicated in a transmission-based precaution policy. **PPE is only recommended for risk prone procedures and should be applied appropriately when dealing with known or suspected infections**.

4.2.3.5 Standard precautions[16]

Standard precautions are designed to reduce the risk of transmission of micro-organisms from both recognised and unrecognised sources of infection in healthcare settings. Standard precautions apply to all patients and in all situations, regardless of diagnosis or presumed infection status. Because all patients may serve as reservoirs for infectious agents, adherence to standard precautions during the care of **all** patients is essential to interrupt the transmission of micro-

---

[16] For details about standard precautions, refer to the NICE clinical guidelines (2003 http://www.nice.org.uk/page.aspx?o=71774); the Epic Project guidelines (2001 https://webarchive.nationalarchives.gov.uk/ukgwa/20100719164623/http://www.dh.gov.uk/en/Publicationsandstatistics/Publications/PublicationsPolicyAndGuidance/DH_4005481); the Royal College of Nursing's working well initiative (2004 http://www.rcn.org.uk/publications/pdf/goodpracticeinfectioncontrol.pdf); the US CDC guideline for isolation precautions in hospitals (1996 http://www.cdc.gov/ncidod/hip/ISOLAT/ISOLAT.HTM) and the WHO guidelines for preventing hospital-acquired infections (2002 https://apps.who.int/iris/bitstream/handle/10665/205187/B0007.pdf?sequence=1&isAllowed=y).

organisms. These precautions apply to (1) blood, (2) all body fluids, secretions and excretions **except sweat**, regardless of whether they contain visible blood, (3) non-intact skin and (4) mucous membranes.

All healthcare workers (including caregivers) should be trained in the appropriate use of standard precautions.

4.2.3.5.1 What are standard precautions?

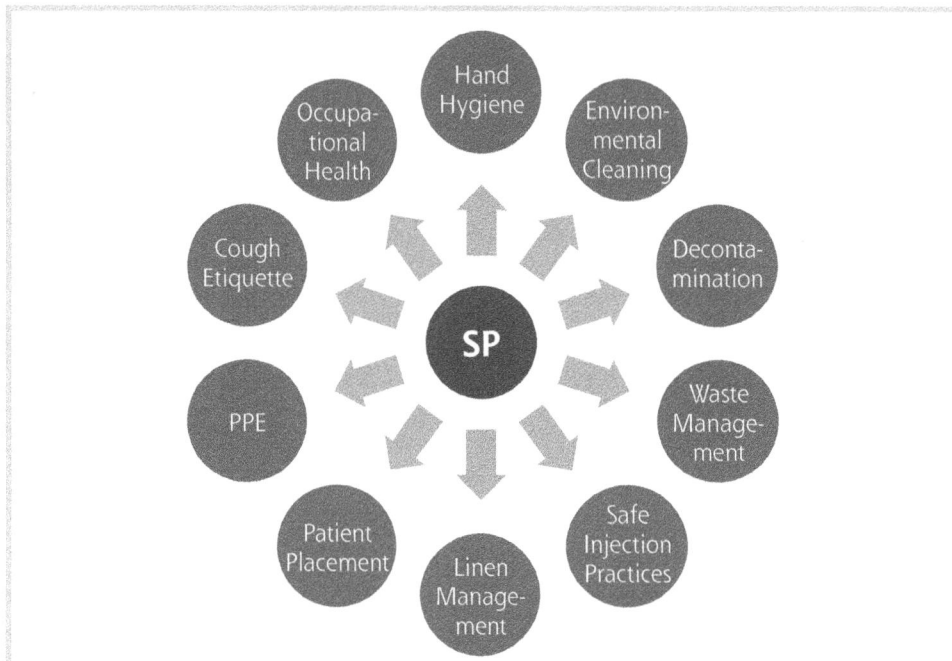

Figure 4.10   A diagram of all the aspects of standard precautions (courtesy Shaheen Mehtar)

A summary is given below:
- optimum hand hygiene – wash or ABHR (see 4.2.2 Hand hygiene)
- use of appropriate PPE (gloves) when exposed to blood and body fluids
- safe injection practices (single-use needle and syringe) (see 4.4.1 on safe injections)
- safe, immediate discarding of used hypodermic needles and sharps (safety box)
- healthcare waste management (colour-coding and disposal)
- maintaining a clean environment (trained cleaning staff)
- handling of used linen
- decontamination (cleaning) and sterilisation of medical devices between patients (see Chapter 3 on Decontamination)
- managing exposure to blood and body fluids – occupational health (also see 7.3 Occupational health)
- respiratory (cough) etiquette.

Education of patients, carers and healthcare workers (see section 1.11 on Education in IPC). Education is an integral part of IPC and is essential to ensure that policies and procedures are clearly understood by all.

Patient placement: There are no special requirements for patients apart from when specifically indicated during transmission-based precautions. However, there must be the recommended distance between beds in an open ward (see section 5.6.2 on Bed spacing).

PPE: Use of gloves (and if necessary, plastic aprons) when dealing with blood and body fluids including intravenous access is the only type of PPE recommended for standard precautions.

Each component of standard precautions will be dealt with under the appropriate section of the book. Here, hand hygiene, appropriate use and application of PPE for transmission-based precautions is discussed.

4.2.3.6 Transmission-based precautions

Transmission-based precautions are applied to reduce transmission of potentially transmissible and epidemiologically important pathogens. These are **always in addition to standard precautions. Remember, there may be more than one route of transmission**. The general recommendations are shown below. Specific recommendations are listed in Chapter 7.

> **Transmission-based precautions are based on the route(s) of transmission irrespective of the pathogen(s) involved.**

4.2.3.6.1 Isolation facilities – patient placement

Isolation facilities are recommended as a precaution for any transmissible infectious disease. Ideally, isolation facilities should be single-person occupancy with en suite ablution facilities and independent ventilation (usually negative pressure ventilation). Readers are referred to the building requirements in Chapter 5 on the Built Environment. It is advisable that experienced and well-trained clinical staff attend to such a patient to reduce the risk of infection and transmission.

Patients with infections caused by the same pathogen, particularly during an outbreak, such as SARS-CoV-2, may be cohorted (nursing several patients together in one area) in a single space such as a ward or the end of a clinical area. This is not uncommon in low-resource settings but certain rules should be followed to ensure best IPC practice.

4.2.3.6.2 Types of transmission-based precautions

Currently, transmission-based precautions consist of contact precautions for direct or indirect transmission; droplet and airborne for those transmitted via the respiratory route. Droplet precautions are aimed at short-range aerosols: larger infectious droplet nuclei which fall through gravity and can settle on surfaces in the patient's zone. Airborne precautions deal with long-range infectious nuclei: smaller infectious particles that are carried on air currents and depend on good ventilation to reduce risk.

Figure 4.11 illustrates the changes in protection for HCW from contact precautions to wearing a medical mask for droplet precautions, progressing to wearing a respirator and negative pressure ventilation for airborne precautions. Depending on the route of transmission, more than one type of precaution may be required.

All health workers and visitors entering isolation rooms must wear appropriate PPE.

Standard precautions, including meticulous hand hygiene following the WHO 5 Moments of Hand Hygiene, will apply to ALL TYPES OF TRANSMISSION-BASED PRECAUTIONS.

Readers should be aware that transmission-based precautions may be modified depending on the type of pathogen involved and as information emerges regarding known routes of transmission.

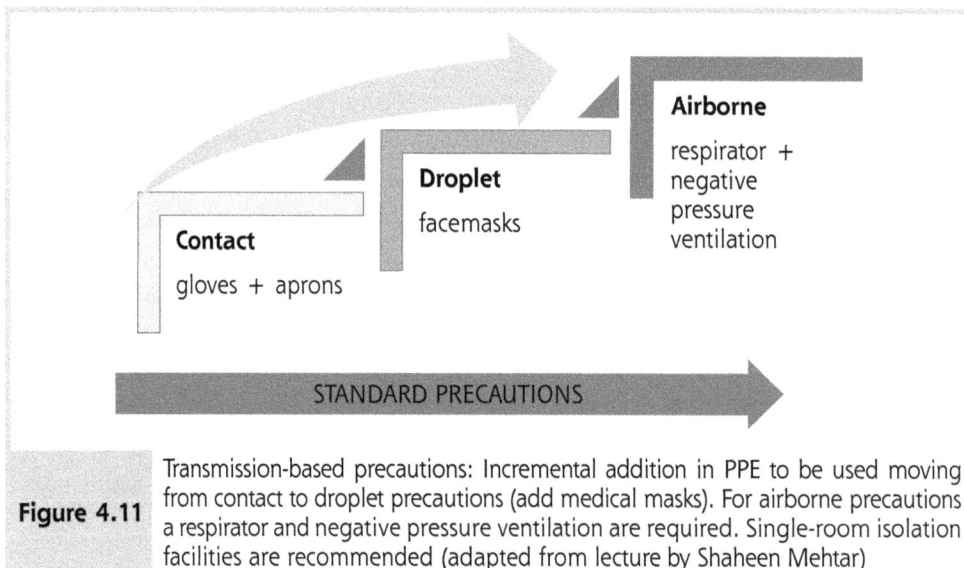

Figure 4.11 Transmission-based precautions: Incremental addition in PPE to be used moving from contact to droplet precautions (add medical masks). For airborne precautions a respirator and negative pressure ventilation are required. Single-room isolation facilities are recommended (adapted from lecture by Shaheen Mehtar)

4.2.3.6.3 Contact precautions

Contact precautions are applied when caring for patients with suspected or confirmed infections or colonisation with microbes transmitted by **direct or indirect contact**. Conditions and/or organisms which require contact precautions include the following:

- Antimicrobial-resistant bacteria transmitted by contact such as, but not limited to, methicillin-resistant *Staph aureus* (MRSA), Vancomycin-resistant enterococci, extended-spectrum- (ESBL) and carbapenem-resistant (CR) gram-negative bacteria (GNB), MDR- and XDR *Ps aeruginosa* and *Acinetobacter spp*, and drug-resistant *Candida spp* such as *C auris*.
- Conditions: skin infections, diarrhoeal diseases.
- In addition, procedures such as wound dressing or where contact with faeces, urine, secretions or excretions is anticipated, necessitate contact precautions.

Specific guidelines for contact precautions are shown in Table 4.4. A poster containing the essential aspects of the precautions should be placed outside the isolation area.

Table 4.4 Guidelines for contact precautions[17]

Patient placement
Ideally single-patient occupancy room. If no isolation facility is available, initiate bed space isolation: place patients approximately 2 m apart.
If dedicated toilet facilities are not possible, consider assigning one or use of bed pan/commode.
Put up isolation sign 'Contact precautions' – it must be clearly visible.
Place clean, unused PPE and ABHR outside patient room/isolation area – IPC trolley.
Clinical notes should stay outside the patient room/zone.
Minimal stock to be placed in isolation rooms to prevent contamination and wastage. Keep the door to the unit closed.

[17] CDC. 2007. Guideline for isolation precautions: Preventing transmission of infectious agents in healthcare settings. Appendix A. http://www.cdc.gov/ncidod/dhqp/pdf/guidelines/Isolation2007_appendixA.pdf; later version: http://www.cdc.gov/hicpac/2007IP/2007ip_appendA.html; Preventing transmission of infectious agents in paediatric in-patients haematology-oncology settings: What is the role of non-pharmacological prophylaxis? http://www.ncbi.nlm.nih.gov/pmc/articles/PMC3103128/; Mehtar S. 2010. *Understanding infection prevention and control*. Claremont: Juta & Co Ltd; Nulens E. 2018. International Society for Infectious Diseases. Guide to infection control in the hospital. https://www.isid.org/wp-content/uploads/2018/07/ISID_InfectionGuide_Chapter7.pdf; Munoz-Price LS, Banach DB, Bearman G, Gould JM, Leekha S, Morgan DJ, Palmore TN, Rupp ME, Weber DJ & Wiemken TL. July 2015. Isolation precaution for visitors. *Infection Control & Hospital Epidemiology* 36(7): 747–58 doi: https://doi.org/10.1017/ice.2015.67.

Hand hygiene
Perform HH according to the WHO 5 Moments of Hand Hygiene. HH must be performed before donning and after removal of PPE.

Personal protective equipment
Masks: not indicated **Aprons:** Worn to reduce contact exposure and splashes from the patient and patient environment. Do not leave the room (or patient zone) while wearing the apron. Discard into HCRW waste container inside the isolation area before leaving the area. Aprons are single use only. **Gloves (keep a box of gloves inside the isolation room – discard box when patient is discharged).** Wear a fresh pair of gloves when in contact with the patient inside the isolation area. Change gloves where applicable. Always perform HH before donning and after removal of gloves.

Maintenance of a clean environment
Daily cleaning Wear appropriate PPE. Use dedicated cleaning equipment (colour-coded cloth and bucket). Clean all surfaces daily with detergent and water and then wipe over using 70% alcohol or hypochlorite solution 1 : 1000 ppm. **Terminal cleaning – after patient has been discharged** Remove bed linen and privacy/inter-bed curtains, place in a bag labelled as infectious and send to the laundry. Clean all surfaces, including walls to hand height **with soap and water and then** wipe over using 70% alcohol or hypochlorite solution 1 : 1000 ppm. Upon discharge, clean and disinfect all equipment in the room or sluice before taking it to the storage area. Remove PPE and perform HH after completion of the task. Discard PPE and other disposable cleaning items in a HCW (infectious) container.

Patient care equipment
Dedicated equipment is preferred. Ideally use disposable equipment (if possible), such as stethoscopes, blood pressure cuffs and thermometers. Should disposable equipment not be available, then decontamination procedures should be applied to the equipment used for infectious patients, including those in isolation. Using equipment between patients poses a risk of transmission – discard disposable items if these were inside the isolation room or area. Any shared equipment is cleaned and then wiped with a disinfectant (e.g. disposable detergent disinfectant-impregnated wipes) after each use.

Management of used linen
Treat all linen as contaminated and infectious. Place in medical/clinical waste plastic bag (colour-coded) inside room, seal and place in linen bag dedicated for contaminated/infected linen in the sluice. Ensure prompt removal. Double bag **only if leakage hazard** exists and ensure safe transportation. Attach list of contents to outside of bag.
Catering
Meal orders, delivery and removal of trays must be performed by nursing personnel. Crockery and cutlery: • Wash in an automated dishwasher. • If manually cleaned, wash in hot water (> 55 °C) and detergent and leave to air dry. • Disposable crockery and cutlery not indicated.
Patient transport
Limit movement outside of room. Wear appropriate PPE when transporting the patient outside the room. Inform receiving department in advance of the infectious status of the patient and maintain precautions. Inform the theatre if the patient is scheduled for surgery. Inform EMS when there is an interfacility transfer, as well as the receiving healthcare facility.
Visitors
Visitors should: • always announce themselves to the person in charge of the unit. • be informed of the reason for isolation. • adhere to the prescribed PPE. • perform HH before entering and after leaving the room.
Duration of isolation and transmission-based precautions
Precautions to be maintained for the duration of stay or until there are confirmed negative specimens where applicable. Decision to be made in collaboration with the IPC practitioner/team and the clinical team.

4.2.3.6.4 Respiratory route transmission

4.2.3.6.4.1 Respiratory precautions

Microbes are released through a cloud of breath from the source which contains varying size of particles ranging from larger droplets to smaller nuclei (aerosols) when people talk, cough or sneeze (respiratory tract activity). How far these travel will depend upon the strength of expulsion from the source, the ventilation rate in the area and the protection worn by both the source and the exposed person.

The number of microbes liberated are:
- Talking: 0–200
- Coughing: 0–3 500
- Sneezing: 4 500–1 000 000

Depending on the air velocity, these can travel 100–300 m/s.[18]

Precautions related to the respiratory route of transmission are based on the particle size and are divided into:

Long range aerosols: These are usually very small infectious nuclei (previously thought to be <5 µm), such as TB, which remain suspended in the air for longer periods of time, particularly in poorly ventilated and crowded areas. Their buoyancy depends on the temperature and humidity of the air into which they are expelled – the drier the air, the quicker they disperse. Airborne precautions (see 4.2.3.6.4.1.2 below) are recommended for these types of aerosols.

Short-range aerosols: These are larger, heavier particles that fall to the ground due to gravity. These can contaminate surfaces surrounding the patient's environment. Currently, droplet precautions are recommended (see 4.2.3.6.4.1.1 Droplet precautions).

4.2.3.6.4.1.1 Droplet precautions

Large droplet nuclei are able to travel only short distances (short-range aerosols) and cannot remain suspended in the air for long periods of time. Transmission occurs when droplets containing microbes generated from an infected person are propelled a short distance before they fall because of gravity, landing on surfaces surrounding the patient, contaminating the environment and coming in contact with another person's conjunctivae or mucous membranes (eyes, nose or mouth). Microbes transmitted by the droplet route include influenza, SARS-CoV-2 and other respiratory viruses, mumps, rubella and *Neisseria meningitidis*, the cause of meningococcal meningitis. Some viruses and bacteria survive outside the body, for short periods of time, in the presence of mucous, serum and organic matter and may be transmitted indirectly via contact with contaminated surfaces.

Transmission from large droplets requires close proximity (approximately 1 m) to the source or through risk-prone procedures causing aerolisation and splashes.

Examples of risk-prone procedures for droplet transmission in hospitals include:
- coughing up or inducing sputum production for laboratory tests

---

[18]   Richard RL & O'Grady F. 1962. Airborne infection: Transmission and control. *Chest*. Downloaded from chestjournal.chestpubs.org by guest on 12 October 2009.

- collecting throat or nasopharyngeal swabs
- endotracheal suctioning (open and closed) of ventilated patients
- chest physiotherapy
- taking chest x-rays from patients who are coughing, especially with poor cough etiquette
- bronchoscopy
- re-use of ventilator circuits and respiratory equipment
- washing and cleaning respiratory ventilation equipment in clinical areas without adequate knowledge or protection.

Recommendations for droplet precautions are outlined in Table 4.5. A poster containing the essential aspects of the precautions should be placed outside the isolation area.

Table 4.5 Guidelines for droplet precautions[19]

Patient placement
Place patient in single room with en suite bathroom. Put up isolation sign 'Droplet precautions'. Place clean, unused PPE outside patient's room. Clinical notes should stay outside patient area.
Hand hygiene
Perform HH according to the WHO 5 Moments of HH. HH must be performed before donning and after removal of PPE.
Personal protective equipment
Surgical mask (well fitting) is to be worn before entering the patient's room. Surgical masks are single-use items and must be discarded in the HCRW container after removal, just before leaving the isolation area. Replace damp, soiled or contaminated masks immediately. Perform HH after removal. A well-fitted respirator must be used if patient has infections such as a novel influenza or SARS (including SARS-CoV-2) during an outbreak or pandemic.
Maintenance of a clean environment
Daily cleaning Wear appropriate PPE.

---

[19] CDC Guideline for isolation precautions: Preventing transmission of infectious agents in healthcare settings, 2007. Appendix A. http://www.cdc.gov/ncidod/dhqp/pdf/guidelines/Isolation2007_appendixA.pdf; later version: http://www.cdc.gov/hicpac/2007IP/2007ip_appendA.html.

Use dedicated cleaning equipment (yellow cloth and bucket).

Clean all surfaces daily with detergent and water and then wipe with a disinfect using 70% alcohol or hypochlorite solution 1 000 ppm.

Terminal cleaning

Remove bed linen and privacy/ inter-bed curtains and place in infectious colour bag and send to the laundry.

Upon discharge, clean and disinfect all equipment in the room or sluice before taking it to the storage area.

Clean all surfaces, including walls, to hand height with soap and water and then disinfect using 70% alcohol or hypochlorite solution 1 000 ppm.

Remove PPE and perform HH after completion of the task.

Patient care equipment

Dedicated equipment is preferred.

Using equipment between patients poses a risk of transmission.

Clean shared equipment (e.g. dynamap, thermometer etc) after patient use.

Correct management of used linen

Treat all linen as contaminated and infectious.

Place in medical/clinical waste plastic bag inside room, seal and place in linen bag dedicated for contaminated/infected linen in the sluice.

Ensure prompt removal.

Attach list of contents to outside of bag.

Catering

Meal orders, delivery and removal of trays must be performed by nursing personnel.

Crockery and cutlery
- Wash in an automated dishwasher.
- If manually cleaned, wash in hot water (>55 °C) and detergent and leave to air dry
- Disposable crockery and cutlery is not indicated.

Patient transport

Limit movement outside of room.

Patient should wear surgical mask when leaving the room for another department.

Inform receiving department in advance of the infectious status of the patient and maintain precautions.

Inform the theatre if the patient is scheduled for surgery.

The patients must be last on the theatre list to ensure adequate cleaning/disinfection and ventilation of the environment.

Theatre staff must wear respirators if patient has infections such as influenza, SARS or TB.

Visitors

Visitors should:
- always announce themselves to the person in charge of the unit.

- be informed of the reason for isolation.
- be restricted. Preferably no children, immune-compromised visitors or those not previously exposed as a close contact of the patient.
- adhere to the prescribed PPE.
- wear a **surgical mask** before entering.
- perform HH before and after leaving the room.

Discontinue isolation precautions

According to diagnosis and infectious period for the condition, immuno-competence and clinical improvement of patient.

Decision made in collaboration with the IPC practitioner/team and clinical team.

4.2.3.6.4.1.2 Airborne precautions

Airborne pathogens are transmitted via very small-sized aerosols (infectious nuclie) and are carried on air currents, particularly in poorly ventilated and crowded rooms. Pure airborne pathogens include the following, but during pandemics, influenza and SARS-Cov-2 may also become 'opportunistic' airborne pathogens:

- measles
- varicella (chickenpox)
- pulmonary tuberculosis (PTB), **and sites such as larynx trachea,**
- patients with extra-pulmonary TB (e.g. TB of the bone) do not require isolation if PTB has been excluded.

Patients with the above infections should be nursed in a negative pressure room, preferably with en suite ablution facilities. The ventilation rate of 6 to 12 air changes per hour (ACH) can be delivered either by an independent AHU or extractor fans which exhaust to the outside air (see section 5.3.6.1 on Ventilation).

In the absence of negative pressure ventilation and in out-patient settings or primary healthcare clinics, a pedestal fan can be used to extract air by reversing it to face outside while extracting from the room. This should achieve around 6–12 ACH. All healthcare workers entering the room of a patient with suspected or confirmed tuberculosis should wear a fit-tested respirator or equivalent (see Figure 4.11). If TB patients are cohorted in one ward, the patients should wear a surgical mask while in the room.

Table 4.6 highlights specific recommendations for airborne precautions. A poster containing the essential aspects of the precautions should be placed outside the isolation area.

Table 4.6   IPC Recommendations for airborne precautions

Patient placement
Place patient in single room with negative pressure ventilation and an en suite bathroom.   If a negative pressure room is not available, put the patient in a room with open windows to increase airflow towards the outside. **Keep door closed at all times.**   Cohort patients with same diagnosis or micro-organism, but use single room for MDR/XDR-PTB cases.   Put up isolation sign 'Airborne precautions'.   Place clean, unused PPE outside patient room.   Clinical notes should stay outside patient area.
Hand hygiene
Perform HH according to WHO 5 Moments of HH.   HH must be performed before donning and after removal of PPE.
Personal protective equipment
All staff wearing respirators must have undergone a fit-test to ensure that the correct size respirator is used to provide optimal protection.   Respirators are to be donned **before** entering the patient's room.   Always perform a facial seal check after donning the respirator, prior to entering.   Never share your respirator with other healthcare workers.   The respirator can be used for the duration of one shift or until damp, contaminated or deformed.   Replace damp, soiled, contaminated or damaged respirators immediately.   Remove respirator **after** exiting the patient room and either store individual respirators in a marked paper bag outside the isolation room or discard in healthcare risk waste container.   Perform HH after removal.   If a respirator does not fit properly, it is unsafe and may provide a false sense of security.   A respirator should **not** be worn by a patient whilst in isolation or during transportation outside the room. A surgical mask is adequate..   Wear gloves when in contact with the patient's secretions.
Maintenance of a clean environment
Concurrent cleaning   Wear appropriate PPE.   Use dedicated cleaning equipment (yellow cloth and bucket).   Clean all surfaces daily with detergent and water and then disinfect using 70% alcohol or hypochlorite solution 1 000 ppm.

Terminal cleaning

Remove bed linen and privacy/ inter-bed curtains and place in an infectious colour-coded bag and send to the laundry.

Clean and disinfect all specialised equipment which will not remain in the room prior to removal to the equipment storage area.

Clean all surfaces, including walls to hand height **with detergent and water and then disinfect** using 70% alcohol or hypochlorite solution 1 : 1 000 ppm.

Remove PPE and perform HH after completion of the task.

Patient care equipment

Dedicated equipment is preferred.

Using equipment between patients poses a risk of transmission.

Clean shared equipment (e.g. dynamap, thermometer etc) after patient use.

Patient-care equipment. Clinical and non-clinical equipment should be dedicated for the duration of the patient's stay if possible. If the equipment is shared, it should be decontaminated thoroughly between each patient.

Respiratory equipment or any items coming into contact with respiratory secretions should ideally be disposable or heat-stable for adequate decontamination and heat sterilisation. If the equipment is heat-labile, chemical sterilisation should be available. Items requiring heat or chemical decontamination should be cleaned thoroughly before being processed.

Other equipment. If the patient is bedbound, bedpans and urinals should be cleaned thoroughly and heat-disinfected. Soaking in chemical solutions is inadequate and not recommended.

Correct management of used linen

Treat all linen as contaminated and infectious.

Place in an infectious colour-coded plastic bag inside room, seal and place in linen bag dedicated for contaminated/infected linen in the sluice.

Ensure prompt removal.

Double bag not necessary, but ensure safe transportation.

Attach list of contents to outside of bag.

Catering

Meal orders, delivery and removal of trays must be performed by nursing personnel.

Crockery and cutlery:
- Wash in an automated dishwasher.
- If manually cleaned, wash in hot water (>55 °C) and detergent and leave to air dry.
- Disposable crockery and cutlery are not indicated.

Patient transport

Limit movement outside of room.

Patient should wear surgical mask when leaving the room for another department or shared common patient areas such as shared bathrooms.

Provide a surgical mask for coughing patients when they are transported in ambulances.

Inform receiving department in advance of the infectious status of the patient and maintain precautions. Inform the theatre if the patient is scheduled for surgery. Theatre staff must wear respirators.
Visitors
Visitors should always announce themselves to the person in charge of the unit. Inform visitors of the reason for isolation. Limit visitors. Preferably no children, immune-compromised visitors or those not previously exposed as a close contact of the patient. Visitors should adhere to the prescribed PPE. Visitors to wear a **surgical mask** before entering (respirators are not recommended for visitors unless they have had a fit test performed). Adequate distance must be maintained. Visitors should perform HH before and after leaving the room.
Discontinue isolation precautions
According to diagnosis, immune status and clinical improvement of the patient. Incubation period of the disease. A minimum isolation period of 2 weeks on effective treatment for sensitive PTB. MDR and XDR PTB must stay in isolation until transfer to a suitable facility as soon as possible; or Until two negative sputum specimens. Decision made in collaboration with the IPC practitioner/team and clinical team.
Specimens
In addition to standard precautions: In the case of a patient with confirmed or suspected PTB, sputum should never be collected in a room shared with other patients or in a communal bathroom. Ensure patient uses a separate area (cough room) to produce a sputum specimen. Ensure that the ventilation is adequate in the area where sputum is collected. Provide sputum pot, tissue and HH facilities.

4.2.3.6.4.1.3 Protective isolation (source isolation)

Severely immunocompromised patients may require being isolated to protect them against exogenous infections including hospital pathogens. Specific precautions are required for some patients because their clinical condition (e.g. a bone marrow transplant) puts them at particular risk of infection from other persons (**protective isolation**). Such facilities should be under positive pressure ventilation and function under astringent conditions. PPE (masks, gowns, gloves and headgear) is worn to protect the patient and meticulous hand hygiene is advised. The food is processed to ensure minimal bacterial counts.

4.3 Personal protective equipment

4.3.1 General rules about PPE

- PPE is placed on a clean surface OUTSIDE the infected patient zone (isolation or bed).
- PPE is put on OUTSIDE the patient zone and before entering the patient zone.
- PPE is removed INSIDE the patient zone followed by hand hygiene (ABHR).
- Wearing the same PPE when moving between patients is not recommended (unless approved by the IPC team).

PPE should be readily available in all healthcare facilities and should be of the best affordable quality. Purchasing inferior quality PPE usually results in overuse because the products are substandard and more items are used. The IPC team should advise on appropriate procurement and use of PPE.

> PPE such as gloves, aprons and medical masks are single-use and must be discarded directly after each patient use!
> Extended use of respirators is permitted under specific circumstances.

4.3.2 Gloves

Gloves are the most commonly used PPE in healthcare to protect healthcare workers and patients. Gloves should be well fitting, intact and of adequate length for the intended purpose. Gloves are often used as a substitute for hand hygiene. It should be noted that up to 20% of gloves sustain minute perforations during manufacture and therefore hand hygiene after removing gloves is essential.

The ideal glove would be:
- puncture-resistant
- allergen-free
- a barrier to microbes
- powder-free
- comfortable to wear
- long enough to provide adequate protection
- thin enough to allow optimum sensitivity when carrying out a procedure.

4.3.2.1 Types of gloves

Natural rubber latex (NRL) is the most commonly used material to make gloves because of its flexibility and barrier properties; however, with reports of increasing latex allergy among healthcare workers and the general population, there are now several alternatives such as nitrile available on the market. It is beyond the scope of this book to discuss details of the types of gloves available. The reader is referred to the latest literature on the subject.

For best practice the following applies:
- Wash and dry hands before wearing gloves and after discarding.
- For optimum protection the glove barrier must be intact throughout the procedures and if a breach occurs, new gloves should be donned.
- Use a pair of gloves for a single procedure only. Ideally gloves should be changed between procedures even on the same patient.

4.3.2.2 Indications for glove use

Not all procedures require gloves and the appropriate use is based on risk assessment (Table 4.7). Surgical gloves should only be used in the operating theatre; sterile latex gloves are used for aseptic ward procedures and non-sterile gloves for examination or taking blood samples.

Table 4.7 Recommended use of the various types of gloves

Type of glove	Indication	Comment
Sterile		
Surgical gloves (latex sterile)	Surgical procedures in OT, vaginal delivery, invasive vascular access, insertion of CVP, preparing total parenteral nutrition (TNP) and chemotherapeutic agents	Use for specific indications only. Gloves are expensive and should not be used on the wards Some surgeons use double gloves for protection or as a strike-through indicator

Latex sterile Latex-free (if indicated)	Invasive aseptic procedures:
	• Vascular access
	• Performing a lumbar puncture
	• Insertion of
	  ○ CVP and TPN lines
	  ○ Urinary catheters
	  ○ Chest drains
	• Preparing TPN and chemotherapeutic agents
		At ward level – routine or emergency
		For protection of patient Sometimes recommended when handling large open clean wounds
		At pharmacy level – preparation of medication

Nitrile sterile	Substitute for latex sterile, becoming increasingly common	Indicated for pharmacy, laboratory and sterile fluid production
Non-sterile (clean) gloves		
Latex non-sterile	Contact with blood or body fluids and items visibly soiled with body fluids	For protection of staff; non-latex cheaper gloves can be used for indirect patient items

Type of glove	Indication	Comment
	Direct patient contact • Taking blood – IV insertion and removal • Wound dressings • Removing urinary catheter • Vaginal examination • Suctioning non-closed system of endotracheal tube **Indirect patient contact** • Emptying patient bowls • Handling waste • Cleaning spillages • Cleaning equipment	
Plastic or nitrile non-sterile	For non-sterile procedure, e.g. • Emptying urine bag • Bedpans • Infectious linen	Nitrile (and polyurethane) is widely used as an alternative to latex gloves
Nitrile gloves	Handling chemicals • Radiotherapy • Disinfectants • Other chemicals Also used in latex allergy	
Other types of gloves		
Domestic gloves	Domestic/housekeeping, e.g. • Washing patient-use items • Contaminated surfaces • Cleaning instruments • Handling linen • Wiping up blood and body fluid spillage	Latex gloves may interact with chemicals used in cleaning, can lead to allergy
Heavy duty gauntlets Heat-resistant gloves	Removal of healthcare waste including sharps containers Stacking and unpacking sterile packs from sterilisers	Not clinical gloves
No gloves required		
	Direct patient exposure • Taking blood pressure, temperature, pulse • Injections: subcutaneous or intramuscular • Bathing and dressing patient • Transporting patients • Care for eyes and ears	There is no risk to staff from routine domestic chores; specific indications for transmission-based precautions only Meticulous hand hygiene (ABHR) after each patient contact is essential

Type of glove	Indication	Comment
	• Manipulation of vascular lines in the absence of blood (changing a fluid bag) • Giving oral medication **Indirect patient exposure** • Telephone calls, writing reports • Oral medication • Handling food trays • Handling non-invasive ventilation equipment • Moving patient furniture	

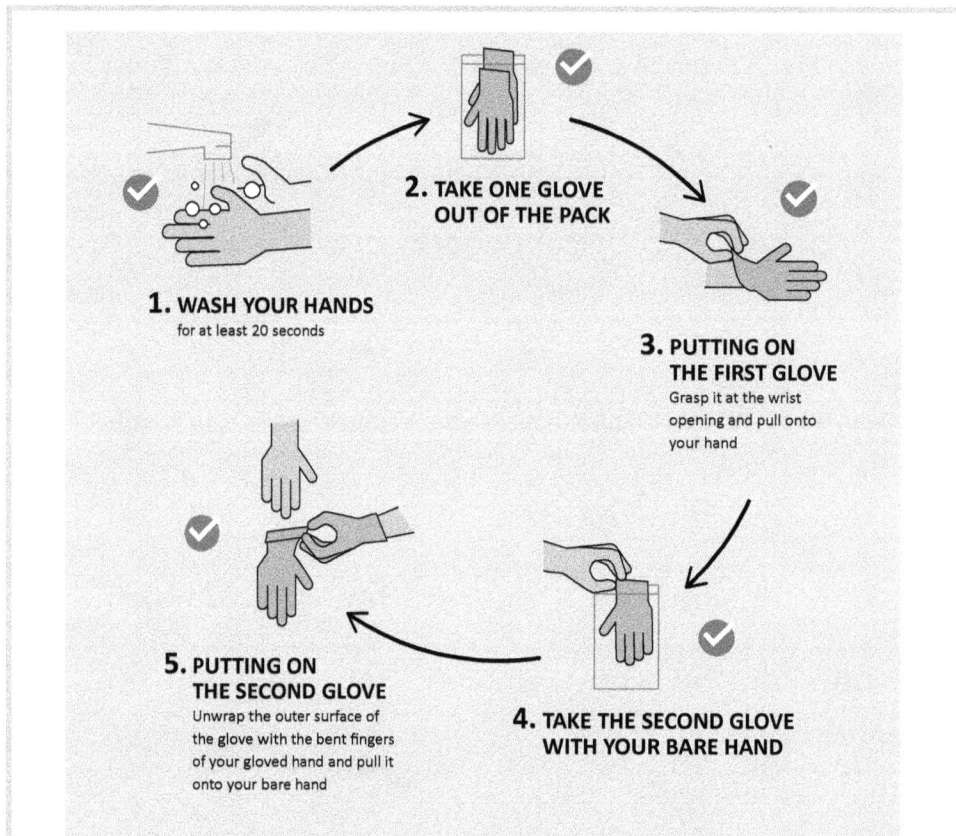

1. **WASH YOUR HANDS** for at least 20 seconds

2. **TAKE ONE GLOVE OUT OF THE PACK**

3. **PUTTING ON THE FIRST GLOVE** Grasp it at the wrist opening and pull onto your hand

4. **TAKE THE SECOND GLOVE WITH YOUR BARE HAND**

5. **PUTTING ON THE SECOND GLOVE** Unwrap the outer surface of the glove with the bent fingers of your gloved hand and pull it onto your bare hand

Figure 4.12 How to wear gloves properly (modified from https://oursafety.info/product/how-to-wear-gloves-properly/)

4.3.2.3 Procedure for handling gloves

Examination gloves come in boxes of 100 single gloves and are non-sterile. The correct procedure for putting on gloves is shown in Figure 4.12.

Sterile gloves, used for surgery or aseptic procedures, come individually wrapped and should be handled with care, ensuring the outer surface does not get contaminated. Some surgeons wear double gloves (of different colours) for added protection as well as making it easier to spot a tear on the outer glove.

Latex allergy.[20] Natural rubber latex (NRL) is a widely used and cost-effective material, with many unequalled benefits, and for the majority of the population does not represent a clinical risk. However, in specific groups with frequent exposure, allergy to NLR has a prevalence of 3% to 64%.[21] Latex allergy is most commonly noted in healthcare workers, rubber industry workers and patients with repeated exposure to latex, such as children with spina bifida.

The importance of risk assessment is to make an informed decision as to whether latex products are essential for the task since suitable alternatives are available.

Powder-free gloves are available, which are known to reduce the incidence of non-bacterial wound infections and latex allergies.

There has been a global move towards latex-free medical devices. Many items of medical equipment contain latex, but are often not labelled as such and this can have a serious outcome. A clear history of allergy to latex, nuts and other materials should be taken from patients and healthcare workers so that latex-free equipment can be provided where necessary. Depending on the level of hypersensitivity, healthcare facilities can still treat or employ individuals who are latex hypersensitive. The occupational health department should be actively involved in managing latex allergy and, with the IPC team, will recommend suitable safe alternatives.

4.3.2.3.1 Types of latex allergy

Natural rubber latex (NRL) is harvested from the rubber tree *Hevea brasiliensis* and processed to make it fit for purpose. The compounds used have been identified as allergens and associated with IgE-mediated reactions.

There are three types of allergy related to NRL. One is caused by the natural proteins (Type I), another by the chemicals that are used to convert the NRL to a usable item (Type IV), and then a mixture of the two.

[20] Bousquet J, Flahault A, Vandenplas O, Ameille J, Duron J, Pecquet C, Chevrie K, Annesi-Maesano I. 2006. Natural rubber latex allergy among healthcare workers: A systematic review of the evidence. *Journal of Allergy and Clinical Immunology* 118(2): 447–54. https://doi.org/10.1016/j.jaci.2006.03.048. (https://www.sciencedirect.com/science/article/pii/S0091674906009468).

[21] Parisi et al. 2021. Update on latex allergy: New insights into an old problem. *World Allergy Organization Journal* 14:100569 http://doi.org/10.1016/j.waojou.2021.100569.

4.3.2.3.1.1 Type I allergy

Type I NRL allergy is an immediate allergic reaction to NRL proteins. Skin irritation and urticaria, hay fever and asthma are commonly reported and can be potentially life-threatening. Some deaths have been reported. Latex allergens attach to corn starch used in powdered latex gloves. The powder acts as a vehicle, making the latex proteins airborne when these gloves are used, and enables the allergens to be inhaled. NRL-sensitised individuals may experience symptoms of an allergic reaction by being in a room where powdered NRL gloves are used, even though they are not in direct contact with the gloves. Clinical manifestations induced by Type I hypersensitivity reactions to NRL vary greatly depending on the route of exposure (cutaneous, percutaneous, mucosal or parenteral), the amount and features of the allergens, the level of sensitisation and individual factors. They may get worse at each following exposure.

Management of Type I allergy. Avoiding the allergen is the best treatment option as there is no cure for Type I NRL allergy. However, medications are available to treat symptoms of NRL allergy once it develops.

4.3.2.3.1.2 Type IV allergy

Some individuals react to the accelerator chemicals used in the manufacturing process of NRL. The reaction is a delayed hypersensitivity that occurs 6–48 hours after exposure.

The main symptom is a red, itchy, scaly rash, often localised to the area of use (wrists and forearms with glove use), but which may spread to other areas.

Management. Occupational health or medical advice should be sought and sensitised individuals should avoid the specific chemicals in future.

4.3.3 Face covers (medical masks and respirators)

Face covers are designed to cover and fit over the nose and mouth to prevent exposure to droplets and aerosols and to protect the wearer's mucous membranes from splashes and larger infectious nuclie. They are also used to protect immunocompromised patients from exposure to respiratory pathogens. It should be noted that in well-ventilated areas the risk of airborne transmission is greatly reduced. During the COVID-19 pandemic, face covers came into prominence as one of the major interventions to prevent the spread in the community and health facilities. However, in clinical practice, the irrational use of masks should be discouraged unless specifically indicated following a risk assessment.

4.3.3.1 An ideal face cover

- fits snugly over the nose and mouth and extends to midway between ear and nose to provide full cover

- has robust ties to the back of the head and a nose clip that can be easily moulded – **ear loops do not provide a firm fit**
- is comfortable and allows easy breathing
- allows passage of air, but filters particles such as droplets and aerosols
- is water-repellent
- lasts as long as the procedure (1–2 hours).

4.3.3.2 Types of face cover

Types of face cover include visors, goggles and face masks of different types. During the COVID-19 pandemic, face covers for the community and healthcare workers were extensively researched and developed – there is considerable variation in standards of production. IPC and procurement teams should acquaint themselves with the available products and purchase the best quality.

4.3.3.2.1 Visors and goggles

Protection can be afforded from splashes by visors and goggles and are indicated where exposure to fluid is anticipated, such as deliveries, suctioning a ventilated patient or in the manual cleaning of clinical equipment. A visor does not offer adequate protection against long- or short-range aerosols without a face mask worn with it.

4.3.3.2.2 Face mask (medical or surgical mask)

The efficiency of any face cover depends upon the fit first and then the make-up of the face cover.

There are several types of face mask:

1. **Paper masks** (Queen Charlotte) are very thin and porous and offer no protection to the user. These have been discontinued by most IPC programmes and are strongly discouraged because they give a false sense of security.
2. **Surgical (medical) masks** are made of several layers with an inner layer of polypropylene spun-bond; the outer layer is fluid resistant with a softer inner layer for comfort. Surgical masks are manufactured to regulated international standards which meet several parameters such as filtration, integrity and breathability. They offer approximately 87% bacterial filtration efficiency (BFE). A face mask has large pores and lacks an air-tight seal around the edges. Surgical masks are indicated in transmission via the respiratory route for HCWs, patients and visitors. They are effective for short periods of time, after which the microbial barrier is breached when the mask becomes moist. Continual wearing of masks does not prevent inhalation but may protect against splashes.

Ju et al provide an excellent review of standards, efficacy and methods of testing masks and respirators and is recommended reading.[22]

A face mask must fit well and cover the nose and mouth; on the side it should cover halfway between the ear and nose. It must be securely fastened around the back of the head to prevent aerosol leaks from the sides during use. Loose-fitting masks or masks worn without the lower ties being fastened do not provide adequate protection.

3. **Surgical masks with an attached visor** are effective in reducing exposure to splashes. However, goggles or visors are preferable where there is a higher risk of droplets.

4. **Fabric or cloth masks.** During the COVID-19 pandemic, when universal masking was required in some countries, the use of fabric or non-medical masks greatly increased. Although there are clear standards in many countries to which the masks should comply, unfortunately, fabric masks are mass produced without any regulation. In April 2020, the South African government published standards on the quality of fabric masks – there should be two layers of cotton or similar material with a layer of polypropylene spun-bond in between. The mask must be well fitting and not dislodge during talking. Fabric masks may be re-used after thorough washing and drying in the sun.

4.3.3.2.3 Indications for wearing masks

The actual indications are part of transmission-based precautions and these are to:
- Reduce exposure of mucous membranes to splashes.
- Reduce exposure in larger infectious nuclei.
- Transportation of patients on droplet or airborne precautions.

4.3.3.2.4 Procedure

To put on a face mask you should:

1. Remove a face mask from the container, holding it by its ties.
2. Place across the mouth and over the nose (stretch to cover both).
3. Tie the top and mould around the bridge of the nose.
4. Pull to cover the lower part of the face under the chin.
5. Securely tie the lower ties.

---

[22] Jerry TJ Ju, Leah N Boisvert & Yi Y Zuo. 2021. Face masks against COVID-19: Standards, efficacy, testing and decontamination methods. *Advances in Colloid and Interface Science* 292: 102435. https://doi.org/10.1016/j.cis.2021.102435 (https://www.sciencedirect.com/science/article/pii/S0001868621000762.

If the mask has elastic ear holders, place on face, mould and pull over face to cover chin.

To remove a mask you should:

1. Untie or break off the lower ties.

2. Untie the top ties.

3. Hold by the ties and discard appropriately.

Points of note

- Do not wear a mask around the neck for re-use.
- Use a mask for one procedure/specific task only and then discard.
- Do not move between patients wearing the same mask. You should change masks between patients.

4.3.3.3 Respirators

A respirator is made up of multiple layers of paper with layers of polypropylene spun-bond in between which are tightly bonded to the outer layers. The efficacy of a respirator relies on an airtight seal around the face of the user. There are several respirators available which reduce chemical, vapour and microbial aerosol inhalation. The one recommended for prevention of aerosol inhalation as part of IPC is a respirator equivalent to N95, KN95, European P2 and P3 respirators. It has a filtration rate of >99.7% and prevents particles of >3 μm from being inhaled. Some respirators come fitted with an expiratory valve, which greatly improves user comfort but should not be used for source isolation.

Engineering and administrative controls are generally regarded as the most effective methods to control exposures to airborne hazardous substances. The US Occupational Safety and Health Act (OSHA) considers the use of respirators to be the least satisfactory approach to exposure control. It holds *that it is not the type of mask **but the fit of it** which is important in preventing airborne transmission.*

Respirators are specialised equipment and should be **fit-tested** to each healthcare worker's facial contours; however, in less well resourced countries this is not always possible. A well-fitted respirator is uncomfortable to use over prolonged periods of time and is known to cause carbon dioxide retention. These should be used only when undertaking risk-prone procedures and removed immediately afterwards.

Respirators are not recommended for HCWs with respiratory insufficiency and should never be used on patients, the public, visitors or caregivers (see section 7.2.6 Transmission of infectious agents via the respiratory route).

The costs of operating a functional respiratory protection programme are substantial – including regular medical examinations, fit-testing equipment, training on its use by the IPC and occupational health staff, and maintaining the programme for all eligible staff.

4.3.3.3.1 Fit-testing respirators

Ideally, it is recommended that all HCWs using respirators are fit-tested to ensure minimal leakage.[23]

1. The HCW wears the respirator and moulds it to his or her face.
2. A closed hood is placed over the HCW's head and various chemicals which leave a taste in the mouth when inhaled are puffed into the hood.
3. The HCW is asked to identify the various tastes.
4. The respirator is adjusted after each chemical is used.
5. The respirator is passed when HCW can no longer taste the chemical.
6. The results are recorded for each HCW, date of testing and type of respirator.

Note
- Ideally each respirator should be fit-tested – it usually takes up to one hour.
- A well-fitted respirator may be used by the same HCW until it is damaged (if short supply).
- Fit-testing is not practical in a busy healthcare facility. Some countries do not have fit-testing systems.
- A respirator can be used with caution without a fit-test, but a face fit is performed instead. Where usage is high, a face fit is acceptable but must be done properly.
- Some types of respirators do not require testing.

4.3.3.3.2 Caring for respirators[24]

Respirators are expensive and may have to be re-used for economical reasons. Although not ideal, the healthcare worker may use the same respirator repeatedly, providing it is not damaged. When removing the respirator, use a disposable paper towel and hold the respirator while the elastic holders are carefully removed.
- Wrap in a paper towel and store safely in a paper bag with the user's name on it.
- Respirators should never be stored in a plastic bag – they absorb moisture and become ineffective.
- Carry out hand hygiene after removal.
- Respirators should be discarded after one week.

---

[23] https://www.osha.gov/laws-regs/regulations/standardnumber/1910/1910.134AppA/.
[24] Dept of Health, South Africa. 2020. National IPC Strategic Framework Implementation Manual.

4.3.3.4 Indications for a face covering

Table 4.8 outlines the indications for use of face coverings for the prevention of transmission by splashes, droplets or aerosols. Other indications such as exposure to gas, vapour or chemicals are not included here.

Table 4.8 Types of face covering and recommendations

Type	Indication	Comment

Surgical/medical face mask	• Routine use by surgical team in the operating theatre
	• Droplet transmission:
	  ○ HCW
	  ○ patients when moved
	  ○ visitors
	  ○ caregivers
	• When entering protective isolation for extreme immunocompromised patient
	• To avoid splashes contaminating HCW mucous membranes
	• When transporting patients with respiratory disease (TB, SARS-CoV-2)
		• Ritual use; no evidence that it reduces infection
		• Effective in reducing risk of droplet transmission by preventing inhalation
		• Protection of patient from HCW
		• Effective in protecting against small-volume splashes

Respirators	• Airborne precautions such as TB to protect the HCW when undertaking risk-prone procedures • Respiratory route transmission for an unknown pathogen • During an outbreak of respiratory viruses such as SARS-CoV-2 or influenza	• Used in conjunction with negative pressure ventilation • Initial encounter with an unknown pathogen of respiratory origin; may be modified later
Fabric/cloth mask	• For community use only	• Not recommended for use in healthcare facilities
Hanky/tissue/cloth	• Patients with known or suspected TB – new cases or those who have had inadequate treatment	• For use by the patient when present in public areas or healthcare facility waiting rooms; tissues are discarded after each use

4.3.4 Aprons

Plastic aprons are widely available in healthcare facilities and are used to prevent contamination of clothing from splashes. These are specifically indicated when there is a potential risk of coming into contact with blood, body fluids and patient secretions.

4.3.4.1   **Indications** for the use of aprons include:
- contact precautions
- minor cutting procedures
- burns dressings
- dialysis units.

Each apron should be worn and secured before patient contact. After use, the apron should be ripped off, rolled inside out and discarded.

4.3.4.2   **Re-use of aprons.** In low-resource countries plastic aprons are scarce and are re-used for transmission-based precaution. In such circumstances a dedicated durable apron such as a plastic butcher's apron can be used provided it maintains its integrity in the face of disinfectant application. The apron is used for only one patient and is wiped down with alcohol (or a suitable disinfectant) after each use (put user's name inside the apron). There should be an area to hang the apron to allow it to dry thoroughly before the next use. If the inner face of the apron is not noticeably different from the outside, it should be labelled as the inside. The cost of HAI, transmitted by contact, far exceeds the perceived savings from re-using aprons!

4.3.5 Gowns and coveralls

Gowns are made of either cotton (which is not fluid resistant) or non-woven material with waterproof lining. The use of gowns is usually restricted to operating theatres, transmission-based precautions or during outbreaks. **Cotton gowns** are not recommended for transmission-based precautions unless they are worn in combination with a plastic apron on the inside to render it fluid resistant.

Non-woven (disposable) gowns of varying lengths are available which have waterproofing of the arms and front to prevent penetration with fluids during a risk-prone procedure and surgery. These are used for contact transmission-based precautions in selected situations.

Coveralls have been recently introduced as part of PPE for outbreaks such as Ebola and SARS-CoV-2. These are expensive but provide a full body protection, particularly if extensive splashing is expected. These are often misused because of a lack of understanding of the actual risk from the pathogen.

4.3.6 Eye protection

All healthcare workers are advised to use eye protection when dealing with blood or splashes. The protection is afforded by the use of goggles for each individual healthcare worker, visors or shields. Some face masks have shields attached, which also afford protection from minor splashes, but are not as effective as goggles.

Eye protection is recommended where splashes from blood or body fluids are expected, such as surgical procedures, dental procedures using high-speed drills, trauma units and when attending deliveries.

Goggles and face shields are reusable and can be cleaned, disinfected and re-used, provided the integrity of the elastic ties is maintained.

4.3.7 Head coverings

Headgear is indicated:
- to prevent hair from falling into a patient's wound
- during processing of sterile equipment
- for sterile fluid production units in pharmacy
- for protection of healthcare worker from splashes of contaminated fluids.

Headgear is also indicated in food processing and pharmaceutical products manufacture. Headgear is available as caps, bandannas or scarves, or full-head and beard-cover hood. Cloth caps have now largely been replaced by disposable paper ones.

In IPC, routine-use headgear is not recommended unless there is a risk of excessive splashes.

4.3.8 Overshoes

There is no evidence for the use of overshoes anywhere in a healthcare facility. If personal footwear requires protection, it is best to change into clogs or similar which can be washed if contaminated.

Overshoes have been implicated in transmission of microbes from the shoes to the hands of healthcare workers.[25]

4.4   Risk-prone (clinical) procedures in healthcare

Introduction

The insertion of devices to provide medical care and surgery are part of everyday occurrences in a healthcare facility. The more the attention and care are given to preparation prior to insertion of device and during the procedure, the fewer HAIs there will be. The Institute of Healthcare Improvement (IHI) recommends applying 'bundles' of care for such procedures. Bundles are a group of up to five 'groupings of best practices with respect to a disease process that individually improve care, but when applied together result in substantially greater improvement. The science

---

[25]   Frederick DJ. 2020. Hospital footwear as a vector for organism transmission. Honors Undergraduate Thesis. 706. https://stars.library.ucf.edu/honorstheses/706.

supporting the bundle components is sufficiently established to be considered standard of care.'[26] Bundles are included at the end of each section below.

4.4.1 Injections

The reader is referred to the WHO guidelines on safe injections[27] and related recommendations.

Injections are widely used to deliver vaccines, medication and for drawing blood for laboratory tests or collecting for blood transfusion.[28] In the community intramuscular injections are more common, while in hospitals intravenous administration is used, especially in highly specialised units such as intensive care or operating theatres. In 2000, contaminated injections caused an estimated 21 million HBV infections, 2 million HCV infections and 260 000 HIV infections, accounting for 32%, 40% and 5% of new infections respectively for a total burden of 9 177 679 disability-adjusted life years between 2000 and 2030.[29]

Injections carry risks of infection to the patient and transmission of blood-borne viruses (BBV) to healthcare workers if the technique is unsatisfactory. Purchasers of such equipment should be aware of products on the market and select the most appropriate ones for their clinical application –'the right tool for the job'.

The choice of route is determined by:
- The type of medication
- The type of patient – emergency or elective
- The speed of action required by the medication
- Convenience for healthcare delivery – community or inpatient
- Available resources.

4.4.1.1 Routes of administration

The parenteral means of delivering drugs or vaccines is by injection, usually with a needle and syringe for small amounts of fluid and intravenous access for larger amounts.

26 Resar R, Pronovost P, Haraden C, Simmonds T, et al. 2005. Using a bundle approach to improve ventilator care processes and reduce ventilator-associated pneumonia. *Joint Commission Journal on Quality and Patient Safety* 31(5): 243–8. http://www.ihi.org/resources/Pages/Publications/UsingaBundleApproachto ImproveVentilatorCareProcessesandReduceVAP.aspx.
27 WHO guideline on the use of safety-engineered syringes for intramuscular, intradermal and subcutaneous injections in healthcare settings (2016).
28 WHO guidelines on drawing blood: best practices in phlebotomy (2010).
29 Hauri AM, Armstrong GL & Hutin YJ. 2004. The global burden of disease attributable to contaminated injections given in health care settings. *Int J STD AIDS* 15(1): 7–16.

Table 4.9 Routes of drug administration to patients

Route of injection	Site	Method	Fluid load
Intradermal	Through the epidermis into the dermis	Needle and syringe	1 ml or less
Subcutaneous	Between the dermis and the subcutaneous tissue	Needle and syringe; rarely slow infusion	Up to 2 ml
Intramuscular	Into large muscles such as gluteus or deltoid	Needle and syringe; deep into the muscle	Up to 5 ml
Intravenous – peripheral	Small to medium-size vein on arms; uncommonly on leg	Cannula connected via an administration set to a source of fluid	Any amount depending on patient's needs
Intravenous – central	Deep central veins such as subclavian vein	Long venous catheter connected via one or more administration systems to fluid source (or measurement system)	Any amount, depending on patient's needs
Portacath	Implanted under skin	Rubber bung for repeated injections	Bolus or medium volume

4.4.1.1.1 Bolus injections

Injection devices include:

- **Hypodermic needle and syringe.** While hypodermic needles and syringes are still widely used in LMICs, development of safety devices has arisen from a need to reduce the risk of occupational needlestick injuries among healthcare workers, the re-use of single-use items and the safe disposal of used sharps.
- **Gauge of hypodermic needle.** The gauge of the hypodermic needle should be appropriate to its use in clinical practice (Table 4.10). The gauge sizes are standardised and have a universal colour coding; however, these should be verified beforehand.
- **Single-use needle and syringes.** Needles and syringes are the commonest means of parenteral administration and drawing blood. Sterile needles and syringes are packed individually and assembled by the user. These are intended for single use and should be discarded as a single unit into a sharps box immediately after use. It is noteworthy that a single-use needle and syringe can be quite safe if used with care and attention.

Table 4.10   Recommended needle gauges for different procedures (WHO)

Needle gauge	Recommendations for procedures
16–18	Blood donation
19	Not often used
20–22	Venous access
23	Subcutaneous/intramuscular injection
24	Intradermal injections
26–27	Paediatric usage
27–28	Neonatal usage

4.4.1.1.2 Safety-engineered devices (SEDs)[30]

There are two types of device:

- **a passive device**, which does not require the user to activate the safety mechanism
- **an active device**, which requires a second manoeuvre from the user.

When activated correctly, safety devices can prevent either re-use or inoculation accidents and needlestick injuries. There is wide recognition that SEDs should be used whenever possible to reduce risk to healthcare workers. Occasionally SEDs are not recommended (Table 4.11). The cost of SEDs is now comparable to a hypodermic needle and syringe. Training in the use of SEDs should be widely implemented.

Table 4.11   The type of injection devices available and their advantages and disadvantages

Device	Advantages	Disadvantages
Hypodermic needle and syringe	• Widely available • Least expensive • Come in wide range of needle lengths and gauges • Do not require special training • Can be safer for drawing blood in paediatric population • For patient with small or difficult veins, drawing blood can be easier	• Require blood transfer creating additional risk for needlestick injuries or blood splashing • Difficult to draw large or multiple blood samples • Risk of being re-used on multiple patients

---

30   World Health Organization. 2016. WHO guideline on the use of safety-engineered syringes for intramuscular, intradermal and subcutaneous injections in health care settings. World Health Organization. https://apps. who.int/iris/handle/10665/250144.

Device	Advantages	Disadvantages
Evacuated tube system (ETS)	• Safer than using hypodermic needle and syringe because do not require blood transfer • Allows numerous blood samples to be collected through single venepuncture	• Requires one to be skilled in its use • Needle holders designed for re-use create additional risk for needlestick injuries • Mixing components from other manufactures can create a problem with compatibility • Requires paediatric ETS with a reduction of vacuum • Higher cost
Winged-steel needles (butterfly)	• Good for drawing blood from paediatric population or patient with small or difficult veins • Allows better precision than hypodermic needle and syringe	• Because of the air in tubing, first tube without additive should be used or discarded • Difference in winged-steel needles for ETS and winged infusion set can create confusion • Higher cost
(a) Passive SEDs		
Auto disable (AD) syringes	• Safety mechanism prevents re-use • Do not require activation of the safety mechanism • AD syringes are NOT needlestick prevention features and are not recommended for drawing blood	• During probing, safety mechanism can be activated • Require blood transfer, creating additional risk for needlestick injuries • Difficult to draw large blood samples • Air in the syringe can affect test results • Require additional training
Lancets	Retractable	
(b) Active SEDs		
Manually retractable syringes	• Safety mechanism retracts the needle into the syringe • reducing the hazard of needle exposure or re-use	• Safety mechanism cannot be activated when syringe is full of blood or during the blood transfer • Require healthcare provider to do an extra step • Require blood transfer, creating additional risk of needlestick injuries • Difficult to draw large or multiple blood samples • Higher cost

Device	Advantages	Disadvantages
Self-re-sheathing needles and syringes	• Sleeve forwarded over the needle provides guard around the used needle, reducing the risk of needlestick injury and prevents re-use	• Needle cannot be covered when syringe is full of blood or during blood transfer • Require additional training • Higher cost
Winged-steel needles with passive or active safety mechanism	• Needle locking mechanism helps to reduce the risk of needlestick injury and prevents re-use • If syringe is used for drawing blood, blood can be transferred in safer way	• If used in connection with ETS, because of the air in tubing, first tube without additive or discard tube • Require additional training • Higher cost
Manually retractable ETS	• Safer than using hypodermic needle and syringe because it does not require blood transfer • Allows numerous blood samples to be collected through single venepuncture • Safety mechanism prevents • re-use and helps reduce the risk of needlestick injuries	• Requires one to be skilled in its use • Needle holders designed for re-use create additional risk of needlestick injuries • Mixing components from the other manufactures can create a problem with compatibility • Requires paediatric ETS as vacuum can be too strong for paediatric population • Requires additional training • Higher cost

SEDs have proven to be effective by reducing the cost associated with occupational exposure to blood-borne pathogens. If the use in all clinical areas is not possible, the use of SEDs in high-risk areas should be considered.

4.4.1.2 Re-use of needles and syringes

Narrow lumen medical devices such as hypodermic needles, administration sets and syringes are single use and should not be reprocessed for further use.

> **The recycling or re-use of any intravenous-related equipment is strongly discouraged.**

4.4.2 Intravenous (IV) systems

Intravenous therapy is the most common invasive procedure in a hospital and it is reported that at any one time between 25 and 40% of patients will have an intravenous cannula in situ. In intensive care, up to 70% of patients will have venous access via a peripheral or central venous pressure (CVP) catheter. Infections from intravenous cannulation range from 7% to 30%, depending on the technique and equipment used. Types of infection range from localised phlebitis to bacteraemia and may result in gangrene or loss of limb.

The adverse events from intravenous systems are anaphylaxis because of drug allergies, adverse drug reaction and incompatibility, haematoma or extravasation fracture of cannula or catheter when dislodged in the venous system and, most importantly, HAI.

Pathogens can enter from either **intrinsic** or **extrinsic** sources. Intrinsic sources of contamination occur during the preparation of fluid, manufacture of the delivery system or unsuitable storage and transportation, while extrinsic sources occur during the procedure and use of intravenous systems.

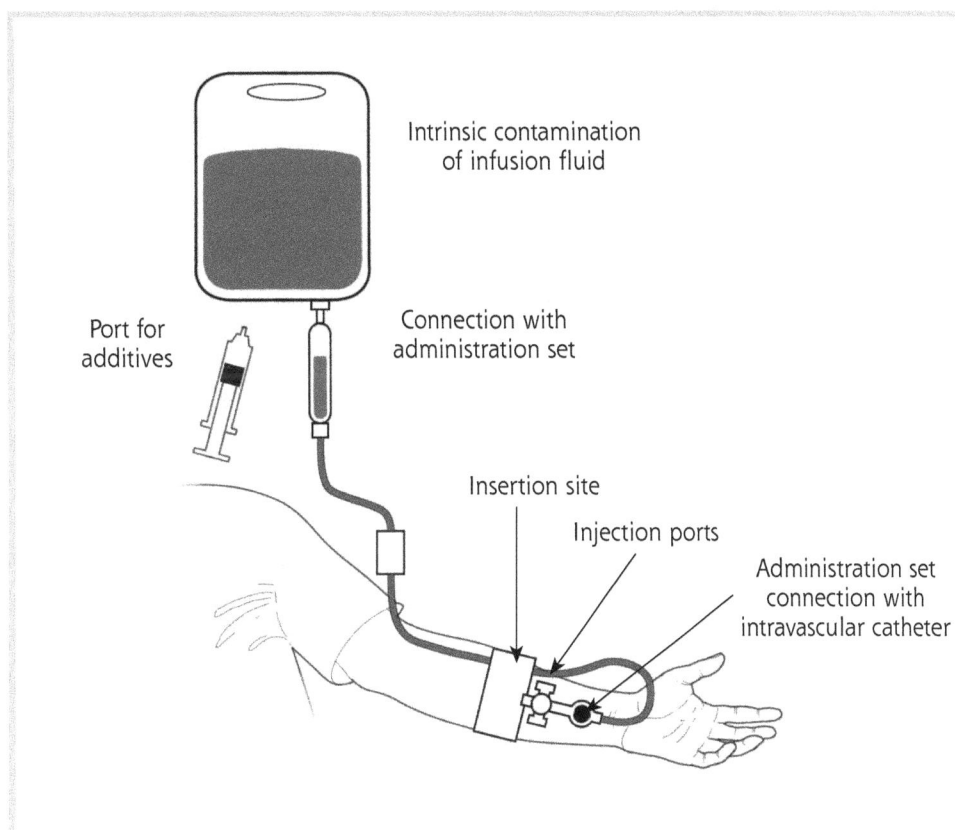

Figure 4.13 Illustration of areas where intrinsic and extrinsic contamination can occur during administration of fluids via a peripheral line

4.4.2.1 Intrinsic sources of infection

4.4.2.1.1 **Fluid bags.** Fluids used for intravenous therapy contain nutrients, which serve as an ideal breeding ground for microbes. If the fluid becomes contaminated, the direct entry into the bloodstream leads to serious consequences in the patient. The contaminants are bacteria and fungi usually found in the environment, especially in wet, warm areas. The release of endotoxin, pyrogens and other toxic substances may also occur in poorly prepared fluids. Quality assurance checks eliminate the problems in the production area, but appropriate storage of fluid bags at the correct temperature after being processed and dispatched from the factory is essential to maintain their integrity.

Entry points in fluid bags:
- During preparation the fluid is contaminated with environmental or human bacteria owing to poor preparation and sterilisation techniques.
- During sterilisation, if the steriliser is not functioning properly and has not been validated.
- During transportation and handling of fluid bags, damage to the structure of the bag can occur.
- During storage at production or clinical areas. Fluid bags left on the floor or at high temperatures in clinical areas are subject to damage.
- Storage in a warm, wet environment promotes degradation of the fluid and contamination from the surrounding environment.
- Changes in the chemical structure of the fluid bag can occur under adverse storage conditions and allow the infusion of bacteria or products to enter the fluid bag by osmosis.
- Addition of extra drugs or supplements through a contaminated port prior to dispatch such as for cancer chemotherapy drugs or total parenteral nutrition.

4.4.2.1.2 **Intravenous equipment.** Contamination of cannulae, administration sets and connections can occur during processing or are due to inappropriate storage such as an unclean environment or damaged packaging. Close inspection of all items to be used should include the integrity of the packaging, absence of stains or water marks and the expiry dates.

4.4.2.2 Extrinsic sources of infection

Extrinsic infections occur during setting up and inserting intravenous access. Essentially, intravenous therapy should be a closed system. Any break in the circuit potentially leads to risk of infection. The addition of drugs should be via a closed port under strict aseptic technique.

Entry points occur:
- During cannulation when the hands of the healthcare worker are not adequately cleaned.

- When the patient's skin site is not adequately cleaned.
- When the junction between the cannula and the administration set is leaking.
- When the injection port is used without cleaning or is leaking.
- Owing to a contaminated intravenous cannula, e.g. from a damaged package.
- During the addition of drugs through damaged or leaking ports or via open ports.
- When a used syringe and/or hypodermic needle is left lying open or exposed in a clinical area to deliver repeated doses to a patient (sometimes seen with multiple dosing).
- Owing to poorly fitting connection between the administration set and the fluid bag.
- When pre-cut adhesive sticky tape is left cut and exposed for use on patients.
- When a hypodermic needle is used as an air vent for fluid bags without such a provision.

4.4.2.3 *Components of intravenous access*

4.4.2.3.1 Selecting a peripheral intravenous device

Devices used for intravenous access should be well designed, robust and appropriate for the purpose they were intended. The IPC practitioner should consider the following points before advising procurement:

- Should be of the appropriate gauge to fit comfortably into the vein (see Table 4.10 in section 4.4.1.1).
- Should be made up of non-reactive and non-pyrogenic material.
- Should be easy to use by the HCW.
- Addition of drugs should be via closed injection ports located on the administration set; the exception is anaesthetic drugs, which require accurate dosing and are delivered via a port on the hub.
- The hub should fit firmly into the administration set, preferably with a Luer lock to avoid disconnection when the patient moves.
- Has a safety device, to prevent inoculation accidents, included in the design.
- A narrow-gauge (neonatal or paediatric) cannula should not fold on itself when introduced.

4.4.2.3.2 Administration sets

Administration sets are used to connect the intravenous cannula or catheter to the infusion bags. There are two types of administration set: (1) fluid and (2) blood transfusion sets. These should have a Luer lock that fits snugly into the intravenous device and can be secured.

The spike should be long enough so that once pushed and fixed into the fluid bag it remains in place without leaking. The drip chamber should be clear and the drops of fluid easily visible for counting delivery.

4.4.2.3.3 Blood administration sets

Tubing is of a wider bore compared to the fluid sets, and the drip chamber contains a small bag to trap particles of fibrin during transfusion.

In paediatrics or where small doses of drugs are delivered by infusion, a burette is integrated into the administration set into which the drug is injected and diluted before infusion.

The administration set tubing should be clear and the contents should be easily visible.

4.4.2.3.4 Addition of drugs

4.4.2.3.4.1   **Injection ports.** Ideally there should be no injection ports on the administration set or the intravenous cannula, but that is not possible because drugs have to be added during therapy. Open injection ports, once used, retain fluid that cannot be removed and provide an ideal breeding ground for pathogens. However, injection ports are necessary for bolus injections or additions; a closed, self-sealing rubber bung that does not leak with repeated use is recommended.

4.4.2.3.4.2   **Three-way taps** are attached to intravenous systems either to deliver drugs or to monitor the patient's medical progress. Open three-way taps contain a residual amount of fluid or blood after use that are open to contamination and become colonised quickly. Closed ports on three-way taps are preferable.

4.4.2.4 Supplementary administration sets

4.4.2.4.1   **Administration sets** (Y-sets) are available which can be inserted into the existing set via a Luer lock connection to the injection port or via a needle at one end which is inserted into the injection port (piggybacking) which increases the risk of introducing bacteria into the blood stream. If an additional line is required, it is safest to add this via a Luer lock rather than piggybacking.

4.4.2.4.2   **Piggybacking** is an additional administration set with an integrated needle which is inserted into the injection port of the main administration line. This contributes to increased infection rates by breaking the closed circuit and allowing access of pathogens.

4.4.2.4.3   **Needleless systems.** Injection ports which accommodate the nozzle of the syringe eliminate the use of needles for mixing or delivering drugs. These are effective in reducing bacterial contamination as well as needlestick injuries. The port is fitted with a non-return valve and prevents backflow and contamination. The system is adaptable to any type of delivery system, but is particularly useful in mixing drugs in multi-dose vials.

4.4.2.5 Multi-dose vials (MDVs)

MDVs are widely used for drugs, vaccines and dry medication which have to be reconstituted before delivery. It is cheaper to purchase drugs in larger volumes, so most pharmacies supply MDVs to the clinical areas. A cleaned and disinfected MDV rubber diaphragm is pierced with a needle and syringe to remove the drug for administration. Blood-borne virus outbreaks have been reported from contaminated fluid, needles and syringes used with MDVs.

Ideally, each injection should have a single-use vial, but this is expensive, and therefore MDVs should be used with extreme care. The surface of the rubber diaphragm should be wiped with alcohol and allowed to dry. The same needle or syringe should not be used from the patient to the vial or vice versa. Closed needleless spike systems with non-return valves are available on the market and have shown to greatly reduce bacterial contamination.

4.4.2.6 Infusion bags

Infusion fluids come in bags which contain from 1 to 5 litres. The bags are prepared under strict and sterile conditions and are usually made of polymers that maintain sterility during transport and storage. Infusion bags should be sealed except for a port for the introduction of the administration set, an air inlet and an injection port for the addition of drugs directly into the bag. All infusion bags must have an integrated air inlet with a filter to prevent contamination. The use of hypodermic needles to release the vacuum in the bag during use is not recommended.

4.4.2.7 Portacaths

There are several methods of accessing the vascular system, such as peripheral venous cannula, arterial lines (A-lines) for monitoring blood gases and CVP lines. Portacaths are intravenous devices with a diaphragm that are implanted under the skin in patients undergoing prolonged intermittent therapy. Only peripheral and CVP access will be discussed here.

4.4.3 Peripheral intravenous access

Peripheral intravenous cannulae are used to deliver medication to a patient (or draw blood) via a vein. They are designed to be flexible and to fit comfortably in the chosen vein. The cannula is secured in place with tape and connected to the administration set.

4.4.3.1 Pathophysiology of peripheral cannulation

When an intravenous (IV) catheter is introduced into the vein, there is direct communication between the bloodstream and potential contamination arising during the procedure. Zhang et al[31] describe the four possible pathways of infection during peripheral cannulation: (1) migration of microbes down the catheter tract; (2) via the catheter hub; (3) by bacteria circulating in the bloodstream (existing infection); or (4) from contaminated infusate. The most frequently isolated bacteria from peripheral catheters are coagulase-negative staphylococci and *Staph aureus* from the skin.

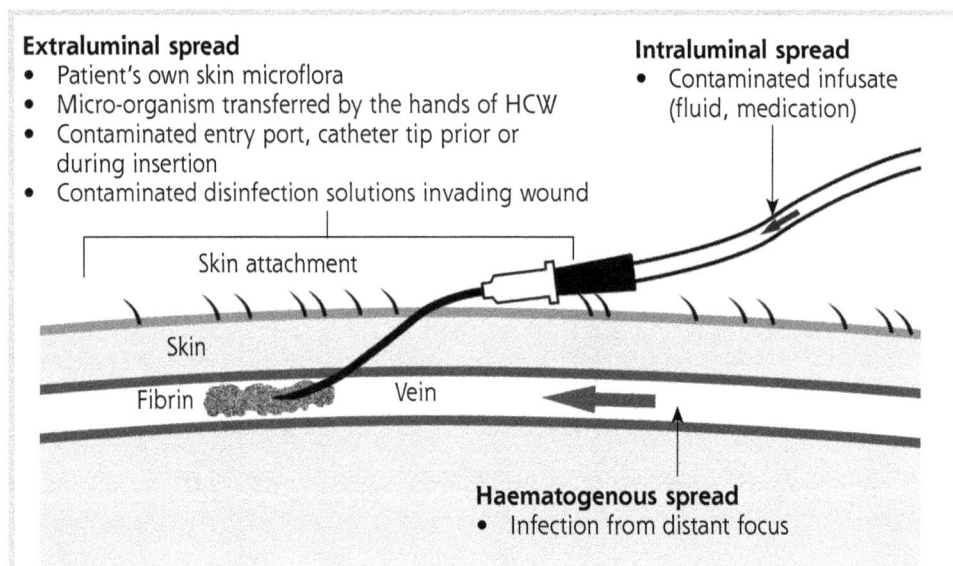

Extraluminal spread
- Patient's own skin microflora
- Micro-organism transferred by the hands of HCW
- Contaminated entry port, catheter tip prior or during insertion
- Contaminated disinfection solutions invading wound

Intraluminal spread
- Contaminated infusate (fluid, medication)

Skin attachment

Skin

Fibrin

Vein

Haematogenous spread
- Infection from distant focus

Figure 4.14 Sources of microbial contamination in patients with intravenous catheter

If the skin has not been adequately cleaned and disinfected, the bacterial load may be significant enough to result in infection. The risk factors for peripheral line infection are inadequate skin disinfection, leakage of blood or fluid around the site of entry, introduction of bacteria via hands and contaminated injection ports.

4.4.3.2 Peripheral intravenous cannulation (PIVC)

Intravenous therapy should be planned in advance; even in an emergency, provisions should be readily available to ensure safety of both the patient and the staff. The correct technique for cannulation can be found in the literature – the key points are outlined here:

[31]   Zhang L, Cao S, Marsh N, et al. 2016. Infection risks associated with peripheral vascular catheters. *Journal of Infection Prevention* 17(5): 207–13. doi: 10.1177/1757177416655472.

- Make sure the patient is comfortable.
- Carry out hand hygiene.
- Identify a site for insertion of the cannula.
- Clean the site thoroughly with 70% alcohol and allow to dry.
- Carry out hand hygiene.
- Put on a pair of gloves.
- Insert the cannula carefully and ensure backflow is established.
- Anchor the cannula.
- Attach the administration set and run slowly to ensure a good flow.
- Observe for any swelling.
- Daily inspection of the site is recommended.
- Remove the cannula when no longer required.

4.4.3.3 *Key elements of the PIVC bundle of care*[32]

The State of Victoria, Australia, recently published its peripheral IV cannulation bundle of care which is the simplest and most comprehensive account.

The bundle of care has five key elements:

1. Assessing the need for a PIVC
2. Maximising first insertion success
3. Maintaining asepsis at insertion
4. Dressing and securing the PIVC
5. Review and removal of the PIVC

Note: If the IV cannula becomes contaminated by contact with any surface, it is preferable to insert a fresh sterile one.

If, after two attempts, the IV cannulation has failed, ask someone else to carry out the procedure. The cannula must be changed for a new sterile one.

If the site looks clean and dry, there is no reason to relocate the IV cannula if it is flowing freely.

4.4.4 Central venous pressure (CVP) catheters

CVP lines are mainly used in intensive or high-care and oncology units for delivery of cancer chemotherapy. The CVP catheters are usually introduced directly into

---

[32]   Peripheral intravenous cannula bundle of care, Change package. State of Victoria, Australia, Safer Care Victoria, March 2022. www.safercare.vic.gov.au.

the large veins in the neck, such as the subclavian vein, but occasionally may be introduced via the brachial vein. They are used to deliver high volumes of a variety of fluids such as drugs, replacement fluids and nutrition. Sometimes the CVP line may be the only venous access and has to be carefully maintained over weeks.

4.4.4.1 Pathophysiology

CVP lines are foreign bodies and may be made of materials which encourage biofilm production in bacteria colonising the CVP line. Most of the invading bacteria arise from the patient's own skin and are usually flushed away by the host's defences. In the presence of a foreign body it is difficult to remove bacteria. They remain on the surface of the CVP catheter and, after some time, multiply and block the channels. The presence of a foreign body in the venous system also splits the blood flow at the point of entry, which results in fibrinogen and minute clots forming around the catheter. These extend gradually, ultimately blocking the eyes or exit channels of the catheter.

Types of central venous pressure catheter

1. **Short-term catheters.** These are introduced directly into the large veins and used for a period of no more than two to three weeks. They are usually used for acute medical care.

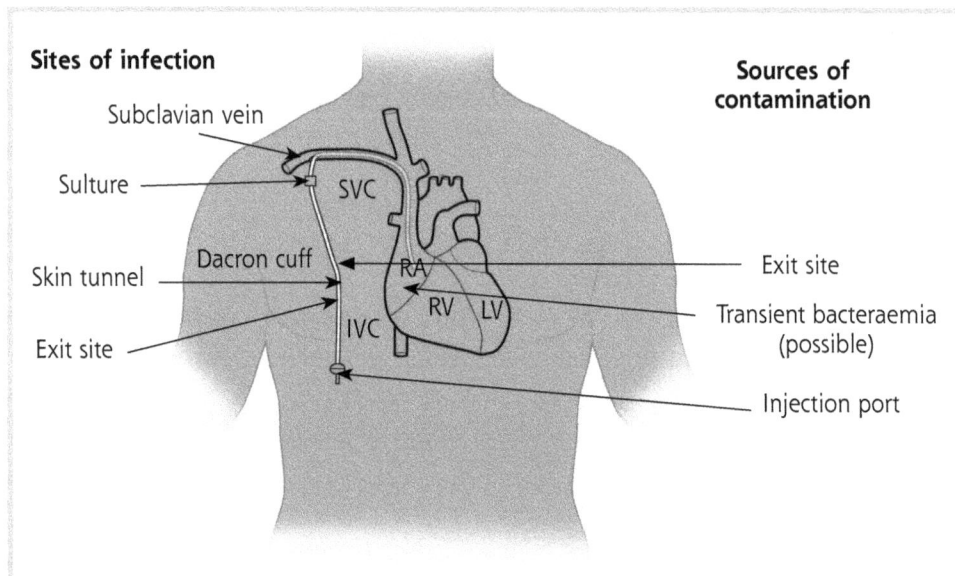

Figure 4.15 CVP line insertion sites and points of infection

2. **Long-term catheters.** These are also known as Broviac or Hickman catheters and are tunnelled under the anterior chest wall. These are usually left in for long periods and are indicated in long-term TPN or medication. Patients can be discharged with a CVP line in situ and care for it themselves.

4.4.4.2 Selecting a CVP intravenous catheter

CVP catheters are available in single, independent double or triple lumen, depending on the needs of the patient, and are a great improvement in reducing HAIs. CVP lines have to be robust and reliable and should be able to survive for weeks without blocking, fracturing or leaking.

The design of the CVP line is influenced by its function. It is advisable to plan ahead and decide on the use before choosing an appropriate CVP catheter for the job. The required specifications for the CVP line are that these are made up of non-reactive material, of adequate length, with minimum dead space, easy to attach to administration sets, well fitting to prevent leakage (Luer locks essential) and should not break off or dislodge.

4.4.4.3 CVP line insertion

The insertion of a CVP line is an aseptic procedure and should be carried out preferably in a clean or sterile environment. This is not always possible because many lines are inserted in the intensive care units.

Sterile drapes, gowns and gloves are recommended. Masks are preferred. Setting up a CVP line usually requires two persons – one to insert the CVP line and the other one to assist. The procedure involves the following:

1. Collect all the necessary equipment and place it on a procedure trolley.
2. Set up a sterile field.
3. Place the patient in the Trendelenburg position (angle of 45°).
4. Inspect the site of insertion. Make sure there are no small abrasions, skin lesions or broken skin in the immediate vicinity. These increase the risk of infection.
5. Surround the site with sterile drapes, but with adequate space for a good visual field.
6. Clean the site with a sustained action antiseptic (usually alcohol-based chlorhexidine) for at least two minutes, making sure the area is well covered. Allow to dry.
7. Carry out aseptic hand hygiene.
8. Wear sterile gown and gloves.
9. Insert the CVP line with minimum trauma and bleeding (depending on whether there is guide wire or direct insertion).
10. Clean the site thoroughly again with the recommended antiseptic (hospital policy) and dry.

11. It is recommended that the CVP insertion site dressing is clear for easy inspection and semi-permeable to reduce collection of fluid around the insertion site. However, some fluid collection is inevitable from the skin.

12. Clean the hub thoroughly with an alcohol wipe before connecting the administration set.

13. All venous entry points, such as three-way taps or 'traffic lights', should have closed ports and be left connected even when not in use to avoid contamination.

14. Each of the ports or entry sites should be labelled with the type of infusion to prevent cross-contamination or adverse drug reactions.

15. Discard all sharps and waste appropriately.

16. Remove protective clothing. Carry out hand hygiene.

17. Record in the patient's notes.

4.4.4.4 Maintenance of CVP lines

In maintenance of CVP lines the following must be carried out:

- The CVP line insertion site should be visually inspected frequently for leakage, redness or fracture.
- It is preferable that the administration sets are changed each day at the same time under strict aseptic conditions.
- Multi-lumen catheters can be shut off individually and changed aseptically when required.
- If heparin locks have to be introduced, these should be done aseptically.
- The CVP line can remain in situ as long as it fulfils its function and should be removed as soon as no longer required.
- The dressing should be changed when it looks moist and should be handled with great care in an aseptic manner.
- All administration sets and ports should be clearly labelled and checked to ensure there is no incompatibility between infusions (particulate matter).
- If there is leakage, accidental disconnection or any break in the system, it should be corrected immediately and noted in the patient's records.
- Blood samples taken from CVP lines can be misleading and are best avoided unless specifically indicated.
- The use of antibiotics to maintain infected CVP lines is not recommended. Antibiotics increase the risk of multidrug-resistant bacterial infections. The CVP line should be removed and replaced under a single dose of the appropriate antibiotic if clinically indicated.

> **Key elements of a CVC or CLABSI bundle[33]**
> - Perform hand hygiene
> - Use maximum sterile barrier precautions
> - Clean skin with chlorhexidine prior to insertion
> - Avoid the femoral site for catheter insertion, if possible
> - Remove unnecessary catheters as soon as possible.

Hyperalimentation (TPN) lines, which are lifelines for some patients, can easily get contaminated and infected because the infusions are highly nutritious. Since some may be tunnelled along the anterior chest wall, the procedure to change these lines is expensive and time-consuming.

- The hyperalimentation line should be dedicated to TPN only and no other substance or fluid should be introduced into the lines.
- A separate CVP line should be inserted for other medication.
- The line should be a completely closed system with no ports, three-way taps or opening for additives. All additives should be put into the fluid bag under strict aseptic conditions in a laminar flow cabinet.
- Both the insertion and exit sites should be inspected daily, kept dry and cleaned every day with sustained-action antiseptic and alcohol solution.

4.4.5 Safe disposal of sharps

Observe the following safety precautions when using and disposing of sharps:

- The sharps box should be placed within arm's reach of the user. It is recommended that a sharps box be placed on the procedure trolley.
- In high-dependency areas, sharps boxes should be placed next to each bed.
- The needle and syringe should be discarded as a single unit.
- If removal of the needle from the syringe is unavoidable, use a sharps box with a needle-removing facility or use forceps, or approach the needle carefully along the barrel of the syringe, using a gloved hand. Take extreme care.
- Sharps should never be passed directly from hand to hand.
- Avoid recapping, bending, breaking or manipulating used needles.
- Discard disposable sharps in an appropriate sharps box (conforming to British Standard 7320, United Nations Standard 3291 or equivalent). (Also see section 6.3 Healthcare waste management.)
- Do not overfill the container.

---

[33] Department of Health, South Africa. 2020. Practical Manual for the Implementation of the National Strategic Framework.

- Drop items carefully into the sharps box; do not push items down.
- **Never** put your hand into a sharps box.

4.4.6 Urinary tract infection

A urinary tract infection is an infection involving part or all of the urinary tract. The effects of the infection depend on the interaction between the bacterium and the host's defence mechanisms.

- **Cystitis** is infection of the bladder. The symptoms are usually of a local nature or a lower urinary tract infection.
- **Pyelonephritis** is an infection involving mainly the kidney or the upper urinary tract. Symptoms tend to be of a more systemic nature, such as fever, chills and a fast heart rate.

4.4.6.1 Pathophysiology

The bladder is sterile; however, the urethra is colonised with bowel flora at its lower end. During sexual intercourse, or in defaecating, bacteria ascend from the perineum to the bladder via the urethra, but are cleared by the protective mechanisms of the bladder. However, when a foreign body, such as a urinary catheter, is in place the local defences are bypassed and bacterial infections occur. These infections may arise from the patient's own flora (endogenous) or from the hands of healthcare workers or be due to bad catheterisation technique (exogenous).

Males have a longer urethra than females and therefore the latter frequently have more cystitis, especially during their sexually active life.

The most common pathogen isolated from the urinary tract is *Escherichia coli* (80%) or coagulase negative staphylococci; however, other gram-negative bacilli such as *Klebsiella spp* and *Proteus spp* also cause infection. Most of these bacteria produce biofilms and are difficult to reach by the body's defences or antimicrobial agents. In the presence of bloodstream infections microbes may enter the kidney directly via the bloodstream. Renal abscesses are attributed to tuberculosis and *Staph aureus* infections. Obstruction from stones or tumours or damage to the genito-urinary tract can lead to risk of infection.

4.4.6.2 Catheter-associated urinary tract infection (CA-UTI)

Infection is the most frequently reported complication of urinary catheterisation and more than 40% of all HAI are catheter-associated. CA-UTIs are associated with substantially increased death rates, especially among the elderly. Although not all CA-UTIs can be prevented, it is believed that a large number can be avoided by proper catheter management.

The indications for catheterisation vary greatly depending on the clinical diagnosis. However, it is evident that the urinary catheter must be removed as soon as it is no longer required. CA-UTI has been identified as a leading source of nosocomial antibiotic-resistant pathogens.

Diagnosis of UTI can be difficult in a patient with a long-term indwelling catheter, because bacteriuria is present in such patients. Therefore colony counts are used to distinguish between colonisation and actual clinical infections. Urine cultures obtained from the drainage bag safe-sampling port that show colony counts of $>10^2$–10^3 cfu/ml are considered to be indicative of a true CA-UTI.

The risk factors for CA-UTI are:
- Prolonged catheterisation (>6 days) – after 30 days of catheterisation, essentially all patients become infected. This is the most important, potentially modifiable, risk factor.
- Female gender.
- Diabetes, malnutrition, renal insufficiency.
- Monitoring of urine output.
- Positioning the drainage tubing below the drainage bag outlet.
- Contamination during insertion (not using an aseptic technique).
- Faecal incontinence (contamination by *E coli* in women).
- Interruption (breaking circuit) of the closed-catheter system.

It is recognised that ultimately all catheterised patients will develop CA-UTI, but certain risk factors increase the probability of infection – the risk of infections is greatest at the time of insertion. Almost all the bacteria isolated from the urinary tract are capable of producing biofilm. Diabetic and immunocompromised patients have a greater likelihood of infection with *Candida albicans*.

4.4.6.3 Components of urinary catheterisation

4.4.6.3.1 Types of urinary catheter

The choice of the urinary catheter is important to prevent or minimise infection and to ensure patient comfort.

Catheter material. Urinary catheters are made up of any of the following material, but latex catheters are by far the commonest but are being phased out:
- **Latex.** The catheter is soft, flexible, conformable and cheap – it is considered the best catheter choice for routine use. Red rubber latex catheters are radiopaque; the addition of barium to the latex also makes these catheters firmer and less likely to kink. Latex allergy may be a problem, especially in children with spina bifida who have repeated exposure to latex (see 4.3.2.3.1 Types of latex allergy). In these cases all items should be checked to ensure they are latex-free.
- **Silicone.** Silicone catheters are available uncoated or hydrogel-coated and these are more biocompatible with urethral tissue than latex, with reduced incidence of urethritis and urethral strictures. The advantage of silicone

catheters is that the thinner walls provide larger internal lumens per external diameter and are less prone to collapse during aspiration. This permits a greater flow and is advantageous for patients with blood clots or sediment in their urine. They can remain in situ longer than latex catheters.

The disadvantage of silicone catheters is the permeability of the balloons, resulting in loss of fluid over time. Silicone balloons should be checked regularly, adding fluid as needed. There is the tendency of the balloons to form creases or cuffs when deflated, which can lead to painful and difficult removal. Patients may complain of discomfort because silicone catheters are firmer than softer latex catheters.

- **Silicone-elastomer.** Silicone-elastomer-coated catheters are sometimes confused with 100% silicone catheters. These are actually latex catheters coated inside and out with silicone. The difference between silicone-coated and 100% silicone catheters is worth noting for two reasons:
    - patients who are latex-sensitive should be managed with all-silicone catheters, not silicone-coated catheters, and
    - patients who are not latex-sensitive may prefer silicone-coated catheters to all-silicone catheters because these catheters combine the strength and flexibility of latex with the durability and the reduced encrustation typical of all-silicone catheters.
- **Hydrogel-coated.** Hydrogel-coated catheters are soft and highly biocompatible. Because they are hydrophilic, they absorb fluid to form a soft cushion around the catheter, thus reducing friction and urethral irritations. While these are more costly, they are of benefit for long-term catheterisation.
- **Antimicrobial-coated.** These urinary catheters are designed to reduce bacterial attachment, colonisation and migration of bacteria. One type of coating combines a thin layer of silver alloy with hydrogel and is reported as being effective in reducing CA-UTI by 30% without causing bacterial resistance. It should be noted that these catheters have not been studied in patients with long-term indwelling catheters to determine efficacy, cost-effectiveness and lack of emergence of resistant bacteria.

Silver-hydrogel-coated catheters are available in latex and silicone, and nitrofurazone-coated catheters (antibiotic) are also available. Studies show that these reduce UTI rates for up to seven days. However, they fail to provide a significant reduction in infections caused by organisms resistant to nitrofurazone. There are concerns that the coating could lead to further selective antimicrobial resistance.

- **Plastic.** These catheters are used mainly for intermittent or self-catheterisation by patients with residual urine in their bladders. They are available in one size and are supplied in packs of multiple catheters.

4.4.6.3.2 Urinary catheter size

The French catheter scale is commonly used to measure the outside circumference (π × diameter) of cylindrical medical instruments including urinary catheters.

It is best to select the catheter with the smallest diameter that will provide good drainage, which is typically a 14–18 French unless the patient has blood clots or sediment that occlude the lumen. Larger catheters are uncomfortable for the patient and can cause urethral erosion and impaired para-urethral gland function (mucus production that protects against ascending bacteria).

Where a patient already has a large catheter (>18 French) in place, the catheter should be downsized with each catheter change until the catheter is within an acceptable size range.

4.4.6.3.2.1 Urinary catheter tip

There are two types of urinary catheter tip – straight or coudé (curved).

For routine catheterisation, a straight-tip catheter should be used. Coudé-tip catheters have a firm, curved tip designed to negotiate the male prostatic curve and may be helpful for difficult insertions. Coudé-tip/catheters should be inserted with the tip pointed upward towards the patient's umbilicus.

4.4.6.3.2.2 Urinary catheter balloons

The balloons are designed to secure the catheter but not occlude the urethra or prevent leakage. When filled, the 30 cc balloon weighs approximately 48.2 g and sits high in the bladder and can lead to bladder spasms and leakage. It may also damage the bladder neck. A large balloon results in stasis because the drainage eyes sit above the balloon and therefore above the urine. It is important that the right size balloon is selected. Pre-testing of catheter balloons is no longer recommended because most companies pre-test them during the manufacturing process.

Long-term catheters are at risk from bladder stones that can puncture the retention balloon. If the patient experiences repetitive spontaneous balloon deflation, she or he should be evaluated by the urologist for the presence of bladder calculi.

For routine catheterisation the common balloon size for paediatrics is either 1.5 cc or 3 cc; for adults a 5 cc balloon is usually adequate.

Filling the balloon. Follow the manufacturer's instructions and use sterile water to fill the catheter balloons. Under- or overinflation can result in an asymmetrical balloon, which can deflect the catheter tip to one side and cause occlusion of the drainage eyes, irritate the bladder wall and lead to bladder spasms. The rule of thumb is that a 5 cc balloon requires about 10 cc of fluid for symmetrical inflation. Normal saline is not recommended because it can lead to crystal formation in the inflation lumen (and difficulty in deflating the balloon). Inflation with air will cause the balloon to float in the bladder.

Silicone catheter balloons can lose fluid over time as fluid diffuses out into the urine. For this reason fluid levels should be checked at least every two weeks and fluid added as needed.

4.4.6.3.2.3 *Urinary catheter drainage systems*

Retrograde bacterial migration from the urine drainage bag outlet tube is a major source of bacterial contamination. The drainage tubing should not be allowed to drop below the level of the drainage bag. Drainage bags are designed with either an anti-reflux valve or anti-reflux chamber to prevent reflux of contaminated urine from the bag into the tubing. The position of the drainage bag should be below the level of the patient's bladder. The drainage bag should be suspended on the end of the bed with the tubing in a straight line, avoiding looping or kinking to promote unobstructed urine flow. It should be clear of the floor.

There is a wide range of drainage systems available and choice will depend on the method of catheterisation and the individual's needs. Most bags are made of non-latex material and the connector to the urinary catheter should have a urine sampling port to avoid disconnection of the urinary catheter during sampling. In medium and long-term bags there should be a tap with a non-return valve to drain the collected urine.

Most common is the **urinary drainage bag**. These can be attached to the leg (at the thigh, knee or calf) and have different capacities (usual for adult, 350–750 ml). **Body-worn bags** are intended for daytime use to enable mobility, whilst larger capacity bags are used for night-time drainage. **Night bags** sometimes have a drainage tap to facilitate emptying and can remain in situ for as long as five to seven days. They should be used with a hanger, either hooked onto the bed or free-standing. It is important to maintain a 'closed' drainage system (that is, connecting the catheter and drainage bag as a continuous unit) to reduce the risk of UTIs.

During transportation of patients with drainage bags, they should **not be** positioned on the abdomen or between the legs. Stainless steel drainage bag holders should be used to anchor the bag to the trolley or bed. The patient can be taught to use a bucket or similar to hang the bag properly.

Maintaining a closed drainage system is essential in reducing infection. Bacteriuria occurs in a closed and open system of drainage after thirty days and four days respectively.

4.4.6.3.3 Procedure for urinary catheterisation

Urinary catheterisation is an aseptic procedure. Before starting, check that all the necessary equipment is present and sterility is maintained:

- sterile gloves
- suitable antiseptic which is non-toxic to humans

- swabs or cotton wool
- sterile paper towels
- anaesthetic lubricating gel
- appropriate range of catheters
- receptacle for urine, or if the catheter is to be left in situ, a urine bag with tube to connect to the catheter
- if a Foley catheter is to be used, a syringe of appropriate size and water or saline for the bulb.

Before starting the procedure, carry out an aseptic handwash (or alcohol rub), dry hands and wear sterile gloves. An IPC practitioner must know the difference between male and female catheterisation procedures in order to recognise infection.

Male catheterisation. With the patient supine and with good light and visibility:
- Use the non-dominant hand to hold the penis – this hand is the 'non-sterile hand' and holds the penis throughout the procedure. Retract the prepuce (where uncircumcised and no phimosis).
- Clean the glans carefully with water and soap or a mild detergent.
- With index finger and thumb behind the glans, stretch the penis straight and slightly upwards to overcome the first curve of the urethra.
- Insert a few millilitres (5–10 ml) of gel (e.g. lignocaine 2%) into the urethra to avoid urethral spasm, using the single-use insertion device, and allow some to spill over onto the surrounding glans to lubricate the catheter's insertion as well as anaesthetise the procedure. Allow some time (2–3 mins) for the anaesthetic gel to take effect.
- To avoid urine spill, a collecting bag may be connected to the catheter prior to the procedure or a small collecting bowl be put in place. Once flow starts the tube is kinked to obstruct the flow of urine and the bag is connected.
- Allow the catheter to slip into the urethra until soft resistance is encountered – the second urethral curve. To overcome this, straighten the stretched penis, while pushing gently against the catheter. Sometimes the penis needs to be turned further downwards, towards the bed, to enable passage of the catheter through the prostate.
- Once urine flow is achieved, push the catheter in as far as it will go or until the 'fork' of the catheter. This is to prevent the balloon from being inflated whilst still in the prostate.
- Inflate the balloon with the appropriate amount of water or saline (usually 5–10 ml).
- Retract the catheter gently until there is a slight tug to indicate that the balloon is resting in the correct position against the bladder neck or prostate. Urine should flow freely.

- Taping the tube to the inner thigh prevents any tug on the tube pulling on the catheter in the bladder.

Note: In an uncircumcised male remember to replace the prepuce – failure to do so will cause paraphimosis.

Female catheterisation. As with male catheterisation, but anatomically the female urethra is much shorter and without the obstacle of the prostate. Identifying the urethral orifice can sometimes be difficult. Again, this is carried out with the patient in the supine position with good visibility:
- Clean the area around the urethra by wiping from front towards the back with warm soapy water.
- Lubricate the catheter tip with gel. Some advocate anaesthetising the urethra in advance of catheterisation. Open the labia with the non-dominant hand and slide the catheter into the urethra.
- Where the urethral opening is not visible, try to palpate for it at the anterior side of the vagina, where it can often be felt as a small horseshoe-like ridge. Guide the tip of the catheter with the index finger into the opening.
- Push the catheter approximately 10 cm into the bladder to ensure that it is properly positioned in the bladder.
- Fill a Foley catheter's balloon with the appropriate amount of water or saline. Then retract the catheter until there is a slight tug to indicate that the balloon now is in position against the bladder neck. Most of the catheter tube usually protrudes from the urethra.

If the urethra is missed and the catheter is accidently placed in the vagina, leave it there as a marker until after the procedure is over and use another catheter to introduce into the urethra.

Key elements of the CA-UTI ('Bladder') Bundle[34]

- Avoid unnecessary urinary catheters
- Insert urinary catheters using aseptic technique and maintain a closed system of drainage
- Maintain urinary catheters based on recommended guidelines
- Review urinary catheter necessity daily and remove promptly.

[34] Department of Health, South Africa. 2020. Practical Manual for the Implementation of the National Strategic Framework.

4.4.6.3.4 Catheter-related procedures

4.4.6.3.4.1 Securing the catheter

All urinary catheters should be secured. Unsecured urinary catheters can lead to bleeding, trauma, pressure sores around the urethral meatus and bladder spasms from pressure and traction.

It is recommended that once connected, the catheter should be secured to the thigh for women and the upper thigh or lower abdomen for men. The lower abdominal position in men decreases the potential for pressure necrosis and urethral erosion at the penile-scrotal junction.

Ambulatory men may find the abdominal site difficult. These patients can be instructed to secure the catheter to the upper thigh in the daytime and to change the position to the lower abdomen for sleep.

There are several devices to secure the catheter, including adhesive and non-adhesive straps and catheter-specific anchors.

A new catheter-specific anchor offers advantages that include a re-closable locking mechanism that swivels as the patient moves and an adhesive comfort pad that can be left in place for up to one week without altering skin integrity. Whichever product is selected, nurses should instruct patients in the proper use and removal of it.

4.4.6.3.4.2 Emptying the urine drainage bag

The drainage bag should be emptied when it is three-quarters full. Do not break the closed drainage circuit by disconnecting the bag from the catheter or drainage tube.

The procedure is as follows:
- Wear a pair of non-sterile gloves.
- Place a clean, dry urine measuring jug below the tap of the drainage bag.
- Release the tap slowly, ensuring neither splashing nor allowing the tap to touch the side of the jug.
- When the bag is completely empty wipe the tap with an alcohol swab.
- Close tap.
- Record urine measurement and take to sluice for testing or discard. Place jug in an automatic washer-disinfector and run machine.
- Remove gloves and carry out hand hygiene.

> **Do not use the same urine jug from patient to patient – it transfers bacteria between patients.**

4.4.6.3.4.3 Urine sampling

Drainage bags have a 'safe sampling' port designed to obtain urine specimens while maintaining the integrity of a closed system.

When collecting a urine sample use an aseptic technique:

- Wear non-sterile gloves.
- The drainage tubing is occluded below the port temporarily, allowing the urine to collect in the tubing (no spigots!).
- The sampling port is swabbed with alcohol and the urine is withdrawn following manufacturer's instructions using a needle, blunt cannula, or Luer-lock syringe.
- Urine for a culture and sensitivity can be obtained from a newly inserted catheter and drainage bag if indicated.
- Do not break the closed circuit to take a urinary specimen.
- Do not send a sample of urine from the urinary bag for microbiological analysis.

4.4.6.4 Catheter irrigation

Catheter irrigation is not recommended unless there is obstruction with clots or mucous plugs are anticipated. Closed, continuous irrigation with a three-way catheter is indicated for patients with repeated obstructions. Breaking the closed system drainage increases the risk of infection and is not recommended. Catheter irrigations should be performed as an aseptic technique with sterile saline and a syringe used each time. Vigorous irrigation and aspiration should be avoided. Bladder instillation with antimicrobial agents should be avoided unless absolutely necessary.

4.4.6.5 Catheter change

It is best to monitor patients closely for signs of blockage or encrustation and the catheter should be changed based on the patient's specific needs. However, removal of the catheter as soon as it is not needed is advised. Bacterial seeding from the urinary catheter is avoided by prescribing a single dose of antibiotic for a prolonged indwelling catheter half an hour prior to change in cases of endocarditis or implants.

4.4.6.6 Catheter removal

Traditionally, the fluid from the balloon is carefully aspirated before removal of fluid. Vigorous suction on the balloon may result in the collapse of the inflation lumen and encourage formation of creases, ridges or cuffing at the balloon area. This will increase the catheter balloon diameter size, resulting in a difficult removal and urethral trauma. It is recommending that the fluid be allowed to return to the syringe by gravity. With a small diameter inflation lumen, this may take up to 30 seconds. It is best to follow the manufacturer's instructions.

4.4.6.7 Care of the catheter–meatal junction

Extraluminal migration at the catheter–meatal junction occurs more often in women. Washing or cleaning the perineum thoroughly before catheterisation it is strongly recommended. Recommendations vary from just soapy water to 10% povidone iodine or 1–2% aqueous chlorhexidine solution.

Although routine perineal care is recommended, catheter manipulation should be avoided because it may contribute to bacterial migration into the bladder around the catheter–meatal junction. Meatal care after catheter insertion is not necessary. It should be noted that petroleum-based creams or ointments can degrade latex catheters and should be avoided.

4.4.6.8 Management of urinary catheter systems

Patients and caregivers should receive instructions regarding the following points:

- Keep drainage bags off the floor below the level of the bladder.
- Do not allow the outlet tube to touch the collection container or floor when emptying.
- Disinfect the urine collection containers after use.
- Empty the drainage bag when half to two-thirds full to avoid traction on the catheter from the weight of the drainage bag.
- Empty each urine bag into an individual jug or container at ward level.
- Use non-sterile gloves when emptying a urinary bag.
- Wipe the nozzle of the tap dry and wipe with an alcohol wipe after use.

4.4.6.9 Complications

Complications associated with catheterisation are:

- Leaks affect 25–65% of patients with indwelling catheters. Constipation, bladder spasm and catheter blockage should be excluded. Use a smaller gauge catheter.
- Encrustation is due to the precipitation of minerals and other materials (e.g. mucus, protein and bacteria) onto the catheter and is a common occurrence (causing recurrent blockage in 40–50% of long-term catheterised patients), exacerbated by *Proteus spp* infection and alkaline urinary pH. Increasing fluid intake, acidification of urine, treating infection, use of larger-bore catheters and irrigation solutions may help.
- Inflammation. Foreign body reaction, exacerbated by infection and encrustation. Try a different type of catheter.
- Bladder spasm. Intermittent clamping of catheters, gradually lengthening time clamped, or the use of catheter valves may help the bladder to regain/maintain its capacity and tone. Antispasmodics may be effective in providing relief from spasm.

- Blockage requires catheter change. Try to determine whether a pattern of blockage can be established, usually towards the end of the lifespan of a catheter, and move to more regular changes.

Note: It is not recommended that extra fluid is added to the catheter balloon, or that the catheter or balloon size is increased, as this can lead to spasm and leakage.
- Trauma during catheterisation – with bleeding, perforation or creating a false passage.
- Infection. The risk of infection is greatest at the time of insertion. About a third of patients with a long-term catheter develop systemic symptoms suggestive of a UTI, but only 5% become bacteraemic. Fever due to a urinary source develops with a frequency of about 1 in 100 to 1 in 1 000 days of catheter use.
- Renal failure occurs in up to 68% of spinal injury patients. This is usually associated with the formation of renal stones.

4.4.6.10 Prophylactic antibiotics

A Cochrane review of antibiotic policies for short-term catheter bladder drainage in adults concluded that there was weak evidence only that antibiotic prophylaxis (compared to antibiotics when clinically indicated) reduced the rate of symptomatic UTI in female patients following abdominal surgery and being catheterised for 24 hours. There was also limited evidence that prophylactic antibiotics reduced bacteriuria in non-surgical patients. Long-term antibiotic prophylaxis against CA-UTI is not recommended

4.4.6.11 Suprapubic catheterisation

Suprapubic catheters have been used in paediatrics and for patients where urethral access is difficult. There are some advantages – a comparison between suprapubic and urethral catheterisation is shown in Table 4.12.

Table 4.12   Comparison between suprapubic and urethral catheterisation

	Suprapubic	**Urethral**
Infection rates	Lower	Higher
Contra-indicated	Sphincter deficiency Chronic unstable bladder	
Complications	Leakage, bladder spasm, infection	Infection, stricture, leakage
Bladder stones	Common	Less common
Secured/anchored	Must be well secured	Less problematic
Catheter removal	Difficult – bleeding and trauma	Easier

4.4.6.12 Intermittent catheterisation

Patients with chronic bladder dysfunction due to neurogenic or other reasons are increasingly being taught to self-catheterise at fixed times during the day to prevent incontinence. It has proven to be relatively safe.

Short, firm catheters are provided in a pack. The patient is taught to carry out catheterisation as aseptically as possible into the toilet or receptacle. As soon as the bladder has been emptied the catheter is withdrawn, washed and cleaned thoroughly before drying.

4.4.6.13 Catheter care at home

Patients with chronic urinary dysfunction can be sent home trained in intermittent catheterisation to manage themselves and thereby reduce infection. There is a close working relationship between the district nurse and the clinic, which provides support and supplies as needed.

The concept of intermittent catheterisation has shifted the emphasis from sterile to clean in the home. This is acceptable since the only flora present is that of the patient and the manipulation is done by him or her. Exogenous infection is rare. It is more economical since the drainage bags and irrigation equipment are cleaned and re-used. However, cleaning medical products can be an added burden to patients or caregivers who may be confused regarding cleaning procedures. Cleaning procedures must be individualised and patient and caregiver needs and their ability to follow the procedure must be taken into consideration.

A recommended solution for cleaning urine drainage bags or irrigation equipment include full-strength vinegar, one part vinegar to three parts water (1 : 3).

Patients might have strong preferences regarding the type of outlet device that works best for them when they have to empty the bags themselves. Patients with disabilities or limited mobility may require a special type of outlet device.

Home-care agencies may have a policy for cleaning and re-use of irrigation supplies – these must be approved by the IPC team.

Closed-system maintenance can be difficult for home-care patients who frequently switch from standard drainage bags at night to leg bags during the day. These frequent breaks in the system greatly increase the risk of CA-UTI.

Leg-bag systems have been designed to hold the volume of urine produced during sleep. A sterile leg bag can be attached to the catheter at the time of insertion and extension tubing used to attach the standard drainage bag to the leg bag at bedtime.

The standard drainage bag is removed and cleaned each morning, maintaining a closed system.

4.5 Wounds

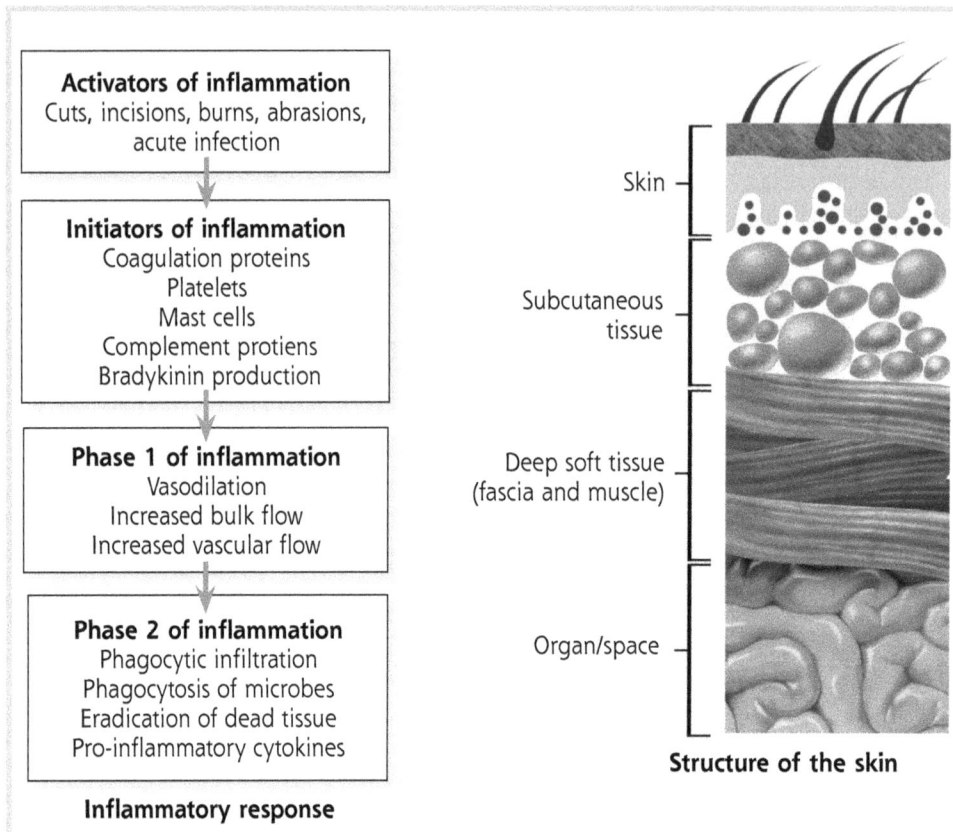

Activators of inflammation
Cuts, incisions, burns, abrasions, acute infection

↓

Initiators of inflammation
Coagulation proteins
Platelets
Mast cells
Complement protiens
Bradykinin production

↓

Phase 1 of inflammation
Vasodilation
Increased bulk flow
Increased vascular flow

↓

Phase 2 of inflammation
Phagocytic infiltration
Phagocytosis of microbes
Eradication of dead tissue
Pro-inflammatory cytokines

Inflammatory response

Skin

Subcutaneous tissue

Deep soft tissue (fascia and muscle)

Organ/space

Structure of the skin

Figure 4.16 Structure of the skin and inflammatory response when skin is breached

Wounds are categorised into two types – those which are purposely made by surgical incisions and those which occur through trauma or co-existing disease such as diabetes or vascular insufficiency.

Non-surgical wounds (pressure and chronic ulcers). Pressure and chronic ulcers (ischaemic) are common and account for up to 30% of admissions in acute care facilities. This section is relevant to IPC because ulcers can be a source of MDRO colonisation and spread.

4.5.1 Pathophysiology

A break in the skin results in a complex repair mechanism being activated. Wound healing is a complex series of events which begins at injury and continues for a long time. The initial **inflammatory phase** is immediate and occurs within 48 hours or may last up to five days – haemostasis is achieved by vasoconstriction, platelet aggregation and clotting. Following this, inflammation occurs with vasodilation and phagocytosis. Next is the **proliferative phase**, which may last from two days to three weeks. Granulation occurs with fibroblasts laying down a bed of collagen, filling defects and producing new capillaries. Contraction of the wound edges occurs to reduce the open wound. This is rapidly followed by **epithelialisation** where cells move across the collagen and fibroblasts (crossing the moist surface) and travel approximately 3 cm from point of origin in all directions. Finally, the **remodelling phase** may take three weeks in a healthy individual to years in the less immuno-competent person. New collagen forms, which increases the tensile strength of wounds, but scar tissue is only 80% as strong as the original tissue.

The repair mechanism is hindered by several factors:
- presence of debris or foreign bodies
- bacteria
- poor immune responses
- malnutrition
- extreme age.

4.5.1.1 Pressure ulcers[35]

Pressure ulcers appear on the dependent parts of the body such as the heels, bottom (sacral area), shoulders and back of the head when a patient is lying supine. These are usually seen in patients who are debilitated or frail and have poor circulation.

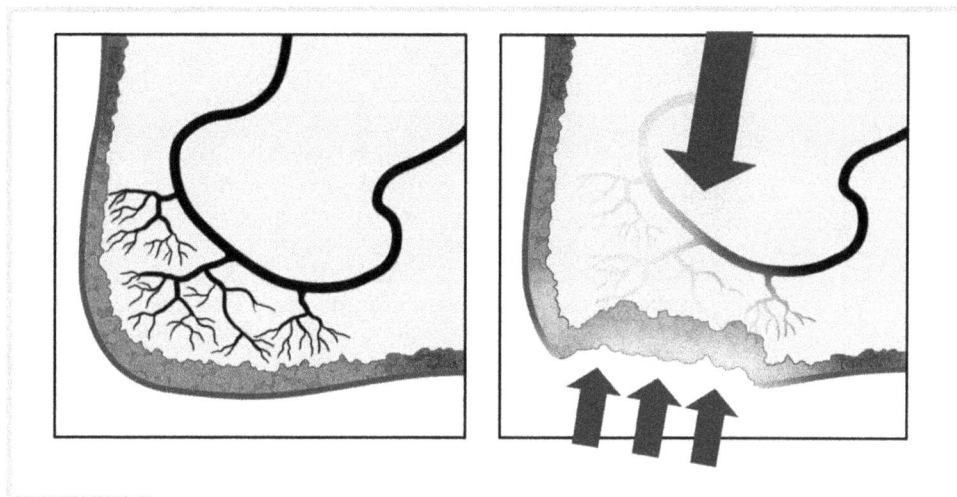

Figure 4.17 Ischaemic ulcers occurring during increased pressure on the area

---

[35] Bergstrom N, Bennett MA, Carlson CE et al. 1994. *Treatment of pressure ulcers –clinical practice guideline No15*. Rochelle, MD: Agency for Healthcare Policy and Research (AHCPR).

4.5.1.1.1 Causes of ulcers

Pressure ulcers arise owing to a combination of situations and factors and usually occur in immobile patients. When there is pressure on the tissue for a prolonged period of time the blood supply is decreased and the soft tissue in between is subject to abnormal pressure, resulting in necrosis. This is usually seen with a bony prominence resting on a hard surface. The tissue closest to the bone is typically the first tissue to undergo necrosis. Therefore, visible skin discolouration or redness may actually be an indicator of underlying adipose or muscular necrosis. The other cause is friction and shearing, which also lead to tissue necrosis.

Ischaemic ulcers (Figure 4.17) usually occur in dependent parts of the body where the blood supply is reduced or static due to poor venous circulation often seen in diabetics and those with chronic disease.

4.5.1.1.2 Assessment of ulcers

In order to manage ulcers, staging is essential (Table 4.13).[36] The following assessment method has been recommended by the National Pressure Ulcer Advisory Panel Consensus Development Conference.[37] The report was revised in 2007 and added two more stages which are deep tissue injury and unstageable injury. For the purposes of this book the original stages have been included.

Table 4.13 Staging of ulcers (taken from the National Pressure Ulcer Advisory Panel Consensus Development Conference 2005)

Staging of ulcer	Description
Stage I	Non-blanchable erythema of intact skin, the heralding lesion of skin ulceration. In individuals with darker skin, discolouration of the skin, warmth, edema, induration or hardness may also be indicators. A stage I pressure ulcer is an observable pressure-related alteration of intact skin whose indicators as compared to the adjacent or opposite area on the body may include changes in one or more of the following: skin temperature (warmth or coolness), tissue consistency (firm or boggy feel) and/or sensation (pain, itching). The ulcer appears as a defined area of persistent redness in lightly pigmented skin, whereas in darker skin tones the ulcer may appear with persistent red, blue, or purple hues.

[36] Shea JD. 1975. Pressure sores: classification and management. *Clinical Orthopaedics and Related Research* 112: 89–100.

[37] Taken from the *NPUAP Report* 4(2), September 1995. From NPUAP Pressure Ulcer Stages. Revised by the National Pressure Ulcer Advisory Panel. 53(3).

Stage II	Partial thickness skin loss involving epidermis, dermis or both. The ulcer is superficial and presents clinically as an abrasion, blister or shallow crater.
Stage III	Full thickness skin loss involving damage to or necrosis of subcutaneous tissue that may extend down to, but not through, underlying fascia. The ulcer presents clinically as a deep crater with or without undermining of adjacent tissue.
Stage IV	Full thickness skin loss with extensive destruction, tissue necrosis or damage to muscle, bone or supporting structures (e.g. tendon, joint capsule). Undermining and sinus tracts also may be associated with stage IV pressure ulcers.

4.5.1.1.3 Reverse staging

Clinical studies indicate that as deep ulcers heal, the lost muscle, fat and dermis are not replaced. Instead, granulation tissue fills the defect before re-epithelialisation. Given this information, it is not appropriate to reverse-stage a healing ulcer. For example, a pressure ulcer at stage III does not become a stage II or a stage I during healing. The progress should be charted by noting an improvement in the characteristics (size, depth, amount of necrotic tissue, amount of exudate etc).

4.5.1.2 Management of ulcers

Once the ulcer has been staged, it is best managed by experts in wound care. The IPC challenge is to ensure that colonising bacteria do not lead to serious infection. A summary of the types of dressing is shown in Table 4.14.

Table 4.14 Wound management products and application

Characteristic/function	Advantage	Disadvantage	Best use
Alginates			
• Soft non-woven fibres derived from seaweed • Come as pads, ropes or ribbons • Absorb wound exudate and form a gel-like covering over the wound, maintaining a moist wound environment • Absorb many times their own weight; Are a dry dressing; extremely lightweight	• Useful for packing exudating wounds • Do not inhibit wound contraction • Highly absorbent	• Require a secondary dressing • Can be too drying if wound has a low volume of exudate	• Wounds with moderate to heavy exudate

Foam dressings			
• Highly absorbent dressings of hydrophilic polyurethane foam • Varied absorption rates for the different foams • Some have adhesive tape surrounding an 'island' of foam • Less frequent dressing change	• Very absorbent, can frequently be left undisturbed for 3–4 days • Comfortable and conformable	• Drying effect if there is too little drainage	• Heavily exudating wounds – following debridement and desloughing • Deep cavity wounds – to prevent premature closure while maintaining a moist environment • Weeping ulcers, such as venous stasis

Hydrogel-impregnated gauze			
1. **Wound gels** create or maintain a moist environment; some hydrogels provide absorption, desloughing and debriding capacities to necrotic and fibrotic tissue	• Hydrating wound surfaces and liquefying necrotic tissue • Non-adherent and can be removed without trauma to the wound bed	• Not too absorptive, so may not be an appropriate choice for moderate to highly exudating wounds • Require secondary dressings	• Provide and maintain a moist wound environment • By increasing moisture content, they clean and debride necrotic tissue • For wounds with minimal or no exudate
2. **Hydrogel sheets** are cross-linked polymer gels in sheet form; some available with an adhesive border	'Soothing' effect promotes patient acceptance		

Transparent films*			
• Semi-permeable membrane dressings; waterproof yet oxygen- and water-permeable • Prevent bacterial contamination • Maintain a moist wound environment, facilitate cellular migration and promote autolysis of necrotic tissue by trapping moisture at the wound surface	• Permit evaluation of wound progress without removal • Usually waterproof and gas-permeable • Help maintain a moist wound environment • Economical	• Potential for causing skin tears if removed improperly • Non-absorptive – overwhelmed by exudate • Tend to roll up in high friction areas such as coccyx	• Superficial wounds • Wounds with light exudate • Wounds on elbows, heels, flat surfaces • Covering blisters • Retention of primary dressing

*Some newer transparent dressings are designed to keep IV sites dry. These films have a higher moisture vapor permeability (MVP) and should not be used.

4.5.1.2.1 *Assessment of the patient.* Assessment is the starting point of ulcer treatment. The entire patient, not just the ulcer, must be assessed. The following aspects should be addressed:
- the medical condition of the patient and control of underlying diseases such as diabetes
- nutritional assessment
- pain assessment
- psychological assessment.

4.5.1.2.2 *Tissue load management.* The goal of load management is to create an environment that enhances soft tissue viability and promotes healing of the pressure ulcer(s):
- The vigilant use of proper positioning and support surfaces are important.
- Avoid positioning patients on a pressure ulcer. Do not use donut-type devices.
- Use devices like pillows or foam to keep the heels off the bed and to keep knees and ankles from touching.
- Maintain the head of the bed at the lowest degree medically necessary.
- No evidence to show that any one support surface consistently performs better than another.
- A patient should avoid sitting if he or she has an ulcer on a sitting surface.
- Move a sitting patient at least once an hour.

4.5.1.2.3 *Ulcer care.* Initial ulcer care involves debridement, wound cleansing, dressing application and possible adjunctive therapy.

Debridement should be performed to remove moist, devitalised tissue. Small wounds can be debrided at the bedside, extensive wounds in the operating room or special procedure room. Stable heel ulcers with eschar **do not** need debridement. The presence of edema, erythema, fluctuance or drainage would necessitate eschar debridement.

Wound cleansing should be carried out with caution. Weigh benefits of cleaning against trauma to the tissue bed caused by the cleaning. Do not use povidone iodine, iodophor, sodium hypochlorite solution, hydrogen peroxide or acetic acid as they have been shown to be cytotoxic. Use normal saline at a pressure between 4 and 15 PSI.

An **ideal dressing** should protect the wound, be biocompatible and provide ideal hydration. The cardinal rule is to keep the ulcer tissue moist and the surrounding intact skin dry.

Electrotherapy has been shown to be effective in pressure ulcer treatment.

4.5.1.2.4   Managing bacterial colonisation and infection. Observe the following:
- Pressure ulcers are colonised with multiple bacteria and fungi from the skin and gut of patients and the environment (exogenous and endogenous).
- Anaerobes play a significant role in pressure and ischaemic ulcers, especially in the presence of necrotic tissue.
- Diagnostic sampling should be carried out with a needle aspiration or tissue biopsy when possible – superficial wound swabs yield little or no valuable information.
- Use sterile instruments and clean dressings during wound care.
- Treat the most contaminated ulcer last in patients with multiple wounds. Change gloves and wash hands between patients.

4.1.5.3 Home-based care

If patients are sent home with chronic ulcers, caregivers, taught by skilled staff, should be trained to manage wounds at home. The patient should be visited periodically to assess progress. Any sign of deterioration or infection should result in a proper medical assessment.

4.5.1.4 Wound care and management

There is a plethora of dressings available on the market, specifically designed for the various stages of ulcers (Table 4.15). The management of ulcers can be prolonged and expensive and new methods may arise which are far more effective, reducing the need for prolonged dressings.

Table 4.15   Types of wound and management recommendations

Wound type	Aim	Dressing
Yellow necrotic with high exudate	Remove slough and absorb exudate	Hydrocolloid with hydrocolloid paste if deep; hydrogels; alginates or enzymatic removal of slough (Elase)
Yellow necrotic with low exudate	Remove slough and absorb exudate	Hydrogels (rehydrate to aid removal of slough); hydrocolloids; enzymatic removal
Cavity wound with high exudate	Absorb exudate, maintain moist environment	Alginate or foam cavity dressings
Cavity wound with low exudate	Hydrate to maintain moist environment	Hydrogel
Malodorous wound	Clear infection, reduce odour, absorb exudate, protect	Systemic antibiotics only if clinical signs of infection seen; foam or alginate with activated charcoal; flagyl gel with caution

4.5.1.4.1 Wound debridement

There are four types of wound debridement.

4.5.1.4.1.1 Autolytic debridement

Autolysis uses the body's own enzymes and moisture to rehydrate, soften and finally liquefy hard eschar and slough. Autolytic debridement is selective because only necrotic tissue is liquefied. It is also virtually painless for the patient. Autolytic debridement can be achieved with the use of occlusive or semi-occlusive dressings, which maintain wound fluid in contact with the necrotic tissue. Autolytic debridement can be achieved with hydrocolloids, hydrogels and transparent films.

Best uses of autolytic debridement are in stage III or IV wounds with light to moderate exudate.

Advantages: It is very selective, with no damage to surrounding skin. The process is safe, using the body's own defence mechanisms to clean the wound of necrotic debris. It is effective, versatile and easy to perform with little to no pain for the patient.

Disadvantages: It is not as rapid as surgical debridement and the wound must be monitored closely for signs of infection. If an occlusive hydrocolloid is used, it may promote anaerobic growth.

4.5.1.4.1.2 Enzymatic debridement

Chemical enzymes are fast-acting products that produce slough of necrotic tissue. Some are selective.

Best uses of enzymatic debridement: It can be used on any wound with a large amount of necrotic debris and for eschar formation.

Advantages are that chemical enzymes are fast acting, with minimal or no damage to healthy tissue with proper application.

Disadvantages: It is expensive and it requires a prescription. It can only be carefully applied to the necrotic tissue and may require a specific secondary dressing. Inflammation or discomfort may occur.

4.5.1.4.1.3 Mechanical debridement

This technique has been used for decades in wound care by allowing a dressing to proceed from moist to wet and then the manual removal of the dressing causes a form of non-selective debridement.

Hydrotherapy is a type of mechanical debridement. Its benefits as opposed to its risks are of issue.

Best uses are for wounds with moderate amounts of necrotic debris.

Advantage is the cost of the actual material (that is, gauze) is low.

Disadvantages are that it is non-selective and may traumatise healthy or healing tissue. It is time-consuming and can be painful for patients. Hydrotherapy can cause tissue maceration. Also, waterborne pathogens may cause contamination or infection. Disinfecting additives may be cytotoxic.

4.5.1.4.1.4 *Surgical debridement*

Sharp surgical debridement and laser debridement under anaesthesia are the fastest methods of debridement. They are very selective. This means that the person performing the debridement has complete control over which tissue is removed and which is left behind. Surgical debridement can be performed in the operating room or at the bedside, depending on the extent of the necrotic material.

Best use is for wounds with a large amount of necrotic tissue in conjunction with infected tissue.

Advantages are that it is fast and selective and it can be extremely effective.

Disadvantages are that it is painful to the patient. It is expensive, especially if an operating room is used and the patient requires transport.

4.5.1.4.2 Support surfaces

The surface upon which a patient lies has a major impact on healing. These are physical forms such as mattress overlay, replacement or specialty beds which support the patient to reduce pressure on the ulcers and improve circulation. The choice depends on the length of patient use and the type of ulcer being treated.

They function as shown below to reduce pressure and improve circulation of the patient:
- static
- alternating/pulsating
- low air loss
- immersion (air fluidised, water, gel)
- turning/rotating/oscillating.

4.6 Surgical site infections (SSI)

4.6.1 What is a surgical site?

A surgical site is the incision or cut in the skin made by a surgeon to carry out a surgical procedure.

The position and size of the surgical site depend on the intended procedure and the type of surgery. For example, laparoscopic surgery (which uses fine instruments and a video camera) requires very small incisions, whereas more complex surgery may require a very large incision.

4.6.1.1 *Primary intention*

Surgical wounds may heal by primary intention, delayed primary intention or by secondary intention.

Most heal by primary intention, where the wound edges are brought together (apposed) and then held in place by mechanical means (adhesive strips, staples or sutures), allowing the wound time to heal and develop enough strength to withstand stress without support.

Wound edges come together after approximately 4–6 days, before granulation tissue is visible.

4.6.1.2 Secondary intention

On occasion, surgical incisions are allowed to heal by delayed primary intention where non-viable tissue is removed and the wound is initially left open. Healing by secondary intention occurs when the wound is left open, because of the presence of infection, excessive trauma or skin loss, and the wound edges come together naturally by means of granulation and contraction.

4.6.2 Surgical wound infection

Surgical wound infections comprise up to 12% of all HAIs. An SSI occurs when bacteria from the skin, other parts of the body or the environment enter the incision made by the surgeon and multiply in the tissues. This results in physical symptoms as the body tries to fight the infection. There may be pus, inflammation, swelling, pain and fever. The infections may arise endogenously (up to 90%) or exogenously (up to 15%), the later is of major concern to IPC practitioners.

The commonest bacterium is *Staph aureus*. Other common causative bacteria include other gram-negative aerobes, *Streptococcus spp* and anaerobes. High standards of asepsis (procedures that reduce the risk of bacterial contamination, for example sterile equipment) in operating theatres are the key to minimising the risk of infection.

The likelihood of an SSI depends on a number of factors related to both the patient and the surgical procedure. In particular, the risk of developing an SSI varies according to the type of surgery, the general health of the patient at time of operation and the length of the operation.

SSIs occur at the incision site, superficial (affecting skin and subcutaneous tissue) or deep (affecting the facia and muscles), or can be an organ space infection affecting any part of the anatomy opened or manipulated during the operation.

Infections **not considered superficial SSIs (by CDC)** include:
- stitch abscesses (minimal inflammation and discharge confined to the points of suture penetration)
- infection of an episiotomy or neonatal circumcision site
- infected burn wounds
- incisional SSIs that extend into the fascial and muscle layers.

4.6.2.1 Risk determinants of SSI[38]

Despite the fact that every surgical site is contaminated with bacteria by the end of the procedure, few become clinically infected. The interplay of four important determinants lead to either uneventful wound healing or SSI: (1) inoculum of bacteria, (2) virulence of bacteria, (3) micro-environment of the wound, and (4) innate and acquired host defences.

4.6.2.1.1   *Inoculum of bacteria.* Bacterial contaminants may enter the wound from the hands of the surgical team, the air in the operating theatre or from the instruments or surgeon(s) that come into contact with the wound. SSIs are generally the consequence of intra-operative contamination.

4.6.2.1.2   *Virulence of the bacterial contaminant.* While the virulence of the microbe is an important consideration in SSI, it represents the one variable that is intrinsic to the procedural site and the types of bacterium that already colonise the patient and cannot easily be controlled by preventive strategies.

4.6.2.1.3   *The micro-environment of the wound.* The micro-environment is a contributing factor. Haemoglobin at the surgical site is a well-known adjuvant substance. Necrotic tissue can act as a haven for contaminants to avoid phagocytic defences of the host. Foreign bodies, particularly braided silk and other permanent braided suture materials can harbour contaminants. Dead space within the surgical site also provides a local environment that fosters infection.

4.6.2.1.4   *Integrity of host defences.* Impaired host defences can be viewed as innate or acquired. Transfusion appears to be immunosuppressive. Similarly, chronic illnesses, hypoalbuminaemia and malnutrition are significant factors. Hypothermia and hyperglycaemia are also recognised as variables that impair the host response, while corticosteroids and other medications may also adversely affect the host and increase SSI rates.

4.6.3 Classification of surgical wounds and risk of infection

Different surgical sites may contribute to the risk of developing clinical infection, as shown in the classification below.[39] For example, clean operations should have a much lower risk of SSI compared with gut operations. The stratification of surgical

[38]   Anderson DJ, Kaye KS, Classen D et al. 2008. Strategies to prevent surgical site infections in acute care hospitals. *Infection Control and Hospital Epidemiology* (SI29): S51–S61.

[39]   Cruse PJ & Foord R. 1980. The epidemiology of wound infection. A 10-year prospective study of 62,939 wounds. *Surg Clin North Am* 60: 27e40.

wounds provides a rough guide to the 'acceptable' infection rates based on the classification,[40] however, recently these classification are being contested.[41] For the purposes of this section, the four categories stand.

4.6.3.1 Clean wounds

The wound is judged to be clean when the operative procedure does not enter into a normally colonised viscus or lumen of the body. Elective inguinal hernia repair or thyroidectomy are examples of a clean operative procedure. SSI risk is minimal and originates from contaminants of the operating theatre environment or from the surgical team, or most commonly from skin. SSI rates in this class of procedures should be 2% or less, depending upon other clinical variables.

4.6.3.2 Clean-contaminated wounds

A clean-contaminated surgical site is seen when the operative procedure enters into a colonised viscus or cavity of the body, but under elective and controlled circumstances. The most common contaminants are endogenous bacteria from within the patient. Vagotomy–pyloroplasty is an example. Infection rates for these procedures are in the range of 4–10% and can be optimised with specific preventive strategies.

4.6.3.3 Contaminated wounds

Contaminated procedures occur when gross contamination is present at the surgical site in the absence of obvious infection. Laparotomy for penetrating injury with intestinal spillage and elective intestinal procedures with gross contamination of the surgical site are examples of contaminated procedures. As with clean-contaminated procedures, the contaminants are endogenous bacteria that are introduced by gross soilage of the surgical field, for example a colectomy. Infection rates will be greater than 10% for this classification of wound, even with preventive antibiotics and other strategies.

4.6.3.4 Dirty wounds

Surgical procedures performed when active infection is already present are considered dirty wounds. Acute bacterial peritonitis and intra-abdominal abscess that have a mixture of aerobic and anaerobic pathogens are examples of this class of surgical site. Pathogens to be expected are the pathogens of the active infection

40 Culver DH, Horan TC, Gaynes RP et al. 1991. Surgical wound infection rates by wound class, operative procedure, and patient risk index. National Nosocomial Infections Surveillance System. *Am J Med* 91: 152S–157S.

41 Stefanou A, Worden A, Kandagatla P, Reickert C & Rubinfeld I. 2020. Surgical wound misclassification to clean from clean-contaminated in common abdominal operations. *Journal of Surgical Research* 246: 131–38. https://doi.org/10.1016/j.jss.2019.09.001.

that are encountered. Unusual pathogens are often encountered in dirty wounds, especially if the infection has occurred in a hospital or nursing home setting, or in patients receiving prior antibiotic therapy.

Risk index

The risk index initially based on the National Nosocomial Infection Surveillance (NNIS) system[42] has been further developed, with a point being added to the patient's risk index for each of the following variables to predict an SSI:

- 1 point – the patient has an operation that is classified as either contaminated or dirty
- 1 point – the patient has an American Society of Anesthesiologists (ASA) pre-operative assessment score of 3, 4, or 5
- 1 point – duration of operation greater than two hours

Physical status classification for surgical patients (ASA)

Class I	A patient in normal health
Class II	A patient with mild systemic disease resulting in no functional limitations
Class III	A patient with severe systemic disease that limits activity, but is not incapacitating
Class IV	A patient with severe systemic disease that is a constant threat to life
Class V	A moribund patient not likely to survive 24 hours

4.6.4 Prevention of SSI

The number of variables that can influence SSI rates is large. Pre-operative planning and intra-operative technique become important in prevention of SSI. In addition, the appropriate use of preventive antibiotics in an appropriate fashion is very important. Finally, new strategies that appear to enhance host responsiveness must be considered as part of prevention.

4.6.4.1 Pre-operative planning

4.6.4.1.1 **Surgical site.** The site of the surgical incision should be managed prior to the actual arrival of the patient in the operating theatre.
- Site of the planned incision should not be shaved or clipped.
- Depilatory agents have been recommended, but will occasionally result in a hypersensitivity reaction.
- Shaving or clipping the surgical site should be reserved for the operating room immediately prior to the skin incision.

---

[42]　Culver DH, Horan TC, Gaynes RP et al. 1991. Surgical wound infection rates by wound class, operative procedure, and patient risk index. National Nosocomial Infections Surveillance System. *American Journal of Medicine* 91: 152S–157S.

4.6.4.1.2 *Surgical team.* The following factors connected with the surgical team and the patient's condition will increase the rate of SSI:

- The presence of open skin wounds on or infection of the hands or arms of the surgeon.
- If the patient has any pre-existing infection, SSI will be more likely.
- If the patient has had an extensive pre-operative hospitalisation (more than four days), colonisation of the patient with hospital-based microbes is likely and appears to increase the rate of SSI.
- Finally, a course of antibiotics leading up to the operation for a pre-existing infection that is independent of or associated with the disease for which the operation is being performed will increase the rate of SSI.

4.6.4.2 In the operating theatre

4.6.4.2.1 *Pre-operative skin preparation.* Prevention in the operating theatre begins with the skin preparation of the operative site. The site is cleansed with chlorhexidine or povidone iodine – some containing 40% isopropyl alcohol. Isopropyl alcohol has excellent antiseptic qualities, but should be used with caution because of its flammability when used with electrocautery. All antiseptics should be allowed to dry before the incision is made to allow optimum antiseptic effect.

4.6.4.2.2 *Personal protective clothing.* Most surgical teams use caps, gowns, masks and sterile surgical gloves. Double gloving has been documented to prevent blood 'strike through' onto the surgeon's hands and is desirable to prevent risks of blood-borne occupational infection.

4.6.4.3 During operations

SSI depends largely on the skill and technique of the operating team and less often on the support provided post-operatively.

4.6.4.3.1 *The length of surgery.* Operations lasting more than two hours increase the risk of infection and exponentially thereafter.

4.6.4.3.2 *Drapes.* Cotton drapes are still in use in many low-income countries despite reports of lint resulting in non-bacterial wound infection. The other disadvantage is that cotton offers no barrier once wet.

Wet drapes on the patient may allow passage of bacteria into the operative area from other unprepared areas. Gowns and drapes that have become soaked should be replaced. Wide areas of skin preparation around the proposed surgical site will reduce the risk of microbial breakthrough into the wound area if towels and drapes become wet.

Non-woven drapes have several advantages, such as lack of linting and a good fluid barrier, but they are expensive and disposable. New non-woven material is available which can be re-used and is lint-free as well as water-repellent.

Adhesive plastic skin drapes should be avoided in clean operations – they collect moisture underneath and increase bacterial colonisation.

4.6.4.3.3   *Sterilisation of surgical devices* (see Decontamination of medical devices, Chapter 3). Sterilisation of instruments after thorough cleansing of any particulate matter is obviously important for infection control. An adequate supply of instruments should minimise the need for the rapid steam sterilisation of dropped or contaminated instruments during the procedure.

4.6.4.3.4   *Surgical technique.* Poor surgical technique is a major risk factor. The team should ensure good haemostasis and minimise tissue injury during operation. Haemoglobin within the soft tissues or within the wound space becomes a potent stimulus to microbial multiplication and infection.

The wound edges should be clean and easily apposed during closure. Maceration of the wound edges and desiccation lead to increased bacterial counts that accumulate within the wound. Poor perfusion of the skin resulting from decreased temperature and hypovolaemia can increase the risk of infection. Soft tissues should be handled gently to avoid crushing that can result in tissue necrosis and increased rates of SSI.

Suture material in the wound can also increase rates of SSI. The likelihood of an infection is greater with braided silk than with an absorbable suture material. For this reason, **absorbable suture material is preferred**. Silk fascial sutures should not be used. If a permanent suture is used for fascial closure, **monofilament alternatives** should be chosen.

Avoid dead space within the surgical wound. The drain should exit through a separate stab wound, and not through the surgical incision itself. Passive drains (Penrose drains) should not be used.

When the surgical site is severely contaminated or, frankly, dirty, the skin and subcutaneous tissues should be left open for topical post-operative management.

4.6.4.4 Post-operative care

The risk of wound infection is generally determined by pre-operative and intra-operative events. Little in the post-operative period will change this. Sterile dressings are placed over the wound, but the fibrin matrix is deposited rapidly at the wound interface, and this creates a biological seal that is affected very little by the surface surgical dressing. Topical ointments on the surface of the closed incision have a minimal role in the prevention of SSI and are discouraged.

4.6.4.5 Preventive antibiotic therapy

Systemic antibiotics given after the contaminating event have had no appreciable effect upon the natural history of infection. Post-operative antibiotics do not affect SSI rates because:

- Microbial pathogens are embedded in the fibrin matrix and antibiotics cannot reach them.
- The inflammatory cascade continues after wound closure and results in ischaemia – antibiotics cannot penetrate.

4.6.4.6 Antibiotic prophylaxis

Systemic preventive antibiotics should be used when:

- There is a risk of infection associated with the procedure (e.g. colon resection)
- consequences of infection are unusually severe (e.g. total joint replacement)
- patient has a high risk index.

The antibiotic should be administered pre-operatively, but as close to the time of the incision as is clinically practical, preferably giving a high blood level at the time of incision. Antibiotics should be administered before the induction of anesthesia in most situations. The antibiotic selected should have activity against the pathogens likely to be encountered in the procedure.

Post-operative administration of preventive systemic antibiotics beyond 24 hours has not been demonstrated to reduce the risk of SSI.

4.6.4.7 Oral antibiotic bowel preparation

The use of oral antibiotic bowel preparation requires appropriate mechanical preparation of the colon. For colon surgery, most surgeons choose to use preventive systemic antibiotics and the oral antibiotic bowel preparation together.

4.6.4.8 Enhancement of host defences

Reducing SSI can be assisted by improving host defences by:

- increased oxygen delivery
- optimising core body temperature
- blood glucose control
- controlling blood volume.

These elements have become a part of the SSI bundle towards reducing infection.

4.6.5 The key elements of an SSI bundle are:

- Appropriate delivery of prophylactic antibiotics – selection, timely administration and stopping
- Appropriate hair removal – only if necessary
- Post-operative blood glucose control
- Normothermia – keep the patient warm

An additional consideration should be to keep access to the operating theatre to a minimum during the operation – opening and closing doors may cause air turbulence in the theatre.

4.6.6 Management of surgical wound infections

The type of surgery (clean, clean-contaminated, contaminated or dirty) will determine the risk level of infection and the likely spectrum of pathogens. If wounds are not grossly infected, they may respond to local measures such as removal of sutures. Frequent cleaning should be undertaken and the wound requires a drain to allow healing. Deep-seated infection related to complicated abdominal surgery may require broad-spectrum antibiotics and investigation for possible surgical intervention.

4.6.6.1 Procedure for dressing a wound

Dressing a wound is an aseptic procedure irrespective of the type of wound:

1. Lay a trolley with a sterile wound dressing pack (contains all the necessary items) or collect up the necessary items.
   - (a) Clean surface with alcohol and allow to dry.
   - (b) Lay out the sterile items so that these are easily accessible.
   - (c) Place a bag for dirty dressings and discarded items.
   - (d) Ensure alcohol rub is available.
2. Remove the old dressing and inspect the wound.
3. Carry out hand hygiene.
4. Wear sterile gloves (standard precautions) if local policy recommends it.
5. Clean the wound thoroughly and carefully using cotton wool or similar soaked in the recommended cleaning solution. Do not leave any fibres behind as these interfere with healing. **Note:** Some procedures recommend the use of forceps and others suggest using hands only. Follow local practice.

6. Take a needle biopsy for diagnostic purposes if necessary. Alternatively, exude any fluid from the infected wound by pressing together with two pieces of gauze held in two sterile forceps. Take a specimen of pus for examination if required.

7. Apply necessary medication and dressings as prescribed.

8. Cover the wound with appropriate dressing.

9. Discard all dirty dressings.

10. Discard gloves (if used).

11. Carry out hand hygiene.

If antiseptics are being used, it is best to have individually packed sachets to avoid cross-contamination. If a multi-use bottle is used to dispense an aliquot into a gallipot, make sure that this is either done when the sterile wound pack is opened or ask a colleague to assist.

Dressing trolleys are still found in some countries, although they are becoming less common. These are covered with communal-use bottles and jars containing disinfectants, which are a major source of contamination to surgical and other wounds. These are a potential source of an outbreak, especially among immunocompromised patient groups. The patient monitoring equipment such as stethoscopes, blood pressure apparatus and dry cotton wool balls also become contaminated through hands and splashes.

The reasons for contamination are:
- Topping up of jars containing cotton wool with antiseptics from multi-use bottles and using these for cleaning injection sites.
- Putting dirty hands or cheatle forceps into the antiseptic containers and contaminating the entire jar.
- Constantly using the dressing trolley, which then does not allow time to change the jars, clean or disinfect them.
- Dressings becoming contaminated by splashing and from the environment on the ward.
- Some antiseptics becoming inactivated in the presence of cotton wool, rayon and other similar material and thus lose their antimicrobial activity.
- Inadequate and infrequent cleaning of the trolley itself between patients or shifts.

Dressing trolleys should be replaced by individual wound packs.

4.7   Ventilator-associated pneumonia

Ventilator-associated pneumonia (VAP) is a subtype of hospital-acquired pneumonia (HAP) which occurs in people who are on mechanical ventilation through an endotracheal or tracheostomy tube for at least 48 hours.

4.7.1 Prevalence

VAP is one of the most common infections acquired by adults and children in intensive care units (ICUs).[43] Previously VAP was reported as affecting 10–20% of patients undergoing ventilation. The NNIS report rates that range from 1 to 4 cases per 1 000 ventilator days, but rates may exceed 10 cases per 1 000 ventilator days in some neonatal and surgical patient populations.[44]

VAP is a cause of significant patient morbidity and mortality, increased utilisation of healthcare resources and excess cost. The mortality attributable to VAP may exceed 10%. Patients with VAP require prolonged periods of mechanical ventilation, extended hospitalisations, a larger number than is usual of antimicrobial courses and increased direct medical costs. Improved IPC initiatives using bundles have been shown to prevent VAP by careful attention to the process of care.

4.7.2 Pathophysiology

VAP arises when there is bacterial invasion of the pulmonary parenchyma in a patient receiving mechanical ventilation. Inoculation of the formerly sterile lower respiratory tract typically arises from aspiration of secretions, colonisation of the upper and lower respiratory tract or use of contaminated equipment or medications. The presence of a foreign body such as the endotracheal tube prevents the natural bronchial defences from functioning optimally. Secretions accumulate in the subepiglottic space and are reported to contribute to increased rates of infection.

When patients are sedated the aspiration of stomach contents has contributed to aspiration pneumonia in ventilated patients.

VAP has been categorised into:

1. **Early onset pneumonia**, which occurs within five days of being incubated. The bacteria are usually community-acquired such as *Haemophilus influenzae*, *Streptococcus pneumoniae* and *Staph aureus* and are antibiotic sensitive. TB should be considered in countries with a high incidence of TB.

2. **Late onset pneumonia** occurs after five days of intubation. It is associated with bacteria from oropharyngeal and gastrointestinal colonisation. These are usually resistant to antibiotics (MDROs) because of the administration of antibiotics, inadequate infection control practices and repeated manipulation by the staff, admission to the ICU and underlying disease or surgical procedures.

[43] Coffin SE, Klompas M, Classen D et al. 2008. Strategies to prevent ventilator-associated pneumonia in acute care hospitals. *Infection Control and Hospital Epidemiology*. 9, supplement 1.

[44] Joint Commission perspectives on patient safety. April 2006. Joint Commission on Accreditation of Healthcare Organizations, 9(4).

The microbiological criteria for VAP are difficult to establish since the mouth and endotracheal tube are colonised with HAI pathogens not necessarily causing infection. Invasive sampling techniques may be more accurate but not routinely possible.

4.7.3 Risk factors

The risk factors for VAP are as follows:

- Admission to an ICU: The ICU environment is often colonised with multiple antibiotic-resistant bacteria. Patients undergo more manipulation than on the wards and therefore there is more contact by the staff. Antibiotics are more frequently prescribed in ICUs and many of these are broad spectrum, which further contributes to resistance.
- Prolonged intubation: Patients who have been ventilated for more than five days are at risk of developing VAP.
- Enteral feeding: The presence of a nasogastric tube depresses the normal host defences.
- Aspiration of stomach contents is common in supine patients and is a risk.
- Paralytic agents reduce the swallowing and cough reflex, resulting in a build-up of secretions and colonisation.
- Underlying illness: Surgical procedures, diabetes or immune suppression increases the risk for VAP.
- Extremes of age: Neonatal and elderly patients are at risk for VAP and have a higher mortality rate from it.

4.7.4 Diagnosis of VAP

The clinical diagnosis is based on a patient who is mechanically ventilated and has (a) an increase or decrease in temperature of 2 °C or more from the norm; (b) an increase in white cell count; and (c) new infiltrates on the chest X-ray. Since these patients are sedated it is difficult to establish other symptoms of pneumonia.

Microbiological evidence of infection would be supported by positive blood culture isolates preferably matching respiratory sputum samples taken by tracheal aspirate or invasive bronchial methods.

4.7.5 Reducing risk for VAP

The prevention of VAP or reduction in the incidence of the disease is based on skilled staff that are knowledgeable about preventing VAP using good IPC practices to reduce the risk factors listed above. The application of a VAP bundle encompasses these risk reducing strategies. The four subsections below set down in detail the practices recommended by IPC specialists in the field:

4.7.5.1 Administrative

- There should be a written policy on how to handle ventilated patients. VAP bundles have been introduced, which have reduced the incidence of VAP dramatically.
- Regular updates and training for all ICU staff should be carried out.
- Enforcement of existing IPC policies.

4.7.5.2 Patient factors

- Orotracheal intubation is preferred over the nasotracheal route because the outcomes are better and it reduces sinusitis.
- Only intubate patients if absolutely necessary and only as long as it is necessary.
- Cleaning the oral cavity has shown to reduce colonisation and VAP.
- Treat the underlying disease.
- Avoid H2 antagonists or protein-pump inhibitors if not indicated for patients with stress ulcers. Acid-suppressive therapy may increase colonisation.

4.7.5.3 Preventing aspiration

- The patient should be placed in a semi-recumbent position (30–45° angle) to prevent aspiration of gastric secretions.
- Avoid distension of the gastrointestinal tract.
- Do not repeatedly intubate and extubate as this increases the risk for VAP. All such procedures should be planned and evaluated daily.
- Subglottal suctioning of secretions is recommended.

4.7.5.4 IPC practices to reduce VAP

- Always carry out hand hygiene before and after patient contact.
- Wear non-sterile gloves during endotracheal suctioning.
- Ensure the patient is in a semi-supine position.
- A new ventilator circuit should be provided for each patient and should be changed once it has become soiled or malfunctioning. There are no fixed schedules for changing circuits.
- Heat- and moisture-exchange filters are recommended if there are no contra-indications such as haemoptysis or when high minute ventilation is required. These filters should be changed weekly.
- It is recommended that closed suction systems are in place and changed for every new patient or as clinically indicated.
- Use a sterile suction catheter each time the patient is suctioned. If re-using the catheter is unavoidable, rinse in sterile water and store in the original packing. Do not allow contamination.
- Open bowls containing sterile water are not sterile after they have been used once. Discard water after each session and store the bowl dry until the next time.

- The endotracheal tube should be cuffed. An inline suctioning port.
- Use sterile water to rinse re-usable respiratory equipment.
- Remove condensate from ventilator circuits. Keep the ventilator circuit closed during condensate removal.
- Ventilator circuits should either be disposed or, if re-used, heat-disinfected. Chemical processing like the use of ethylene oxide is not recommended.
- Store and disinfect respiratory therapy equipment properly.

4.7.6 Key elements of a VAP Bundle[45]

The following key elements are contained in the VAP bundle

- Elevate the head of the bed to 45 degrees when possible, otherwise attempt to maintain the head of the bed greater than 30 degrees
- Daily evaluation of readiness for extubation
- Subglottic secretion drainage
- Oral care and decontamination with chlorhexidine (0,5%)
- Initiation of safe enteral nutrition within 24–48 hours of ICU admission.

4.8 Bundles of clinical risk-prone procedures

4.8.1 What is a bundle?[46]

Bundles were developed by the US Institute of Healthcare Improvement to help healthcare providers to deliver more reliably the best possible care for patients undergoing particular treatments with inherent risks. A bundle is a structured way of improving processes of care and patient outcomes. It is a short, straightforward set of practices (usually three to five) which, when performed collectively, reliably and continuously, have been proven to improve patient outcomes. Data from these frequent measures fed back to those involved in the procedures has also been shown to result in improvement to the process and a reduction in negative actions.

The power of a bundle comes from the evidence behind it and the method of execution, which must be completely consistent. It is not that the recommended changes in a bundle are new. Indeed they are well-established best practices, but they are often not performed uniformly, making treatment unreliable and even at times idiosyncratic. **A bundle ties the changes together into a package of interventions that people know must be followed for every patient, every single time.**

---

[45] DOH South Africa. Practical Manual for the Implementation of the National IPC Strategic Framework, 2020 https://www.ihi.org/resources/Pages/ImprovementStories/WhatIsaBundle.aspx.
[46] Institute of Healthcare Improvement. https://www.ihi.org/Topics/Bundles/Pages/default.aspx.

4.8.2 How are bundles produced?

Each bundle is based on the best available scientific evidence. In order for this evidence to be assessed for transfer into practice, a 'cause and effect chart' is produced. A 'cause and effect chart' is an industrial-quality improvement tool which describes a system under the key headings: people, environment, methods and equipment. From this, the key bundle criteria are identified. The model for improvement suggests a series of small tests until there is non-person-dependent reliability in the system.

4.8.3 How can a bundle be used in practice?

The goal is to make a process more reliable, and that is done by improving habits and processes. The effectiveness of the bundle comes from the guidelines and the way the work is organised. A bundle has specific elements that make it unique, but the changes are **all necessary and all sufficient**. This means that if there are four changes in the bundle and any one of them is removed, the results are not the same.

A bundle focuses on how to deliver the best care – not **what** the care should be. The changes in a bundle are clear-cut and straightforward; they involve **all-or-nothing measurement**. Successfully completing each step is a simple and straightforward process. It is a 'yes' or 'no' answer; there is no in between. Bundle changes also occur **in the same time and space continuum**: at a specific time and in a specific place, no matter what. This might be during morning rounds every day or every six hours at the patient's bedside, for instance. It usually takes two people to ensure the bundle is properly implemented.

Each bundle pack contains:
- The bundle
- A statement of commitment for the clinical team to sign
- A cause and effect chart describing the evidence for optimal practice
- SOP for the bundle, including criteria
- A data collection sheet
- A digital slide presentation to explain the bundle to your staff.

4.8.4 Difference between a bundle and a checklist

A checklist can be very helpful and an important vehicle for ensuring safe and reliable care. A bundle is a small but critical set of processes all determined by robust evidence. Because some elements of a checklist are nice to do but not required, there may be no effect on the patient if they are not completed. When a bundle element is missed the patient is at much greater risk of serious complications.

There is also a level of accountability tied to a bundle that is not always present with a checklist. An identified person or team owns it. A checklist might be owned by everybody on a floor or a team, but we know that, in reality, when it is owned by everyone nobody owns it! A bundle is a person's or a team's responsibility and it is their job at a certain point and time. It is very clear who has to do what and when, within a specific time frame. The accountability and focus give a bundle a lot of its power.

Summary

A bundle is a specific tool with clear parameters. It has a small number of elements that are all scientifically robust, which when taken together create much improved outcomes. There is no need to convert helpful checklists into overloaded bundles. If the concept of a bundle becomes so broad and loses in meaning, its power will start to diminish.

- Bundles provide a set of consistent evidence-based guidance and a common approach for the management of patients.
- The availability of the bundle should reduce duplication of effort.
- The reporting nature of the bundles system allows you to demonstrate the quality of your clinical team's work.
- Improving the quality of the clinical team's work will **save time**.

Appendix A

Antiseptics used in hand hygiene

Antiseptics are safe to use on the skin (living tissue), while **disinfectants** are used on inanimate objects and surfaces because they have adverse effects on living tissue. Although these two terms are often used interchangeably, the products should not be. Antiseptics are used for hand hygiene and skin preparation during surgery. Some antiseptics are combined with others to increase efficacy and sustain antimicrobial effect. The concentration of antiseptics may differ in different formulations and the regulations of a country, but all antiseptics have optimal antimicrobial activity only at the recommended dilutions. The two commonly used antiseptics are chlorhexidine gluconate, either 2% or 4% w/v, or povidone iodine, which has replaced tincture of iodine for safety reasons. Both are formulated as aqueous or combined with alcohol – the alcohol concentration ranges from 70% for hands to 40% used for skin preparation in surgery to prevent diathermy burns.

Other antiseptics such as triclosan are used for specific indications such as reducing colonisation of MRSA.

An ideal antiseptic

- is non-toxic to human tissue
- has a broad spectrum of antimicrobial activity
- can be combined with other antiseptics without losing activity
- is not readily inactivated by (cationic or anionic) detergents
- is not readily inactivated by organic matter
- has a rapid, sustained action
- can accumulate in the epidermis without harm to humans
- does not produce toxic residue when used over a period of time.

Antimicrobial activity of antiseptics. An effective antiseptic should have a wide spectrum of activity to cover all possible microbes that hands of healthcare workers come into contact with during clinical activities. Some antiseptics have proven to be toxic for human use and have been withdrawn.

Table 1 Antimicrobial spectrum of antiseptics

Note: Hexachlorophene 3% and tincture of iodine are no longer recommended

Group	GPC	GNB	MTB	Fungi	Viruses
Alcohols	Good	Good	Good	Good	Good
Chlorhexidine 2% and 4% (aqueous)	Good	Good	Fair	Fair	Good
Iodophors	Good	Good	Fair	Good	Good
Parachlorometaxylenol (PCMX)	Good	Fair	Fair	Fair	Fair
Triclosan	Good	Good	Fair	Poor	Good

The speed of killing microbes without being inactivated by organic matter is one of the criteria when choosing an appropriate antiseptic. Table 2 outlines these characteristics.

Table 2 Properties of antiseptics

Group	Speed of kill	Inactivation of organic matter	Use	Comment
Alcohols	Fast	Moderate	Hands; surgical site prep	Best at 70–90% strength with emollients (glycerine or Ceryl ROH – less drying)
Chlorhexidine 2% and 4% (aqueous)	Medium	Minimal	As above	Persistent effect; not near mucous membranes; toxic to eyes and ears; inactivated by non-ionic surfactants
Iodophors	Medium	Moderate	As above	Less irritating; rapidly neutralised by organic matter
Parachlorometaxylenol (PCMX)	Medium	Minimal	Hands	Neutralised by non-ionic surfactants
Triclosan	Medium	Minimal	Chlorhexidine substitute	Plasmid-mediated cross-resistance with MRSA

5   The built environment

Shaheen Mehtar

Learning outcomes

What you should know after reading this chapter:
- Role of IPC in hospital design
- IPC requirements in designing healthcare facilities
- Infrastructure requirements for IPC
- Layout of general and specialised units

Introduction

Hospitals have been in existence in one form or the other for more than two centuries. Classical examples are 'fever hospitals' in Europe, tuberculosis sanatoriums, cholera hospitals and infectious diseases hospitals in the tropics. The working principles at the time were good ventilation, wide open wards with lots of natural light and low occupancy, but this was not always possible.

Changing disease profiles and increased urbanisation occurred over the years, causing existing health facilities to expand or contract to accommodate these changes. Specialised areas such as operating theatres, intensive care units, neonatal units and sterile services were introduced, or modernised, to keep abreast of developments in healthcare. As more evidence emerged relating to the role of surfaces and fomites in transmission of pathogens, particularly when directly in contact with patients and staff, designs and material used in health facilities improved. New health facilities were built in confined available urban spaces and were designed to serve an ever expanding population. The re-emergence of infectious diseases has posed an infection prevention and control (IPC) dilemma because, without a hierarchy of controls (administrative, engineering and personal protective IPC precautions) in place, transmission of pathogens such as *Mycobacterium tuberculosis* and SARS-CoV-2 is exacerbated by crowded and poorly ventilated healthcare facilities.

Modernisation of health facilities requires the combined knowledge and expertise of engineers, architects, facility managers, project managers, designers and infection control personnel. Many countries have building regulations and several documents are available which specify requirements for building or renovating hospitals. The COVID-19 pandemic changed the perspective on ventilation and recognised (or established) routes of transmission. In the past five years, new scientific evidence and developments have taken place regarding IPC and the built environment.

This chapter discusses the role of IPC as part of the project team designing hospitals to support good infection control practices. particularly in low- to middle-income (LMIC) settings, to reduce transmission in facilities.

5.1 Role of IPC in a project team

When planning a new healthcare facility or considering renovations, a project team is established. A project manager is appointed who ensures regular meetings to update the team of experts, monitors progress and sees that the required specifications are met. As a reminder to the reader, the role of IPC is to reduce the number of infectious particles, reduce the number of people exposed to the infectious source and apply the routes of transmission of pathogens to design. In order to achieve this, *the built environment must accommodate for light, ventilation and space between beds*. The IPC aspects to be considered are:

- workflow relating to patients, staff, equipment and removal of waste
- layout of clinical areas that allows for good natural ventilation and adequate bed spacing (air movement)
- adequate number of isolation rooms with en suite ablution facilities for the population
- natural ventilation and temperature control in the clinical environment with mechanical ventilation for certain specialist areas
- ensuring constant supply of good quality water and power
- adequate space for staff administration, restrooms and recreation
- movement of supplies and removal of waste in and out of the facility
- adequate space allocated to staff offices, restrooms and activities to ensure the clinical areas on the wards are not taken over for these purposes.

In some countries, building regulations include IPC recommendations, recognising that IPC can contribute significantly to a project team by advising on the main areas to reduce transmission of HAI and other pathogens. The project team should consider the following:

- Timely and collaborative partnerships to successfully achieve IPC goals specific for each phase of construction planning

- Understanding and assessing the risk of infection relating to construction projects and the built environment particularly during renovations
- Stakeholders to understand the basic principles of 'designed-in' rather than 'add on' infection control measures
- Good project management in relation to IPC considerations in all building projects and renovations
- Quality control throughout the duration of the project
- Continually monitoring progress and implementation of IPC principles.

For this to happen, the IPC teams must be trained and knowledgeable about current trends and evidence in workflow, building layout and ventilation.

5.2   Renovations

During renovation of existing structures there is a risk from fungal spores, such as *Aspergillus spp*, and moulds causing infection.[1] These are dispersed from the plaster and dust created during building works and enter the host via the respiratory tract or can be directly imbedded into surgical wounds,[2] particularly in highly immunocompromised patients (principally bone marrow transplant patients). Patients should be relocated to safe temporary accommodation during renovations. The same applies to operating theatres (OT) where operations, especially implant surgeries, are undertaken. Even minor works (removing ceiling tiles) can release spores; the OT must be closed for that period of time, cleaned and commissioned by the engineers and IPC team prior to opening. IPC should conduct a post-renovation assessment to ensure the area is fit for purpose and patients are safe. Any interference with the ventilation system, for example, should be preceded by notification and planning to minimise risk to patients.[3]

5.3   Designing a new healthcare facility

There are several considerations in the design of a healthcare facility. All are concerned with the need to accommodate multiple demands made on a modern hospital to provide safe, quality healthcare.

1   Donna Haiduven. 2009. Nosocomial aspergillosis and building construction. *Medical Mycology* 47 Supplement 1: S210 S216. https://doi.org/10.1080/13693780802247694.
2   Tabbara KF & Jabarti AA. 1998. Hospital-construction-associated outbreak of ocular aspergillosis after cataract surgery. *Opthalmology* 105: 522–6.
3   Talento A, Fitzgerald M, Redington B, O'Sullivan N, Fenelon L & Rogers TR. 2019. Prevention of healthcare-associated invasive aspergillosis during hospital construction/renovation works. *JHI*. 103: 1–12.

5.3.1 Population and disease profile

The primary principle when designing should be the size and disease profile of the population to be served as this influences the structure and layout of the healthcare facility. Inevitably these parameters will change in subsequent years, and healthcare facilities must be flexible enough to reflect this change. The impact on health facilities is also influenced by the age, gender and social status of the surrounding community and referral patterns to and from primary healthcare to inpatient facilities.

5.3.2 Design elements

In the past ten years or so, there is increasing evidence in the field of Water Sanitation And Hygiene (WASH) and ventilation. Guidelines on natural ventilation for infection control in healthcare settings, drafted by the World Health Organisation,[4] provide a useful background for IPC practitioners involved in designing healthcare facilities and some aspects of these have been incorporated into this chapter. More recently, during the COVID-19 pandemic, a roadmap to improved indoor ventilation (2021)[5] has brought the latest evidence to bear on ventilation in enclosed spaces and is recommended reading for all. The WASH elements must be a priority for IPC when designing a health facility.

5.3.3 Choosing a site

When selecting a location, bear in mind an expanding urban population and make sure that the projected 10 years allow for expansion if necessary. Site design should integrate the buildings within the existing topography and surrounding buildings. Minor modifications may be permitted, within the limits of environment and wildlife protection. The healthcare facility should be conveniently placed within easy reach of the population it serves, being accessible by public and private transportation. Ideally, it should be integrated into the existing environment and buildings, using existing facilities such as electricity, water and, sometimes, steam supply. If these are inadequate, provision must be made to provide a sustainable supply in both the quality and quantity required. Where these elements are overlooked, this oversight impacts negatively on the optimum functioning of the facility and the project team is made aware of these facts prior to starting building.

---

[4]   World Health Organization. 2009. *Natural ventilation for infection control in healthcare settings*. Geneva: World Health Organiation.

[5]   Roadmap to improve and ensure good indoor ventilation in the context of COVID-19. Geneva: World Health Organization; 2021. Licence: CC BY-NC-SA 3.0 IGO.

5.3.4 Climatic considerations

Countries with moderate winter and summer temperatures should consider the use of natural ventilation. Where mechanical ventilation is supplied to the entire hospital, the system must be maintained and be able to keep the areas served at the required temperatures.

In warmer climes, particularly in poorer settings, the use of large windows and doors serves well to ventilate[6] and can be effective in reducing airborne transmission in crowded healthcare facilities. In LMICs the cost of installing mechanical ventilation may be excessive and therefore systems should be established to make maximum use of natural ventilation in general areas. Mechanical ventilation, whether negative or positive pressure ventilation, should be applied to specific areas according to recommendations and should be supplied via independent air handling units.

5.3.5 Building design

The essential elements when designing a health facility are:
- flexibility
- easily cleanable surfaces, furnishings and fittings
- constant supply of good quality water, sanitation and power supply.

Building designs change frequently from high-rise to low-rise buildings, with services conveniently structured to minimise long walks between clinical and utility areas. It is estimated that 30–45% of a nurse's time could be spent walking between the patient areas and the utilities. This should be taken into account when considering workflow.

For simple buildings, Priolo[7] recommends attention to building, roof design, aspect ratios and the use of overhangs, wind walls and recessed spaces. Care should also be taken to ensure pedestrian comfort at the ground level outdoors.

5.3.5.1 *Internal distribution of space and its effect on ventilation*

The internal layout will affect the workflow and movement of patients, staff, equipment and services. It is best to cluster clinical specialities that require similar facilities and infrastructure together. For example, the maternity unit should be close to the neonatal and paediatric wards with easy access to kangaroo care, rooms for mothers to express breast milk (EBM room) and storage. The burns

6   Escombe RA, Oesar CC, Giman RH, et al. 2007. Natural ventilation for the prevention of airborne contagion. *Public Library of Science Medicine* 4(2). Available at www. plosmedicine.org.
7   Priolo C. 1998. Design guidelines and technical solutions for natural ventilation. In: Allard F. *Natural ventilation in Building: A Design Handbook*. London: James & James, pp 195–254.

unit should be close to the other surgical wards and the operating theatre. Service provision such as kitchens, waste disposal and laundry services, if provided on site, should be carefully planned.

Tall buildings (10 floors or more) can be laid out by clinical specialty per floor, which helps to consolidate services and resources. However, these have an effect on the wind direction and can produce an up-and-down draft which may carry airborne pathogens from one area of the facility to another. Wind direction will also affect mechanical ventilation if it is placed incorrectly, particularly in a tall building. This is because there is a 'blow-back' effect, or entrainment, when the air which has been exhausted outside is drawn back into the building at the level of another floor. This is particularly dangerous when negative-pressure ventilation is applied to airborne pathogens.

A central atrium in tall buildings acts as a flue, drawing the air up from the clinical areas towards the top of the building. It can also cause air currents to float from one floor to the other on its way up to the top of the building, causing infection if the airflows are not correctly balanced.

Short buildings have the advantage of a better workflow, movement of staff and patients and the use of natural ventilation. They do, however, require more blocks to distribute the clinical specialities, unlike a tall building, which can house all the specialities in one major block.

5.3.5.2 Layout and design of wards

The layout of wards has changed over the years. Acute specialities have moved to smaller 4–6 bed units with an increase in the number of toilet and ablution facilities and a larger proportion of isolation rooms. Chronic disease patients require more space for socialising and rehabilitation for an aging population. Below are examples of the various types of wards that can be found in hospital buildings today, some dating back several centuries.

5.3.5.2.1 Dormitory (Florence Nightingale) wards

These were one of the first type of wards designed for hospitals. It is a single open space with beds lined on either side of the ward usually placed under large openable windows. The offices and isolation rooms are located towards the entrance of the ward, while all the amenities, clean and dirty utilities, are at the far end (Figure 5.1). The advantage of such a ward is that the patients are visible to the nursing station usually positioned in the centre of the ward. The disadvantages are the lack of privacy, that it facilitates transmission of infection, particularly airborne pathogens, and has few patient toilets.

If there are isolation rooms, these are usually located outside the main ward area.

office	WD		patient toilet & bath
	NIGHTINGALE WARD	sluice	
		clean store	
		cleaners cupboard	
office & tea	WARD		patient toilet & bath

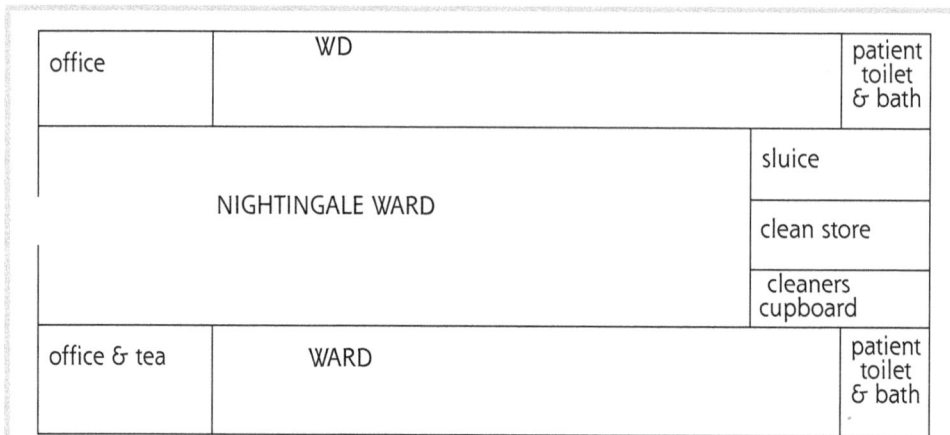

Figure 5.1   Diagrammatic representation of a dormitory or Nightingale Ward – open plan

5.3.5.2.2 Racetrack ward

Racetrack wards were laid out around a central nurses' station and clean and dirty utilities, while the patient beds occupied the whole floor (Figure 5.2). Each unit contained 4–6 beds, but did not usually have en suite facilities. The isolation rooms were on the far side of the ward.

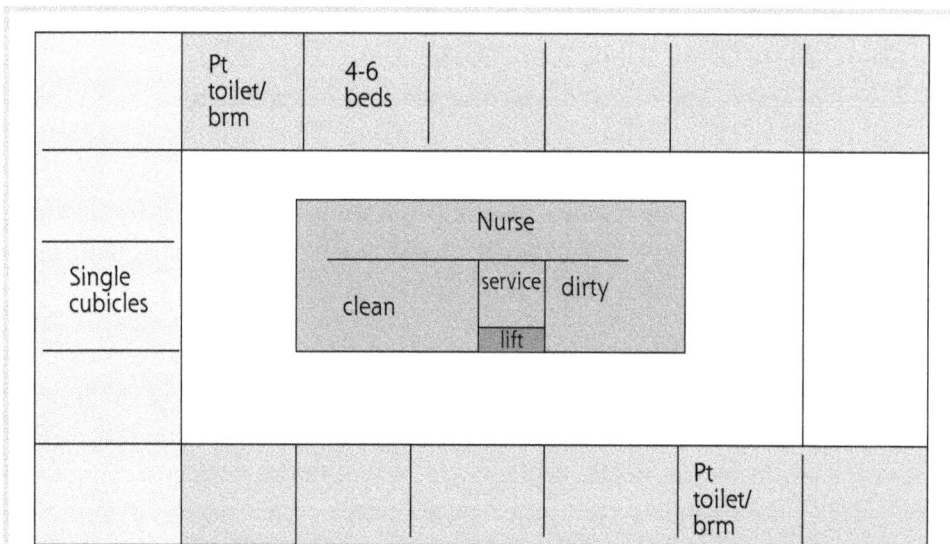

Pt toilet/ brm	4-6 beds				
Single cubicles		clean	Nurse / service / dirty / lift		
				Pt toilet/ brm	

Figure 5.2   Racecourse ward which runs around the nurses' station. The isolation rooms are located on one side.

In some designs the lift came up into this central pod, which was the only entrance to the ward apart from the fire escape. If there was more than one such ward on a floor, then the lift came into the corridor, allowing access to several wards.

The advantage of this layout ward was the reduced time of walking between the utilities and the clinical areas. The isolation rooms had an outside wall, which allowed negative-pressure ventilation to be installed. Most of these rooms also had en suite ablution facilities. The disadvantage was the lack of flexibility of the layout. If the lifts opened in the centre of the ward, there was a piston effect and airborne transmission from other wards, such as MRSA outbreaks had been reported. Finally, the beds behind the nurses' station could not be monitored constantly.

5.3.5.2.3 Bay wards

Bay wards have been designed using separation of clean and dirty areas. The corridor runs the length of the ward with the patient beds on one side, usually arranged in 4-6 bedded units and some single isolation rooms. The utilities and provisions are situated opposite the ward areas across the corridor. Staff facilities are usually at the entrance of the ward. The isolation beds are also located at the entrance of the ward (Figure 5.3). The advantage is this type of ward is that the bays can easily be cordoned off in case of an outbreak or cluster of HAIs. Cohort isolation is possible. The disadvantage is the long distance between the beds and utilities and there is considerable pressure on the already overworked staff to move up and down the corridor.

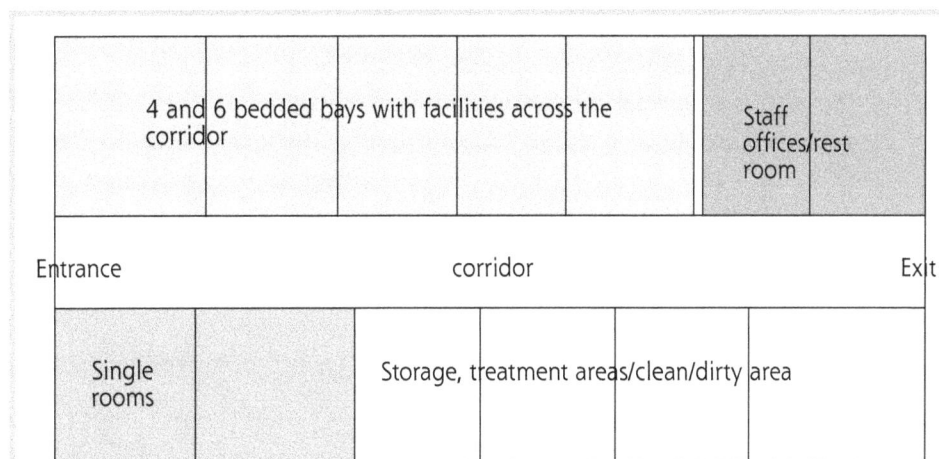

Figure 5.3 Bay wards with smaller units on one side and the utilities across the corridor

5.3.6 Infrastructure requirements

The health facility should receive maximum natural light during the day. If natural ventilation is considered, the wind direction should be taken into account. In countries with extreme temperatures, the effect on natural ventilation must be balanced to prevent overheating or overcooling.

From an IPC perspective, good ventilation is essential to improve patient safety and reduce airborne transmission. A light and airy environment adds to the patient's sense of well-being. Healthcare facilities in high-income countries rely almost entirely on controlled (mechanical) ventilation providing neutral, negative or positive ventilation as needed. In LMICs, health facilities usually have either natural or mixed ventilation. This chapter covers both natural and controlled ventilation. Other IPC requirements are a constant supply of good-quality water, sanitation facilities and an uninterrupted supply of power.

5.3.6.1 Ventilation

Generally, neutral ventilation, supplied either naturally or mechanically, is sufficient for most general areas in health facilities. Specialised areas such as the operating theatre, isolation rooms and pharmacy will require positive pressure-controlled ventilation while negative-pressure ventilation is indicated for airborne transmission (isolation rooms) and dirty areas (SSD) of the facility.

The resurgence of tuberculosis, and recently the COVID-19 pandemic, have led to a renewed interest in ventilation and airborne transmission. Convincing new evidence has emerged which has changed thinking around airborne and droplet transmission. The cloud produced by a person during speaking, coughing, sneezing or shouting is made up of a range of size of particles. These are now classified as *short- and long-range aerosols* which are released, travelling varying distances depending upon the temperature and humidity – the concept of <5 μ no longer applies. The heavier ones (short range) will succumb to gravity and fall relatively quickly, contaminating surfaces in the environment. The lighter ones (long range) will float on air currents to considerable distances of up to 3 m or more. Both these, short- and long-range aerosols, depend on ventilation – the better the ventilation, the quicker these particles will be removed from the environment and reduce transmission.

5.3.6.1.1 Types of ventilation

There are three ways to ventilate a building (Table 5.1), and they are summarised below.

Table 5.1   Types of ventilation (adapted from WHO natural ventilation, 2009)

	Mechanical	**Natural**	**Mixed**
Advantage	Suitable for all climates and weather Can be controlled	Suitable for mild and moderate climates Low costs and maintenance Capable of high ventilation rates Controllable by occupants	Suitable for all climates and weather Energy-saving Flexible

Disadvantage	Expensive to install and maintain, especially negative-pressure	Affected by climate Difficult to design Reduces comfort level if hot, humid or cold Inability to provide negative pressure in isolation areas	Expensive Difficult to design

Mechanical ventilation is best suited to extreme temperatures and is expensive to install and maintain – a skilled group of engineers is required. Natural or mixed is best suited to temperate climes, but require considerable skill to install and maintain.

5.3.6.1.1.1 *Natural ventilation*

Natural ventilation uses summer and winter winds to provide a sufficient number of air changes to deliver comfort and fresh air in the building (Figure 5.4). It can be used effectively for reducing transmission of airborne pathogens such as *M tuberculosis* and SARS-CoV-2. The healthcare facility should be constructed to maximise this capability.

- A major objective is to use natural airflow patterns on the site to increase the potential of natural ventilation such as summer cooling and winter minimum ventilation by studying prevailing wind directions and locating the building accordingly.
- The driving wind pressure is not just the positive pressure at the windward openings but also the negative pressures at the leeward openings. Building form and orientation should be such as to increase the negative pressures in the wake of airflows.[8]

The planning for use of natural ventilation starts with the architectural design. Its planning includes the system layout and component selection, vent sizing and design control strategy and is concluded by detailed design drawing. Instructions on the use of open windows should be available for the patients and healthcare workers.

The WHO (2009) recommends the following when developing the design concept for a naturally ventilated building for infection control. The three basic steps are:

Step 1. Specify the desired airflow pattern from the inlet openings, through the wards and other hospital spaces such as corridors, to the outlet openings.

Step 2. Identify the main available driving forces which enable the desired airflow pattern to be achieved.

---

[8]   World Health Organization. 2009. Natural ventilation for infection control in health care settings. World Health Organization. https://apps.who.int/iris/handle/10665/44167.

Step 3. Size and locate the openings so that the required ventilation rates can be delivered under all operating regimes.

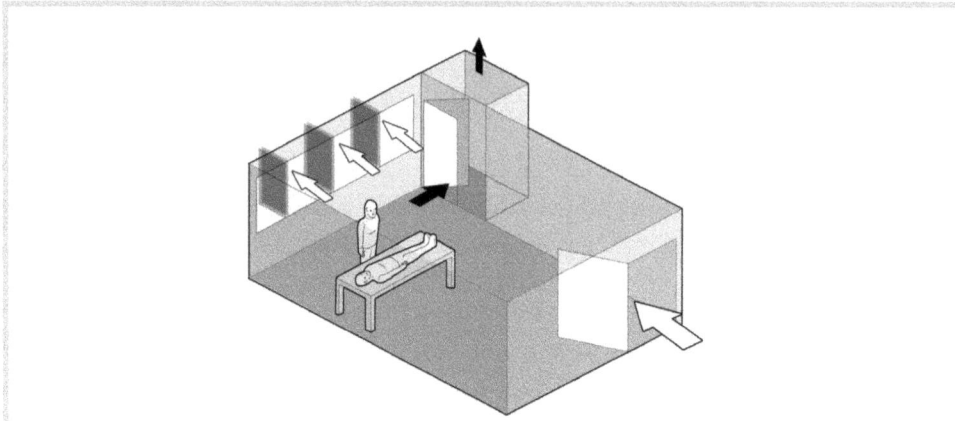

Figure 5.4 Natural ventilation achieved by opening the windows and the door to the corridor in the isolation room

5.3.6.1.1.2 Neutral ('balanced') ventilation

Most areas in the hospital will only require neutral ventilation where equal volumes of air are delivered to and removed from an area in equal proportions. This would apply to all wards and common areas in the healthcare facility. Open windows are used to deliver such ventilation since the rate of air movement is not an issue, but at least 6 ACH is expected. In LMICs, especially where transmission of tuberculosis within the healthcare facility is a concern, patient areas should have windows constructed with a larger section at the bottom that can be opened in the summer and closed during the winter. The upper section (skylight or similar) could remain open with louvres so that when a heater is placed below the window, hot air rises and flows out of the upper windows (Figure 5.5). Extractor fans can be installed for exhausting air.

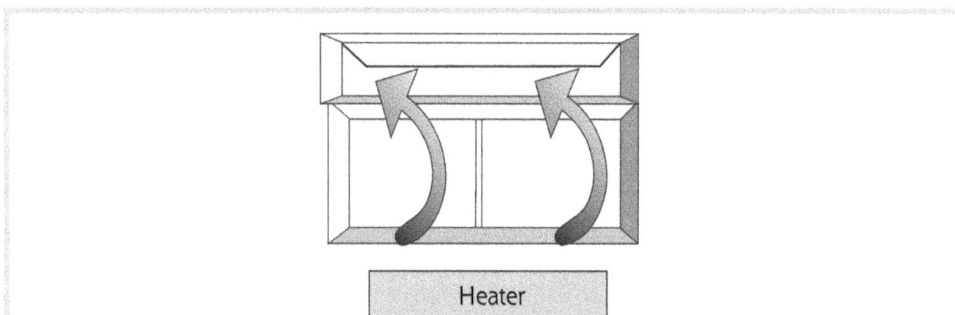

Heater

Figure 5.5 A smaller open window above with the heater placed below so that hot air can rise and remove some of the airborne particles; useful when nursing TB patients in cold climates

5.3.6.1.1.3 Controlled (mechanical) ventilation

Air handling units are designed to deliver a predetermined airflow and temperature into a particular area (Figure 5.6).

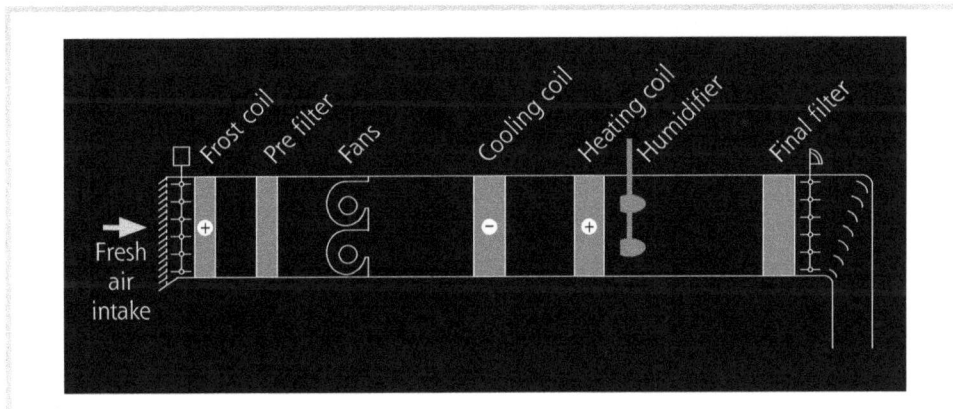

Figure 5.6 Layout of an air handling unit and delivery system to clinical areas

Air is drawn in through a set of coarse particle (dust) filters, also known as the pre-filter, by a fan. The air is moved through a cooling or heating coil, depending on what is needed, then through a humidifier and finally a fine filter (approximately 70–80% efficacy) to remove any particles and is pushed into the healthcare facility areas via ducts which are regulated to deliver air as specified. Usually in hospitals no special ventilation requirements are necessary unless indicated by type of work or disease of the patient, and this will be addressed under each section. Mechanical ventilation is necessary in order to deliver specific air pressure ventilation, allowing control of requirements and maintenance of the air handling unit (AHU) to ensure the highest efficiency. A point of note is that later additions of interior partitions and furniture in clinical areas should not block airflow or ease of access. Vents should be appropriate for balancing the ventilation.

5.3.6.1.1.3.1 Negative-pressure ventilation (NPV)

NPV is indicated where airborne precautions are required, such as for TB, measles and chickenpox, acute respiratory disease isolation (SARS-CoV-2) and the dirty area in the sterile services department. *The air extracted from the area greatly exceeds the volume supplied* (Figure 5.7). The air is drawn into the room from surrounding spaces such as doors and corridors into the isolation room (*leaks inwards*). It is removed at a rate which prevents the movement of contaminated air to leak backwards into other areas. For NPV, the air volume is accurately balanced and the windows in the room must remain closed at all times as opening them will disturb the airflow.

Negative-pressure ventilation can be delivered by the following means:

- Controlled ventilation where air is removed by mechanical means, exhausted to the outside air to ensure maximum dilution after removal.
- Extractor fans installed in outer walls or windows. These are less accurate but suffice in low-resource countries.
- Wind turbines or 'whirlybirds', which are usually placed in the roof and work on the same principle as extractor fans, but do not need electricity.

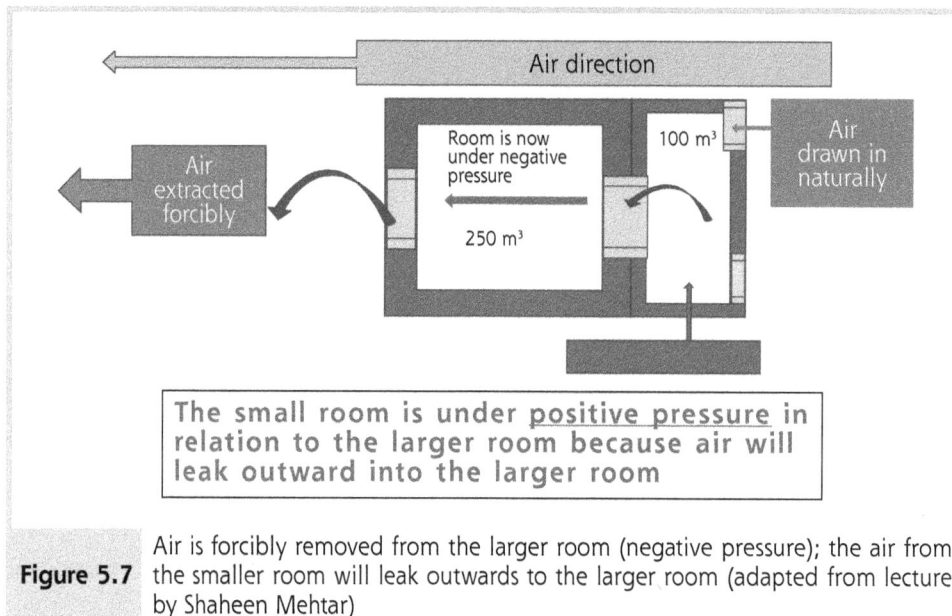

Figure 5.7 Air is forcibly removed from the larger room (negative pressure); the air from the smaller room will leak outwards to the larger room (adapted from lecture by Shaheen Mehtar)

5.3.6.1.1.3.2 Positive pressure ventilation

This is the opposite of negative pressure in that *the air will constantly leak outwards*. There are a few areas in the hospital which require positive pressure ventilation. These are the bone marrow transplant unit, operating theatre, clean area of the sterile service department and clean preparation areas of the pharmacy.

The operating theatre requires a constant supply of positive pressure-controlled ventilation to ensure a constant supply of clean air. Air is removed from the OT at a rate which reduces the level of bioburden at the wound site during operation.

Patients who are extremely immunocompromised (for example, bone marrow transplant cases) require positive pressure ventilation with HEPA filtration to prevent inhalation of fungal spores found in outdoor air. Clean air will pass outwards, preventing unfiltered air from returning inwards. Positive pressure without air filtration does not provide protection.

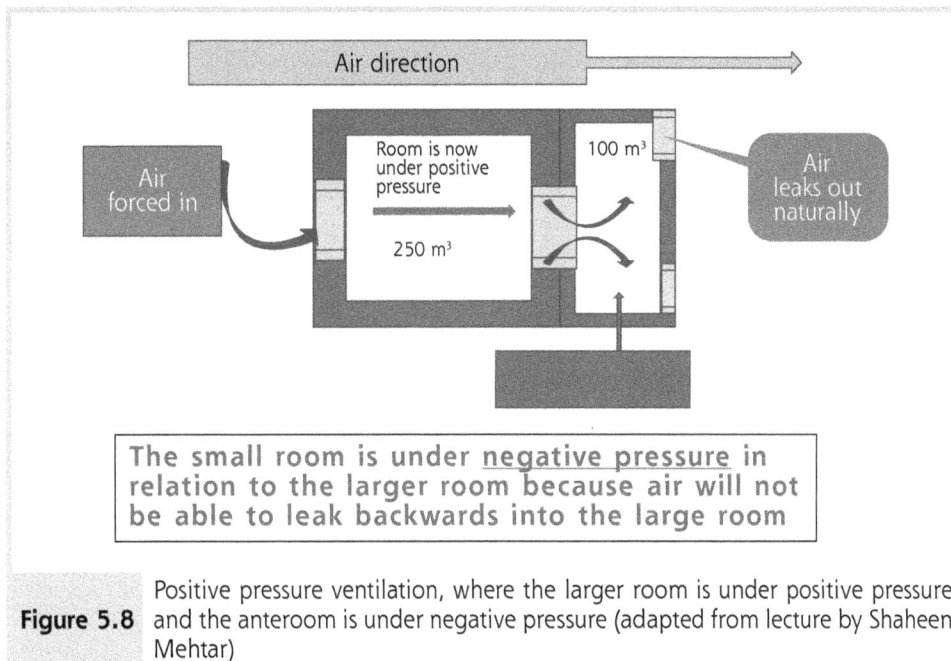

Figure 5.8 Positive pressure ventilation, where the larger room is under positive pressure and the anteroom is under negative pressure (adapted from lecture by Shaheen Mehtar)

The latest WHO document on a roadmap to improved ventilation[9] clearly lays out what should be considered for improving ventilation in a health facility and at home – it is recommended reading.

Building ventilation has three elements:
- **Ventilation rate** (m^3/h, l/s, or ACH): volume of outdoor air provided into a space
- **Airflow direction:** the overall airflow direction, which should flow from clean to dirty
- **Air distribution or airflow patterns:** The external air should be delivered to each part of the space in an effective and efficient manner and pollutants should be removed in an effective and efficient manner.

5.3.6.2 Air changes

An **air change** is defined as occurring when a volume of air equivalent to the volume of the room has been supplied to or removed from that room (whichever airflow is the greater). The rate of air change is usually given as ACH and is derived from the volume of a room and the ventilation rate.

---

9   Roadmap to improve and ensure good indoor ventilation in the context of COVID-19. Geneva: World Health Organization, 2021.

Ideally, the number of air changes should be determined by the engineers at commissioning and thereafter annually or when problems with the ventilation are suspected. The way to calculate air changes is based on a formula relating to the volume of air in the room and the rate of air supplied.

The formula for calculation ACH

The formula to calculate ACH is 60 multiplied by the cfm of your air exchange device, divided by the volume of air in the room.

The ACH formula as an expression is

$$ACH = \frac{60Q}{Vol}$$

ACH = number of air changes per hour
Q   = Volumetric flow rate of air in cubic feet per minute (cfm)
Vol = Space volume L × W × H, in cubic feet

To calculate the volume of air in a room multiple the length (L), width (W), and height (H) to get your total cubic air volume.

The formula for air volume as an expression is: Vol = L × W × H

5.3.6.3 Ultraviolet germicidal irradiation (UVGI)

The use of UVGI is being extensively researched as an adjunct to negative-pressure ventilation, especially for tuberculosis isolation facilities. There are considerable differences of opinion as to its use in an uncontrolled environment. The UV light used in this context is of a specific wavelength (254 nanometres) and is measured in microwatt-seconds per square centimetre. It is known to kill tiny microbes carried in respiratory nuclei; however, it does not affect larger droplet particles. UVGI (Table 5.2) will not affect larger micro-organisms such as mould and fungi, but it is effective against viruses and vegetative forms of bacteria.

Table 5.2 Microbiological activity of ultraviolet germicidal irradiation

Types of micro-organisms	Mw sec/cm²
Vegetative bacteria	2–4 000
Spores	12 000
M tuberculosis	10 000
Yeast	6–8 000
Mould/spores	13–44 000

UVGI works by altering the DNA of the cell and will destroy cells where it can penetrate by striking them directly. The kill ratio will depend upon time, exposure and intensity of the UV rays. It is also affected by relative humidity, temperature and distance from the microbe. Therefore UVGI is less effective if there is interference because of dust, the distance is **too far** or the speed of air removal is increased.[10] The UV lights should be installed at 3.5 m, above eye level, and not be visible from 10 m across the room. The problem arises in LMICs where the use of UVGI is considered the solution to dealing with a high case load of TB patients, without the presence of any other type of provision. The disadvantages of UVGI for LMICs are that it is expensive, requires specialised knowledge for monitoring and requires maintenance. If it is not properly installed or monitored, patients may develop skin conditions such as keratitis or dermatitis from overexposure.[11] There are reports that UVGI can cause squamous cell carcinoma in experimental conditions[12] and it has now been classified as a co-carcinogen.

UVGI has been effectively used in sterilising laboratory safety cabinets which are in an enclosed defined space with clear parameters for use. Its use in sterilisation of air in pandemics has been promoted as free-standing systems.

5.3.7 Water, sanitation and hygiene standards

The quality and quantity of water for a healthcare facility will depend upon the type of services provided. An excellent account has been published by the WHO,[13] summarising the minimum requirements for water sanitation and hygiene in healthcare facilities (Table 5.3). These guidelines have evolved into full-blown programmes; the WHO WASH programme has laid out tools to measure progress in improving WASH in healthcare facilities.[14]

---

[10] First M, Rudnick SN, Banahan KF, Vincent RL & Brickner PW. 2007. Fundamental factors affecting upper-room ultraviolet germicidal irradiation – Part I: Experimental. *Journal of Occupational and Environmental Hygiene* 4(5): 321–331.

[11] Talbot EA, Jensen P, Moffat HJ & Wells CD. 2002. Occupational risk from ultraviolet germicidal irradiation (UVGI) lamps. *International Journal of Tuberculosis and Lung Disease* 6(8): 738–741.

[12] Richard B & Gammage B (eds). 1996. *Indoor Air and Human Health*. Florida: CRC Press LLC, p146.

[13] Adams J, Bartram J & Chartier Y. 2008. *Essential Environmental Health Standards in Health Care*.

[14] WHO. 2022. *Water and Sanitation for Health Facility Improvement Tool (WASH FIT): A Practical Guide for Improving Quality of Care through Water, Sanitation and Hygiene in Health Care Facilities*. 2nd edition. Geneva: World Health Organization.

Table 5.3   WHO standards on water, sanitation and hygiene at health facility level (WHO 2008, 2018)

Item	Recommendation	Explanation
Water quantity	5–400 l/person/day	Outpatient services require less water, while OT and delivery rooms require more water Upper limit is for VHF (Ebola) isolation centres)
Water access	On-site supplies	Water should be available in all treatment wards and in waiting rooms
Water quality	< 1 *E coli*/thermotolerant total coliforms/100 ml	Drinking water should comply with WHO guidelines on drinking water quality for microbial, chemical and physical aspects Facilities should adopt a risk management approach to ensure water is safe
Sanitisation quantity[15]	1 toilet per 20 users for inpatients At least 4 toilets per OPD Separate toilet for staff and patients Separate toilet for males and females	Sufficient number of toilets available for patients, staff and visitors
Sanitisation access	On-site facilities	Sanitation should be in the facility grounds and accessible to all users
Sanitisation quality	Appropriate for local technical and financial conditions Accessible to all users including those with disability	Technical specification should ensure that excreta is safely managed
Hygiene	A reliable water point with soap and drying facilities OR ABHR available in all treatment rooms, waiting areas and latrines for patients and staff	Hand wash and ABHR should be available at all key areas of the facility, ensuring safe hand hygiene practices

5.4 Workflow and healthcare delivery

The facility should be user-friendly for staff and patients, with a comfortable work environment and clearly defined areas of delivering health safely. A smooth workflow is essential and should consider

---

[15]   WHO. 2018. Guidelines on sanitation and health. Geneva: World Health Organization.

- movement of patients
- movement of staff (healthcare workers)
- movement of supplies
- movement of equipment
- proximity of specialist areas
- support areas.

In the Venn diagram below (Figure 5.9) the interaction between these three elements comes together at the intersection which is the **point of care** – the most vulnerable point in patient care and where IPC must actively prevent or control transmission of pathogens.

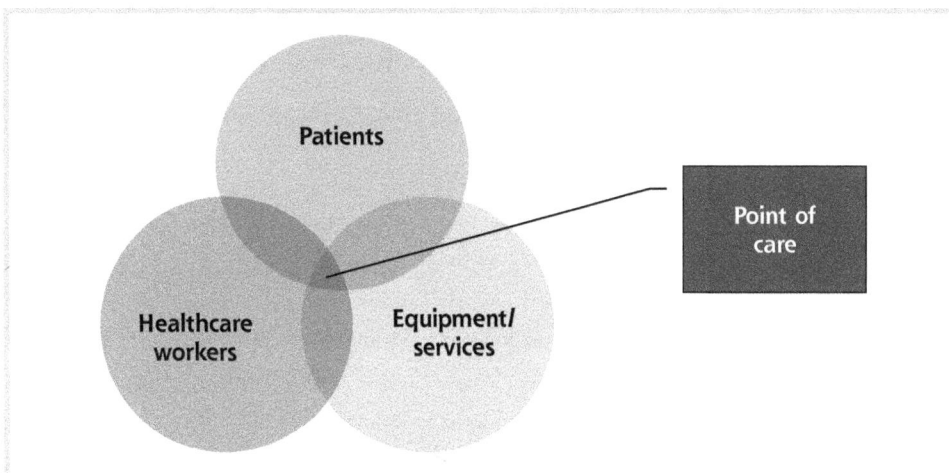

Figure 5.9 Venn diagram showing the interaction between patient, healthcare worker and service delivery at point of care (courtesy Shaheen Mehtar)

5.4.1 Movement of patients

There are usually three types of patient that come to a healthcare facility:

1. Ambulant, or walk-in patients who come to the outpatient department.
   - referred or for consultation
   - for investigation
   - for minor operations
2. Emergency cases, which usually arrive by ambulance or private transport
3. Inpatients admitted for a medical or surgical procedure.

5.4.2 Signage

Access by ambulance or private transportation should be easy and clearly marked. All services rendered to patients must be clearly visible and labelled, with easy accessibility, particularly for disabled or elderly patients with difficulty of movement, such as pharmacy, laboratory and x-ray departments.

Access for wheelchairs, patient trolleys and delivery systems for sterile services and medical provisions should be considered; ramps rather than stairs serve such a population better, with wider corridors and a minimum number of links and other corridors leading off to the various departments.

5.4.3 Movement of staff

Healthcare workers should have access to all the areas they work in and to service areas. In specialised areas such as the OT, access to changing rooms, donning and doffing areas for PPE and rest rooms should be easily accessible. Administrative staff should have easy access to their place of work, preferably away from the clinical areas.

5.4.4 Movement of equipment and supplies

Healthcare facilities require a constant supply of medical products, linen and non-medical stores.

There should be provision for access for delivery systems to the healthcare facilities as well as removal of waste and repair items from clinical areas. Wide peripheral roads which do not impinge on patient-care areas should be provided which lead directly to the main stores and delivery areas.

In the clinical areas, clean supplies are delivered and dirty or used items are removed. It is important that these elements are considered during planning. Ideally, the 'clean' deliveries can take place from within the healthcare facility, while the 'dirty' items should be removed from the sluice or similar 'dirty' areas to the outside without traversing the clinical areas.

5.5   Layout of a healthcare facility

The public, staff and trade will need access to different parts of the healthcare facility and to allow for this some areas are open while others are restricted to certain personnel only.

5.5.1 Administration (offices) non-clinical areas

The non-clinical areas should be located on the ground and within easy reach of the public. There should be adequate space to accommodate the needs of the administrative staff in either an open-plan office or individual offices. Handwash basins or ABHR should be provided in each office area. The administration block should ideally have an independent ventilation system from the patient-care areas.

Entry to the administration block should be secured to minimise theft and to restrict access to records. There should be small meeting rooms, a boardroom and areas for conferences and meetings. A tea room or small kitchen should be provided.

5.5.2 Furnishing of clinical areas

As discussed previously, the type of ward design does affect IPC practices and therefore advice from the IPC team is needed during renovation or building of new facilities.

All clinical areas should have hard-wearing floor coverings and wall finishes which are easy to clean. In specialised units such as the OT, there may be additional requirements.[16]

5.5.2.1 *Floor coverings*. All clinical areas should have continuous washable floor coverings such as vinyl or epoxy resin, which are water- and stain-resistant, not adversely affected by detergents, disinfectants or cleaning materials, and they should dry quickly. The flooring should be coved up to the wall to a minimum of 2.5 cm and sealed to allow for easy cleaning and reducing dust traps. If this is not possible, the floor should be sealed at its junction with the wall. Wooden floors are not recommended in clinical areas, but if these do exist, they should be sealed. Carpets are not recommended for health facilities, but particularly not in clinical areas.

5.5.2.2 *Walls* should be smooth, covered with paint or materials that are water impermeable and easily washable. Wall tiles are not recommended as these collect dirt, carry fungal spores and are difficult to clean.

5.5.2.3 *Ceilings* should have a homogenous plastered surface with flush-mounted recesses for lights, ventilation grilles and other ceiling fixtures. Access to services should be through a hatch which is sealed to prevent dirt from falling into the patient areas. Removable grid tiles may be used in general ward areas but they are not advisable in isolation rooms. The ceiling joints should be sealed to prevent dust and leakage from entering the clinical areas.

5.5.2.4 *Light fittings*. Apart from ceiling lighting, examination angle-poised lamps should be positioned for convenience of use and regular cleaning. Frequently wipe with detergents or, in exceptional situations, disinfectants may be used. The lamps should be able to withstand these chemicals.

5.5.2.5 *Surfaces*. All ledges, surfaces, cabinets and cupboards should be smooth, without crevices or open joints and should be made of material that can be easily cleaned and regularly wiped with a detergent or disinfectant.

5.5.2.6 *Doors*. The corridor doors should be one and a half panels with a large vision panel and a privacy curtain. The door surfaces should be smooth

[16] NHS Estates. 2002. *Infection Control in the Built Environment: Design and Planning*. London: The Stationery Office.

and the door handles made of material that can be easily cleaned with detergents (or disinfectants). Baffle plates should be provided in the doors to help with balance of airflow and ventilation.

5.5.2.7   *Windows* should be lockable if mechanical ventilation is used, but can also be opened if necessary. In some healthcare facilities the open and closing mechanisms are complex so that the patients are unable to open the windows when the ventilation is turned on.

5.5.2.8   *Window covers.* Washable curtains are preferable to blinds since the former can be removed frequently for cleaning, especially in isolation rooms and high-risk areas. Blinds retain dust and are difficult to clean. They also break easily and look unsightly.

5.5.3 Temperature control

In well-established hospitals, temperature control is provided via mechanical ventilation (AHU) which can be regulated to either heating or cooling the air to ensure comfort for the patients. Independent temperature control for specific units such as the burns or neonatal units can be provided. Alternatively, independent units can be used.

5.5.3.1   *Heating* may be provided by single hot-air units, radiators linked to the hot water system or via temperature control on mechanical ventilation. All systems should be easily accessible for cleaning. The grilles on the heating system should be removable and cleaned frequently. The heater itself should be placed where there is sufficient space to clean behind and under it. It is recommended that heaters be placed underneath the windows, especially where there are skylights to promote the upward movement of air.

5.5.3.2   *Cooling.* Fans or single cool air units (air conditioners) should be cleaned regularly and maintained. The filters must be inspected, washed or changed regularly, especially in dusty and warm climes to ensure maximum efficiency.

5.6   Layout of a general ward

5.6.1 Risk of transmission

With adequate ventilation and good bed spacing, transmission of pathogens can be reduced dramatically in a general ward.

The main risks arise from:
- Overcrowding. The beds are too close to each other and cross-contamination from droplets and splashes can occur.

- More than one patient in a bed can result in cross-infection.
- Inadequate space to work with individual patients results in cross-contamination during procedures.

5.6.2 Bed spacing

Building regulations (NHS, UK)[17] specify a layout for a general ward. A summary is provided here:

- Beds, centre to centre, should be a minimum of 2.5 m apart to allow for bedside tables, equipment, procedure trolleys and bed curtains for each bed. If the distances are less, the risk of transmission is increased. However, the WHO recommends 1 m edge to edge of the beds.
- Beds should be grouped in the smallest number, such as single rooms or four-bedded units, but no more than six beds per unit. Each room should be equipped with en suite toilet facilities and handwash basins located at the entrance of the unit.
- It is recommended that there should be an adequate number of single rooms. The recommendation varies from 33% to 40% of acute beds, depending on the disease profile.
- Permanent partitions (usually glass) should be placed between each grouping of beds to reduce access and transmission of infective agents.
- All bed areas should be easily accessible for cleaning and maintenance.
- Spacing should take into account equipment around the bed and access to handwashing facilities.
- If en suite toilets are not provided, toilet and ablution facilities should be calculated based on the number of beds. The toilets should not be more than 12 m from the day room or bed area.

5.6.3 Provisions for hand hygiene

A clinical handwash basin should be provided with adequate facilities for handwashing and drying. The handwash basins have been found to be a major source of MDRO and therefore the current recommendation is that the handwash basin should be located at the entrance of the ward, preferably in the corridor, and away from the patient zone to minimise splashing of patients and the environment. This is a major change in placing of hand wash basins in recent buildings.

ABHR should be provided – at least one bottle per each four-bedded section, but preferably one per bed. It should be located close to the patient's bed or mounted on the wall at the entrance of the ward. It is **not advisable** to place ABHR at the handwash basin.

[17]   Ibid.

5.6.3.1 Clinical handwash basin

A clinical handwash basin is especially designed to minimise splashing.

The design of a clinical handwash basin includes:
- Taps should be elbow (or foot) operated mixer taps which are activated by the user. The handles are usually moved forward to turn on and backwards to turn the water off. Automatic hand detection systems go on when the hands are placed under the water nozzle and shut off automatically when the hands are removed. Single taps are still found in many hospitals. The tap can be turned off with the paper towel used for hand drying before discard. The taps **should not be aligned** to run directly into the drainage aperture to minimise splashing.
- The bowl should be deep to avoid splashing and have no overflow outlet or recesses where the water may collect, There should not be a drain-hole plug so that water is always free-flowing. Waterproof splash backs should be used for all handwash basins and should be properly sealed.
- The number of handwash basins per bed is difficult to determine, but one recommendation is:
  - Low-dependency units should have at least one handwash basin per six beds.
  - Outpatients and clinical examination and treatment rooms should have one handwash basin per room.
  - All toilet facilities should have handwash basins, soap and hand drying facilities.
- The location of the clinical handwash basin must fulfil the following stipulations:
  - The handwash basin should be visible and within easy reach of all staff and visitors, preferably near the entrance of the ward but away from patient areas.
  - The handwashing liquid soap and/or antiseptics should be wall-mounted and hand drying facilities should be provided close by with an ample supply of paper towels (or similar) for drying hands.
  - A bin for disposal of paper towels or single-use cloth towels should be placed next to the handwash basin.
  - There should be clearly displayed signs on the steps of carrying out hand hygiene.
- The handwash basin should be dedicated for washing hands only. Separate facilities for washing patient equipment or emptying patient bowls should be provided.

5.6.4 Dirty utility (sluice) area

The dirty utility area carries a high load of MDRO and is a high-risk area for transmission of pathogens. It should be kept clean and dry. Separate hand hygiene facilities should be provided. **Always** wash and dry hands before leaving the dirty utility room.

The area is used for:
- bedpan, urinal and bowls for washing and disinfection
- testing urine
- disposal of liquid waste
- temporarily holding items that go for reprocessing or disposal
- commodes, sani-chairs, bedpans, urinals and patient bowls for inpatient areas
- used linen bags.

The sluice area should not be used for
- sluicing linen
- washing and soaking medical devices
- storage of sterile or other laboratory specimen containers.

The routine use of disinfectants is not recommended, as it encourages anti-microbial resistance, but may be used as advised by the IPC team.

5.6.4.1 Risk of transmission arises from:
- wet areas which increase the risk of MDROs
- contaminated equipment, such as bedpan and urinals, used for patients directly after removal from the sluice
- leaks in the sluice and slop hopper
- non-functioning bedpan washer-disinfector.

5.6.4.2 Ward washer-disinfector

Each acute ward should have at least one functioning bedpan washer-disinfector to cope with the number of bedpans, urinals and jugs required for patient care. Usually the cycle starts with pressure jet cleaning of the bedpan followed by thermal disinfection achieving 80 °C for 60 seconds or 90 °C for 6 seconds (NEN-ISO 15883-3).

Provision must be made for storage of clean bedpans, urinal and patient bowls to ensure these remain dry. There must be handwash facilities, a functioning slop hopper for disposal of body fluid waste and a sink to wash urine jugs or similar equipment. Waste disposal system should be in place.

5.6.5 Clean utility area

There is little risk of transmission in this area unless there is gross violation of IPC practices. The storage areas should be well ventilated, dry and clean. The area is used for:

- storage of drugs and preparation of lotions
- storage of clean clinical equipment
- storage of sterile supplies
- cleaning and laying up of procedure trolleys.

Provision must be made for the following:

- There should be adequate storage space either in cupboards or on shelves to prevent dust and splash contamination.
- Sterile services department (SSD) supplies should be placed on racks to allow good air circulation.
- Surfaces fitted with materials which can be easily cleaned, to prepare drugs and lotions.
- Clinical handwash basin.

In outpatients or primary care clinics this room should be adjacent to the treatment area and should be easily accessible for cleaning.

5.6.6 Treatment room

Most healthcare facilities have a separate treatment room for inpatients and outpatients, but the clean room often doubles up for both. The use of such a room will dictate its layout. There must be good ventilation, facilities for hand decontamination (handwash basins and ABHR), flooring and surfaces must be easily cleaned and adequate space must be provided to manage patients.

5.6.7 Disposal room (waste holding room)

There is risk of transmission if this room is overfilled, The room should be cleared and cleaned at least daily; it should be well ventilated. The area is used as temporary holding area before removal of

- waste containers
- sharps boxes
- used linen
- used clinical equipment destined for the SSD
- used items for disposal.

Provision must be made for the following:

- Adequate space and storage areas to house containers, especially on weekends if there is no collection.

5.6.8 Staff areas

There should be provision for the staff to rest, take a tea break and relax during their shifts.

Staff areas should take priority during the planning stage. If these areas are neglected, single (isolation) rooms and other smaller non-clinical areas may be taken over by staff to provide these facilities. There should be comfortable seating with facilities such as kettles, fridges, microwave ovens for the preparation of hot beverages, warm food and a supply of cold water in the tea room. The floor covering should be made of an easily washable impervious surface The area must be well ventilated to ensure no transmission of respiratory or other pathogens occurs during breaks.

A handwash basin and facilities should be provided for each of these areas.

5.6.9 Patient waiting areas/day rooms

While this area has to be comfortable and inviting, the floors should be covered with material that can be easily cleaned and therefore carpets are not advisable. The chairs should be comfortable but covered with a washable surface that can withstand disinfectants and dries quickly. Televisions, food dispensers and other similar items should be cleaned in the usual way. In countries like South Africa, where there is a high prevalence of tuberculosis, this area should be spacious and naturally well ventilated; if the weather permits, the patients can go and spend the day outside in the fresh air under trees.

5.6.10 Play area

The room or area should be open and airy. In warmer countries an outside facility may be provided. The floor should be covered with mats that can be cleaned or laundered. The furniture should be covered with waterproof material for easy cleaning. Soft toys must be machine washable at reasonable temperature; hard toys must be easy to clean.

5.6.11 Visitors' toilets

These are a high-use areas and therefore there should be high-grade finishes to maintain a good standard of hygiene. All toilets must have lids, which should be closed during flushing. Handwash basins with handwashing and drying facilities should be provided. Sanitary bins should be stationed in each female toilet and there should be at least one bin in the basin area.

In countries where squatting toilets are used there should be adequate provision for frequent cleaning and drying of these toilets. Squatting toilets are not recommended from an IPC point of view because of the difficulty in maintaining a clean and dry environment. It is also not patient friendly for pregnant women and the elderly.

The toilets must be cleaned regularly and maintained.

5.7   Specialised areas of care

Advances in medical care have resulted in several specialised units of care that require more attention from the IPC team to help reduce HAIs. The inpatient facilities are discussed here, and, in addition, facilities for isolation of patients during outbreaks such as Ebola or SARS-CoV-2 are described.

IPC recommendations to prevent infection relate to the differences between general and specialised wards.

- Layout should allow for more staff and patient movement and more bed space to accommodate more equipment.
- Isolation facilities with ensuite facilities; more single rooms required, possibly 40% of total beds, depending on the disease profile.
- Ventilation (usually mechanical) either negative or positive pressure as needed.
- Water quality. Drinking quality in general areas; high-quality water in dialysis units and SSDs.
- Medical-grade air delivered to OTs and ICUs.
- Increased frequency of cleaning and disinfection.
- More PPE used compared to general wards.
- Healthcare waste management needs to be better – more frequent collection.
- Linen and laundry demand is higher.

As a general rule, the higher the level of medical interventions and care, the greater risk there is of infection transmission, and IPC takes this into account.

5.7.1 Isolation facilities

Isolation means 'to keep a patient, or group of patients, in conditions that prevent their infection transmission to others, or to keep the isolated patient free of infection'. While this is a good prevention strategy, it can be psychologically quite traumatic and depressing, particularly if the person is isolated over a long period of time, for example with MDR TB. Provision should be made to keep the patient occupied during the isolation period.

Each clinical ward should have isolation facilities adjacent to the main ward(s) for infectious patients. Here, transmission-based precautions are usually indicated and can be implemented under controlled conditions. It is suggested that 33–40% of the beds should be isolation rooms, depending on the disease profile of the community. Some countries may require more isolation beds.

While the siting of isolation rooms differs by facility, it is wise to locate the isolation room with an outside wall should an extractor fan be required to be installed. There should be large windows with skylights that can be opened. There should be a handwash basin within the room and en suite toilet facilities to prevent the patient from leaving the room. There should be provision for a bedside locker, a feeding table and a small cupboard for patient-care articles. An anteroom is desirable to store PPE and other provisions and help to balance the ventilation pressure. It houses the following:

- handwash basin and hand hygiene facilities such as soap, paper towels and ABHR
- PPE based on appropriate transmission-based precautions
- clinical notes and charts
- treatment trolley (if required)
- storage of linen and facilities
- provision for removal of waste and used clinical items
- storage of cleaning equipment.

Each isolation room should be fitted with a door with a large vision panel; the door should remain closed at all times. A holder for a sign instructing the type of transmission-based precautions in force should be placed on the door. In some isolation rooms an intercom system may be fitted to communicate with the patient or visiting clinical staff. This will prevent the constant opening and closing of doors. If caregivers are allowed to stay with the patients, facilities for them must be considered.

If cohort isolation is required in the event of an outbreak or epidemic, four-bedded units can be converted into isolation facilities provided they have appropriate facilities (as detailed above for single isolation facilities) to cater for a larger number of patients.

5.7.2 Operating theatre (OT) complex

The OT unit is usually made up of a complex of rooms and is often a self-contained unit. It provides surgical support for emergency, elective and trauma cases. The design should be appropriate to its function. The dynamics of the OT is where staff, patient and equipment come together at the **'point of care'**, which is the site of incision which must be protected (Figure 5.10). The OT is laid out in zones to ensure the prep room (layup area) and operating theatre are the cleanest, then the scrub and anaesthetic rooms, followed by the sluice and outer corridors. This is achieved by positive pressure ventilation, temperature and pressure difference across the zones.

Risk of transmission

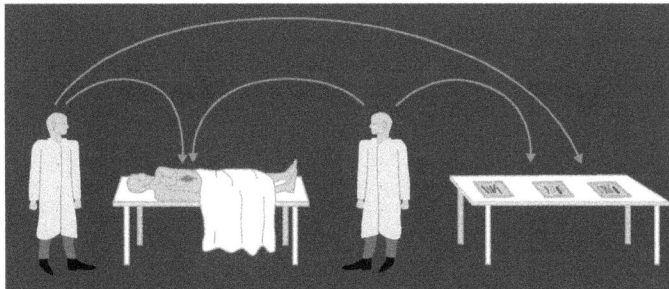

Figure 5.10 Figure 5.10 Contamination of wound from various sources in the OT (adapted with permission from a lecture by Christina Bradley and Peter Hoffman)

Most surgical site infections are endogenous, but the OT environment can increase the risk of infection:

- From the lack of adequate ventilation
  - skin scales contaminated with bacteria from the operating team can enter the wound
  - skin scales can land on the open surgical devices
  - aerosols created can spread microbes
- From poorly processed surgical equipment including
  - transmission of healthcare acquired pathogens
  - transmission of blood-borne viruses
  - transmission of respiratory pathogens
  - transmission of skin disease related pathogens
- From lack of hand hygiene and aseptic procedures
  - increase in the risk of surgical site infection as well as the above
  - poor outcome and patient morbidity and mortality.

5.7.2.1 Location

The OT complex may be either purpose-built or converted hospital accommodation. These are busy units and require careful planning to avoid expensive mistakes. The OT complex should be located away from the main flow of hospital traffic and corridors, but within easy access of surgical, accident and emergency, and burns clinical areas.

5.7.2.2 Layout

The OT complex is zoned and should be clearly recognisable by staff working in the OT and visitors. This is easier to achieve in a purpose-built unit with physical barriers to restrict access. Access for maintenance staff should be considered. An example of a layout is shown in Figure 5.11.

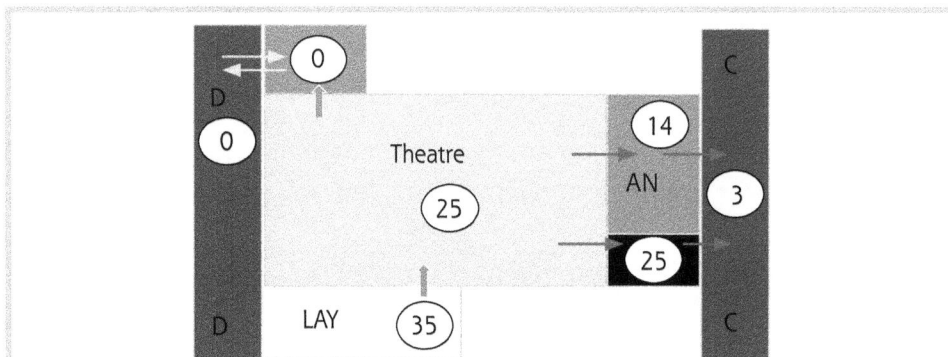

Figure 5.11 Zoning of operating theatre complex. Lay = layout room with the highest ventilation pressure (35 ACH), followed by the theatre (25 ACH) allowing air to flow towards the anaesthetic room (14 ACH), scrub area and then to dirty utility (neutral) and corridors (3ACH). The arrows indicate the direction of air flow reflecting movement from higher to lower pressure areas (adapted from a lecture by Shaheen Mehtar)

5.7.2.2.1 Outer zone

The outer zone is considered the **non-sterile zone** and entry into this area does not require a change of clothing. There should be no direct access into the clean zone, but there should be access to the main hospital. This area contains:

- main access door
- accessible area for removal of waste and used surgical instruments to the SSD
- sluice
- storage for medical and surgical supplies
- entrance to changing facilities
- access for maintenance such as engineers, plumbers and electricians.

> **There should be a physical barrier between the non-sterile zone and the clean zone.**

5.7.2.2.2 Clean zone

This is the restricted area and is accessible to OT staff only. It does require a change into theatre garb but not the wearing of PPE. The movement from the clean zone should be unidirectional into the aseptic zone, preferably via the scrub area, and exit to the non-sterile (outer zone).

This area includes:

- sterile supply stores
- anaesthetic room
- recovery
- scrub room
- clean corridor
- rest room for staff.

There should be a partial physical barrier between the clean zone and the aseptic zone.

5.7.2.2.3 Aseptic zone

The aseptic zone is **restricted to the working OT team** only and includes the operating theatre (surgical suite) and the layout room. Older designs include access to sterilisers for dropped instruments, but this is no longer encouraged. Staff working in this area should wear a mask, a gown and sterile gloves. The OT should have smooth, washable walls and floors.

The ventilation, temperature and humidity of the OT is controlled, creating a controlled environment. There should be a scavenging system for anaesthetic gases.

The patient, operating team and surgical equipment come together at the operating table – the wound site which should have the **lowest** bacterial counts of all.

5.7.2.3 Air delivery systems for operating theatre[18]

The basic mechanics of mechanical ventilation has been previously discussed (see section 5.3.6.1.1.3). The IPC team must understand ventilation in the operating theatre and advise accordingly during the building or renovation project. Air conditioners as a sole means of ventilation are not recommended if clean air is required as these only deliver partially filtered clean air.

5.7.2.3.1 Conventional ventilation

Conventional ventilation is the most common ventilation system used in most general and some specialised operating rooms.

5.7.2.3.1.1 Design features

Parameters to have in place if possible based on available resources are:
- **Air changes.** Maintenance of 20–24 air changes per hour (ACH). If recirculation is used, at least 3 ACH should be fresh air from outside and recirculation must take place via a fine filter such as EN779 F7.
- **Filtration.** Filter all air with appropriate coarse pre-filters (e.g. filtration efficiency of 30%) followed by final filter (e.g. EN779 F7).
- **Air supply (Figure 5.12).** Air should enter at the ceiling or high up on the walls and then pass from the theatre into the surrounding less clean areas. **(Furniture or other portable items placed against a wall exhaust at floor level will inhibit the air changeover in a theatre and therefore the placing of these items should be monitored and prohibited if necessary.)**
- **Doors.** Keep OT doors closed (self-closing) except as needed for passage of equipment, personnel and the patient.
- **Traffic.** Limit the number of personnel entering the OT to only those necessary for the surgical procedure. The microbial level in the OT is directly proportional to the number of people moving about in the theatre.

The air is propelled through the ducts by a fan calculated to deliver at least 20–24 ACH in the operating room and is usually delivered from the ceiling with a downward flow (Figure 5.12). The air is under positive pressure with respect to the corridors and adjacent areas when delivered to the layout room and operating theatre. The

---

[18]   Taylor E. & Hoffman P. 2008. Prevention of infection in special wards and departments – Operating theatres. In Fraise A & Bradley C. (eds). *Control of Healthcare-associated Infection.* 5th ed. London: Hodder Arnold.

air is exhausted from the sterile zone via the aseptic zone into the outer zone or via the corridors and sluice to the outer atmosphere in a unidirectional flow via carefully balanced dampers and grills which prevent reversal of airflows when doors are opened. Routine maintenance of the AHUs is essential. The ventilation may be turned off if not in use, but it must be turned on 60 minutes before use.

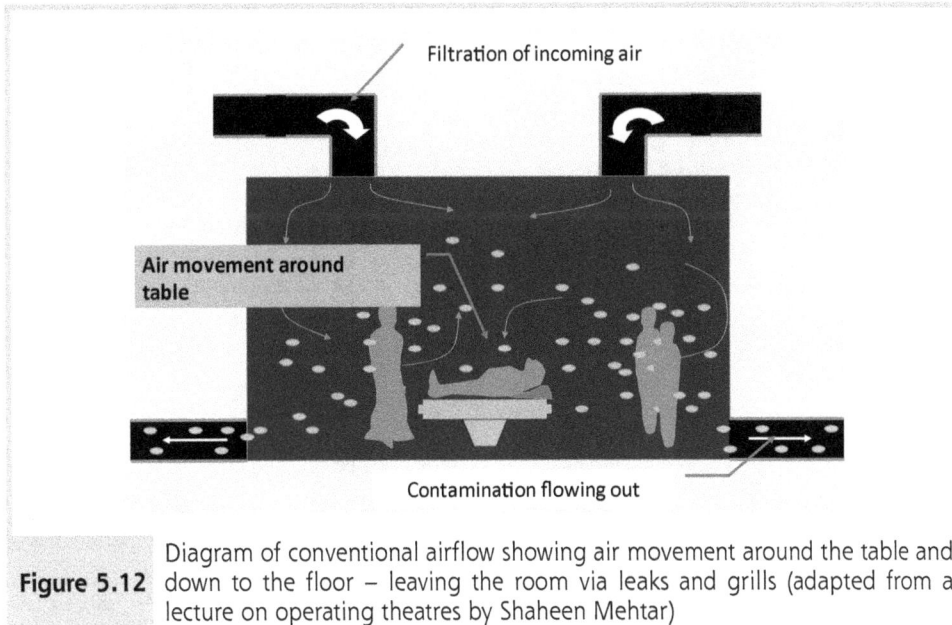

Figure 5.12 Diagram of conventional airflow showing air movement around the table and down to the floor – leaving the room via leaks and grills (adapted from a lecture on operating theatres by Shaheen Mehtar)

5.7.2.3.2 Ultra-clean ventilation

Ultra-clean ventilation is designed to move particle-free air over the aseptic operating field in one direction. It flows vertically or horizontally and is usually combined with high-efficiency particulate air (HEPA) filters. HEPA filters remove particles > 0.3 µ in diameter.

A bacterial count of 10 cfu or less per cubic metre at the wound site should be achieved. Air is drawn from the atmosphere and passed through a conventional AHU and is delivered to a canopy over the operating table to form a curtain of clean air around the operating field. Approximately 80% of the air in the room is recycled through the canopy and passed through HEPA filters to remove skin scales and particles generated by the surgical team.[19] The air may be delivered vertically or horizontally. The former is preferred.

---

[19] ISO 14644 specifies the approved airflow speed limits in laminar flow systems. This standard basically specifies that to obtain accurate laminar flow, the airflow speed needs to be 0.45 m/s within a 20 cm distance of the HEPA filter's surface (with a 20% tolerance, so minimum flow of 0.3 m/s and a maximum of 0.54 m/s).

Ultra-clean ventilation used to be recommended for implant surgery (especially orthopaedics), but recent studies suggest a SSI bundle intervention (refer to section 4.6.5) with conventional airflows is as effective in reducing SSIs. Ideally, all necessary equipment and personnel remain inside the curtain of air until the end of the operation, but this is not always possible and the air curtain is frequently interrupted.

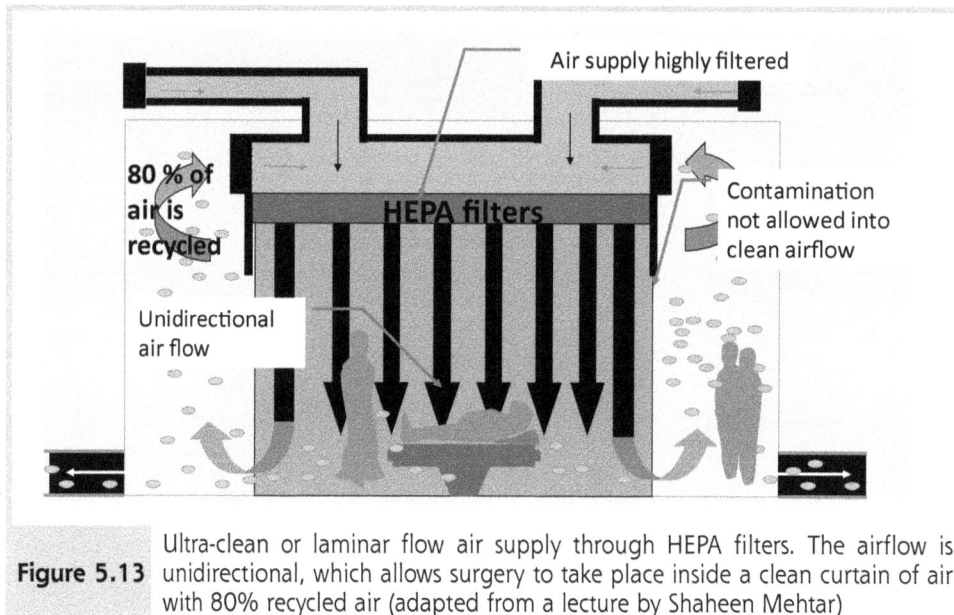

Figure 5.13   Ultra-clean or laminar flow air supply through HEPA filters. The airflow is unidirectional, which allows surgery to take place inside a clean curtain of air with 80% recycled air (adapted from a lecture by Shaheen Mehtar)

5.7.2.3.3 Wall-mounted air conditioners

Air conditioners are installed in warm countries, more for comfort than for clean air delivery. It must be clear that these *do not provide clean air* because there is only a coarse filter in place to remove larger dust and debris particles. The units are usually mounted on the outside wall and the air is directed downwards and drawn back onto the unit itself (towards the wall). The operating table (wound site) does not receive any significant air changes and the bacterial air counts remain unaffected.

5.7.2.3.4 Free-standing air conditioners

As noted above, these are cooling units with no filtration of air and therefore do not fulfil the criteria for air delivery systems, especially for an OT.

5.7.2.4 Temperature and humidity

The temperature and the humidity (not less than 55%) play an important role in maintaining staff and patient comfort in the OT. They must be carefully regulated and monitored. In low humidity there is a danger of the production of electrostatic sparks, especially in low-resource countries. Temperature should be controlled and maintained between 18 °C and 24 °C for safety and comfort of the patient and staff and to prevent hypothermia in patients, which is linked to increased SSIs.

5.7.2.5 Equipment

Patient monitoring. Equipment such as suction apparatus and ventilators must be fitted with bacterial filters in order to prevent contamination of the machines. All equipment should be serviced regularly and a register of dates and fault findings should be kept.

Surgical devices (see Chapter 3 on Decontamination of medical devices)
The following precautions and recommendations promote safe usage and maintenance:

- Used instruments should be counted, handled minimally, and then sent for sterilisation. Point-of-use rinsing to remove coarse organic matter before being sent to the SSD is recommended. Soaking in any disinfectant is not recommended.
- Clean and sterile supplies taken to the operating room should be transported in a covered cart. The dust cover should be removed when the cart enters the surgical suite.
- Supplies entering the suite should be removed from their shipping or transport containers prior to transport to the OT.
- Soiled items should travel in covered containers from the operating room to a decontamination area where soiled items are stored until they are transported to the reprocessing area.
- All soiled items should be contained and not stored in the same area with clean or sterile items.

5.7.2.6 Storage areas

There should be adequate storage area for large patient-monitoring equipment, such as x-ray machines or similar.

- A store for sterile services should be available next to the lay-up area.
- A store for linen and consumables should be available.
- A secure ventilation-controlled area to keep medical supplies should be provided.

5.7.2.7 Waste management

Most of the waste generated in the OT is clinical or infectious waste and should be treated as such. Several sharps boxes should be present in the anaesthetic, OT and recovery rooms – all sharps should be safely discarded after use.

5.7.2.8 Cleaning programme (see section 6.4 on environmental cleaning)

There should be a simple, clear policy which can be easily followed. The cleaning team for the OT should be dedicated and equipment should be stored separately.

Daily cleaning. The following routine cleaning is carried out daily:
- Cleaning should be carried out after each operation session.
- All the surfaces are wiped with water and detergent and dried. Disinfectants are not recommended unless specifically indicated. Walls should be wiped to hand height (up to 3 m) every day at the end of each operating day.
- The floors are scrubbed with warm water and detergent and dried.
- The operating table is wiped clean to ensure removal of all visible signs of organic matter. Equipment is damp dusted and dried.
- The sluice is cleaned with warm water and detergent and dried.

Weekly cleaning. Weekly cleaning involves tasks not covered by the daily routine:
- All areas inside the OT complex should be cleaned with water and detergent and dried.
- Shelves and racks should be emptied, wiped dry and restacked.

Disinfectants. The routine use of environmental disinfection is not recommended unless there is a specific indication such as spillage of blood or after operating on an infectious case.

5.7.2.9 Maintenance

The maintenance of the OT complex must be rigorous and thorough and a record of maintenance should be kept. It necessarily involves the services of IPC and engineering personnel as well as the OT staff.
- Equipment should be checked weekly and sent for repairs, if necessary. A register of equipment inspection should be maintained for each item.
- Ventilation should be checked regularly and the filters should be monitored by a pressure differential across them and changed should the pressure differential fall.
- An annual maintenance programme is essential in which the IPC team works closely with the engineers. The OT complex is relocated for a week and the entire complex is thoroughly checked and cleaned. All major maintenance is carried out. The IPC team will check the airflows once the engineers have completed their work.

5.7.2.10 Other points to consider

The complex and varied technology of the OT and the number of dedicated areas all require specialised maintenance. These include:

- suction
- piped gases
- scavenging systems for anaesthetic gases
- water supply
- storage of large equipment, e.g. x-ray machines, ECG monitors etc
- changing areas
- anaesthetic rooms
- recovery area
- scrub-up area
- sterile preparation area
- sterile service storage for packs, sterile gowns and surgical equipment.

5.7.2.11 Staff health

The main concern here is ensuring that staff do not become a source of infection or endanger safety in the OT:

- OT staff with open skin lesions or cuts should not be allowed to work directly with patients. All open lesions should be covered with a waterproof dressing.
- Staff with coughs and colds should not be allowed in the sterile area, but they may work in the outer zone.
- All staff should be offered hepatitis B immunisation.
- Theatre staff work intensively for long hours and should be provided with adequate rest facilities with refreshments inside the OT complex to prevent them from going out in theatre garb.

5.7.2.12 Commissioning an operating theatre

Commissioning an OT is critical before surgical activity begins.[20] The IPC team should be involved in planning and commissioning of OTs as part of the project team and also after the annual maintenance and change of filters. The IPC team should have regular meetings with the project team during construction to ensure that the layout, ventilation system and facilities comply with specifications.

Testing of OTs is done on a specified date after thorough cleaning and are ready for use, but **before** becoming operational. The quality of air is sampled as part of the commissioning and is carried out in an empty OT. The air sampling results take 48 hours and the OT should not be used until the test results are available. An annual record of airflows for each operating room should be kept for later comparisons.

---

[20] Hoffman PN, Williams J, Stacey A et al. 2002. Microbiological commissioning and monitoring of operating theatre suites – A report of the Working Party of the Hospital Infection Society. *Journal of Hospital Infection* 52: 1–28.

5.7.2.12.1 Methods of air sampling – IPC team

5.7.2.12.1.1 *Air sampler*

An air sampler is used by the IPC team to sample the air for bacterial contamination, based on a template of sampling sites for bacteriological clearance. The results usually take 48 hours and the OT should not be used prior to the results being released. Acceptable levels in an empty OT are 10 cfu/m^3 for conventional ventilation.

5.7.2.12.1.2 *Settle plates*

Open agar plates are placed over an area and left open to pick up any microbe contamination. After a given time, approximately 12–24 hours, the plates are incubated and the colonies counted. Settle plates are subject to much variation, are inaccurate and therefore have limited use when commissioning OTs.

5.7.2.12.2 Airflows

The general direction of airflows is unimportant, but should provide generally turbulent ventilation with no stagnant areas.

Checking direction of airflows. There are two methods:

1. **Smoke pencil or vapour-producing gadget.** The instrument is held under the inlet grill and the air movements are followed through the room.
2. **Tissue paper.** A very simple way is to hold a piece of tissue paper against the vent and this gives an idea whether it is an inlet or exhaust air grill. However, it cannot be used to determine airflows within the room.

5.7.3 Burns unit

The burns unit delivers highly specialised services to a very vulnerable population. The nature of the condition of patients admitted to the unit increases the likelihood of colonisation and infections with microbes that are difficult to treat. The patient's defences are lowered, and there is frequent direct contact with staff and equipment. Patients in the burns unit are temporarily immunosuppressed, have lost their primary defence because of loss of skin and have large, moist wounds that can easily become colonised. The environment is constantly wet or damp. In many units there is sharing of equipment between patients. Transmission of pathogens is facilitated by these conditions. While hands are the most important source of transmission, environmental factors also play an important role.

5.7.3.1 *Risk of transmission*

To minimise the risk of transmission the following factors must be kept in mind:
- Environmental ventilation should be mechanically controlled where possible, especially in high-care burns areas.

- The patients are very ill – and sometimes critical – and they are immunologically incompetent. Particularly in developing countries, they are at higher risk of acquiring pathogens and becoming infected from hands of staff, equipment or the environment.
- The equipment used is easily contaminated if good IPC practices are not followed.
- The changing of dressings and soaking in a bath also carry risk of bacterial contamination of the wounds.

5.7.3.2 Design and layout

The unit should be purpose-built: self-contained with a number of single rooms. The ratio of single rooms to multi-bedded bays should be higher than in regular wards. The following precautions apply:
- If possible, the burns unit should be separated from other high-risk areas such as ICUs.
- There should be a dedicated and controlled entrance to the burns unit.
- The offices and changing areas should be towards the entrance to reduce street traffic in patient areas.
- The clean areas, such as offices, changing rooms for staff and stores for clean linen, drugs and sterile supplies, should be well separated from the dirty areas.
- Transportation of dirty equipment and linen should ideally be carried out in closed containers to prevent aerosols in the corridor and the dispersing of bacteria during transit.
- Where possible, highly compromised patients should be housed in single cubicles until they have received a skin graft.

The most important aspects in the layout of the burns unit are:
- spacing between beds should be 3–3.5 m
- minimum equipment and clutter – trolleys are most effective
- ventilation with adequate circulation
- good facilities for soaking and dressing of the patients
- adequate resources to manage long-stay patients
- isolation facilities for infected patients
- handwash facilities
- transport of infected waste and soiled linen.

5.7.3.3 Ventilation

The burns unit should have a separate air delivery system (or AHU) which is filtered for particles. Air is delivered to the main ward areas in the burns unit and is extracted into the corridor. For isolation rooms, negative-pressure ventilation is recommended to contain the inevitable infections and co-infections with airborne diseases. Designated patient treatment and burn bath areas should be under normal ventilation, directed away from the busy patient areas. The ventilation should be checked every six months to ensure the filters are working properly, especially in countries with high dust levels.

5.7.3.4 Temperature and humidity

The temperature of the burns unit is expected to be higher than other hospital wards and should be controlled. Humidity control is desirable, although the environment is usually quite moist.

5.7.3.5 Prevention of transmission

5.7.3.5.1 Hand hygiene

Provision of hand hygiene, handwashing and ABHR must be provided for each patient. The handwash basin must be situated away from patients, preferably located outside the entrance to each ward area.

5.7.3.5.2 Personal protective equipment

PPE include gloves and gowns or aprons as indicated following risk assessment. Do not use gloves as a substitute for hand hygiene.

5.7.3.5.3 Care of equipment

The care of equipment is repeated here for emphasis (see section 6.5 Patient care articles). Ideally, bowls and bedpans should not be shared. If these are communal, thorough (heat) disinfection after each patient use is recommended.

5.7.3.5.4 Baths

These are in frequent use and should be cleaned frequently after each patient use with an ammonia-based detergent and dried. Wipe over with hypochlorite if recommended.

5.7.3.5.5 Mattresses

The mattress covers should be waterproof and intact and the covers replaced if any puncture or tear is noted. The mattress covers should be wiped with warm water and detergent and dried. Because of excessive leaking from burn wounds, the mattresses may be wiped over with disinfectant if indicated. The mattress covers should be removed and laundered between patients. The mattresses **must** be dry and clean.

5.7.3.5.6 Bedpans and urinals

Bedpans are a frequent source of gram-negative contamination. After patient use the bedpan or urinal must be sluiced and clean and processed above 80 °C for one minute to kill most vegetative bacteria. Store inverted to dry.

5.7.3.5.7 Ventilators

Ventilators must be cleaned and disinfected between patients. Ideally, self-humidification filters are advisable. These protect the equipment and prevent the use of humidifiers. Internal filters to prevent the machines from contamination are advisable. High-level disinfection with heat (80 °C) is preferred, but appropriate chemical disinfection may be considered.

5.7.3.6 General cleaning

Daily damp mopping of furniture, bedside tables and door handles should be carried out. All areas should be dried immediately. Follow cleaning recommendations.

5.7.3.7 Visitors

Anyone entering the burns unit must follow the protocol and should be advised by the nurse-in-charge. They should be asked to:
- wash and dry their hands if there is to be or has been any contact with the patient
- not sit on patients' beds.

The number of visitors should be limited and they should be informed of the dangers of infection.

5.7.3.8 Staff education

All staff must be trained in infection control practices and updated regularly. There should be a written infection control policy for the burns units with detailed procedures. Compliance with hand disinfection and infection control should be monitored.

5.7.4 Bone marrow transplant unit

Bone marrow transplants require high-dependency nursing. Patients are immunosuppressed over a long period of time, which increases their susceptibility to different pathogens, depending on the stage of their immune suppression. The patients have to be protected from infections until they have recovered sufficiently to protect themselves. IPC practices have to be implemented from the start and maintained throughout the patient's illness.

5.7.4.1 Risk of transmission

Immunosuppressed patients are at risk from endogenous pathogens but also from airborne transmission and hands of staff. They are prone to bacterial, viral and fungal infections at different stages of their immune state.

5.7.4.2 Design and layout

The unit should be purpose-built, sited away from construction areas or where environmental contamination with fungal spores is possible.

- Doors and windows should be well sealed.
- Single rooms with en suite toilet facilities should be provided. Ideally these units should have an anteroom to store patient-care articles and PPE for staff.
- Hand-hygiene facilities are essential inside (ABHR) and outside the single room (handwash basins).
- Clinical equipment should ideally be kept outside the single room if not constantly in use.
- There should be a dedicated area for pharmacy preparations with a laminar flow cabinet.
- Adequate staff facilities should be provided.
- The room should be at positive pressure with an air supply filtered through HEPA filters.

5.7.4.3 Prevention of transmission

The following precautions should be taken to prevent transmission of infections to highly at-risk patients:

- Hand hygiene should be frequent and facilities should be provided for this.
- PPE is recommended based on procedures.
- Equipment (clinical) should be heat-sterilised or disposable.
- Non-clinical equipment such as bedpans or urinals should be heat-disinfected.

5.7.4.4 Cleaning

Cleaning, as in other units, is a critical consideration. In the bone marrow unit it involves:

- Daily cleaning of all surfaces with a dedicated, clean damp cloth (disposable preferred). The environment should be kept as dry as possible.
- Environmental disinfectants are not necessary unless specified by IPC team.
- Toilets are cleaned daily and the toilet seat wiped with an appropriate disinfectant.
- Domestic staff should wear recommended PPE when entering the isolation rooms.

5.7.4.5 Food preparation

Food and liquid preparation needs to be carefully controlled to reduce the risk of infection that may be transmitted by food and water.

- During the initial period of total neutropenia, patients may be given a special diet of canned foods heated up in a microwave.

- Uncooked foods, such as fruits and salads, are not recommended during the neutropenic stage.
- Later, cooked food can be prepared with meticulous attention to cleanliness. Crockery and cutlery should be heat-disinfected in a dishwasher.
- Drinking water should be carefully prepared.
- Milk and dairy products should be carefully controlled.

5.7.4.6 Pharmaceutical products

Pharmaceutical products should be administered with particular care:
- All medication should be prepared in a laminar flow cabinet.
- The person handling the drugs should wear sterile PPE.
- Delivery systems such as intravenous and enteral feeding systems must be sterile. Re-use is not recommended.
- Left-over products must be discarded.

5.7.4.7 Microbiological screening

Microbiological screening is subject to certain restrictions.
- The frequency of patient screening depends on the unit policy.
- Investigation of an infective episode is according to unit policy.
- Environmental screening is not recommended routinely unless there is an outbreak or the ventilation system has broken down.

5.7.4.8 Staff

The staff must observe the following precautions:
- The immune status of the staff should be established and necessary vaccination should be offered.
- Staff with any illness, cough, cold, diarrhoea or skin lesion should not be allowed to work for the duration of symptoms.

5.7.4.9 Visitors

Visitors should follow the same precautions as the staff. Children should not be allowed to visit unless specifically required.

5.7.5 Intensive therapy units

Intensive therapy units (ITUs) house extremely sick patients in need of urgent surgical or medical attention. They use some of the most sophisticated equipment and advanced medical practices. Because of their nature, ITUs contribute to more HAIs than any other unit. Patients may become infected or colonised with healthcare-associated pathogens. High-dependency nursing leads to much more contact between the staff and patient and a greater chance of transmission. Antibiotics are used extensively in ITUs and for prolonged periods of time. The result of this is multidrug-resistant bacteria and fungi in the environment. Any break in IPC procedures usually results in transmission and therefore IPC policies for ITU should be clear and meticulously implemented.

5.7.5.1 Risk of transmission

As the risk of transmission of infection is high and the outcome serious for patients in this unit, IPC procedures for the following must be meticulously observed:
- hands of staff and attendants
- assisted ventilation and equipment
- suction and drainage systems – re-used suction tubing
- device related infection
- increased use of disinfectants
- non-clinical devices
- dressing trolleys.

5.7.5.2 Location and layout

The ITU should be located close to the clinical areas it serves. Larger hospitals may have more than one ITU with step-down facilities to high-dependency units. The running costs of such units are high and often there is an effort to try to cut costs by taking shortcuts. However, such cost cuts are really not cost-effective in the long run.

The design of an ITU differs depending on the available floor space, size of population it serves and location. Usually there are several beds in one open space with a nursing observation station located centrally to improve observation of patients. Some units have single rooms with glass partitions and privacy curtains and these are also visible from the main nursing station.

Single rooms in an ITU are essential and should be carefully considered during planning. This is one area that the IPC team must visit regularly to support to the staff.

5.7.5.3 Prevention of transmission

The following IPC precautions should be taken to prevent the transmission of infections as far as possible in this high-dependency unit:
- Bed centres should be a minimum of 3.5 m apart to allow for easy movement of staff, equipment and procedures.
- Handwashing facilities should be placed outside the direct patient care area, e.g. in the corridor.
- ABHR should be available next to each patient bed, on the procedure trolley, clinical notes trolley and any area where hand contact is expected.
- Staff should be dedicated and skilled in ITU procedures. They should understand IPC procedures and implement them. Frequent training and refresher courses are essential.

- Visiting staff such as doctors, physiotherapists and x-ray technicians should be aware of IPC practices in the ITU and follow them meticulously.
- A sharps box must be placed next to each patient's bed – the frequency of injectable medication is higher in high-dependency units.

5.7.5.4 Ventilation

The ITU should preferably have independent, controlled positive-pressure ventilation with negative pressure in the isolation rooms, especially in areas with endemic TB. The windows must be sealed. Ideally, airflows should be away from the patients, exhausted out towards the atmosphere. This is not always possible and most ITUs are linked into the main hospital ventilation system.

5.7.5.5 Admission policy

Any patient with a communicable disease should be *admitted directly to a single room*. This includes patients with diarrhoea, skin lesions or a recognised communicable disease or HAI pathogen. The patient may be moved to the open ward when there is a confirmed negative report.

5.7.5.6 Disinfection of the environment

The routine use of disinfectants in the ITU is not recommended unless specifically indicated. Warm water and detergent are sufficient for damp dusting, followed by drying. In case of outbreaks or high rates of infection, a suitable hospital-approved disinfectant may be used.

5.7.5.7 Personal protective equipment

These have been detailed elsewhere. However, appropriate PPE is indicated as a supplement to other more effective practices.

5.7.5.8 Procedures

In ITUs, patients are on several types of medical intervention, which are risk-prone procedures and also increase the risk of infection in these critically ill patients. It is essential that the staff are highly skilled and qualified in dealing with the patient's clinical needs while being aware of safe IPC protocols.

5.7.5.9 Decontamination of clinical equipment

Clinical equipment should not be decontaminated in the ITU because there is risk of spreading pathogens. All equipment should be sent to the SSD for decontamination and sterilisation if required. In exceptional cases, if there is a shortage of ventilators and equipment has to be processed in the unit, a designated area should be earmarked and equipped with all the necessary items to carry out decontamination. However, this is not recommended.

5.7.5.10 Some recommended policies for the intensive therapy unit

The following IPC policies should be implemented in the ITU unit:

- antibiotic policy
- environmental cleaning and disinfection policy
- decontamination policy
- visitors' policy
- waste disposal
- sharps disposal
- aseptic procedures.

5.7.6 Dialysis unit

The activity in a dialysis unit is part of a routine where known or new patients are treated as outpatients. Most of these units are self-contained and not necessarily linked directly to the renal unit. The infrastructure should be independent.

5.7.6.1 Risk of transmission[21]

The main risk is of transmission of blood-borne viruses such as hepatitis B and C and HIV via the haemodialysis machines and other equipment. Bacterial infections from device-related infections and less commonly from surfaces of the machine and control panel may occur. Multi-dose vials (MDVs) are known sources of both virus and bacterial transmission and should be avoided.

5.7.6.2 Layout of dialysis units

The dialysis unit should be a self-contained area where stations for dialysis patients are laid out to provide maximum comfort and safe procedures.

There should be a general patient treatment area, isolation facilities for infectious patients (HBsAg-positive), an administrative area ('nurse's station') and areas for medication preparation, storage of clean supplies and equipment, cleaning and disinfection of equipment and processing of dialysers.

Each station is considered a potentially contaminated space and any equipment, supplies, charts or staff entering that patient zone must be dealt with carefully. There should be sufficient space between stations to allow accessibility for cleaning and staff to move freely. The area should be free of clutter and arranged in an orderly fashion. Excess lengths of tubes, hoses and wires should be removed from the floor.

---

[21] Morbidity and Mortality Monthly Report (MMMR). 27 April 2001. Recommendations for preventing transmission of infections among chronic hemodialysis patients. 50 (RR–5).

5.7.6.3 Drug preparation area

All medication and fluids, especially where MDVs are used, should be prepared in a separate area away from the patient areas. Single-dose medications should be prepared at the patient's bedside. Carrying MDVs from one station to another is not recommended because of possible accidental contamination of the MDV.

5.7.6.4 Trolleys

Each station should have a dedicated trolley with all the necessary provisions for a patient. The trolley should not be moved between patients without being cleaned and disinfected as required. Unused supplies from a dialysis station should not be re-used or taken back to the clean supply area. These items should be discarded.

5.7.6.5 Patient selection

All patients should undergo hepatitis B and C and HIV testing prior to starting dialysis. If possible, they should be immunised against hepatitis B. If a patient is found to be HbsAg-positive, he or she should be isolated.[22]

5.7.6.6 Staff

The staff should be skilled, well trained and knowledgeable about haemodialysis. Staff should be immunised against hepatitis B and offered post-exposure prophylaxis whenever blood exposure occurs (see section 7.3 Occupational health).

Staff members caring for HBsAg-positive patients should not care for HBV-susceptible patients at the same time (e.g. during the same shift or during patient changeover).

5.7.6.7 Blood-borne virus exposure

The transmission of hepatitis B and C and HIV is higher in a dialysis unit than other high-dependency areas. A factor is the considerable exposure to blood and sharps and sometimes spillage. The proper use of sharps should be a priority and all needles and syringes and products in contact with blood must be carefully discarded.

5.7.6.8 Prevention of transmission

The main route is from contact with blood and body fluids and therefore contact precautions should be in place. The use of gloves and plastic aprons is recommended. Facilities for both handwashing and drying as well as ABHR should be provided and used frequently by the staff and patients.

---

[22]   Tokars JI, Arduino MJ & Alta MJ. 2001. Infection control in haemodialysis units. *Infectious Disease Clinics in North America* 15(3): 797–812.

5.7.6.9 Waste management

There should be an ample supply of waste containers for both infectious and non-infectious waste. A sharps box should be placed next to each station and changed as soon as three-quarters full.

5.7.6.10 Other IPC precautions

- Items used at a dialysis station should either be disposed of or dedicated for use only on a single patient, or cleaned and disinfected before being taken to a common clean area or used on another patient.
- Non-disposable items that cannot be cleaned and disinfected (e.g. adhesive tape, cloth-covered blood pressure cuffs) should be for single-patient use.
- Unused medications (including MDVs containing diluents) or supplies (e.g. syringes, alcohol swabs) should be discarded once the patient has completed his or her treatment.

5.7.6.11 The dialysis process

5.7.6.11.1 **Maintenance of dialysis machines** depends on the type of machine used. However, it should be noted that an intact dialysis membrane does not allow the passage of pathogens (acts as a bacterial filter).

5.7.6.11.2 **A single-pass machine** can be rinsed and disinfected at the beginning and end of the day or session since the internal pathways are safe from blood contamination. For a batch recirculating machine the system has to be drained, rinsed and disinfected after each use. These machines are also fitted with filters to prevent transfer, which are essential to prevent transmission of pathogens. Both types of machine should be cleaned and disinfected if blood leakage occurs because the dialysis fluid becomes contaminated with blood.

5.7.6.11.3 **Pressure transducer filter protectors** are used primarily to prevent contamination and preserve the functioning of the pressure monitoring components (i.e. arterial, venous, or both) of the haemodialysis machine. Haemodialysis machines usually have both external (typically supplied with the blood tubing set) and internal protectors, which serve as a backup.

5.7.6.12 Disinfectants

The use of disinfectants in a dialysis unit is recommended. These are used for the equipment and sometimes for the environment, especially in the case of spillage or blood leakages. Not all disinfectants are appropriate and local protocols and recommendations should be followed. Some recommendations are hydrogen peroxide, peracetic acid and ozone. Heat disinfection by pasteurisation (>80 °C) is a reasonable alternative.

5.7.6.13 Monitoring dialysis fluids

Fluids used in dialysis should be carefully monitored according to local protocol. Contamination of fluids can occur during use or storage and should be checked regularly to ensure sterility.

5.7.6.13.1 Types of fluid. There are several types of fluid used in the dialysis unit and these have to be monitored regularly to ensure sterility, osmolarity and appropriate content. These are:

- water used to prepare dialysate
- dialysate itself
- bicarbonate concentrate.

The frequency of and indications for testing the fluids are shown below:

- at least monthly for established water treatment systems
- at least weekly for new water treatment systems
- after a suspected pyrogenic reaction
- after a suspected bacteraemia
- after any modification to the water treatment system.

The results of these tests on the fluids should be within the standards of microbial limit or their products (such as endotoxins):

- Dialysis water should have a bacterial count of no more than 200 cfu/ml and there should be no endotoxins (0 EU/ml).
- Bicarbonate concentrate should have a bacterial count of no more than 200 cfu/ml with 5 EU/ml of endotoxin.

5.7.6.14 Cleaning

There are no particular recommendations except that the cleaning staff should be aware of the work environment. They should be provided with appropriate protective equipment. The main risk is from needles and sharps or spillage. They should be trained in these aspects.

5.7.7 Neonatal units[23]

The neonatal unit (NNU) is a highly specialised unit caring for premature, low-weight babies and those with congenital or acquired disease. Often, neonates stay in the NNU for a long time and are exposed to HAI like any other high-dependency or intensive care unit. The difference is that these infections frequently result in death. The staff working in the NNU should be highly trained and aware of good

---

[23] Recommended Standards for Newborn ICU Design. Report of the Seventh Census Conference on Newborn ICU Design. Committee to Establish Recommended Standards for Newborn ICU Design. 1 February 2007. Available at: www.nd.edu/nicudes/.

IPC practices at all times to ensure safety of these patients. The NNU must be freely accessible to mothers and immediate families; policies should take this into account.

From an IPC perspective, the requirements in an NNU are similar to adult intensive care, with a few exceptions.

5.7.7.1 Risk of transmission

The risks are similar to adult ICUs, but the effect of infection is usually higher morbidity or mortality in neonates.

5.7.7.2 Design and layout

Neonates, particularly premature babies, who are extremely vulnerable, are usually transferred from intensive care to a high-care ward and then to a normal ward before discharge. It is not practical to place every neonate in a single room, but those with transmissible infections can be housed in single facilities provided the staffing levels allow for individual nursing.

5.7.7.2.1   **Siting.** The NNU should be located in a self-contained unit close to maternity and labour wards if possible, with controlled access and ventilation. An appropriate number of air, oxygen and vacuum outlets should be provided with an emergency electrical supply of high quality.

5.7.7.2.2   **Spacing.** It is recommended that there is a minimum of 2.4 m between cots, bassinets or incubators. This may not be feasible in low-resource countries, but an adequate distance should be considered which can comfortably house the necessary critical care equipment and care items. It is noteworthy that an incubator is closed and acts as an isolation cubicle.

5.7.7.3 The layout of neonatal intensive care

The ward is usually divided into bays housing up to ten incubators. Incubators provide a closed, controllable environment, and contact with the neonate can be regulated. Incubators are partially effective in containing infections because the neonate is enclosed.

Neonates requiring UV light therapy should be placed in open bassinets with the UV lights above them. The nursing station should be located so that vigilant care can be provided at all times. The neonates are often ventilated and provision should be made to ensure safe endotracheal suctioning and ventilator maintenance. Single-patient-use ventilator equipment is recommended.

Hand decontamination with ABHR should be provided at the entrance of each ward, each bay and on each incubator to ensure good hand hygiene compliance. There should be at least one handwash basin located at the entrance of the bedded bay.

5.7.7.3.1 The high-care nursery

The layout is usually similar to the intensive care area; however, there is usually less critical care equipment present. The neonates may be housed in open cots, so special care should be taken to provide for ABHR hand hygiene.

5.7.7.3.2 The main ward

The room layout is similar to that of an ordinary neonatal ward. There must be adequate space between the cots or bassinets to accommodate medical devices and support equipment. Sometimes the wards are divided into smaller units for ease of nursing management.

5.7.7.3.3 Isolation facilities

Infected neonates can be isolated in the individual incubator, or if there are several cases, in a separate section of the ward.

5.7.7.3.4 Family area

Members of the family should have a separate waiting area and have immediate contact with the ward staff upon arrival so that they can be advised of procedures.

5.7.7.4 Ventilation and temperature

Temperature regulation is essential in the NNU and the ambient temperature is usually kept more or less constant at 26 °C (22–26 °C), which is higher than adult units. The humidity should be controlled to between 30% and 60% without causing condensation on the walls and windows.

Ideally, the NNU is kept under positive-pressure ventilation with a minimum of 6 ACH. The ventilation pattern (airflows) should be designed to allow controlled filtered air into the unit and exhausted through outlets, doors and windows without creating a draught near the neonates. However, this is not always possible and most NNUs have mechanical ventilation without much attention to air changes. As long as the NNU is warm, well ventilated and reasonably comfortable for the neonates, there is no contravention of IPC principles.

5.7.7.5 Kangaroo care or private family facilities

Kangaroo care is becoming increasingly popular for low birth weight infants. The mother or father carries the infant in direct contact with his or her skin, usually on the chest. They stay in the hospital and should have appropriate facilities to support them and their baby.

Facilities include:
- Room or rooms offering some privacy for the parent to nurse and carry the infant; these rooms away from the clinical area. There are separate rooms

where the parent and child can be together. This allows privacy and reduces cross-infection to others.

- Overnight wards for post-natal mothers who are enrolled in the kangaroo programme should be available.
- Ablution facilities.
- Access to NNU and staff at all times.

Screening of parents. In countries such as South Africa where tuberculosis is common, outbreaks in kangaroo units have been reported among mothers.

Parents are screened to make sure they are fit to kangaroo or provide adequate skin-to-skin care for the infants.

It would be prudent to take a clinical history from the mother if the kangaroo unit is a shared facility, detailing a history of:

- cough, weight loss or night sweats in the past month
- diarrhoea, abdominal upset, vomiting
- cold or flu-like illness
- contact abroad or travel abroad
- drug usage.

5.7.7.6 Milk preparation area

The milk kitchen should be housed separately with facilities for preparing feeds, sterilising bottles and storing prepared formula feeds for up to 24 hours. Equipment and facilities include:

- plastic aprons
- weighing scales
- provision to boil or sterilise water
- mixing containers, measures and equipment
- addition of supplements (in conjunction with dieticians)
- facilities for washing-up equipment
- disposal area for liquid waste
- high level disinfection facility for all equipment and bottles used
  - chemical disinfection (hypochlorite) (see section 6.5 Patient care articles)
  - heat disinfection
- pasteurisation facilities
- register for milk with an identification system for neonates
- handwash basin
- waste disposal area.

Expressed breast milk (EBM)

A private room should be provided for mothers to express breast milk. There should be provision for sterile bottles for each mother to express milk into. The bottle should be labelled either by the mother or by a member of staff in the presence of the mother after the milk has been expressed.

EBM can be brought in from home in bottles supplied by the hospital or sterile bottles purchased if not supplied.

The bottles must be clearly **labelled** with:
- name of the mother
- name of the infant
- hospital number of the infant
- date and time of expressing milk.

EBM and formula milk must be **stored** in the refrigerator at 4 °C and no more than 6 °C. Each infant should have its own rack which holds labelled bottles for 24 hours, and no more.

Pooled breast milk. Donated breast milk can be pooled, but must be pasteurised at 70–75 °C for three minutes or 90 °C for less than one minute before being stored or frozen.

Supplements are added after the milk has been removed from the freezer and thawed.

5.7.7.7 Procedure areas in neonatal units

If a procedure or operating room is situated inside the NNU, it should comply with all the recommendations of adult operating rooms except that temperature and humidity are higher.

5.7.7.8 Specialised equipment (see also section 6.5 Patient care articles)

All high-care areas have specialised equipment and NNUs are no exception. The babies are placed on ventilators, intravenous therapy is started and nasogastric feeds and sometimes total parenteral nutrition are given. They are constantly monitored. All the items needed are specifically designed for neonates and small babies and can be very difficult to clean and decontaminate. Neonates are placed in a controlled environment of an incubator or in a bassinet if indicated.

The processing of neonatal equipment to render it safe for use is highly specialised and requires skill because the items are small and delicate. The NNU environment should be clean and dry.

Respiratory (ventilator) equipment. Equipment used in mechanically ventilating the baby has the same risk as that used for adults, except that the difference is that the neonates are very vulnerable. There are several items of equipment that are used to support respiratory function in a neonate. Some of them are mentioned below.

5.7.7.9 Care and use of equipment in the neonatal unit

Incubators. Incubators need to be cleaned regularly and thoroughly. The incubators are usually cleaned after a baby has been discharged and the process of cleaning must be meticulous. A written protocol is essential.

The incubator is removed from the main ward area. In some hospitals, a red sticker is attached to it to indicate it has not been cleaned. The mattress and contents of the incubator are removed and cleaned thoroughly with warm water and detergent, paying special attention to corners, hinges and areas where mucus and dirt may become trapped. It must be wiped dry. The inside of the incubator should be wiped with a large 70% isopropyl alcohol-impregnated swab (other chemicals such as chlorine may be toxic when inhaled by neonates). The incubator is plugged into the electrical supply and all gauges are checked. A green sticker shows the incubator has been cleaned and is ready to return to the ward.

Humidifiers are a necessity, and inline humidification is preferred. Open-circuit humidifiers are not recommended. If these are used, the humidifier is emptied after 24 hours of use. They should be washed thoroughly and dried. The use of chemical disinfection is not advised. Humidifiers should be sent for sterilisation to the SSD. The humidifier should be filled with sterile water just before use.

Resuscitaires. All circuits and connections are disconnected. All areas need to be washed, especially the thread on the connectors with a soft brush (held below the water level). Resuscitaires should be sent to the SSD for sterilisation if heat-stable, or ethylene oxide if heat-sensitive.

5.7.8 Other essential units in the health facility

When designing a healthcare facility, provision should be made for all support units to function optimally and should be integrated into the working structure of the healthcare facility. When these units are considered the principle remains the same, only the scale is adjusted according to the size of the facility and the population it serves. All individual units should be provided with staff facilities such as tea rooms, toilet facilities and rest areas. Although these are discussed in detail under support services, this list should serve as a reminder when designing a healthcare facility:

- **Engineering unit** supports the healthcare facility, particularly the SSDs, with engineers, plumbers and electricians. These personnel should be catered for with a separate workshop to carry out small repairs and to send and receive repaired items. They should also service storage and staff-changing facilities and rest areas.

- **Laundry and linen** management areas should be provided. Even if there are no onsite facilities for laundry, there should be a linen management room to send and receive linen (see section 6.2 Linen and laundry).
- **Healthcare waste** is segregated into infectious and non-infectious waste and there should be storage facilities for both before being collected. There should be an administration office for the waste manager or similar (see section 6.3 Healthcare waste management).
- **Housekeeping unit** should have a separate area with stores for cleaning equipment, such as gloves, mop heads, buckets and detergents. There should be an area for keeping records (see section 6.4 Environmental cleaning).
- **Kitchen** should be located in a separate area with provisions for good hygiene and access to the clinical areas (see section 6.1 Kitchens and food preparation).
- **Sterile services unit** is strictly speaking not a support unit because it is a specialist unit in its own right. The SSD should be located outside the operating theatre suite but close to it for ease of transportation of equipment. The SSD also provides services to wards and other clinical areas and therefore should be easily accessible (see section 3.5 The sterile services department (SSD)).
- **Pharmacy** should be located close to clinical areas but also have access to delivery and temperature-controlled storage for drugs, vaccines and fluids.

5.8 Mortuaries

Hospital mortuaries house deaths from infective and non-infective causes. There are special requirements in mortuaries for the storage of bodies and facilities for performing post-mortems. The environment should be safe for mortuary healthcare workers. Their main work is not unlike an OT, although the regulations are less demanding. The role of IPC is to ensure that the environment of the mortuary is made as safe as possible for the people who work there and that precautions against infection are known and practised.

5.8.1 Risk of transmission

Given the fact that post-mortems may be performed on infectious bodies, there is considerable risk of transmission of infection to healthcare workers if they are not adequately protected. The following are ways in which infection can be transmitted during a post-mortem:

- piercing injuries from sharp bony fragment and sharp instruments such as scalpels and saws
- aerosols from cutting bones and opening the cadaver to investigate cavities
- respiratory aerosols from opening the lungs
- splashes from blood and body fluids

- more recently, handling bodies of people who died from Ebola has a high level of risk.

5.8.2 Design and layout

The mortuary should be situated away from the main hospital area and should be accessible to motor vehicles and undertakers' transportation.

The mortuary should be divided as follows:
- **Changing and showering area.** All staff should change out of their outdoor clothes and wear work clothes with covered footwear. Facilities for showering should be provided.
- **Refrigerator for bodies.** Refrigeration for bodies should be compartmentalised and held at a temperature of no more than 6 °C (4–8 °C). These special refrigerators should be emptied and cleaned regularly. The cooling system must also be checked and maintained regularly by the engineers.
- **Operating or post-mortem examination area.** The staff should be protected during post-mortems, especially from blood and body fluids (piercing injuries) and airborne transmission. The post-mortem room should ideally be under controlled negative-pressure ventilation, especially in countries with airborne-disease transmission. After the post-mortem the area should be cleaned with warm water and detergent and wiped over with hypochlorite.
- **Storage of body parts.** Body parts are preserved in formalin, which poses a risk to staff from exposure to chemicals. Appropriate protective clothing is advised.

5.8.3 Personal protective equipment

As the need for protection from formalin is clear, fully protective clothing is essential in the mortuary. This comprises heavy plastic aprons, gloves for light and heavy work and gumboots. Masks and visors or goggles (face protection) should also be worn as they provide protection from splashes.

5.9 Healthcare clinics

Primary healthcare for the majority of the populace is catered for by a system of clinics in Africa. These comprise primary healthcare clinics, community clinics and day hospitals. Since patients who attend these facilities usually have either very limited means or virtually no means at all, many have often ignored the early symptoms of disease and arrive for treatment in an advanced state of infection. In addition to this, the patient load is very high. Waiting rooms are invariably crowded with sick people waiting for treatment. Clinics pose a particular set of challenges to IPC teams. In this section the role of IPC in minimising the transmission of infection in clinics and day hospitals is described. The scope of this role is considerable, taking into account all aspects of the difficult task of providing adequate and sensitive healthcare to large numbers of patients with widely different medical needs.

5.10 Community-based clinics

Primary healthcare clinics (PHCs) are the first interface between the public and healthcare delivery systems. They are located as stand-alone buildings in the community and provide both curative and preventive services to the public.

PHCs deal with walk-in patients, who are usually ambulant, and do not provide overnight-stay facilities. In some countries there are fixed days (with appointments) for specific groups of the public for immunisation or preventive care, but the clinics also operate a curative service on a walk-in basis. In LMICs the clinics provide both curative and preventive services as part of a comprehensive service and there are no appointments – patients are seen as they present, crowded into small waiting areas. This can pose a problem for containment of infectious diseases like tuberculosis.

Community Health clinics offer a wider range of services and may have a small maternity unit with a few beds attached to them. The load on community clinics is often enormous, with up to 200 consultations per nurse per day!

Day hospitals offer a comprehensive service including blood sampling, dispensing chronic medication, providing counselling services, performing some investigations such as chest x-ray and minor operations. They usually have a few beds for maternity cases.

5.10.1 Risk of transmission

The risk of transmission of infection to both other patients and healthcare workers in clinics is high. The list below summarises the reasons why this is so:
- exposure to suspected or known cases of respiratory infections such as influenza or TB
- mixed population of vulnerable and immune patients in a crowded waiting area.
- excessive patient load puts severe pressure on the services so that inadequate IPC precautions are often undertaken.
- inadequate decontamination of clinical equipment, which facilitates the transmission of blood-borne pathogens.

5.10.2 Design and layout

The clinics should be easily accessible by public transport to walk-in patients and those who are wheelchair-bound. They should be accessible to ambulances, private vehicles and delivery vans.

The clinic should be laid out with open spaces around it to allow patients to sit outside if they wish. There should be good natural light and ventilation. There should be adequate water and electricity available to run the facility. Solar panels are being used in some clinics to provide heating.

5.10.2.1 Waiting area

The waiting area should be:

- Large enough to accommodate the patients waiting to see healthcare workers.
- Well ventilated. In warmer countries, natural ventilation is used by means of large windows that can be opened.
- Patients could be seated outside in a shaded area.
- Close to a reception area where the patient presents first. This helps with triaging patients who have contagious respiratory diseases. Such patients can then be separated from the rest before they enter the main waiting room.
- Close to the amenities in the clinics such as consulting rooms, testing and counselling areas.
- Provided with facilities to sit comfortably while waiting.
- Provided with water for the patients' use.
- Provided with toilet facilities.
- Provided with waste baskets for disposal of used tissues.

The waiting area could be used to provide health information for the public with posters and information pamphlets.

5.10.2.2 Ventilation

Proper ventilation is essential in reducing the transmission of infection. The temperature and humidity rapidly increase in a crowded, poorly ventilated room and this facilitates the transmission of airborne pathogens. The waiting room can be be under negative-pressure ventilation with increase airflows by:

- opening windows and allowing natural cross-ventilation
- use of 'whirlybirds' to extract the air
- extractor fans can also be used if required.

However, it is best to remove patients with coughs and colds from the main body of the waiting patients (triaging). If possible, a separate facility should be provided for such patients while they wait.

5.10.2.3 Patient consulting rooms

There should be adequate consulting rooms to see the patients. Ideally, the curative and preventive patients should be seen in different areas of the clinic, but if they are seen in the same consulting rooms, adequate precautions should be taken to prevent transmission.

The consulting rooms should have large windows that can be opened, a handwash basin, hand hygiene facilities and good light.

It is advisable for the consultation and examination to take place with the patient sitting **downwind** from the healthcare worker in case the patient coughs or sneezes.

There should be adequate PPE such as gloves and surgical masks should these be needed.

The examination couch should be covered with clean sheets or wiped down after each patient.

5.10.2.4 Counselling rooms

An adequate number of counselling rooms, particularly for HIV patients, should be provided which are discreet and private. This is difficult to achieve in an overcrowded clinic, but arrangements can be made to ask patients who have come for blood tests to go directly to the phlebotomy room. From there the patient can be directed to the counselling facilities that are close by.

5.10.2.5 Phlebotomy

Patients requiring blood tests should have a separate area provided for phlebotomy. The room should be clean, airy, with adequate blood sampling equipment, a sharps box and hand hygiene facilities. There should be a table and chair for both the phlebotomist and the patient to be comfortable when taking blood.

5.10.2.6 Cough room

In countries where there are a large number of TB cases, cough rooms or areas have been provided. These can be simple structures with good ventilation. Sputum sample pots should be provided and there should be hand hygiene facilities available. Instruction sheets on how to produce a sputum sample should be given to each person when she or he enters the cough room.

- **Outdoors.** A small open cordoned-off area outside with a large cover to protect the patient from rain and sun can be provided. It should have large openings between the walls and the roof for adequate ventilation. The patients should be asked to wait 10 minutes between each patient.
- **Indoors.** A separate room from the waiting area, with negative-pressure ventilation and handwash facilities should be provided.

5.10.2.7 Laboratory or sample storage area

Some clinics have facilities to carry out rapid HIV tests or other simple tests. If these facilities do not exist, a designated area to store patient samples prior to collection should be available.

5.10.2.8 Storage

Medical drugs including vaccines should be stored appropriately with refrigeration to maintain temperatures between 4 °C and 6 °C. Other drugs should be stored in cool and controlled storage areas. This is not always possible in hot, dry countries. Sometimes intravenous fluids are also kept at clinics.

Medical supplies, such as bandages, protective equipment and other medical supplies, should be stored separately from drugs.

5.10.2.9 Clinical equipment

All equipment should be stored clean and dry. Any items requiring heat-disinfection or sterilisation should be sent to the nearest SSD. Alternatively, items should be manually cleaned thoroughly and then disinfected with the appropriate disinfectant and left to dry. In some institutions, boiling sterilisers are used to disinfect equipment like vaginal specula.

5.10.2.10 Offices and staff areas

There should be adequate facilities to allow staff to rest and carry out their administrative duties.

5.10.3 Dental clinics

Dentistry is high-risk because there is a high risk of contamination by blood when working with teeth and gums. There have been several reports of blood-borne virus transmission to patients and from patients to staff. This section points out the main risks to dental staff and patients and ways of minimising these risks. As with other medical facilities there is a need for thought and care to be put into the planning of facilities and equipment.

5.10.3.1 Risk of transmission

The main risk in dental services is that of blood-borne virus transmission. This can occur when:
- instruments and equipment are poorly sterilised or not sterilised at all.
- dental anaesthetic syringes are used to deliver local anaesthetic to several patients from the same vial.
- needlestick injuries occur while delivering an anaesthetic injection into the mouth.
- the patient bites or spits.

- high-speed drills are used that cause splashes and droplets.
- water tanks are used to cool the high-speed drills and equipment.

5.10.3.2 Design and layout

The dental facility should be close to the main clinical area and should have the following:
- a waiting area
- individual cubicle for each patient
- a separate area to wash, clean and sterilise dental instruments
- a storage area containing adequate medical supplies
- staff facilities.

5.10.3.3 Ventilation

Good natural ventilation is sufficient. No special type of ventilation is required for dental clinics, but, as with other clinics, care must be taken to see that waiting rooms are adequately ventilated.

5.10.3.4 Dental work stations

The space should be adequate to accommodate the dentist, dental assistant, equipment and a functioning dental chair. There should be adequate storage space. The work stations should afford privacy. There should be a comfortable working chair for the dentist.

There must be provision for a constant supply of electricity, air pressure, water (ideally with high pressure) and good lighting. Natural light is helpful, but must be accompanied by a good examination light.

5.10.3.5 Dental equipment

All dental equipment must be such that it can undergo steam sterilisation. Most dental clinics have a small desktop steriliser that can adequately sterilise open instruments (121 °C for 15 minutes). Previously, the sterilisers were filled with water and when steam was generated, the exposure time was noted. The modern ones are equipped with gauges and proper sterilisation cycle monitoring. Soaking cleaned instruments in a chemical disinfectant alone is not recommended.

There should be an adequate number of dental trays for the number of patients; re-using pre-used dental trays between patients is unacceptable. The rule is usually one in use, one in the steriliser and one being cleaned.

There should be an adequate number of dental syringes. One vial of anaesthetic per patient should be used and then disposed. The needle must be changed between each patient and the vial holder disinfected.

The nozzles of the sprays and jets must be changed and cleaned between each patient. The water-holding tank should be checked and cleaned at the end of each day and replenished with clean water.

High-speed drills are notoriously difficult to clean. These have to be cleaned meticulously before processing in the steriliser, preferably using an ultrasonicator.

5.10.3.6 Personal protective equipment

The dentist should wear non-sterile gloves and a surgical mask, preferably with a visor, as minimum protection.

5.10.3.7 Staff health

All dental staff should be offered hepatitis B immunisation. It is helpful for the staff to know their own HIV and hepatitis B status.

Needlestick and sharps injuries must be reported and post-exposure prophylaxis given. A record should be kept of all injuries.

5.11 Patient facilities during outbreaks and pandemics

5.11.1 Ebola treatment centres

During the Ebola epidemic of West Africa in 2014, several rapidly assembled designs for patient areas were put in place. All of them had the same principles, but with different facilities afforded to these units.[24]

5.11.2 Transmission risk

Ebola virus disease is a blood-borne virus and spreads mainly via contact with human blood and body fluids. Additionally, dead bodies are a source of infection because the virus continues to survive in fresh dead bodies – transmission during burials have been well documented.[25]

PPE is required to prevent exposure of staff. This will require a body cover including cover for the arms and neck, a double pair of gloves, face mask and visor. Recommendations regarding the use of full coveralls vs fluid resistant gowns will depend on the finances.

Putting on and taking off PPE is paramount and therefore a designated area for both must be available. Spraying of humans with chlorine is not recommended.

---

[24]   WHO. 2015. Manual for the Care and Management of Patients in Ebola Care Units/Community Care Centres.

[25]   Centers for Disease Control and Prevention https://www.cdc.gov/index.htm; National Center for Emerging and Zoonotic Infectious Diseases (NCEZID) https://www.cdc.gov/ncezid/index.html; Division of High-Consequence Pathogens and Pathology (DHCPP); Viral Special Pathogens Branch (VSPB) https://www.cdc.gov/ncezid/dhcpp/vspb/index.html; https://www.cdc.gov/vhf/ebola/.

5.11.3 Ventilation

No special ventilation is required, but a good natural airflow is recommended to keep the staff and patient comfortable and safe.

5.11.4 The layout of the Ebola unit

The Ebola unit (Figure 5.14) is divided into a triage area, admission for suspected cases and a 'wet' and 'dry' ward for patients with confirmed diagnosis of Ebola virus disease. The additional areas include a donning area, staff passage, an exit with a doffing area, storage for medical devices, laboratory, waste management system and a mortuary. For details, the reader is referred to the latest WHO guidelines for Ebola as these are updated regularly (www.who.int).

Patient flow starts with the triage area where patients are vetted for possible Ebola signs and symptoms. If suspected of being infected with Ebola, the patient is admitted to a holding ward for investigation. Once the results of the investigations are available, those found to be infected and are symptomatic are admitted to the inpatient facility, which is separated based on the symptoms of the patient. Patients are discharged from the clinical area on the opposite side of the ward (Figure 5.14).

The **staff** entrance is in an anteroom where donning is carried out. After clinical activity, the staff exit from the opposite side of the ward, having passed through the doffing area. Spraying of staff is not recommended.

Medical devices, waste and other material used in the Ebola ward are removed from the clinical areas through a separate exit. All healthcare waste is sent directly to the end point disposal system available.

Ventilation

No special ventilation system is required. Natural ventilation or mechanical ventilation is needed for the comfort of staff and patients.

Mortuary

Management of dead bodies has to be well thought out and executed because of the high risk of transmission to the handlers.

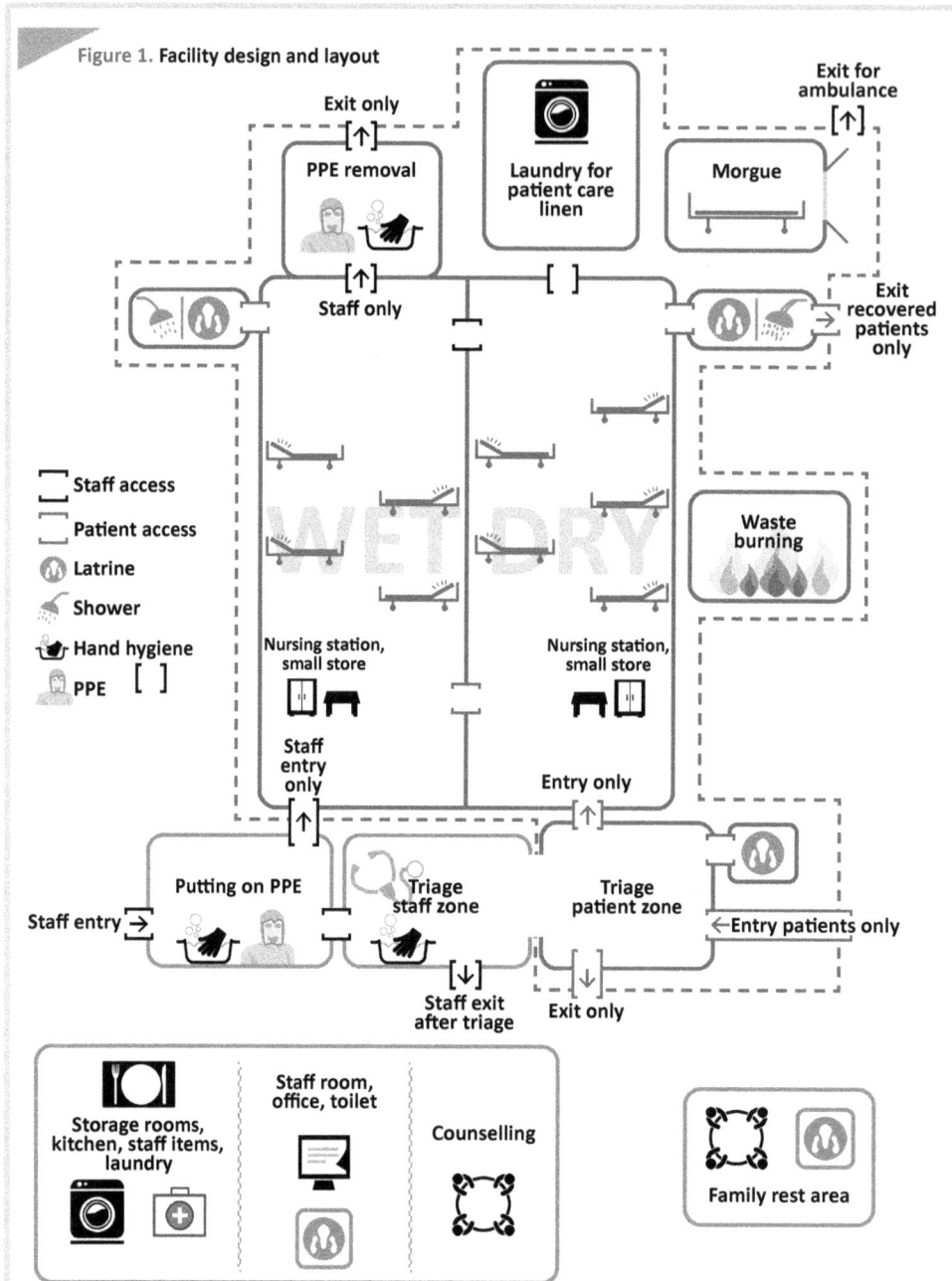

Figure 1. **Facility design and layout**

Exit only

PPE removal

Laundry for patient care linen

Morgue

Exit for ambulance

Staff only

Exit recovered patients only

Staff access

Patient access

Latrine

Shower

Hand hygiene

PPE

Nursing station, small store

Nursing station, small store

Waste burning

WET DRY

Staff entry only

Entry only

Putting on PPE

Triage staff zone

Triage patient zone

Staff entry

Entry patients only

Staff exit after triage

Exit only

Storage rooms, kitchen, staff items, laundry

Staff room, office, toilet

Counselling

Family rest area

Figure 5.14 Ebola facility design and layout (WHO, 2015)

5.12 Acute respiratory infection treatment centre

The other recent pandemic has been SARS-CoV-2 spreading globally with rapid speed. The principle of these units remains the same, with a triage area, a short-stay observation ward awaiting results, and a staff changing room. The clinical areas are divided into a separate severe case ward and a critical case ward (Figure 5.15). A crucial requirement is negative-pressure ventilation for the clinical areas, including the observation ward.

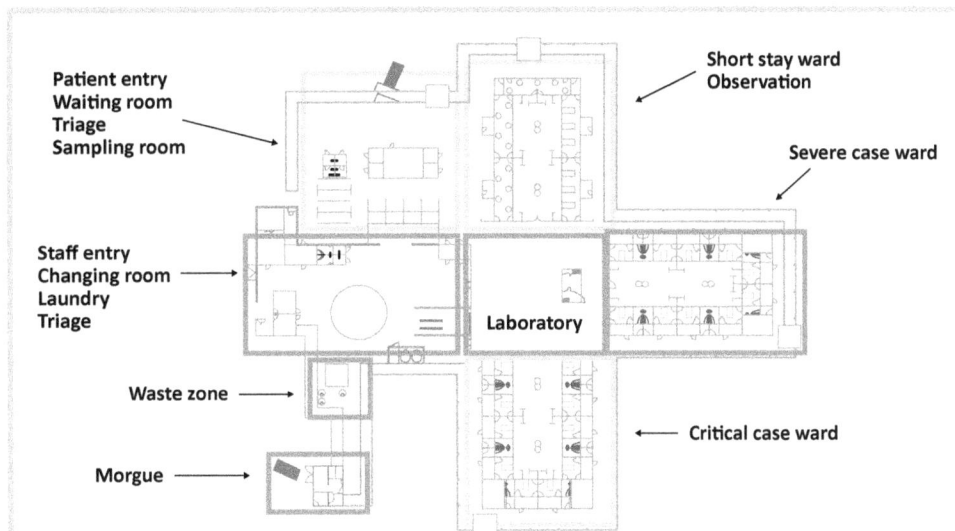

Figure 5.15 Layout for an acute respiratory disease treatment centre[26]

5.12.1 Personal protective equipment

Face covers such as surgical masks or respirators should be worn. During an outbreak respirators are indicated, preferably in combination with a visor. In addition, gloves and aprons may be worn. No other PPE is required. Recycling of respirators is a possibility, but must be done under controlled and well-organised conditions.

---

[26] Severe acute respiratory infections treatment centre: practical manual to set up and manage a SARI treatment centre and SARI screening facility in health care facilities. Geneva: World Health Organization; 2020 (WHO/2019-nCoV/SARI_treatment_center/2020.1). Licence: CC BY-NC-SA 3.0 IGO.

5.12.2 Ventilation[27]

In this treatment centre, ventilation is crucial and must be well thought out and executed. Negative-pressure ventilation is essential in all clinical areas, irrespective of the patient's status (see section 5.3.6.1.1.3.1 Negative-pressure ventilation).

5.12.3 Environment

The environment is usually contaminated with patients coughing and generating aerosols. Regular cleaning with water and detergent, followed by a wipe with a disinfectant, is recommended.

27   WHO. 2021. Roadmap to improve and ensure good indoor ventilation in the context of COVID-19. Geneva: World Health Organization. Licence: CC BY-NC-SA 3.0 IGO.

6 Support services, including environmental cleaning

Briette du Toit Ludick, Buyiswa Lizzie Sithole-Mazibuko & Shaheen Mehtar

Learning outcomes

What you should know after reading this chapter:
- IPC support for catering services
- Waste management and source segregation
- Linen management programme
- Environmental cleaning and domestic services

Introduction

Support services are integral to the functioning of the hospital and are often not given the recognition they deserve for their contribution to the smooth running of healthcare facilities. Inadequate provision for hazard control of food, healthcare waste management or linen has a serious, negative impact on IPC practices. The role of the IPC team is to be part of the quality assurance monitoring and implementation programme by maintaining constant vigilance to ensure that each support system functions optimally.

6.1 Kitchens and food preparation[1]

Healthcare facilities house vulnerable populations who have to be provided with safe, nutritious food that will not cause harm – this can be challenging when dietary needs are diverse. Food must be tasty, familiar and appealing to all cultural and social backgrounds.[2]

---

[1] https://www.theific.org/wp-content/uploads/2016/04/25-Food_2016.pdf; https://isid.org/wp-content/uploads/2018/04/ISID_InfectionGuide_Chapter18.pdf.

[2] International Health Facility Guidelines. Part B: Health Facility Briefing & Design Catering Unit © TAHPI Version 5 June 2017 p 4.

Kitchens and food preparation areas are potential sources of food poisoning, and outbreaks can occur which originate from the staff, preparation and storage of food, transportation of prepared food and during distribution.[3]

Food for the patients and staff is prepared either off or on site. Staff canteens usually have separate kitchens, but the same rules of hygiene apply. Milk preparation for neonates and paediatrics in patient facilities requires strict control and clearly written policies, which are often monitored by IPC and environmental health officers.

The role of IPC is to ensure that workflow and practice ensure safe preparation and delivery of food in healthcare facilities. This section provides a summary of essential IPC aspects for containing the transmission of food-borne pathogens.

6.1.1 Layout and workflow[4]

Kitchens should be located in an independent unit from the main hospital area but should be easily accessible for easy deliveries and removal of waste. There should be adequate space for equipment receiving, preparing food items and delivery. Generally, there are no special ventilation requirements, but provision to remove steam from the cooking area is recommended. The main areas are summarised below – the reader is referred to the International Health Guidelines[5] for details.

The main areas of the catering department should be clearly defined as follows:
- **Staff facilities:** Changing areas for staff when coming on duty and leaving work should be provided with lockers, hand hygiene area, toilets and showers.
  - rest areas and staff dining room
  - cleaners' room
  - office and workstation for managers
- **Receiving and delivery areas:** In the main storage area of the kitchen there should be a separate area for the reception of raw products.
- **Storage areas:** There must be provision for cold storage (4 °C) and freezers (–20 °C).
  - The storage facilities should be adequate for both cooked and uncooked food.

3   Ayliffe GAJ, Fraise AP, Geddes AM & Mitchell K. 2000. *Control of hospital infection: A practical handbook.* 4th ed. London: Arnold. p 243.
4   Afrooz Moatari-Kazerouni, Yuvin Chinniah & Bruno Agard. 2015. Integration of occupational health and safety in the facility layout planning, part II: design of the kitchen of a hospital. *International Journal of Production Research* 53(11): 3228–3242. DOI: 10.1080/00207543.2014.970711.
5   International Health Facility Guidelines. Part B: Health Facility Briefing & Design Catering Unit © TAHPI Version 5 June 2017.

- **Preparation and handling areas:** Preparation areas for cooked and uncooked food should be segregated and preferably should have staff dedicated to working at one station per shift.
  - In compliance with religious requirements, designated areas for different religions must be catered for.
- **Cooking facilities:** blast chillers for cook-chill processing.
  - Cooking, reheating and thawing facilities for cook-chill.
- **Cleaning and washing area:** washing of cooking utensils, cutlery and crockery from the wards.
- **Serving and delivery of meals** will require a holding area for hot/cold food trolleys with electric points.
- There must be a **constant supply of hot and cold water** for washing of utensils, serving equipment and crockery.
- **Adequate handwash and toilet facilities** for staff should be available.
- There should be **rest areas** for the staff.

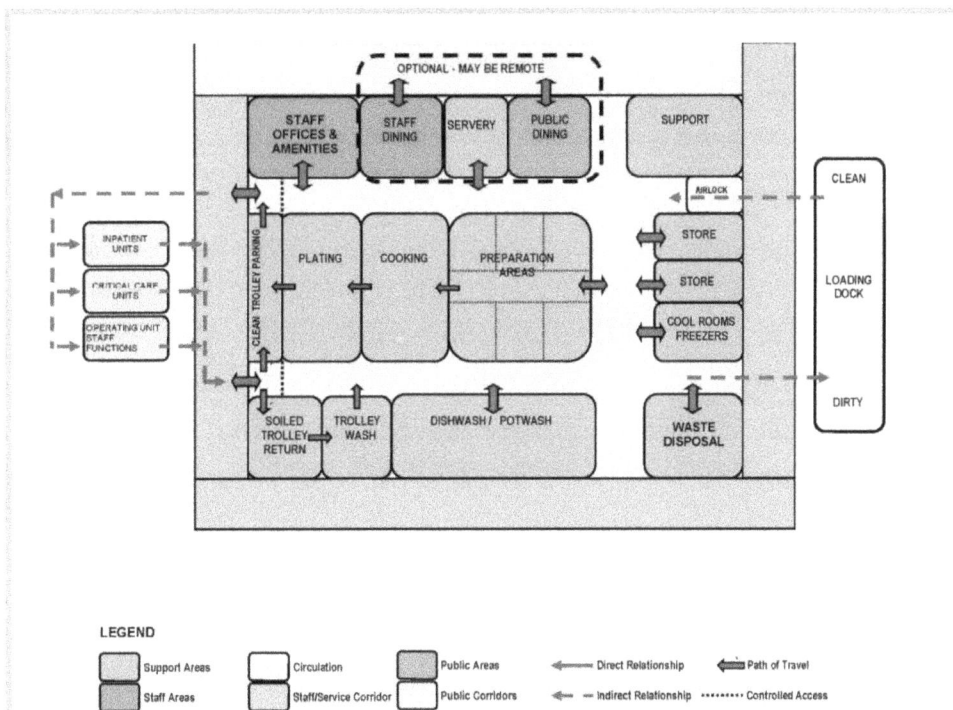

Figure 6.1 Workflow in a catering unit[6]

---

[6] International Health Facility Guidelines. Part B: Health Facility Briefing & Design Catering Unit © TAHPI Version 5 June 2017).

6.1.2 Sourcing raw produce

The purchasing of food produce should be from a reliable source that does not use human sewage in its production of raw vegetables. Meat should be bought from a reputable dealer. Transportation of food from the factory or production area to the healthcare facility should be under controlled sanitary conditions.[7] Bacterial multiplication occurs between 10 °C and 63 °C; some bacteria such as *Listeria monocytogenes* can multiply at 4 °C. Therefore safe transport and storage of fresh and frozen food is paramount

- Frozen foods should be transported and stored at temperatures between –13 °C and –18 °C.
- Meat products should be transported and stored below 4 °C.
- Cold food should be transported and stored at no more than 3 °C.
- Raw vegetables should be kept cool but not refrigerated.

6.1.3 Storage of raw produce before preparation

6.1.3.1 Reception of raw produce

The preparation of food really begins at reception and storage. Food must be delivered in good condition and be fit, in this case, for human consumption by vulnerable patients. This means that it must be delivered and then stored at the correct temperature and in places free of contamination. Raw produce deliveries should be made to a designated area that has adequate space to separate the various items and prepare them for storage. Examples of raw produce are uncooked vegetables, meats, eggs and dairy products. Tinned products and dry rations such as flour and pulses should be stored in airtight containers in a cool storage area.

6.1.3.2 Storage

- Storage should be in a clean, cool and airy space that can be secured.
- Any food capable of supporting bacterial growth should be stored below 6 °C (± 2 °C).
- Various food groups can be stored in similar conditions.
- An expiry date should be clearly visible.

Vegetables should be placed in racks and stacked to allow adequate air movement between the racks. Use a system of 'first in first out'.

Meats, both cooked and uncooked, should be refrigerated and kept separately in different sections.

Dairy products should be refrigerated as soon as possible.

---

[7]   Department of Health, NHS Executive. 1996. *Management of food hygiene and food services in the National Health Service*. London: Department of Health.

Dry rations such as pulses, flour and legumes should be stored in airtight containers in a cool store.

Tinned products should be checked for dents, bulges or leaks. Check expiry dates.

6.1.3.3 Storage temperatures

Freezers should be kept at a minimum temperature of –18 °C and refrigerators at no higher than 4 °C. Temperatures should be monitored and recorded daily and any abnormalities reported to the supervisor.

6.1.4 Food preparation

Food presents many dangers to patients in the form of microbial and chemical contamination such as salmonella food poisoning or heavy metal poisoning. To ensure that hospital food is safe, extensive guidelines for hospital staff involved in the preparation of food have been published. Behind these guidelines is a great deal of research into food and food technology. One of the most useful systems is the American Hazard Analysis and Critical Control Point (HACCP).[8] In either a direct or modified form it is used in most modern hospitals.

HACCP is a structured system that identifies and assesses microbiological and other hazards in production, processing, preparation, storage and distribution of food. This system analyses potential hazards at points at which these may occur, implementing changes and periodically reviewing the systems. A critical area is a point in the process where control can be exercised to eliminate or minimise a hazard such as temperature of food, time spent at room temperature and refrigerator temperatures. HACCP should rapidly detect any failure in the procedures.

The following subsections on food preparation summarise the way modern hospitals carry out food preparation. The emphasis is on safety and the minimisation of the physical, chemical and microbial hazards inherent in food preparation.

6.1.5 IPC measures in catering

When designing a new kitchen or refurbishing an old one, IPC input is invaluable to ensure safe production and distribution of food. Some countries require controlled ventilation in the kitchen to control the steam and reduce heat and this should be considered during refurbishment. The kitchen should have the following provisions:

---

[8]   Richards J, Parr E & Riseborough P. 1993. Hospital food hygiene: The application of hazard analysis critical points to conventional hospital catering. *Journal of Hospital Infection* 24: 273.

6.1.5.1 Handbasins

Staff handwash basins shall be provided in all clean-up, preparation, cooking and serving areas of the unit. Staff in food preparation and serving areas should not be more than 6 m from a handwash basin. Basins should be hands-free operation with paper towel and soap dispensers. Mirrors should not be installed over basins in food preparation areas because contamination from touching hair is possible.

6.1.5.2 Temperature controls

All food storage areas must have functioning temperature gauges which are clearly visible. A log of daily temperatures is recorded and visibly displayed on the fridge or freezer for inspection.

6.1.5.3 Food samples

Every day a small sample of the food prepared and distributed is kept for microbiological analysis, for at least 48 hours in case of an outbreak.

6.1.5.4 Pest control

In new hospitals, the kitchen should not open directly to the outside; an air lock shall be provided between the kitchen and external areas. A section of hospital corridor may be used as an air lock.

In existing kitchens being refurbished, any door leading directly from the kitchen to the outside shall be fitted with a fly screen door with a self-closer.

6.1.6 Designated preparation areas

Raw food products contain micro-organisms that can cause food poisoning if not properly prepared and processed. If uncooked and cooked food are prepared in the same area, using the same knives or utensils and surfaces, cross-contamination occurs and can result in transmission during cooking or food distribution. Cold foods and salads are prepared separately for the same reasons. Milk, cream and other dairy products and cold desserts can become contaminated by the surfaces or from the hands of food handlers. To reduce the risk of cross-contamination, each type of food should be prepared in a separate demarcated area with distinct colour coding if possible.

6.1.6.1   *Uncooked food.* The designated area for preparing uncooked food such as salads should be made of an impervious surface that can be easily cleaned.
- The equipment should be colour-coded to ensure the items are kept separate.
- There should be a washing-up area for items requiring cleaning.
- The equipment used should be kept separate from the areas for cooked food.

- The equipment should be taken to the area for washing up utensils and returned.

6.1.6.2   *Cooked food.* The surfaces of the area in which cooked food is prepared should be made of impervious material and allow cleaning with water and detergent and wiping over with bleach. They should be heat-resistant.

Food should not be left unrefrigerated for more than two hours, especially in warm countries, and must be stored appropriately and immediately on receipt. The following precautions should ensure that the food is safe for human consumption:

- Meat and poultry should be cooked right through.
- Reheated food should be taken up to at least 70 °C.
- Food may be reheated in the microwave. Take care to ensure that the centre of the food is well heated through.
- Liquids should have reached boiling point.
- Cooked food is stored below 5 °C within 90 minutes of cooking and never more than two hours after cooking.
- Food should be thawed slowly.
- Food should not be refrozen after thawing.

Food cooked in the main kitchen is be transported to the wards and distributed safely.

6.1.6.3   *Cook-Serve* refers to the process where food, fresh or frozen is prepared, cooked, plated and served immediately. The food can either be prepared in bulk and then plated on the ward, or it can be pre-plated and taken to the ward on trolleys. This method requires a lot of space to prepare, cook and serve food.

6.1.6.4   *The cook-chill method* is used in several countries.[9] The food is pre-packed, maintained at the required temperatures and distributed as individual meals under carefully controlled conditions.

The processing is according to strict guidelines and there are minimum standards on:

- Bacterial colony counts
- Temperature at which food is stored
- Temperature at which food is served.

The other method is where food is prepared and transported to wards in food trolleys which are warmed up at ward level. The system has to be carefully controlled and monitored regularly.

---

[9]   Department of Health. 1989. *Chill and frozen. Guidelines on cook-chill and cook-freeze catering systems.* London: Department of Health.

6.1.6.5   ***Off-site preparation*** happens on a remote site on the hospital premises. The equipment must be meticulously clean and the food freshly prepared and served. Thorough cleaning and sanitising of equipment is essential. This practice is liable to contamination if the food delivery trolleys are not protected from the weather and dirt.

6.1.7 Food delivery to wards

Food for hospital patients usually includes both cooked and uncooked food and is transported in trolleys. There are two systems which operate, depending on the available resources.

1. The trolley is wheeled to the ward with pre-laid trays and the food is distributed directly to patients. This is not very satisfactory since the food temperature may alter and encourage the growth of bacteria.

2. Food is transported in large containers and dished out on plates in the ward kitchen. This too is open to contamination from the kitchen utensils, during transport to and from the ward kitchen since generally cleanliness cannot be guaranteed.

3. The trolleys are loaded in the kitchen and each portion distributed on trays and plates and then transported to the ward. In the ward the food trolleys are plugged in when they arrive at the ward kitchen and allowed to warm up to required temperatures. The food is distributed to individual patients on trays and the used dishes are reloaded in the trolley and returned to the kitchen to be cleaned. This is the most satisfactory method.

Recommendations for food transportation are shown below:

- Food should be transported to the wards and other areas in cleaned closed food trolleys and not open containers.
- Hot food should be transported over 63 °C.
- Cold food should be transported below 10 °C.

6.1.8 The washing of crockery and cutlery

The washing of crockery and cutlery is of critical importance to minimise the possibilities of infection. The following listed points give the precautions that should be taken to prevent this contamination:

- Containers for food transportation should be taken to the washing-up area for cleaning.
- Utensils should be washed at a minimum temperature of 65 °C, ideally 80 °C (automated washing).
- Eating utensils washed at ward level or in the kitchen should be washed in very hot water and dried thoroughly before storage.

6.1.8.1 *Manual washing.* If crockery and cutlery are washed manually, a pair of domestic gloves should be worn. Clean water should be used as hot (55 °C) as can be tolerated by gloved hands, with liquid detergent. It is preferable to use a two-sink system, but, if not available, then use running water to rinse. All food and kitchen utensils should be air-dried (that is, naturally) after washing.

Tea towels should not be used because there is a risk of cross-contamination.

6.1.8.2 *Automated dish washers.* These machines should reach a minimum temperature of 80 °C for one minute. Crockery and cutlery are best washed in a central area so that the dishwashers can be maintained for optimum use.

6.1.9 Recommendations on the use of cutlery and crockery

To ensure crockery and cutlery are safe, the IPC team recommends as follows:
- Disposable crockery and cutlery are not recommended for routine use.
- All utensils should be examined regularly and replaced if damaged, chipped or cracked.
- Disinfectants are not routinely recommended.

6.1.10 Cleaning of the catering area

Environmental cleaning of the catering areas must be carried out by skilled cleaning staff who are familiar with the protocols of the kitchen.

The cleaning programme in the kitchen and related areas is vital to ensure a clean and dry environment.
- Food must not be left outside the appropriate storage areas at any time, especially at night.
- All the drains should be covered with vermin-proof wire mesh. Some kitchens have special drains that prevent any access except from inspection ports, which are also sealed.
- The service areas, floors and surfaces should be washed daily with a neutral pH detergent and wiped over to dry.
- The floors should be cleaned at least twice a day.
- The surfaces must be wiped clean and disinfected with chlorine after each food preparation session.
- Surface disinfection with a chlorine-releasing agents containing 250 ppm of available chlorine or other accepted disinfectants should be applied after thorough cleaning.
- Spillages should be cleared up immediately.

- It is preferable that the kitchen has its own colour-coded cleaning equipment for clean and dirty areas.
- Kitchen equipment must be dismantled, cleaned thoroughly (manually or mechanically) and inspected for removal of all organic matter and stored dry.
- Pest control is essential.

6.1.11 Staff health

- All diarrhoeal disease, skin lesions or family history of gastroenteritis should be reported to the occupational health department for advice and treatment.
- Work programmes should be planned so that staff remain in a designated area per shift and do not cross over.
- Uniforms for the kitchen staff should be provided.
- Personal protective equipment includes:
  — overalls or plastic aprons
  — boots
  — headgear
  — footwear (boots or similar)
  — non-sterile disposable gloves.
- Food serving equipment such as tongs should be provided.
- Immunisation should be offered to the catering staff.

6.1.12 Education and training

All food handlers should be trained in personal hygiene and safe practices in food preparation. Written instruction should be provided to each food handler. Posters on the aspects of hygiene should be strategically displayed around the various kitchen areas. The training should cover all aspects of food preparation and disposal. Refresher courses should be provided when systems change or are upgraded.

Special training should be given to the milk kitchen and food preparation for paediatric patients.

6.1.13 Kitchen waste

The catering manager is responsible for ensuring that kitchen waste is packaged and stored properly in closed containers. Returned cooked food ideally should be discarded. The practice of sending swill to farms has been discontinued in most countries for health and safety reasons.

6.1.14 Inspection of the premises

Regular inspections of the premises and catering practices may be carried out by the environmental health officer, pest control officer or the hygiene inspection team. An audit tool can be used to evaluate the kitchens and offer advice on improvement.

When investigating an outbreak of food poisoning in a healthcare facility, the following areas should be inspected and documented

- staff hygiene – hand hygiene facilities in the workplace, personal cleanliness
- layout of food preparation – segregation of cooked and uncooked food preparation areas, separate utensils, knives and equipment
- storage temperatures of refrigeration, freezer and other units
- separate storage of various food types such as diary, meat, vegetables
- removal of food waste
- cleaning protocols and regimes, use of surface disinfectants
- vermin proofing
- cases of sickness among staff, particularly with diarrhoeal disease, skin rashes or jaundice.

Samples of food are taken from each meal, clearly labelled and stored for 72 hours. In case of food poisoning, these samples are sent for microbiological investigation.

The environmental health officers may take swabs routinely and also send samples of food and milk for analysis.

6.2 Linen and laundry

Laundry is an integral part of a hospital service and a regular clean supply is essential. Linen and patient clothing is a potential source of infection to staff during handling, transportation and processing of laundry. Several outbreaks of scabies due to low-temperature washing of patient linen have been reported. There should be a clear policy on how linen should be handled.[10] The safe handling of linen reduces the risk of transmission to staff and patients.[11] Linen management has a dual purpose – to prevent clean linen from becoming contaminated before it is used in patient care and to prevent dirty (used/soiled/infectious/infested) linen from contaminating patients, staff, the environment and clean linen.

This section discusses safe handling practices for laundry from categories of laundry to type of treatment appropriate to the degree of contamination.

6.2.1 Types of laundry

Laundry should be sorted into its respective category at the bedside The local policy should state which category the linen falls under; however, the following terms are commonly used.

---

[10] Department of Health, NHS Executive. 1995. *Hospital laundry arrangements for used and infected linen*. Heywood, UK: Health Publishing Unit.
[11] Health Protection Scotland. Feb 2009. *Safe management of linen policy and procedures (an element of standard infection control precautions*. Scotland: National Services.

6.2.1.1 Used linen

This is linen that has been used in patient care but is not visibly soiled.

6.2.1.2 Soiled linen

Includes linen that is visibly contaminated with blood, body fluids, secretions or excretions and potentially contains a high bioburden of micro-organisms.

6.2.1.3 Infectious linen

This category of linen is from patients with a specific infection that can potentially infect staff and other patients. Such patients are usually in isolation with transmission-based precautions in place. The risk of handling such linen is minimised by the use of appropriate protective equipment worn by the handler.

Infested linen

Includes linen used in the care of patients with parasites, such as lice, fleas, bedbugs and scabies.[12]

6.2.1.4 Theatre linen

This category includes processed non-wovens and wovens such as cotton drapes and gowns, which are laundered and sent to the SSD for sterilisation. Theatre scrubs do not need to be sterilised.

6.2.2 The laundry cycle

The movement of clean and dirty linen from the point of use to the processing area and back is shown in Figure 6.2. The lighter and darker sections denote used or dirty areas and clean areas respectively.[13]

6.2.3 Laundry collection

Bed linen is changed regularly in most healthcare settings. Making beds should be carried out by two members of staff but, owing to staff shortages, one person often has to work alone. The linen should be removed carefully without creating aerosols and placed directly in a designated linen bag.

Bed curtains are considered part of linen and should be changed after each patient discharge. Where patients bring in their own linen, the washing is usually done in a designated area of the hospital or sent back home.

---

[12]   Aucamp M. 2016. Housekeeping and linen management. *IFIC Basic Concepts of Infection Control.* 3rd ed. International Federation of Infection Control. Chapter 23. https://www.theific.org/wp-content/uploads/ 2016/04/23-HkpgLaundry_2016.pdf.

[13]   South African DoH. 2020. Implementation of the National Infection Prevention and Control Strategic Framework. https://www.knowledgehub.org.za/system/files/elibdownloads/2020.10/National%20 Infection%20Prevention%20and%20Control%20Practical%20Manual%20%28Web%20version%29.pdf.

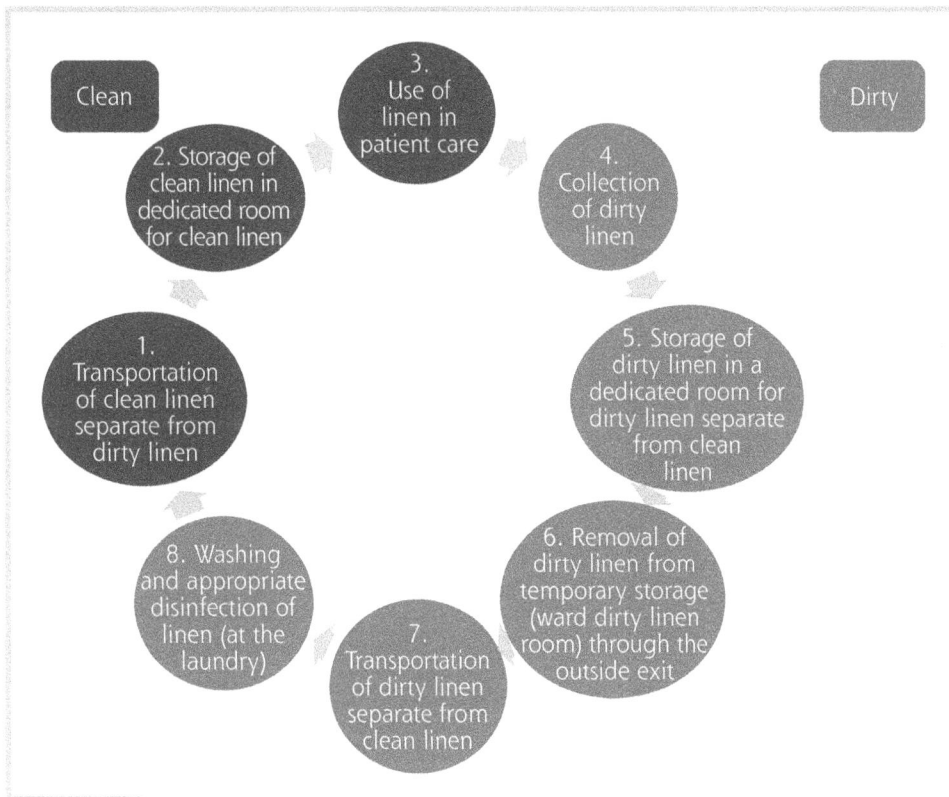

Figure 6.2 Laundry cycle for healthcare facilities[14]

6.2.4 Safe handling of linen

Bed linen should be carefully rolled up and folded when being removed from the bed. Linen should not be shaken because skin scales and bacteria can be dispersed into the air and infect other patients and staff. The clean linen is carefully spread out and tucked in. Pillows should follow the same procedure. All linen should be placed into laundry bags immediately and, once full, closed and labelled.

Linen should not be sorted or handled once it has been removed and collected. If the laundry does not accept soiled linen, there should be a separate area, away from the clinical area but close to the laundry room, where the laundry is sorted and sluiced prior to dispatch to the main laundry area. Appropriate PPE must be available for the person who is responsible for this task.

---

[14] Adapted from South African National Strategic Framework IPC Implementation Manual, 2020.

6.2.5 Disadvantages of sluicing linen in clinical areas

It is not recommended that any linen be washed or sluiced on the wards because there is a danger of transmitting microbes during sluicing and transportation of wet linen:

- There is a risk of splashing to staff who are sluicing, especially if adequate protective clothing is not worn.
- Storing wet linen in bags over a long period of time increases the risk of bacterial multiplication, especially from infectious patients, and contributes to outbreaks.
- The linen deteriorates if kept in closed bags for long periods of time, especially in the heat. Some linen gets mouldy and has to be condemned at considerable financial loss.
- Sluicing unnecessarily increases the workload of the staff.

6.2.6 Storage of used linen

Used linen should be stored in a separate collection area, in sealed and labelled laundry bags. The door of the dirty linen room must be kept closed and access to the room must be restricted.

- The storage period must not exceed 24 hours except over weekends.
- The frequency of collection of linen depends on the volume of laundry:
  - once a day in the mornings from the wards
  - three times a day from the trauma and labour ward
  - up to four times a day from the operating theatres.

6.2.7 Infested linen

Infested linen should be clearly colour-coded or labelled to ensure safety during collection. For infested linen, wear gloves and plastic apron, place linen directly into a transparent plastic bag at the bedside of the patient, close and label the bag with the unit/health facility name and date and mark as infested linen. Inform the pest control department (if one exists) to deal with the linen. Then send directly to the laundry.[15]

6.2.8 Linen transportation from the wards

Linen should be transported dry in closed containers around the hospital. If linen has been sluiced, it should be placed in plastic bags to avoid leakage after

15   South African DoH. 2020. Implementation of the National Infection Prevention and Control Strategic Framework. https://www.knowledgehub.org.za/system/files/elibdownloads/2020. 10/National%20 Infection%20Prevention%20and%20Control%20Practical%20Manual%20%28Web%20version%29.pdf.

collection, and placed in a separate compartment if possible. Used linen from several wards may be collected at the same time, provided the linen is not wet.

6.2.9 Processing of laundry

Linen can be washed either manually or in automated systems. Infected linen should always be washed in an automated system. The following IPC guidelines on procedures ensure safety for the laundry staff and a supply of clean, safe linen.

6.2.9.1 Manual cleaning

Used linen may be washed manually.
- The laundry staff should wear domestic gloves.
- The linen should be placed in large tubs or sinks.
- Hot water (50 °C) and detergent is added and mixed in with the linen and left for 10 minutes.
- Rinse thoroughly.
- A disinfectant such as bleach or ozone may be added to disinfect the linen as well as improve its look.

6.2.9.2 Infected linen

Infected linen should not be washed manually if possible. However, in circumstances where automated systems do not exist, the following is recommended:[16]
- Wear gloves, plastic apron and eye protection – visor (and a mask if indicated).
- Soak infected linen in warm water (not boiling) for several minutes to remove the debris before handling.
- Drain the water.
- Refill with hot water (80 °C) and add detergent. Bleach may be added at this stage.
- Wash carefully, preventing aerosols by holding the linen below water level when rubbing or scrubbing.
- Drain and rinse the linen.
- A second soaking in bleach may be required.
- Cotton items can be boiled for 10 minutes if recommended.

6.2.9.3 Automated methods

Linen is transported from the clinical areas in a dry laundry bag. The laundry bag is hooked onto a conveyer belt system, which turns the bag with its opening facing down. When the laundry passes over a large slop or a shute, the bag is opened automatically or manually and the contents released into the washing system.

---

[16] NHS England and NHS Improvement. March 2019. Standard infection control precautions: national hand hygiene and personal protective equipment policy.

Inspection of linen by the laundry staff can take place once the automated cycle has been completed. The washed linen is moved to the driers and then further for pressing and packing.

- There are two types of automated washing machines: **individual-cycle** machines or **continuous-batch** washing machines. Infected linen must be washed in an individual-cycle machine. Linen should not be left in a machine overnight. Remove and dry before leaving the laundry areas.
- When linen is being pre-washed (sluiced) the cycle should not exceeds 50 °C. This is to prevent coagulation of proteinaceous material onto the linen.

6.2.10 The cycle

Once the machine has been loaded, it interlocks to prevent re-contamination of laundry while rinsing after the thermal cycle. During the thermal cycle, it is essential that the drum rotates to ensure full contact with clothing for the correct length of time, so do not overload the machine.

6.2.10.1 Washing cycle temperatures

Washing temperatures may differ between various machines but the recommended temperatures are:[17]

- 65 °C for 10 minutes **or**
- 70 °C for 3 minutes **or**
- 80 °C for 1 minute.

- Mixing time for disinfection and water penetration 4–8 minutes. A sluice cycle should be available on machines used in smaller units for foul/infected linen.[18]
- Add sluice cycle for fouled linen.
- Add bleach or ozone to final rinse in temperatures not exceeding 60 °C (do not add to hot water as it will damage the linen).
- All machines are fitted with heat sensors, which must be checked every 6 weeks.
- Tumble-dryer should be set at 65–70 °C for 20 minutes.
- Steam pressing for cottons should be at 95 °C.

6.2.10.2 Heat-sensitive clothing

Clothes that will be adversely affected by temperatures over 65 °C should be washed at no more than 40 °C.

- Add bleach to final rinse to give 150 ppm available chlorine. No more than 5 minutes exposure time. Do not use bleach on fire-retardant material.

---

[17]   Safe management of linen. July 2020. Version 2.00. Community IPC policy for care home settings p 8. © Harrogate and District NHS Foundation Trust.
[18]   NHS England and NHS Improvement (March 2019) Standard infection control precautions: national hand hygiene and personal protective equipment policy.

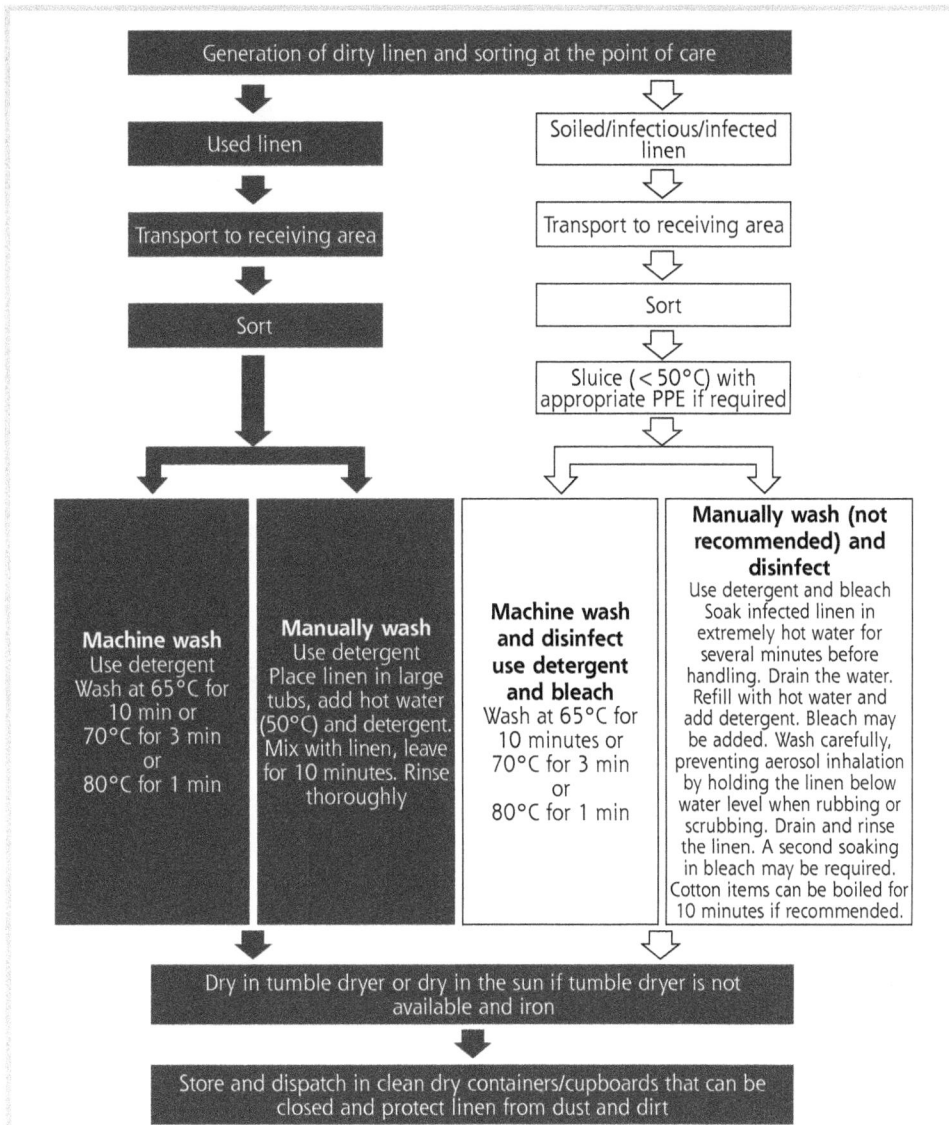

Figure 6.3 Schematic diagram of the different types of linen and their method of processing[19]

6.2.11 Ozone

Ozone is used in many commercial laundries and some healthcare facilities in developed countries. The initial capital outlay is high, but the returns are good over a period of time.

---

19   South African DoH. 2020. Implementation of the National Infection Prevention and Control Strategic Framework.

It has several advantages:
- good bleaching and antibacterial quality
- lowers the consumption of detergents and energy
- can be used for heat-sensitive clothing (cold wash)
- is biodegradable.

The different methods of processing various types of linen is summarised in Figure 6.3.

6.2.12 Laundry equipment

All the equipment should undergo periodic checking and inspection to ensure optimum functioning. Challenge tests of bacterial loads and spores are used by engineers to ensure adequate temperatures have been reached and maintained.

6.2.13 Returning clean laundry

Ensure that linen is completely dry before it is sent back to the wards.

Clean laundry and used linen must be transported separately. The carrier should be divided into two separate non-interlinking compartments for clean and dirty linen. The route should be to bring in the clean linen in the morning and take out the used linen on its return. The laundry should be placed on racks to avoid contamination.

The transportation vehicle should be cleaned daily after the day's delivery with warm water and detergent and dried.

6.2.14 Storage in the clinical areas

Clean linen, pillows, duvets and blankets must be stored on slatted shelves in a designated clean storage area (clean linen room or cupboard) that is kept closed.

When beds are being made the clean linen to be used is stacked on a linen trolley and the trolley parked outside the patient room.

The clean linen must not be left on these trolleys for long periods because the linen will become contaminated, particularly in busy and open areas like the passages.

In order to prevent contamination, linen should not be stored at floor level.
- Staff are reminded to carry out hand hygiene before handling clean linen.

External contractors for laundry services should follow the same IPC policy for linen management as the hospital laundries. The IPC practitioner should inspect the external laundry annually to ensure compliance to IPC policies and procedures as detailed in the service level agreement between the hospital and service provider.[20]

---

20   Ibid.

Curtains

Records must be kept of when window and bed curtains are changed.

- Window curtains must be changed every three months or immediately when they become visibly soiled or after discharge of a patient in transmission-based precautions.
- Inter-bed/privacy curtains are considered part of the patient's linen because they are handled often and can easily become contaminated.
- Change inter-bed curtains:
  - after discharge of an infectious patient
  - every four weeks if the patient(s) are non-infectious
  - immediately when they become visibly soiled.[21]

6.2.15 Staff

The laundering process involves certain hazards to staff. These personnel should therefore take care to avoid scalding or burning from hot water or steam by adhering to the following precautions recommended by IPC:

- Wear plastic aprons, domestic gloves and eye protection (if possible).
- Face masks are not necessary unless indicated when dealing with infected linen.
- Changing areas and rest areas must be provided for staff.
- All skin lesions should be covered.
- Immunisation against polio, tetanus, hepatitis B and TB is advised.
- Report all skin and diarrhoeal disease to occupational health.

Laundry staff must receive at least annual training on standard precautions and routine practices, including hand hygiene, PPE, exposure to blood and body fluids, sharps safety and decontamination.

Laundry staff must be aware they can expect discarded sharps in all types of linen. A system must be in place where incidents of exposure are reported and followed up.[22]

6.2.16 General

The effectiveness of the laundering process depends on many factors, including:

- time and temperature
- mechanical action
- water quality (pH, hardness)
- volume of the load

---

[21] Ibid.
[22] Aucamp M. 2016. Housekeeping and linen management. *IFIC Basic Concepts of Infection Control*. 3rd ed. International Federation of Infection Control. Chapter 23. https://www.theific.org/wp-content/uploads/2016/04/23-HkpgLaundry_2016.pdf.

- extent of soiling
- model/availability of commercial washers and dryers.

Always use and maintain laundry equipment according to manufacturer's instructions.[23]

6.3   Healthcare waste management

Hospitals produce more than 5 million tons of waste each year,[24] of which 85% is general non-hazardous waste; 15% maybe infectious, toxic or radioactive and will require special treatment.[25] It is estimated that each of the 1 500 hospitals in the UK produces 2 250 tonnes of PVC waste that could be recycled.[26] The Global Fund recommends the '5 Rs' – **refuse, reduce, re-use, repurpose** and **recycle**. Open burning and incineration results in toxic gases and carbon dioxide pollution, with serious environmental consequences.[27]

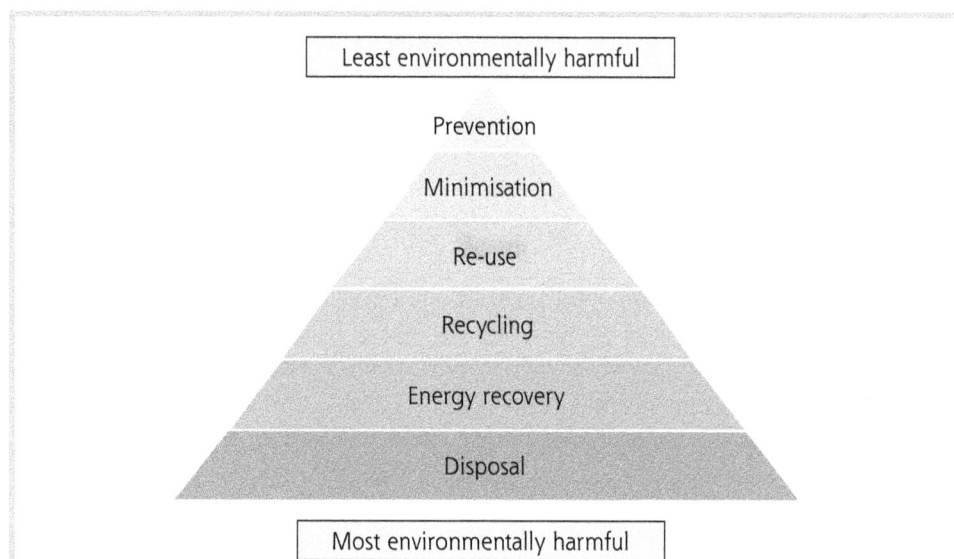

Figure 6.4   Healthcare waste management hierarchy[28]

23   Centre for Disease Control and Prevention & Infection Control Africa Network. 2019. Best Practices for Environmental Cleaning in Healthcare facilities: in Resource-Limited Settings. V1. https://www.cdc.gov/hai/pdfs/resource-limited/environmental-cleaning-RLS-H.pdf.

24   https://practicegreenhealth.org/topics/waste/waste.

25   https://www.who.int/news-room/fact-sheets/detail/health-care-waste.

26   Royal College of Physicians: Less waste, more health: a health professional's guide to reducing waste. www.rcplondon.ac.uk.

27   The Global Fund. 2020. The Technical Brief, Sustainable Healthcare Waste Management. https://www.theglobalfund.org/media/9356/core_healthcarewastemanagement_technicalbrief_en.pdf.

28   WHO https://cdn.who.int/media/docs/default-source/wash-documents/wash-in-hcf/training-modules-in-health-care-waste-management/module-11---classification-of-health-care-waste.pdf.

The WHO reports that 16 billion injections are administered worldwide and not always properly disposed of. In countries where waste is not disposed of properly, all of it is dumped on the municipal waste sites and poses a risk to the public. Many low-resource countries have families that scavenge these waste dumps to earn a living and are at great risk from infection.[29] Measures to ensure the safe and environmentally sound management of healthcare wastes can prevent adverse health and environmental impacts, thus protecting the health of patients, healthcare workers and the general public.

Responsible healthcare waste management requires a critical look at what can be recycled. In some European hospitals, safe recycling has reduced infectious waste to less than 15%, thus reducing cost of end point disposal, reducing greenhouse emissions and saving a considerable amount of money. In other facilities, the heat generated from the incinerator used as end point disposal of infectious and anatomical waste is recycled to produce steam, hot water and heating for the healthcare facility.

It is our collective responsibility to reduce carbon emissions, reduce plastic pollution and save our planet. Strategies for getting rid of healthcare waste must be reconsidered very carefully.

The healthcare waste stream is shown in Figure 6.5. All steps of the stream are relevant to IPC and should be part of the healthcare waste management audit.

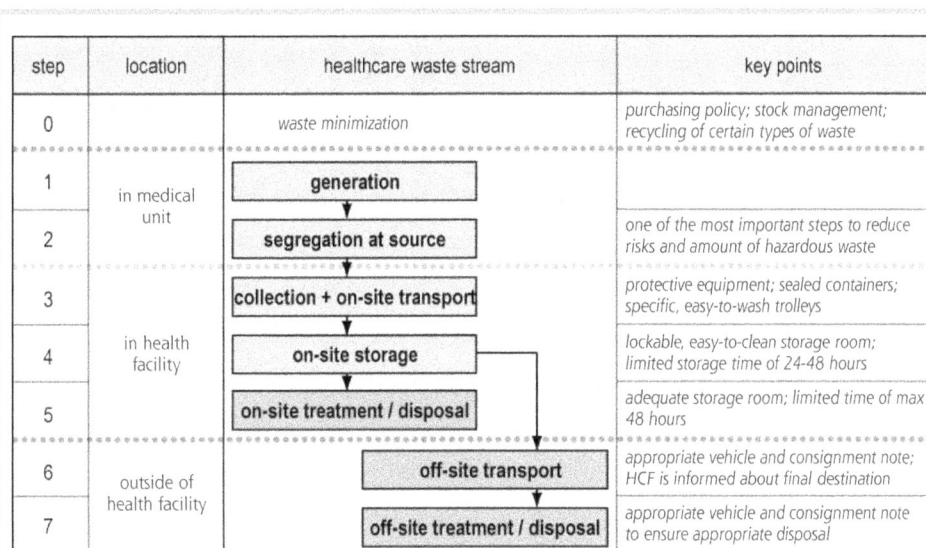

step	location	healthcare waste stream	key points
0		waste minimization	purchasing policy; stock management; recycling of certain types of waste
1	in medical unit	generation	
2		segregation at source	one of the most important steps to reduce risks and amount of hazardous waste
3	in health facility	collection + on-site transport	protective equipment; sealed containers; specific, easy-to-wash trolleys
4		on-site storage	lockable, easy-to-clean storage room; limited storage time of 24-48 hours
5		on-site treatment / disposal	adequate storage room; limited time of max 48 hours
6	outside of health facility	off-site transport	appropriate vehicle and consignment note; HCF is informed about final destination
7		off-site treatment / disposal	appropriate vehicle and consignment note to ensure appropriate disposal

Figure 6.5 Healthcare waste generation and disposal[30]

29 Ibid.
30 Secretariat of the Basel Convention and World Health Organization. 2005. Preparation of national health-care waste management plans in Sub-Saharan countries: guidance manual.

6.3.1 Establish a healthcare waste management plan

Poor waste management is not only a risk to staff and waste handlers but increases the risk of vermin and pests, which may spread disease. All hospital waste should be disposed of safely without risk to handlers or the public and the environment. Waste processed as clinical waste is more expensive than non-clinical waste and source segregation can greatly reduce the cost for the healthcare facility.

With increasing awareness of the detrimental effects of healthcare waste, most countries have comprehensive legislation regarding the generation, segregation and disposal of clinical and non-clinical waste.[31]

Waste arising from healthcare sites includes:
- wastes which are special by virtue of their level of infectivity
- wastes which contain hazardous pathogens
- non-prescription medicines which may have hazardous properties
- photographic chemicals (e.g. x-ray fluids)
- batteries
- oil/solvents
- chemicals.

6.3.2 Responsibility for healthcare waste management[32]

The overall responsibility lies with the CEO of the hospital to ensure the waste management policy of the hospital is complied with (Figure 6.6). This duty may be delegated to the waste manager.

The waste management policy is carried out in the following way:
- The waste manager is responsible for ensuring that the waste policy is being implemented. She or he is also responsible for ensuring adequate supplies of containers, transportation trolleys and protective clothing for the staff.
- All accidental injuries such as sharps injuries or splashes should be recorded in an accident book and reported to occupational health.
- The IPC team is responsible for monitoring the waste policy application in relation to patient and staff safety.

---

31   World Health Organization. 2004. Safe healthcare waste management: A policy paper. Available at: www.who.int/entity/water_sanitation_health/medicalwaste/hcwmpolicy/en/.
32   SANS 10248-1 (2008) (English): Management of healthcare waste – Part 1: Management of healthcare risk waste from a healthcare facility.

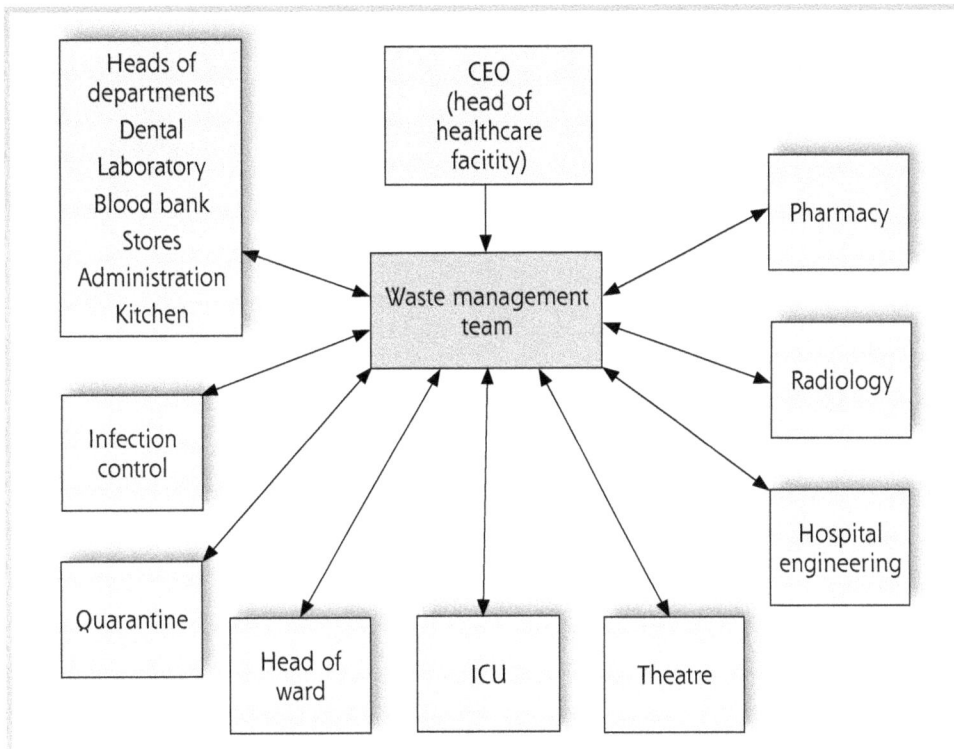

Figure 6.6 The healthcare waste management team[33]

6.3.3 Types of waste[34]

For the purposes of this section the WHO classification of waste has been used. It is the responsibility of the IPC team to ensure that the disposal of waste conforms with the regulations.

6.3.3.1 Infectious waste

Infectious waste is: any waste which consists wholly or partly of human blood or animal tissues, blood or other bodily fluids, excretions, drugs or other pharmaceutical products, swabs or dressings and syringes, needles or other sharp instruments, which unless rendered safe, may prove hazardous to any person coming into contact with it.

It is also: any other waste arising from medical, nursing, dental, veterinary, pharmaceutical or similar practice, investigation, treatment, care, teaching or research, or the collection of blood for transfusion, being waste which may cause infection to any person coming into contact with it.

---

[33] WHO https://cdn.who.int/media/docs/default-source/wash-documents/wash-in-hcf/training-modules-in-health-care-waste-management/module-11---classification-of-health-care-waste.pdf.

[34] Krisunas E. 2007. Healthcare waste management. In C Friedman & W Newsom *Basic Concepts of Infection Control*. Portadown: International Federation of Infection Control; WHO. 2018. Health-care waste. https://www.who.int/news-room/fact-sheets/detail/health-care-waste.

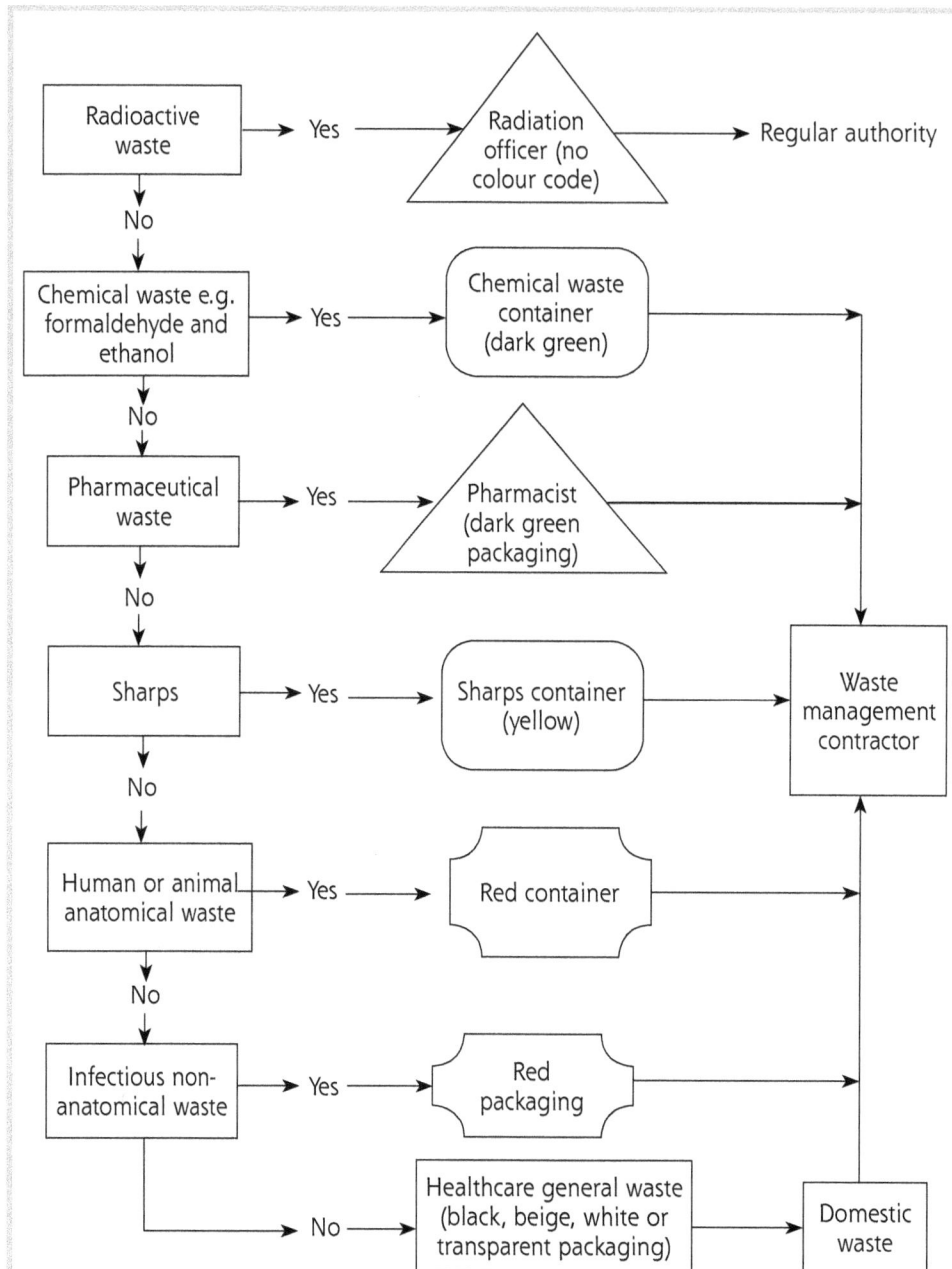

Figure 6.7 Healthcare risk waste flow diagram[35]

---

35   SANS 10248-1: Management of healthcare waste – Part 1: Management of healthcare risk waste from a healthcare facility. South African Bureau of Standards.

Some examples are
- soiled dressings
- body fluids
- intravenous needles and syringes that have been used on a patient
- drainage bags from wounds
- blood products.

PPE used routinely, such as gloves, aprons and face masks that are not contaminated with organic matter, can be disposed of as non-clinical waste. However, this is controversial since gloves and aprons on landfill sites are considered clinical waste and their disposal in this manner is often a bone of contention with the municipalities that are responsible for these sites.

6.3.3.2 Pathological waste
Pathological waste comprises body parts (anatomical waste), human tissues, organs or fluids, and contaminated animal carcasses. Most of this type of waste originates from laboratories, abattoirs or operating theatres.

6.3.3.3 Sharps waste
These objects can cause penetrating injuries to humans and must be disposed of in a manner that renders them safe. These must not be sent to the municipal waste dump because scavengers can get injured and infected. Examples: syringes, needles, disposable scalpels and blades, broken glass ampoules, trocar.

6.3.3.4 Laboratory waste
Most clinical laboratories deal with human tissues and microbes. This is considered **high-risk** waste and should preferably be processed by steam sterilisation before leaving the laboratory premises.

6.3.3.5 Kitchen waste
This includes swill, left-over food and dirty water. It is a potential source of pests and vermin and poses an indirect hazard to staff and patients in a hospital.

6.3.3.6 Radioactive waste
This is not an IPC issue, but should be included in the waste policy to ensure safe disposal of radioactive materials by specialists. The contracts should specify how the waste is to be disposed of, such as products contaminated by radionuclides, including radioactive diagnostic material or radiotherapeutic materials.

6.3.3.7 Chemical waste
This includes waste from pharmacies, laboratories, engineering workshops and all other areas where chemicals are used. The disposal of chemicals into the sewerage

system is not acceptable as it seriously affects the waterways and biodiversity of the country. A contract with a chemical disposal company must contain precise instructions on how to process such waste. Examples are mercury, batteries, disinfectants, sterilants and heavy metals.

6.3.3.8 Pharmaceutical waste

These consist of expired, unused or contaminated drugs and vaccines and should follow a similar path as other chemicals.

6.3.3.9 Cytotoxic waste

This is waste containing substances with genotoxic properties (i.e. highly hazardous substances that are mutagenic, teratogenic or carcinogenic), such as cytotoxic drugs used in cancer treatment and their metabolites. These have to be treated very carefully and managed by a reputable company.

6.3.3.10 Non-clinical waste (non-infectious)

This is mainly waste generated from administrative work or patient contact which is not contaminated with blood or body fluids. Although the risk is **low**, this type of waste is bulky and sometimes difficult to dispose of.

Non-infectious waste is made up of:
* office paper
* domestic waste
* hand-drying paper towels
* paper wrapping of clinical items that is not contaminated with blood or body fluids
* used gloves that are not contaminated with blood or body fluids (contentious)
* sanitary towels
* babies' nappies (from normal clinical areas, NOT infectious disease wards); nappies of babies with diarrhoeal disease are considered infectious and therefore discarded as clinical waste as part of the transmission-based precautions.

6.3.4 Source segregation[36]

The most important step in organising a healthcare waste management programme is to separate infectious and non-infectious waste at the point of generation/source segregation. By separating waste in an organised manner, the amount and type of waste generated in a healthcare facility can be calculated, end stage disposal costs can be reduced and environmental pollution and risk to humans can be minimised or avoided.

---

[36]   Draft Guidelines on Separation of Waste at Source. 2018. Environmental Affairs, South Africa.

It has been considered that any article coming into contact with patients should be regarded as infectious waste. There is no evidence for this. It is unrealistic and results in a large load going for disposing as infectious waste. For example, babies' nappies from an ordinary paediatric ward may be discarded as non-clinical waste since the risk of infection is no greater than in a domestic environment. Similarly, sanitary towels should be treated in the same way since these are discarded in domestic waste in the community.

Source segregation is best achieved by **colour-coding** clinical (infectious) and non-clinical (non-infectious waste). It is a matter or re-educating the staff until the practice becomes second nature.

A simple colour-coding system should be adopted. There is a universally accepted colour-coding system, which recommends **red (or yellow)** for infectious and **black** for non-infectious waste (as per the WHO guidelines). Other colours are chosen based on national or local recommendations.

There should be clearly visible charts showing what goes into which colour bag or container. If a container and a plastic bag are used, then both must be of the same colour to avoid confusion.

6.3.5 Clinical areas

The management of healthcare waste differs from one healthcare facility to another, but it is usually the job of the housekeeping staff to assemble waste containers and position the waste containers at appropriate stations. When three-quarters full, the waste containers are closed and removed to a secure location on the ward for collection by the porters.

6.3.5.1 Waste containers

Each clinical area (ward, investigation or consulting room) should have at least two waste containers, one each for infectious and non-infectious waste. The containers should be clearly marked and identified by colour so that waste can be segregated effectively. In clinical areas with a heavy workload, such as emergency departments, more than one container should be available in each area.

The design of the waste container will depend upon the service provider, but should have the following characteristics.
- Be clearly labelled as infectious or non-infectious waste and colour-coded.
- Have a visual display instruction (poster) to indicate the type of waste to be disposed of.
- Be robust, leak-proof and stand firmly without tipping over.
- Be operated by a non-touch method.
- Either be disposable or be able to withstand cleaning at a hot temperature (90 °C). Containers should contain and hold the recommended weight and volume.
- Once it has reached its capacity, it must be securely fastened and stored, ready for transportation.

If plastic bags are used, these should be colour-coded and robust enough to carry the weight of the contents when lifted. The recommendations are 55 μ of low-density or 25 μ of high-density plastic. In high-risk areas a minimum gauge of 200 μ if low-density plastic or 100 μ if high-density) should be considered.

The container's capacity should match the area of use. In a low-use areas a smaller capacity while in a higher-use area a larger capacity container can be used. Containers must be removed frequently, depending on the HCW management policy.

6.3.5.2 Sharps container

There should be at least one sharps container in each clinical area; usually there are more than one. The container should be located as close to the point of use (at arm's length) as possible, such as the procedure trolley, next to a patient's bed in a high-care area and a treatment room where medication is prepared.

The sharps container should be used only for the immediate disposal of sharps after use and nothing else. It should:

- Be clearly labelled as a sharps container, preferably with a biohazard label on it.
- Be firmly secured in a holder or, if free-standing, should not fall over during use.
- Be robust with a well-fitting lid that cannot be opened once in use.
- Have an opening for discarding the needle and syringes that is wide enough to take the items but not to allow the entry of a hand.
- Have handles that allow the container to fall away from the body during transportation.
- Be for single use and discarded once it is three-quarters full.
- Not able to be opened once it is sealed closed.
- Be leak proof.

6.3.6 Non-infectious waste

This type of waste arises from administrative activities in non-clinical and clinical areas. Often there is confusion about what can go into a non-infectious (black or municipal) waste container. However, the items that are used and discarded from domestic households give an indication as to what items can be regarded as non-infectious waste.

The non-infectious waste container may be left until full if it does not contain any organic material such as food stuff, but will depend on the climate of the country. The container bags should be tied, labelled and removed via the internal transportation system.

6.3.7 Ward storage

Once the containers are full they are securely closed, labelled and stored in a separate area (dirty utility), ready for collection. The storage area should be dry, washable in case of leakage and well ventilated, especially in warm climes. The labels should contain detailed information about the ward of origin and the date the container was sealed and ready for collection.

6.3.8 Collection of waste

Waste should be collected daily and in high-use areas, such as the operating theatre (OT) suite, collections may be more frequent. The collection will depend on the size of the waste containers. It should be noted that **it is not the responsibility of the waste handlers to segregate waste**. If any type of waste has been placed in the wrong colour bag, it will be disposed of accordingly.

Staff should wear uniform, heavy-duty gloves and covered footwear when handling waste containers.

6.3.9 Transportation

In the hospital the waste handling staff should transport waste on trolleys which are robust, well ventilated and clean. Before collection the staff should ensure:
- the container is secured and labelled
- any container which is contaminated on the outside should be double bagged with a clean plastic bag of the same colour before removal
- there are no protruding sharps or devices.

Ward trolleys ideally should have two sections – one for infectious and the other for non-infectious waste. The waste trolley is unloaded at the appropriate destination awaiting collection by a contractor.

6.3.10 Storage

Once the waste has been removed from the wards it is stored in a secured area. Non-infectious waste is collected by the municipality and sent for landfill. Infectious waste will go through a different end point disposal system.

The storage area should be well ventilated with a protected security system. It should be clean, vermin-proof and large enough to accommodate the number of waste containers ready for collection.

If infectious waste is to be incinerated on site, there should be secure facilities provided, especially for sharps boxes.

6.3.11 Final (end point) disposal of waste[37]

6.3.11.1 Non-infectious waste

Non-clinical waste is taken to the local municipality dump for disposal by landfill. The waste is dumped in a designated **landfill site**, which is periodically covered

---

[37] WHO. 2005. Preparation of national health-care waste management plans in Sub-Saharan countries: guidance manual. Secretariat of the Basel Convention and World Health Organization.

over with earth. Once a landfill site is full, it is permanently covered and used for other purposes. A new site is then established.

- All infectious waste destined for landfill must be rendered safe and treated prior to its disposal.
- All waste with a high infectious load is banned from landfill.
- Waste medicines must be incinerated before being sent in the form of ash for landfill.
- Sanitary towels and nappies should be treated as non-infectious waste, unless specifically from infectious patients, and do not require to be treated prior to landfill.

6.3.11.2 End disposal of infectious waste

Infectious waste in most LMICs is incinerated, but this is done poorly. Incinerators can be located at the healthcare facility or at a distant site for use by a district or municipality. The advantage of incinerators is that most of the waste disposed of by this means is rendered completely safe. The little residue and heat from the incinerators can be recycled to reduce costs of producing heating for the healthcare facility or for producing steam.

6.3.11.2.1 Incineration or burning

The most commonly used method is burning or incineration. In some countries the heat from the incinerator is recycled to heat water and provide steam and central heating for the healthcare facility.

6.3.11.2.1.1 Incinerators

There are several different types of incinerator, but all of them require a mix of wet and dry loads for maximum efficiency. The incinerators should meet the required standards as below:

- Minimal post-burn environmental pollution.
- Temperatures to reach 900 °C for the pre-burn and 1 400 °C for the after-burn chambers to ensure the disintegration of steel and the reduction of toxic gas emissions.
- Ashes may be sent for landfill.
- Recycling of at least 60% heat.

Note: Anatomical tissues, infectious matter, medicines and special substances should be only incinerated.

Not all these technologies can be used for the treatment or the disposal of all categories of HCW. The suitable treatment and disposal technologies according to the different categories of HCW are presented in the table below.

Chapter 6: Support services, including environmental cleaning

Table 6.1 End point disposal of infectious or clinical waste

Waste catagory	Rotary kiln	Two chambers pyrolytic incineration	Single chamber incineration	Wet thermal treatment (autoclave)	Chemical disinfetion	Microwave irradiation	Sanitary landfill
A non-risk HCW	N/A	N/A	N/A	N/A	N/A	N/A	N/A
B1 Human anatomical waste	Yes	Yes	Yes	No	No	No	No
B2 Waste sharps	Yes	Yes	Yes	Yes	Yes	Yes	Yes for small quantities with encapsulation
B3 Pharmaceutical waste Classes B32 and B33	Yes	Small amount only	No	No	No	No	No
B4 Cytotoxic pharmaceutical waste	Yes	No Yes for modern ones	No	No	No	No	No Yes for small quantities with inertisation
C1 Infectious waste	Yes	Yes	Yes	Yes	Yes	Yes	Yes
C2 Highly infectious waste	Yes	Yes	Yes	Yes	Yes	Yes	No Yes only after pre-treatment
D Other hazardous waste	Yes	No	No	No	No	No	No Yes only if specially designed
E Radioactive health-care waste	No	No	No	No	No	No	Yes Specially designed

6.3.11.2.1.2 Pit burning

This method is still used in LMICs and is unsatisfactory because of incomplete burning and toxic fumes generated that are detrimental to healthcare workers.

6.3.11.3 Other methods of disposing of clinical waste

Recently, technologies have been developed where clinical waste is first processed through a microwave or heat sterilisation or shredded using electromagnetic systems before disposal to landfill. These technologies are expensive, require an adequate supply of electricity, water and steam, and require good engineering maintenance.

Key elements from the WHO in improving healthcare waste management are:[38]
* promoting practices that reduce the volume of waste generated and ensure proposer waste segregation
* developing strategies and systems along with strong oversight and regulation to incrementally improve waste segregation, destruction and disposal practices with the ultimate aim of meeting national and international standards
* where feasible, favouring the safe and environmentally sound treatment of hazardous healthcare wastes (e.g. by autoclaving, microwaving, steam treatment integrated with internal mixing and chemical treatment) over medical waste incineration
* building a comprehensive system, addressing responsibilities, resource allocation, handling and disposal; this is a long-term process, sustained by gradual improvements
* raising awareness of the risks related to healthcare waste, and of safe practices
* selecting safe and environmentally friendly management options to protect people from hazards when collecting, handling, storing, transporting, treating or disposing of waste.

6.3.11.4 Recycling of health facility waste

In the current climate of eco-friendly healthcare facilities, the recycling of paper, glass, plastic and other items is possible if a good waste management system exists. It is suggested that up to 50% of paper can be recycled and the recovery costs reinvested in the waste management programme.

---

[38] WHO Healthcare Fact Sheet 8 February 2018. https://www.who.int/news-room/fact-sheets/detail/health-care-waste.

6.4 Environmental cleaning in health facilities

The association between environmental contamination in healthcare facilities and healthcare-associated infections (HAI) has been well documented.[39] A clean environment forms the basis of sound IPC practices. The purpose of cleaning the environment is to remove visible dirt, reduce the level of micro-organisms or bioburden and minimise the dissemination of infectious agents in the healthcare facility, thereby providing an aesthetically pleasing, sanitary and relatively contamination-free environment for patients, staff and visitors. Dust contains large numbers of skin scales, particles and micro-organisms, such as bacilli and staphylococci as well as the dried nuclei of bacteria such as *Mycobacterium tuberculosis*. These are dispersed during dry dusting or sweeping. The cleaning programme should be based on evidence and the IPC team should provide information and support. Environmental cleaning is a pivotal IPC intervention. It forms part of a multimodal implementation strategy that has to be implemented together with other elements such as leadership support, training, monitoring and feedback.

6.4.1 The rationale

The cleaning services may be provided in-house or contracted out. Either way the principles should remain the same. Domestic supervisors, cleaners and managers should be aware of schedules, materials and special requirements of the cleaning programme. Cleaning can be monitored against the expected standards and a checklist can be produced, which ensures cleaning of all areas in the health facility is carried out to optimal levels. Specialised areas will have additional cleaning requirements based on the risk of transmission.

Legal requirements will depend on the laws or regulations of the individual country. Every healthcare facility should have a written cleaning policy clearly outlining the frequency, indications and means of cleaning. A terminal cleaning policy should also be available.

6.4.2 The cleaning programme

Adequate resources and the engagement of various stakeholders are essential for the implementation of environmental cleaning programmes in healthcare facilities. Stakeholders include administration, IPC, WASH and facilities management. A standardised and multi-modal approach, including strong

---

[39]   Centre for Disease Control and Prevention & Infection Control Africa Network. 2019. Best practices for environmental cleaning in healthcare facilities: in resource-limited settings. V1. https://www.cdc.gov/hai/pdfs/resource-limited/environmental-cleaning-RLS-H.pdf. Accessed 5 March 2022.

leadership and supervision, is important for the effective implementation of a cleaning programme.[40]

The cleaning programme encompasses the training of the staff, including alerting them to dangers of infection, and lays down how the programme is to be monitored, the cleaning protocols, the type of clothing they must wear in different areas, the type of cleaning and the frequency of cleaning of the different areas.

6.4.3 Education and training

The cleaning team should be trained in appropriate use of cleaning equipment, PPE, contents of cleaning materials, scheduled cleaning of various areas and additional cleaning requirements to minimise transmission of infection. Additionally, the unnecessary frequency of cleaning in areas such as outside corridors should be reduced.

6.4.4 Cleaning protocols

The cleaning policy should be clear, in writing, widely accessible and adhered to. Protocols should be updated depending on the hospital's requirements and new evidence. It is best to ensure nothing is added or taken away from the written policy, especially the unnecessary introduction of environmental disinfectants.

6.4.5 Monitoring the cleaning programme

Monitoring of environmental cleaning through structured programmes ensures adherence to cleaning protocol and that cleaning is conducted according to best practices. Organisational support and resources are important to address shortcomings identified during the monitoring process. It is important to use standardised methodology that is applied routinely and that timely feedback is given to the cleaning staff and management teams.

Various methods of monitoring are shown in Table 6.2. The first two methods are subjective, while the fluorescent marker is a more useful objective indicator of cleanliness. More sophisticated methods are available in high-income countries, using bioluminescence and carrying out microbiological cultures, the latter being more applicable during outbreaks.

[40]   Ibid.

Table 6.2 Methods of monitoring cleanliness available in most settings[41]

Monitoring method	Monitoring staff	Monitoring frequency
Performance observation	Cleaning supervisor	At least weekly or more frequently depending on the following: • Newly appointed staff • Part of a quality improvement project • During an outbreak
Visual assessment of cleanliness	Cleaning supervisor IPC practitioner	• Using a checklist based on local policy • Random checking daily • Checking of isolation rooms upon discharge of patient
Fluorescent markers (e.g. UV lights)	Cleaning supervisor IPC practitioner	• Using a checklist based on local policy • Random checking at least weekly • Monitoring cleanliness of isolation rooms upon discharge of patient
Microbiological swabs	IPC practitioner	• Suspected or known outbreaks • Random testing if other tests fail

A simple check list based on local policy should be created for random inspection of cleaning.

6.4.6 Staff awareness

- Domestic staff should be presentable, clean and have good personal hygiene. Most staff have uniforms, which should be changed whenever these are soiled or wet.
- Staff working in all hospital units, but particularly in infectious areas such as isolation wards or single rooms, are responsible for making themselves aware of the proper precautions required before entering that area. They are within their rights to refuse to work in a hazardous environment if proper training and PPE is not provided.
- Staff should receive adequate training on the following:
  - cleaning policies and protocols
  - methods of cleaning
  - risks involved in the management of healthcare risk waste, cleaning of contaminated areas, handling of infectious waste, cleaning of equipment and the use of PPE.

---

41   Centre for Disease Control and Prevention & Infection Control Africa Network. 2019. Best practices for environmental cleaning in healthcare facilities: in resource-limited settings. V1. https://www.cdc.gov/hai/pdfs/resource-limited/environmental-cleaning-RLS-H.pdf

- Hand hygiene must be carried out according to the hand-hygiene policy of the hospital, but particularly:
  — at the beginning and end of each shift
  — after handling contaminated items
  — before and after meals or smoking
  — after using the toilet
  — after removing gloves
  — if hands are potentially contaminated with blood or body fluids.
- No eating, drinking or smoking is allowed except in specific designated areas.
- Staff working in **specialist areas**, such as the OTs, must adhere to the specified dress code for those areas.
- Staff must attend in-service infection control training.

6.4.7 Personal protective equipment

6.4.7.1 Routine cleaning equipment

Cleaning staff should wear:

- **Domestic rubber gloves** (examination or clinical gloves should not be worn by domestic workers) for normal cleaning duties. The domestic gloves are more protective against chemicals and also withstand heavier work. The gloves must reach up to mid-arm and offer protection against chemicals and direct contact with organic matter. Gloves must be changed or washed thoroughly with detergent after cleaning each bathroom, each patient room and whenever soiled. Domestic gloves are re-usable but should be discarded if torn or having developed a leak.
- **Heavy-duty gloves** if there is contact with chemicals which may harm the skin. Heavy-duty gloves are usually re-usable and must be washed with detergent after use.
- **Plastic aprons** for cleaning activity that may generate splashes. They must be worn by covering the front of the uniform. An apron should be changed at the end of each shift or if torn during the shift.

6.4.7.2 Equipment in specialised areas

Domestic staff working in infectious areas such as isolation wards or single rooms where transmission-based precautions are implemented should wear the protective gear in line with the recommendations. The choice and selection of this gear should be guided by the nursing staff.

Environmental cleaning staff working in specialised areas such the operating theatre (OT), sterile service department, pharmacy, kitchen or high care areas should follow the recommendations of what to wear, how and what to clean, and how to manage their cleaning equipment.

6.4.8 Cleaning schedules

> The routine use of a disinfectant in the environment is strongly discouraged.

6.4.8.1 Frequency of cleaning

All areas of the healthcare facility should be cleaned daily, including weekends. Areas open to the general public should also be cleaned daily and sometimes they will need to be cleaned twice a day after the outpatient department has closed.

Specialised areas will require cleaning at least once a day, if not more often, depending on the current conditions. The OT complex should be cleaned daily. The OT itself should be cleaned at the end of each case and thoroughly cleaned at the end of each session. Some specialised areas have dedicated staff who are well trained in the cleaning requirements.

Cleaning procedures must be planned so that:
- Cleaning progresses from cleanest to the least clean areas of the wards.
- All rooms must be cleaned in the same manner to prevent missing areas.
- A hospital-approved detergent should be used for cleaning unless specified by the IPC team.
- All solutions must be diluted as specified by the manufacturer. This is essential for maximum effectiveness. Increasing the strength does not necessarily increase the antimicrobial activity **and might be harmful to the environment, surfaces and equipment and contribute to the development of antimicrobial resistance.**
- **The use of soap, water and friction (action of washing/scrubbing – 'elbow grease') is effective, cheap and simple and is the first step in the cleaning process.**
- All surfaces should be left dry.
- There is no evidence to 'block' or keep a room empty after thorough cleaning. Rooms can be occupied as soon as all surfaces are clean and dry.

6.4.9 Cleaning methods

The use of cleaning equipment that creates dust or dispersal of dust particles, such as sweeping with a broom, is discouraged.
- **Dry dusting** is not recommended since it only displaces dust from one area to another and increases the dispersal of skin scales.
- **Sweeping.** Sweeping with brooms is not recommended for healthcare facilities for the same reason.
- **Damp dusting.** Dusting or wiping of surfaces must always be done with a damp cloth. The cloth must be dampened in water that contains a detergent.

The detergent breaks the surface tension of the water, allowing the dust particles to cling to the cloth. The cloth is then wrung tightly to remove excess water before being used to wipe down surfaces. Make sure all the surfaces are covered and wiped carefully.

- **Mopping.** A damp floor mop must be used to mop floors. Clean water and detergent must be placed in one bucket and the mop is then rinsed off in the other (dirty) side. The mop must be damp rather than sopping wet and the water must be changed frequently.
- **Spraying.** This method is not advised for health facilities as it creates aerosols that can be inhaled and is detrimental to the patients and staff.

6.4.10 Procedure for cleaning

A daily cleaning routine of all horizontal surfaces and toilet areas is necessary to ensure that optimal cleanliness of the environment is maintained. For specific indications see section 6.5 Patient care articles. For in-depth procedure please refer to published literature.

6.4.10.1 Floors

All floors must be mopped daily with water and detergent; the floors must be polished frequently as required.

6.4.10.2 Patient rooms

The routine for daily cleaning of patient rooms is as follows:
- All waste baskets must be emptied at least daily and relined with new impervious plastic liners to prevent soiling of the waste basket if indicated in the policy.
- High dusting (including difficult to reach areas) must be performed at least weekly using a clean duster.
- Walls must be damp-wiped or spot-cleaned as needed.
- Horizontal surfaces such as window sills, chairs, over-bed tables and bedside cabinets must be damp-wiped daily with a hospital-approved detergent.
- Bathrooms must be cleaned daily with a hospital-approved detergent. Special attention must be given to the toilet, sink, fixtures and the floor. Towel and toilet paper dispensers must be refilled. Soap cartridges must be replaced as needed.
- Surfaces contaminated with blood or body fluids, soil or debris must be removed and wiped over with a cloth containing hypochlorite if indicated.
- High-touch surfaces are those that people frequently touch with their hands, and which become easily contaminated with micro-organisms that can be picked up by others on their hands High-touch surfaces should be cleaned more frequently. These include, but are not limited to, the following:

— bedrails
— IV poles
— sink handles
— bedside tables
— patient monitoring equipment
— transport equipment (wheelchairs)
— call bells
— door knobs and push plates
— light switches.

6.4.10.3 *Cleaning of isolation rooms*

Domestic cleaners must be notified by the nurse-in-charge or by an isolation sign on the door of a patient requiring transmission-based precautions.

- Staff must wear the appropriate transmission-based precautions PPE while cleaning the room and observe the IPC recommendations.
- **Linen and waste bags** must be closed and tagged **inside** the isolation room before removal.
- All equipment used in the room must be cleaned thoroughly prior to storing in equipment storage room.
- **Isolation signs** are not to be removed until terminal cleaning is completed. Return the sign to the nursing station when cleaning is completed.
- High-touch surfaces should be cleaned more frequently.

6.4.10.4 *Terminal cleaning*

Terminal or discharge cleaning refers to cleaning and disinfection of the room after the patient is discharged or transferred. It includes the removal of organic material and reduction and elimination of microbial contamination.[42]

Once the patient is discharged from an isolation area, the following cleaning procedure is recommended:

- Wear appropriate PPE before undertaking terminal cleaning.
- All linen (including bed curtains and window coverings) should be removed, bagged and sent for laundry. It should be labelled as **clinical (infectious)**.
- All the waste should be collected, closed and labelled appropriately.
- All equipment used in the room must be cleaned thoroughly prior to storing in equipment storage room.
- Routine cleaning procedures (outlined above) must be performed.
- Wipe all the surfaces including walls to hand height with warm water and detergent if indicated in the policy. Allow to dry.

---

[42] Centre for Disease Control and Prevention & Infection Control Africa Network. 2019. Best practices for environmental cleaning in healthcare facilities: in resource-limited settings. V1. https://www.cdc.gov/hai/pdfs/resource-limited/environmental-cleaning-RLS-H.pdf.

- All surfaces of the bed frame, mattress and pillow must be damp-wiped with a hospital-approved detergent before the bed is made. Wipe the mattress with warm water and detergent. Dry with a paper towel. Wipe over with hospital-approved disinfectant if indicated (ask IPC team).
- Complete task, remove PPE, wash and dry hands thoroughly before leaving.
- **The room can be occupied as soon as all surfaces are adequately cleaned and allowed to dry properly.**
- **If unsure ask IPC Team for advice.**

6.4.11 Blood spillages

Usually blood spillages are cleaned up by the ward or domestic staff and should be part of their training. However, this might differ based on local policy and prior agreement. Irrespective of who cleans up a spillage, the steps should be carefully followed:

- All spillages must be cleaned up immediately.
- A pair of domestic gloves must be worn.
- A pan and brush are to remove glass or any other solid material mixed in with the blood.
- Place contaminated bits of glass carefully in newspaper and wrap tightly, ready for disposal.
- Confine the spill and wipe it up immediately with absorbent (paper) towels, cloths or absorbent granules (if available) that are spread over the spill to solidify the blood or body fluid (all should then be disposed as infectious waste).
- Surfaces visibly contaminated with blood or body fluids should also be cleaned immediately with water and a detergent.
- Disinfect by using a facility-approved intermediate-level disinfectant such as chlorine at 500–5 000 ppm free chlorine (1 : 100 or 1 : 10 dilution of 5% chlorine bleach).
- Take care to allow the disinfectant to remain wet on the surface for the required contact time (e.g. 10 minutes) and then rinse the area with clean water to remove the disinfectant residue (if required).
- Inspect to ensure no signs of spillage remain.
- Immediately send all re-usable supplies and equipment (e.g. cleaning cloths, mops) for reprocessing (i.e. cleaning and disinfection) after the spill is cleaned up.

6.4.12 Cleaning equipment

Cleaning cloths should be used and confined to specific areas according to the approved colour-coding system. Separate colours should be assigned to clean and 'dirty' areas (such as toilets) and sluice, baths and isolation rooms.

- Change cleaning cloths and mop heads daily. Used cloths and mop heads must be washed with warm water and a detergent before re-use. (If washed in a washing machine, the water must be 60 °C or more.)
- Empty pistol-grip spray containers should be washed prior to refilling if these are re-used.
- Cleaning carts and buckets must be constructed of rustproof material that is easily cleaned and is free of cracks and crevices. All equipment, carts and accessories used by domestic cleaners must be cleaned at the end of each day or if they become grossly soiled or contaminated.
- Following such cleaning at the end of the day, cleaning equipment must be stored dry in a designated storage area or cleaning closet.
- These closets must be kept neat, clean and free of clutter. All equipment must be routinely maintained and kept in good repair or replaced.
- Scrubbing and floor polishing machines should be emptied and cleaned daily and stored. The pads should be checked regularly to ensure optimal efficiency.

Note: For handling of waste that may be a part of cleaning see section 6.3 Healthcare waste management.

6.4.13 Pest control

Cockroaches, rats, flies, ants, maggots, mosquitos and mites are some of the pests that can become vectors in disease transmission in healthcare facilities. They are often found in hospital kitchens, cafeterias, waste holding areas, drains, and drain pipes, where they can find food, water, warmth and shelter. Regular inspection (forming part of environmental cleanliness checks) must be performed to detect the presence of these pests. Any sign of infestation must be dealt with promptly by removing food and water sources, cleaning up in a timely fashion, using pesticides if required, and blocking points of intrusion, such as broken tiles, unsealed areas around pipes or cracks in woodwork.[43] A pest control contract with a company that deals with pests and vermin should exist. Depending on the contract, the pest controllers should visit the healthcare facility as required. Treatments should use an approved insecticide. Assistance may be obtained from a commercial pest control agency when necessary (for example, in the case of rodents). Only approved insecticides and other poisons may be used. A large-scale problem with insects and rodents must be reported to the IPC team.

---

[43] Aucamp M. 2016. Housekeeping and linen management. *IFIC Basic Concepts of Infection Control*. 3rd ed. International Federation of Infection Control. Chapter 23. https://www.theific.org/wp-content/uploads/2016/04/23-HkpgLaundry_2016.pdf.

6.4.14 The ward environment

The ward environment plays a major role in ensuring a high quality of patient care. There are several aspects which influence this environment, such as cleanliness, decontamination of patient care articles and the quality of the beds and mattresses.

The items used routinely for patients should be visibly clean and where possible decontaminated by heat. Several articles such as blood pressure apparatus and thermometers may be shared, but these too must be clean. Computer keyboards and clinical records should be clean and well maintained.

The key word in the ward environment is **dry**. A moist and warm environment increases the risk of gram-negative bacilli (GNB) colonising and infecting vulnerable patients. Much of this happens with inadequate care of patient care articles. The risk assessment should ensure these areas are rendered safe.

6.4.15 Risk assessment for determining environmental cleaning methods and frequency

It is important to do a risk assessment when the decision is made about environmental cleaning procedure for individual patient care areas. This includes the frequency of cleaning, the method and the process and should be based on the risk of pathogen transmission. The following should be used to determine the risk:

- probability of contamination
- vulnerability of the patients to acquire an infection
- potential for exposure (e.g. high-touch surfaces vs low-touch surfaces).

The three elements are combined to determine low, moderate and high risk. The higher the risk, the more frequent and rigorous a cleaning method is required. Risk determines cleaning frequency, method and process in routine and contingency cleaning schedules for all patient care areas.[44]

6.5 Patient care articles

This section deals with the method of cleaning and decontamination of routinely used items (clinical and non-clinical). The recommended method of decontamination for each article is outlined in the table below.

---

[44]   Centre for Disease Control and Prevention & Infection Control Africa Network. 2019. Best practices for environmental cleaning in healthcare facilities: in resource-limited settings. V1. https://www.cdc.gov/hai/pdfs/resource-limited/environmental-cleaning-RLS-H.pdf.

Table 6.3 Methods of decontaminating routinely used items

Items or site	Preferred method	Alternative methods/comments
Airways and endotracheal tubes	• Single-use disposable	• Heat sterilisation. Use disposable for airborne diseases.
Ambu bags	• Send to SSD for heat disinfection.	• Ethylene oxide
Ampoules	• Wipe with 70% isopropyl alcohol and allow to dry before opening.	• **Do not** immerse in disinfectant.
Bath water	• **No** addition of antiseptic routinely unless burns patient	• Antiseptics increase GNB colonisation.
Baths	• Clean with detergent and non-abrasive cream cleanser. Rinse and dry.	• Infected patients. As previous column. Wipe over with chlorine-based agent. Do not soak.
Bed and cots	• Wipe with warm water and detergent to remove all visible signs of dust and dirt. Dry.	• Disinfectant unnecessary for routine cleaning
Bed frames	• Wipe with warm water and detergent. Dry.	
Bed locker	• Wipe with warm water and detergent. Dry. • Clean inside locker once patient has been discharged.	
Bedpans and urinals	• Wear non-sterile gloves. • Empty contents directly into ward washer-disinfector (80 °C × 1 min). Inspect for cleanliness after removal. Clean if necessary and store inverted to dry.	• Macerators with paper-mâché bedpans and urinals • Manual cleaning: • Empty into sluice. Clean bedpans thoroughly with a scrubbing brush and detergent. Rinse. Invert to dry. • **Never soak bedpans**.
Blankets and bed covers	• Change after each patient has been discharged or when visibly soiled. Send to laundry to wash at 80 °C.	• Do not allow bedding from home; these may be infected with bedbugs or carry scabies.
Bowls (dressing, surgical)	• Return to SSD	• Disposable

Items or site	Preferred method	Alternative methods/comments
Bowls (patient wash)	• Wash with detergent, rinse and store inverted to dry.	• Modern ward washer-disinfectors can also wash bowls. • Use fresh water and towels for each patient.
Carpets	• Daily vacuum (vacuum cleaner fitted with a filter) • Shampoo periodically and extract.	• Not recommended in clinical areas
Commodes	• Wash seat daily with detergent and hot water and dry with a disposable paper towel. • Wipe the commode seat with a large alcohol wipe after each use.	• If visibly contaminated, remove soil with tissue. Wash with warm water and detergent. Dry. • Enteric disease: Viral – wipe the commode with hypochlorite (1 000 ppm av Cl2)
Computer and keyboards	• Damp dust daily. • Wipe keyboard carefully to remove visible dirt.	• Use a keyboard cover which is changed frequently.
Crockery and cutlery	• Wash at 80 °C in dishwasher. • Manual cleaning: Wear gloves and hand wash in detergent and hot water (60 °C). Rinse and dry.	• Wear domestic gloves for manual cleaning. • Infected patients: Unless instructed by IPC team, treat as routine. • Disposable crockery is rarely used – except rabies.
Curtains	• Change curtains frequently. • Isolation room curtains should be changed with each terminal clean.	• Blinds: both vertical and horizontal are difficult to clean and wash regularly.
Drains	• Clean regularly.	• Chemical disinfectants are not recommended.
Dressing trolleys*	• Remove all items daily and wipe surface with warm water and detergent. Dry. Wipe over with 70% isopropyl alcohol. • Discard all previous contents of open jars and bottles. Replace with unopened containers.	• If open jars are used, keep the volume small so that the containers can be heat-disinfected when empty. • **Do not top up open disinfectant containers.**
Duvets	• Washable duvet cover and inner, which allows good circulation of air, should be used and changed after each patient.	• Dry-clean or launder after each patient use.

Items or site	Preferred method	Alternative methods/comments
Endotracheal suction catheters	• Disposable – can be used for 24 hours on the same patient • Flush with sterile water after each use. Bowl is washed and dried after each suction and filled with sterile water only before use.	• Decontaminate hands thoroughly before carrying out suction. • Do not share suction catheters between patients.
Feeding bottles (baby)	• Heat-sterilised in SSD.	• Wash thoroughly. Rinse and soak in a fresh hypochlorite solution (125 ppm available chlorine × 30 min). Remove, rinse and dry.
Floor cleaning • Dry • Wet	• Use dust-attracting mop. • Use water and detergent only.	• Sweeping is not recommended. • Disinfectants are not recommended.
Humidifiers	• Empty daily and heat disinfect after each patient use. • Clean with warm water and detergent. Dry. Fill with sterile water only.	• Not recommended. Use heat exchange filters.
Infant incubators	• Wash all removable parts and clean thoroughly with detergent. Dry with paper towel.	• Infected: After cleaning, wipe over with 70% isopropyl alcohol or hypochlorite (125 ppm av Cl2). Leave incubator to stand unused for 6 hours (aeration).
Instruments (surgical)	• To SSD	
Kitchen cloths	• Daily: disposable • Wash in detergent and dry.	• Disposable preferable
Lamps (examination)	• Wipe with damp cloth daily.	
Laryngoscopes	• Disassemble before cleaning. Heat disinfection preferred.	• Disassemble before cleaning. • Wash with detergent, rinse and dry. Wipe over with alcohol.
Linen (see section on Laundry)	• Automated methods	

Items or site	Preferred method	Alternative methods/comments
Mattresses	• Removable and washable mattress covers. • Use water if impermeable cover. Clean with warm water and detergent. Dry thoroughly. • Never admit patients to soiled, stained or damaged mattress. • If rubber covers are uncomfortable, cover with absorbable paper or cotton sheet. Change frequently. • If soiled with blood and body fluids, wipe with a paper towel, clean with warm water and detergent and disinfect with hypocholorite solution 1 : 1 000 ppm or 70% alcohol.	• Major source of cross-infection • Replace torn mattress covers immediately. Soggy mattresses should be discarded. • Horse-hair and cotton-filled mattresses are not recommended.
Mop bucket	• Daily: Wash in warm water and detergent and store inverted to dry.	• Disinfection unnecessary
Mops	• Daily: Detachable head sent to laundry for heat disinfection and dried. • Manual cleaning: Wear rubber gloves. Rinse thoroughly under running water. Wash in hot water and detergent until clean. Store inverted to dry.	• Colour-coding of mops is useful to reduce cross-contamination between clean and dirty areas and infectious isolation rooms. • Sunlight can be used in warm countries.
Nail brushes	• Not recommended	• Single use and heat disinfection only
Nasogastric (feeding) tubes	• Disposable	• Cannot be recycled
Nebulisers	• Single-patient use • Wash and dry the container and mask after each patient use. Store dry and protected from dust. Discard after patient is discharged.	• Heat disinfection if necessary
Oxygen masks	• Disposable	• If re-usable: Wash thoroughly until visibly clean. Dry. Wipe with alcohol or use heat disinfection (SSD).

Items or site	Preferred method	Alternative methods/ comments
Patient toiletries	• Patients should bring their own soap, towels, shaving equipment and other personal items, which should never be shared.	
Pillows (see Mattresses)	• Use waterproof cover. • Clean with a detergent and water after patient is discharged.	
Rectal thermometer	• Single-patient use • Wash in detergent after each use. Wipe with alcohol and store dry.	
Scissors	• Clean if visibly soiled. • Wipe over with 70% isopropyl alcohol before and after use.	
Scrubbing machine	• Drain reservoir after use. Wipe with a damp cloth and store dry.	
Shaving brushes	• Not recommended	• If absolutely necessary, pre-operative skin shaving should only happen in the operating suite – never in the ward.
Sheepskin	• Synthetic: Launder in machine. • Natural: Hand wash in detergent and dry.	• Not recommended for routine use unless clinically indicated. • Restrict to one-patient use only.
Soap (handwashing)	• Tablet: Store dry. • Liquid: Single-use sachets preferred. Send wall-mounted dispenser for thorough cleaning after it is empty and refill under aseptic conditions.	• Tablet soaps are not recommended. • **Never top up** – increases risk of GNB colonisation.
Shower head	• Should be removed and cleaned thoroughly each week. • Soak in descaler if necessary.	• Replace rubber washer with plastic ones to prevent legionnaires' disease.
Sputum container	• Disposable only	
Suction machines	• Empty the reservoir in the sluice after use, wash with warm water and detergent and store dry. • Single-use tubing. • Clean the surface and cover after each use.	• PPE: non-sterile gloves and apron • Never leave fluid (secretions or disinfectant) in the reservoir if not in use.

Items or site	Preferred method	Alternative methods/ comments
	• Reservoirs with single-use liners are available. • Remove lid and carefully remove inner liner containing fluid. Dispose of in either infectious waste container or sluice. • Wash and clean the outer cover, dry and replace bag.	
Surfaces and ledges	• Damp dusting daily. Dry.	
Thermometer (oral) Electronic	• Wash and dry after each patient use. Wipe with 70% isopropyl alcohol and store dry. • Change sleeve after each use.	• **Never** soak thermometers in disinfectants. • Never use without sleeve.
Taps	• Elbow-operated • Clean daily and keep dry.	• Replace rubber with plastic washers to prevent legionnaires' disease.
Toilet seats	• Wash at least daily with detergent and dry.	
Tooth mugs	• Disposable or send to SSD between patients.	
Toys	• Soft: Machine wash, rinse and dry • Other: Wash with detergent, rinse and dry. Wipe with 70% alcohol if made of plastic.	• Do not share toys in an infected ward. Heavily soiled toys may have to be destroyed.
Tubing	• Disposable	• Pre-processed in SSD • **Never** use glutaraldehyde to disinfect respiratory equipment.
Ultrasound	• Disinfect with 70% isopropyl alcohol between each patient use. • Intravaginal: Cover probe with a fresh condom for each patient.	
Ventilators	• These are complex and should be cleaned and disinfected according to manufacturer's instruction. • Sometimes there are technicians in the facility who do the maintenance. • Single-patient-use tubing is preferred, which is discarded.	• Remove tubing and send for heat disinfection to SSD (80 °C × 3 min) or chemical disinfection. • Clean all inspiratory and expiratory connections. • Change both sets of filters. • Check efficiency of air movement.

Items or site	Preferred method	Alternative methods/comments
		• Reassemble. • Clean outside of ventilator. • Register in logbook.
Washbasins	• Clean with warm water and detergent, cream cleaner for stains. • Disinfectants not recommended.	
Wound suction (closed drainage)	• Remove lid and carefully remove inner liner containing fluid. Dispose of in either infectious waste container or sluice. • Wash and clean the outer cover, dry and replace bag. • Check that the valves and connectors are clean and functioning.	• Send for heat disinfection after each patient use.
X-ray equipment	• Damp dust only.	• Wipe with 70% isopropyl alcohol if disinfection required.

*Open containers are a high-risk area for transmission from hands of staff and contamination from the environment and should be avoided.

7 Communicable disease and public health

Shaheen Mehtar

Learning outcomes

What you should know after reading this chapter:
- Notification systems for communicable diseases
- General public health regulations
- Appropriate transmission-based precautions applied to mode of transmission of communicable diseases
- Management of communicable disease patients in healthcare facilities
- Management of communicable disease patients in the home
- Occupational health and IPC

Introduction

Infection prevention and control (IPC) teams traditionally work in healthcare facilities, but often they are required to advise on, and work, on public health and communicable disease programmes, particularly during outbreaks and pandemics like the recent COVID-19 pandemic. More recently, IPC teams have been involved in managing community-based institutions and home-based care mainly for patients suffering from HIV and tuberculosis but other diseases as well. It is more cost-effective to care for chronic patients in the community rather than in hospitals, it allows them to be with their loved ones and they can take control and responsibility for their own treatment and medication.

There are additional benefits of having community IPC teams on hand. First, there is a constant exchange of patients to and from hospitals who could be colonised with healthcare-associated infection (HAI), particularly those with chronic disease. Secondly, in the community the indiscriminate use of antibiotics to treat minor non-bacterial infection that increases the risk of multidrug-resistant bacteria (MDRO) can be monitored and reduced. Thirdly, poor cleanliness and hand hygiene in the homes facilitate the transfer of pathogens between the patients and their household occupiers; this can be improved by support from community IPC teams. Finally, treatable communicable diseases such as tuberculosis, which require meticulous IPC practices to reduce transmission within the community, can be well supported. The IPC teams are also instrumental in increasing awareness among the community, educating patients and caregivers and providing training for home-based carers and voluntary staff, as was significantly noticeable during the COVID-19 pandemic.

This chapter is by no means a comprehensive account of communicable diseases but a summary of relevant factors such as transmission and prevention. Here, communicable diseases are grouped by their main mode of transmission, with the most effective IPC containment measures and appropriate public health measures to be applied. IPC principles and precautions can be instituted more confidently for patients falling within a particular group when dealing with an outbreak in the community; for example, respiratory infection outbreaks should have respiratory precautions in place which are simple and much more manageable at a community level. Caregivers, once trained, can understand and follow the instructions given to them on how to safely manage the patient and the household. Communicable diseases that are more transmissible will have additional precautions, at home and in healthcare facilities.

The reader is also referred to the section on risk management and transmission-based precautions for an in-depth account (see section 4.2.3.6).

7.1 Communicable diseases

A **communicable disease** is defined as an illness that arises from transmission of an **infectious agent** or its toxic product from an infected person, animal or reservoir to a **susceptible host**, either directly or indirectly through an intermediate plant or animal host, vector or environment. The terms 'communicable' and 'infectious' diseases are used interchangeably. The essential factors are a source, a vehicle of transport or transmission and a susceptible host.

7.1.1 Control of communicable disease

In order to set up an effective prevention programme, especially in LMICs, the focus needs to be on those illnesses that have the highest rates of morbidity and mortality in a community. The following general approach to a disease control programme is suggested:

1. **Prevent communicable disease outbreaks.** Many common outbreaks respond to public health measures to control the source such as:
    - improving the quality of drinking water
    - improving sanitation
    - education on hand hygiene
    - controlling vectors
    - waste management, including waste water and human excreta.

2. **Interrupt the transmission by treating and isolating infected persons.**
3. **Remove the vehicle(s) of transmission.**
4. **Improve the population's immunity by promoting better nutrition and a robust vaccination programme.**

After the Ebola outbreak in West Africa (2014–2016) outbreak response teams have been established in most countries – these include clinical, epidemiological, IPC, environmental cleaners, biomedical engineers and social workers.[1] IPC teams working together with these colleagues put measures into place following the hierarchy of controls[2] to isolate the infected cases and institute transmission-based precautions as soon as possible and reduce transmission via contact with humans and the environment (and air). However, the IPC team should reinforce proper precautions not just for healthcare workers but also the patient's caregivers and the community in the event of an outbreak. It is also an opportune moment to re-issue policy documents or write up new ones if these do not exist and monitor implementation. Provisions for the implementation of the policy should be provided – this requires commitment and engagement of political structures particularly the departments of health, environmental health and sanitation, and occupational health.

7.1.2 Notifiable communicable diseases

The national health authority has to be notified of **any condition with the potential to result in serious public heath consequences,** and it is its responsibility to report to the WHO about certain diseases, according to the International Health Regulations (2005).[3]

7.1.2.1 International Health Regulations (2005)

The International Health Regulations (2005) or 'IHR (2005)' make up an international law which helps countries working together to save lives and livelihoods endangered by the international spread of diseases and other health risks. The IHR (2005) aims are:

- To prevent, protect against, control and respond to the international spread of disease while avoiding unnecessary interference with international traffic and trade.

---

[1]   Outbreak response. National Institute of Communicable Diseases, South Africa. https://www.nicd.ac.za/our-services/outbreak-response/.

[2]   Hierarchy of Controls, NIOSH. 2022. https://www.cdc.gov/niosh/topics/hierarchy/default.html.

[3]   World Health Organization. The International Health Regulations (IHR). 2008. www.who.int/topics/international_health_regulations/en/.

- To reduce the risk of disease spread at international airports, ports and ground crossings.
- To support the existing global outbreak alert and response system.
- To improve international surveillance and reporting mechanisms for public health events.
- To encourage countries to strengthen their national surveillance and response capacities.
- To increase the confidence of countries in reporting significant and/or unusual disease events by linking early disclosure to prompt support and accurate information dissemination about the nature of the event.

The list of formidable infectious diseases has been replaced by the concept of a public health emergency of international concern (PHEIC), which refers to an extraordinary public health event that is determined, under specific procedures:

(a) to constitute a public health risk to other states through the international spread of disease; and

(b) to potentially require a co-ordinated international response.

Decisions need to be based on the following criteria:

(a) seriousness of the public health impact of the event

(b) unusual or unexpected nature of the event

(c) potential for the event to spread internationally, and/or

(d) the risk that restrictions to travel or trade may result because of the event.

The WHO regulations aim to help the international community to prevent and respond to acute public health risks that have the potential to cross borders and threaten people worldwide, such as the recent SARS-CoV-2 pandemic, monkeypox and Ebola in Africa. The IHR aim to limit interference with international traffic and trade while ensuring public health through the prevention of disease spread.

The IHR, which came into force on 15 June 2005, require countries to report certain disease outbreaks and public health events and to strengthen their existing capacities for public health surveillance and response. The WHO works closely with countries and partners to provide technical guidance and support mobilisation of the resources needed. The notification might change depending on the public health requirements. The IHR (2005) is currently being updated.

7.1.2.2 National notification systems

The list of diseases notifiable to the national health authorities varies from country to country. These lists are updated if the prevailing disease profiles in a country change.

Categories of notifiable diseases in South Africa

A. **Active surveillance (report in 24 hours):** Acute flaccid paralysis, measles and neonatal tetanus

B. **Urgent response:** Cholera, viral haemorrhagic fever (any) including yellow fever

C. **Rapid response:** Anthrax, diphtheria, hepatitis A, legionella disease, meningococcal disease, plague, poisoning, food poisoning affecting more than four people, pesticide poisoning, rabies (risky bite and case), paratyphoid and typhoid fever

D. **Routine:** Acute rheumatic fever, brucellosis, congenital syphilis, *Haemophilus influenzae* (B), leprosy, malaria, tuberculosis, trachoma, viral hepatitis, whooping cough

In South Africa categories A to C should be initially notified by telephone – and all categories of disease should also be informed in writing by filling in the required form (GW 17/5), within seven days, at the local district health office. The Provincial and National Health Department offices should publish a regular up-to-date summary of these notifications.

7.1.3 Factors affecting the spread of communicable diseases

Factors affecting the spread of communicable diseases are multi-faceted, which is why the containment of diseases in the community is usually difficult – the main one being the human factor.

7.1.3.1 **The domestic environment** in LMICs presents major challenges owing to:
- *Overcrowding*, where sometimes up to twelve people will be living in two rooms
- *Poor ventilation* because either the building is inadequately ventilated or the weather is inclement
- *Movement of people*, mainly relatives, who come and go frequently
- *Cleanliness* and personal hygiene, especially where there is overcrowding and a lack of toilet and ablution facilities
- *Shortage* or *lack of clean running water* for drinking and ablutions
- *Communal toilets*, pit latrines or night soil buckets, which are still present in some rural areas of South Africa.

7.1.3.2 **Heads of households.** To manage infections in the community, identify the head of the household or community and work with them as a priority to build trust. Advise families on how to protect themselves, particularly keeping the children safe, including through vaccination programmes. This is usually achieved by frank and open discussion, education and awareness and supplying provisions to reduce transmission if necessary. Health support is provided, especially to the designated caregiver. The role of the social worker is a major one when dealing with families with little in the way of provisions available to them.

7.1.3.3 **Control of social movement.** It is difficult to keep infected patients away from their families and friends, especially in rural areas, where people socialise extensively on every possible occasion.

Traditional behaviour plays a major part in transmission of communicable disease and should be considered.

- Visitors from far must come to see sick relatives and friends – to do otherwise is considered impolite.
- Overnight guests or visitors in transit must be given a bed, otherwise the family is considered inhospitable.
- Sharing beds with children or adults is common in overcrowded housing and a sign of affection.
- Socialising areas such as pubs, shebeens, clubs and community halls are frequented for long periods of time in a closed and stuffy environment.
- Rituals during gatherings such as feasts, death and birthing rituals are generally dominated by female members of the society, but men also play a major role in some of these events.

7.1.3.4 **Work with traditional leaders and healers**

Seeking medical advice from traditional healers is a priority in rural cultures. In Africa, traditional healers are highly respected and both rural and urban dwellers from all social strata will visit them for their health-related problems – they must be recognised as part of the solution. There is considerable indigenous knowledge in most rural societies who have been dealing with communicable diseases for a long time, which must be acknowledged and where possible, used to contain outbreaks. Traditional healers are trusted and given priority over health clinics because they are more sympathetic and understand the culture – they belong to the same community and are highly respected. They can be your greatest ally!

Here are some of the areas which cause mistrust between healthcare workers and traditional healers, but there may be others:

- Scarification and other treatments as part of traditional medication – as long as it does not interfere or increase the risk of infection, should be allowed.

- Indigenous knowledge is ignored. There a plethora of experience and information that can be used but is not.
- Lack of trust and referral systems between traditional and healthcare establishments.
- Visiting medical teams have been known to be rude, dismissive and demeaning of the local population.

7.1.3.5   **Public awareness** campaigns are run, but they may be alien to the beliefs and traditions of the population they are aimed at:

- Education of the public with campaigns in local languages using common media helps, but the means of spreading the word needs to be public-friendly.
- Promoting general hygiene and improvement within the existing systems is done, but often these systems are not interconnected and therefore not understood adequately.

7.1.3.6   **Notification of suspected or confirmed infection.** Systems should be put into place which will encourage the community to report communicable diseases. Increasing awareness in the community starts with a simple information programme that includes education on how to reduce transmission. The public should be educated to recognise certain signs and symptoms of disease, especially during outbreaks. Those with these suspicious symptoms should attend the nearest healthcare facility as soon as possible. This is not always easy since many communities do not trust healthcare facilities. Nevertheless, healthcare workers must win the trust and co-operation of patients enough to enable them to take a careful history and establish the likely route and cause of the infection. Ensure that traditional healers and heads of the community are included in health delivery programmes.

7.1.3.7   **Reporting sickness** in the poorly informed (and suspicious) communities has always been a major obstacle to early detection. It is considered a sign of weakness and there is stigma attached if there is an illness within the family. Only when a patient is seriously ill do the relatives consider taking him or her to the hospital because there is a fear that when people go to hospitals they die. Usually patients are brought in so late that there is not much that can be done to help them, so the myth lives on.

7.1.3.8   **Vaccination programmes** and other preventive measures should be encouraged, especially for children. It is one of the most important pillars of IPC.

7.1.4 Public health

Public health has been described by Winslow as 'the science and art of preventing disease, prolonging life and promoting health through the organised efforts and informed choices of society, organisations, public and private, communities and individuals'.[4] Public health is concerned with threats to the overall health of a community based on population health analysis. The population in question can be as small as a handful of people or as large as all the inhabitants of several continents (for instance, in the case of a pandemic). Public health typically deals with epidemiology, biostatistics and health services in populations in respect of preventive measures. The goal of public health is to improve lives through the prevention and treatment of disease. The WHO defines health as 'a state of complete physical, mental and social well-being and not merely the absence of disease or infirmity'.

There are several challenges to containing communicable diseases outside hospitals, especially in LMICs – these countries usually bear the brunt of the disease. Diseases such as tuberculosis (TB) create a high burden on the health delivery system. Although it is treatable, TB is one of the diseases of poverty and transmission has usually occurred within the social structures before it gets diagnosed and treated. In South Africa the First National TB Prevalence Survey (2018) reported an overall comorbidity of 28.8% with HIV and an overall TB prevalence rate of 737 per 100 000 of the population (2018).[5] This has reduced since 2009, but transmission is still ongoing, particularly among males.

When epidemics occur in rural areas there are usually inadequate immediate structures in place to contain the spread of diseases. There is an increase in movement from the rural areas to peri-urban areas because of fear and panic where overcrowding and poverty promote the transmission of a pathogen – a classical example is the rapid spread of Ebola virus disease in West Africa (2014) when people moved from the rural to the urban areas. Prior to that, EVD did occur sporadically but remained confined to the rural areas. The vectors play a major role in viral haemorrhagic fevers, and these are difficult to control. In urban areas, dengue, a viral haemorrhagic fever is spreading rapidly in the Middle and Far East countries, while in Africa yellow fever is common on the outskirts of urban communities.

[4]   Winslow CEA. 2002. *Encyclopedia of public health*. In L Breslow (Gale Group ed), eNotes.com. 2006. 24 March 2008. http://www.enotes.com/publich-health-encyclopedia/ winslow-charles-edward-amory.
[5]   The First National TB Prevalence Survey, South Africa 2018.

7.2   Applying IPC principles in the community

> The IPC principles should be simple and easy to follow with practical application of procedures which will contain or, at the very least, reduce transmission.

IPC principles for the community are the same as for hospitals and should be based on interventions aimed at the routes and risk of transmission. Precautions can be modified and applied to home-based care.

Pathogens with the same routes of transmission, such as respiratory viruses, seasonal influenza and pandemic influenza, occurring simultaneously in a community can be managed with the same type of precautions since the route of spread is similar. Provisions for containment of mild or moderately infected cases within the household are possible with some care and re-organisation of the available facilities. Seriously sick patients can be transferred to hospitals for more advanced healthcare and support.

The IPC measures, which are based on risk assessment, will be addressed within each section along with the relevant public health measures and recommended transmission-based precautions. If necessary, additional IPC measures for specific communicable diseases in hospitals will be mentioned. Readers are referred to the *Control of Communicable Disease Manual*[6] for comprehensive descriptions of communicable diseases.

7.2.1 Mutual trust between health workers and the community

In order to establish a robust IPC programme in the community, it is essential that there is a close working relationship between the community and the health delivery facilities for that community. There must be mutual trust and respect. For this to happen, some structures in the community are necessary. It is advisable to win over the head of the tribe/clan or community so that there is a good rapport between the community and the healthcare delivery system. The leaders of the community can facilitate reaching the right people.

7.2.2 Designated caregiver(s)

If healthcare has to be delivered at home to a bed-bound or semi-mobile patient, there should be a named caregiver (or two) within the affected household who is responsible for the care of the patient. These caregivers must be advised on safe practices to reduce risk of transmission to themselves and the family when managing the patient at home. The visiting healthcare worker should demonstrate

6   Heymann DL. 2008. *Control of communicable diseases manual.* 18th ed. American Public Health Association.

the procedures and make sure the caregiver is comfortable with carrying them out. This person can also be the contact person for the healthcare worker and give a progress report at subsequent visits or can contact health authorities in the event of the patient deteriorating or further cases occurring within the household or social circle.

The information should be given by a community healthcare worker to the caregiver and patient in the form of a short leaflet with pictograms which are self-explanatory, but these should be discussed to ensure clarity. The caregiver should communicate the essentials of containment (IPC) to all visitors and be clear about the consequences of breaching these suggestions. It also helps to transfer information within the community by word of mouth and improve preventive measures.

7.2.3 Routes of transmission for communicable diseases

The routes of transmission for communicable diseases are:

7.2.3.1   **Oro-faecal route**, which results from the ingestion of contaminated water or foodstuff.

7.2.3.2   **Inoculation of infected blood and body fluids** contaminated with blood-borne viruses. The inoculation of contaminated blood can occur via vectors (insects) or hypodermic needles and other medical devices.

7.2.3.3   **Respiratory route.** Transmission can occur when someone sneezes or coughs a cloud of mixed-size particles (infectious) that are dispersed into the surrounding atmosphere, which transmit to the surfaces or directly to other humans (see section 4.2.3.6 Transmission-based and section 5.3.6.1 Ventilation). Common diseases are respiratory viruses, TB and *Strep pneumoniae*.

7.2.3.4   **Skin and mucous membrane contact.** Direct or indirect contact occurs when there is overcrowding or in institutions. The proximity to an infected source goes unnoticed until the infection manifests itself. Scabies, impetigo and fungal infections are common examples, but viruses can also spread via this route.

7.2.3.5   **Sexual contact** can result in several types of infection. Most often contact with the genital fluids results in the spread of blood-borne viruses, such as HIV and hepatitis B, and sexually transmitted disease such as syphilis, gonorrhea and trichomonas infections, and, more recently, monkeypox.

7.2.4 Oro-faecal route of transmission

The oro-faecal route of transmission is the most common cause of communicable diseases in most parts of the world. In LMICs it is usually because of contaminated food or water supply. In the summer months there is an increase in diarrhoeal disease, especially among children. Outbreaks of cholera, typhoid fever and dysentery occur when water and food become contaminated. In the domestic environment, pathogens are introduced into food and water by poor hand hygiene, lack of appropriate education and inadequate public health facilities. The source is usually difficult to establish unless there is an outbreak in an institution like a nursery. Adults working in abattoirs or farms or visitors from an endemic area may become carriers and introduce pathogens into the household. In some communities the use of communal night soil buckets contributes to the spread of infectious diseases within the community. Disease transmission may occur via either water or food, or both.

7.2.4.1 Water-related diseases

Water is essential for all life. Water for human consumption is drawn from natural sources such as rivers, streams and wells. In an urban environment it is usually stored in tanks prior to distribution. In the rural environment there may be a shortage of water, lack of piped water or no infrastructure to provide clean water to a population. The availability of good-quality, clean water is directly related to the level of health.

7.2.4.1.1 Diseases associated with water

These diseases mainly affect the gastrointestinal tract, resulting in acute diarrhoea and vomiting. Pollution of waterways with chemicals, especially close to industrial sites, can lead to chronic poisoning. Parasitic diseases are common from drinking contaminated water. Some examples are shown in Table 7.1.

7.2.4.2 Safe water supply – public health

Domestic water supply. The WHO defines domestic water as 'water being used for all usual domestic purposes including consumption, bathing and food preparation'.[7] The minimum requirement is 15 litres per person per day, of which 5 litres is recommended for drinking, cooking and sanitation.[8] Water contaminated by microbes or chemicals may affect large populations, especially in developing countries that lack the infrastructure to provide safe water. The burden of disease is usually carried by children.[9]

---

[7]   Howard G & Bartram J. 2003. *Domestic water quality, service, level and health.* WHO/SDE/WSH/03.02. World Health Organization.

[8]   WHO and UNICEF. 2002. *Global water supply and sanitation assessment 2000 report.* Geneva/New York: WHO/UNICEF.

[9]   WHO. 1993. *Guidelines for drinking water quality.* Vol 1. *Recommendations.* 2nd ed. Geneva: WHO.

Table 7.1 Water-associated diseases (from IFIC Basic Concepts in Infection Control)

Type	Means	Disease
Water-borne	Consumption of contaminated water	Diarrhoeal disease Hepatitis A Typhoid Cholera
Water-washed	Inadequate volumes for personal hygiene	Diarrhoeal disease Impetigo Group A streptococcal infection Trachoma
Water-based	Require an intermediate aquatic host	Schistosomiasis Guinea worm
Water-related vector	Spread by insects associated with water	Malaria Dengue Yellow fever

7.2.4.2.1 Problems with rural water supply

In remote and rural areas there are major challenges in providing fresh, clean water to a population.

- Distance from the water source. In urban areas piped water is delivered into the houses and dwellings. In peri-urban areas poor maintenance of sewage and drinking water pipes has led to water-borne disease outbreaks affecting the community. In rural areas the water supply is not piped and families often have to carry water in unclean plastic containers for long distances from rivers and dams.
- Carrying the water over a long distance increases the temperature of the water to near body temperature. This is an ideal environment for biofilm formation and microbial growth.
- The source is usually a river or a well used for multiple purposes, such as drinking, bathing and washing clothes; some waterways are used as toilets.
- Livestock share the same water source and contaminate the water supply.

7.2.4.2.2 Treatment of water

Clean water must be supplied to all areas via a well-established piped system of delivering a safe and constant supply of water. However, where piped water does not exist it requires working closely with the communities and the heads of those communities to safe guard the water source from contamination and pollution. Water brought in large hygienic carriers is particularly effective during outbreaks of water-borne diseases.

7.2.4.2.3 Water channels for drinking purposes only

Another effective way of providing clean water comes from the community itself managing their water effectively. From a high point above the level of human population a water channel is drawn from the main stream and is planted with water-filtering grasses. The water channel is slowly filtered over stones to fill a secured waterhole. The overflow from the waterhole is returned to the main stream or used for irrigation. The entire system is protected and monitored by the community to ensure livestock and humans do not enter or use the water **above the designated point**. It is an effective way of segregating water for drinking from domestic use. There may be specified times for water collection, which are closely monitored.

7.2.4.2.4 Water containers

Various recommendations exist, but it is inevitable that water can only be collected in the containers available. The use of plastic containers is common and most are reclaimed from other uses such as pesticide or chemical bulk supplies. The danger is when the containers are not properly cleaned and residual chemicals result in poisoning – of note are pesticide containers on farms. Plastic containers also increase microbial growth and promote the production of biofilm. In the rural villages in India, copper water containers were preferred as these inhibited bacterial multiplication, but now these have been replaced by plastic containers, which sadly allow the formation of biofilm on the surface quite quickly.

7.2.4.3 Rendering water safe for consumption

Most of these methods apply to making the water safe after it has been collected.

7.2.4.3.1 Natural sunlight

In hot countries, sunlight has been used to increase the temperature in the water containers to over 60 °C and then be allowed to cool before use. This is a form of pasteurisation and can kill most vegetative forms of bacteria and non-enveloped viruses.

7.2.4.3.2 Boiling

Water should be boiled at 100 °C or more; the water should be observed to be bubbling for three to five minutes before being considered safe to drink or use. Heating water to 75 °C will remove most vegetative bacterial forms, but not spores or parasites. Water should be left in the container it was boiled in and not decanted or contaminated with dirty hands.

During outbreaks of cholera or typhoid, households are further advised to manage water distribution within the household. A named person (usually the mother) is made responsible for distributing the drinking water. The person is asked to wash his or her hands (or use alcohol rub (ABHR)) before using a dedicated container to dispense water into a glass or mug for a household member. Any water left over in the main container is put into a separate receptacle to be used for domestic purposes. The main water container is kept covered and filled daily and boiled. Alternatively, two containers could be used for water, one in use and the other one boiled and cooling.

7.2.4.3.3 Chemical disinfection

Chlorine is widely used as a water purifier. Individual storage tanks should contain 0.5 parts per million (ppm) available chlorine at the end of the chlorination process. It is recommended that river water and borehole water should not be used for one hour and 30 minutes respectively after chlorination.

7.2.4.4 Food and water-borne diseases

Most food- and water-borne diseases that spread by the oro-faecal route are associated with unhygienic conditions or incorrect handling and storage of food. These are more common in water-deprived areas where hand hygiene is limited by the water supply. All food should be treated with care, stored at the correct temperatures, distributed carefully and the crockery washed clean and stored dry.

7.2.4.4.1 Transmission of food-borne diseases

Pathogens are transmitted via:
- The hands of food preparers or handlers. Poor hand hygiene, especially in children, is a common source of transmission of food-borne pathogens.
- Incorrectly prepared food. If a large piece of meat is cooked for too short a time, the inside remains at a much lower temperature compared to the outside, and allows multiplication of bacteria.
- Contaminated cold foods are prepared together with cooked foods. The bacteria from the cold food can contaminate the cooked food and the temperature is right for multiplication of bacteria.
- Lack of cold storage conditions of perishable goods. A classic situation is street vendors or small businesses unable to maintain cold refrigeration during power cuts.
- Flies and pests may contaminate food lying exposed.
- Contaminated water used to prepare foods is a source of disease.

7.2.4.4.2 Public health measures for food-borne diseases

The general recommendations (WHO) to reduce food- and water-borne transmission are outlined below. These measures include what individuals as well as government structures can do to improve water delivery and reduce contamination of food. They apply to all communicable diseases transmitted by the oro-faecal route as outlined below from the *Communicable Diseases Control Manual* (APHA).[10]

1. **Educate** the public regarding the importance of handwashing. Provide suitable handwashing facilities, particularly for food handlers and attendants involved in the care of patients and children.

2. **Dispose of human faeces** safely and maintain fly-proof latrines. Under field conditions, dispose of faeces by burial at a site distant and downstream from the source of drinking water.

3. **Protect, purify and chlorinate public water supplies.** Provide safe private supplies and avoid possible backflow connections between water and sewer systems. For individual and small group protection, and during travel or in the field, treat water chemically or by boiling.

4. **Control flies and other pests** by screening and use of insecticidal baits and traps or, where appropriate, spraying with insecticides. Control fly breeding through frequent garbage collection and disposal and through fly-control measures in latrine construction and maintenance.

5. **Use scrupulous cleanliness in food preparation and handling.** Refrigerate as appropriate. Pay particular attention to the storage of salads and other foods served cold. These provisions apply to home and public eating places. If one is uncertain about sanitary practices, select foods that are cooked and served hot. Fruit should be peeled by the consumer.

6. **Pasteurise or boil all milk and dairy products.** Supervise the sanitary aspects of commercial milk production, storage and delivery.

7. **Enforce suitable quality control procedures** in industries that prepare food and drink for human consumption. Use chlorinated water for cooling during canned food processing.

8. **Limit the collection and marketing of shellfish** to supplies from approved sources. Boil or steam (for at least 10 minutes) before serving.

9. **Instruct the community, patients, convalescents and carriers in personal hygiene.** Emphasise handwashing as a routine practice after defecation and before preparing, serving or eating food.

10. **Encourage breastfeeding throughout infancy.** Boil all milk and water used for infant feeding.

11. **Encourage appropriate vaccination** when indicated.

---

[10]   Heymann DL. 2022. *Control of communicable diseases manual.* 21th ed. American Public Health Association.

7.2.4.5 Diseases transmitted by the oro-faecal route

Some of the diseases transmitted through the oro-faecal route (contaminated fingers, food and water consumption) include food poisoning, hepatitis A and E, amoebic dysentery and cholera. Transmission occurs when infected faecal matter is ingested.

7.2.4.5.1 Food poisoning

Common-source outbreaks usually occur at social gatherings when the food is prepared and stored incorrectly. Such outbreaks may occur within healthcare facilities or in households. Food poisoning brings an acute onset of nausea vomiting, diarrhoea, fever and abdominal cramps. The duration of illness is short-lived, usually lasts a couple of days, is localised and self-limiting and usually does not require hospitalisation. However, in the immunocompromised person (HIV-infected) it may last much longer or become invasive and cause bacteraemia.

Some examples of microbes causing food poisoning are shown in Table 7.2.

Table 7.2 Bacteria causing food poisoning with mechanism and method of spread

Bacterium	Mechanism	Method of spread	Incubation period (hrs)	Food affected
Salmonella spp	Multiplication	Hands, surfaces, raw to cooked food	12–36	Poultry, meat, eggs
Clostridium perfringens	Toxin produced during multiplication	Spores activated during cooking	22–36	Raw meat, dehydrated products
Staph aureus	Toxin	Hands/nose to food	1–6	Dairy products
Bacillus cereus	Multiplication	Inadequate heating, moist storage	1–6	Cereals, rice
Campylobacter	Multiplication	Inadequate cooking temperatures, careless handling	1–10 days	Poultry, meat, water

7.2.4.5.2 Systemic diseases transmitted by the oro-faecal route

The diseases listed below are spread via the oro-faecal route by the ingestion of contaminated food or water. Of these cholera, typhoid and hepatitis A and E are of IPC importance – the public health and IPC measures mentioned previously apply to most diseases associated with the oro-faecal route of transmission as shown in Table 7.3. For further information the reader is referred to the *Communicable Disease Control Manual*, 21st Edition (2022).

- amoebae*
- cholera
- diarrhoea
- dysentery
- giardia*
- hepatitis A, E
- parasites: round/hookworm*
- typhoid

* not an immediate priority for IPC

7.2.4.6 IPC precautions for oro-faecal route of transmission

These are to reduce the risk of food and water contamination:

- Meticulous hand hygiene by food preparers and handlers whenever dealing with food or water.
- Prevent contamination of water and foodstuffs from faeces and urine of carriers.
- Safe food preparation and storage away from pests.
- Keep water and containers free from contamination. Change water regularly and add bleach if recommended by the health authorities.
- Keep food preparation dishes clean and dry.

7.2.4.6.1 Home-based IPC for patients infected by oro-faecal route

The pathogens responsible for infection are sensitive to heat and can easily destroyed with good hygiene.

7.2.4.6.1.1   **The patient**. The person should understand the mode of transmission (contact precautions) and should assist in containing its spread, especially among children.

- Place the patient in a single room if possible. He or she should not share a bed with others, especially if he or she has diarrhoea.
- The door should remain closed. If this is not possible, then restrict visitors.
- Handwash with soap and water or ABHR should be available for use.

7.2.4.6.1.2   **Caregivers**. Caregivers must fully understand the need for hygiene and reduce the risk of contamination by observing the following IPC instructions in all aspects of their care:

- Undertake meticulous hand hygiene (either handwashing with soap and water followed by drying or ABHR) before and after each patient contact. In this situation 'contact' means the following and should be clearly defined in written instructions:

- — feeding the patient
- — cleaning the patient's perineal area
- — washing or bathing the patient
- — changing soiled clothing of the patient
- — changing soiled sheets and bed linen
- — removing faecal matter and urine
- Gloves and aprons are not mandatory (but advisable) if hand hygiene is meticulously followed.

7.2.4.6.1.3 **Healthcare workers.** Healthcare workers visiting patients at home must take the following precautions to avoid contamination:
- Wear non-sterile gloves when examining the patient.
- Discard gloves in the domestic waste after each patient use, especially if soiled with organic matter (bringing the used gloves back to the clinic is not necessary unless there is no waste management in place).
- ABHR should be used immediately before and after patient contact.

7.2.4.6.1.4 **Toilet and ablution facilities.** The caregiver must be aware of keeping the toilet and washing facilities clean and dry to reduce the risk of transmission of infection.
- If there is a flushing toilet and the patient is mobile, the toilet should be cleaned thoroughly after each use.
- Bedpans and urinals can be emptied into the toilet before washing them thoroughly in hot water (gloves should be worn when washing bedpans and urinals).
- Outside communal toilets are to be used by the patient with care, ensuring there is no faecal contamination of the surroundings. The toilet should be cleaned after the patient has used it.
- Meticulous hand hygiene is essential for all those coming into contact with the patient's excretions.
- The patient should have a dedicated towel, which is dried after each use. The towel should be changed frequently.
- The bathing facilities should be kept clean and dry.
- The patient can be given a wash in bed provided the water is discarded immediately and carefully.
- Any spillage of vomit or faeces on the floor of the patient's room should be cleaned up immediately and wiped over with hypochlorite (bleach).
- The caregiver should change his or her clothes if these become wet.

7.2.4.6.1.5 **Food preparation.** Contaminated food presents a considerable danger to the patient and the person preparing the food must observe the following instructions:
- The person preparing the food must make sure that hands are washed and clean before starting preparation.
- Food should be well cooked and served soon after preparation while still hot.
- Fresh vegetables and salads should be washed thoroughly in clean water, but it is best not to offer the patient uncooked food until after recovery.
- Avoid raw seafood such as shellfish.
- Avoid raw milk – all milk must be boiled and cooled prior to use.

7.2.4.6.1.6 **Crockery and cutlery.** The patient's crockery and cutlery can be kept separate for the duration of the illness and washed in very hot water and allowed to air dry.

7.2.4.6.1.7 **Washing the patient's clothes.** Careful washing of the patient's clothes must be done separately from the rest of the household's laundry. All articles soiled by the patient's urine and faeces should be rinsed in ordinary tap water and then washed in very hot water. The articles of clothing can be placed in a bowl and boiling water poured over them and left for 10 minutes, after which detergent may be added and the clothing washed thoroughly and rinsed. Bleach may be added during the final rinse, if it is available, but is not necessary.

7.2.4.6.1.8 **Waste.** In the home environment it is vital that the patient's waste is very carefully managed and disposed of. All items of waste generated in the house can be placed in a separate plastic bag, tied and put into the domestic waste bag. If there is no waste collection in the area, then it should be secured well and taken to a municipal handling area. If none of these options is available, then the least satisfactory is to dig a pit of approximately 1 m deep and put soiled and contaminated waste into it and place a heavy cover to avoid access by animals, vermin or humans. In some countries the waste is placed in a shallow pit and burnt – this is not recommended.

7.2.4.6.1.9 **Social contact.** Social contact should be minimal or avoided until the patient has clinically recovered.

7.2.4.6.1.10 **Visitors.** Visitors should also understand the risk of the transmission of infection to themselves and observe the following restrictions:
- Visitors should be restricted to only a few adult visitors during the early period of infection.

- Instruct visitors, especially children, not to sit on the patient's bed.
- Children should not be allowed to visit unless under strict supervision.
- All visitors should maintain a safe distance of approximately 1 m.

7.2.4.6.1.11 Aftercare. To reduce the risk of further spread it should be remembered that some patients may carry on excreting the bacterium or virus for several weeks after they are clinically improved and therefore the following is recommended:

- Once the patient has recovered, the bed linen should be changed, soaked in bleach (optional) and washed in very hot water.
- All the patient's clothes should be washed thoroughly as well as any other soft furnishings that came into contact with the patient during the illness.
- The room should be cleaned and aired thoroughly before using again
- The toilet and bathroom should be cleaned thoroughly, dried and wiped over with bleach.

7.2.5 Blood-borne virus transmission

The transmission of blood-borne viruses may occur when infectious blood is accidentally passed on to a human, via a bite or inoculation, from an insect vector.

The other common means (non-vector) are when an infected human, either accidentally or deliberately, injects another human being or passes on the virus to him or her via sexual intercourse. This is more often seen among intravenous drug users. Patients admitted to healthcare facilities are accidentally exposed to sharps or poorly sterilised medical devices used during surgery or endoscopy. The IPC practices for both these routes of transmission are similar, with additional precautions for viral haemorrhagic fevers (VHFs) because of their high infectivity during acute disease.

7.2.5.1 Inoculation of contaminated blood by insect vectors

Diseases spread by vectors of major importance such as VHF usually occur in remote or rural areas where there is close proximity between humans and animals. The vector is usually a tick or another insect which bites and injects viruses or parasites into the bloodstream of the person, resulting in devastating consequences. The person-to-person spread occurs within close households and communities, either directly or from a common-source vector. The latter has only been recorded when accidental exposure to blood and body fluids has occurred in healthcare facilities owing to the lack of robust sterilisation and infection control practices – an important fact to remember.

Table 7.3 Some examples of common oro-faecal diseases which result in outbreaks or epidemics

Disease	Infecting agent	Incubation period	Diagnosis	Reservoir	Communicability	Immunisation
Typhoid	Salmonella enterica serovar typhi	8–14 days	Blood culture: 1st week Urine and faeces – 2nd week Bone marrow	Human	While excreting in faeces 5–15% carriers	Not routinely recommended
Paratyphoid	S paratyphi A and B	1–10 days	Faeces and blood culture	Human	While excreting in faeces	Not routinely recommended
Cholera	V cholerae: serotype O1 & O139	2–3 days	Faeces – rapid methods available	Human	While excreting in faeces	Not recommended
Hepatitis A (HAV)	Picornavirus RNA virus	28–30 days	IgM anti-HAV ab in serum; 5–10 days post-infection	Human; primates	Latter half of incubation period and early jaundice	For high-risk groups and travellers
Hepatitis E (HEV)	Non-enveloped single-strand RNA virus	15–64 days	IgM anti-HEV ab in serum	Human; primates	Not known	None

VHFs are a large group and some of them are of particular IPC relevance. They require immediate attention and intervention because of their high morbidity and mortality outcome. The main route of spread is via inoculation or injection of contaminated blood or direct contact with infected primates and humans. Prodromal symptoms of VHF are vague, with a flu-like illness before the haemorrhagic stage of the disease starts, and thus can reach outbreak proportions before being recognised.

Contact precautions with protection of all mucous membranes (droplet precautions) are advised because of the possibility of exposure to minute blood splashes during coughing or intubation from a bleeding respiratory tract.

When there is an outbreak of haemorrhagic fever prompt action must be taken at the local site where the first case has been suspected or confirmed. This is usually done by public health staff:

- Authorities should be notified immediately if a suspected or diagnosed patient has been identified, especially during an outbreak.
- The area is usually quarantined and the residents are not allowed to travel out of the area until there is clearance from the health authorities.
- There should be widespread awareness campaigns, education and support for the community.
- The healthcare facilities should be equipped to handle VHF, and care is usually provided in special isolation facilities.
- The staff should be trained and skilled in patient management.

The 2014 Ebola outbreak has highlighted the rapid spread of the disease due to fear, ignorance and lack of confidence in the healthcare systems. Rapid triage diagnosis and treatment of such patients can save lives. The IPC measures require extra vigilance when putting contact precautions with droplet precautions in place particularly for Ebola, where bleeding into the lungs can result in transmission via coughing or sneezing. The use of heat disinfection is recommended where possible, but the judicious use of disinfectants may be considered if heat is not possible.

7.2.5.1.1 Diseases transmitted by vectors

The recommendations discussed above should be applied for blood-borne viruses which are transmitted by vectors as explained earlier (see above). The diseases that fall into this category are listed below, but it is by no means a comprehensive list. Those of particular relevance to IPC are the VHFs in this group because of the highly infectious nature of some of them. Others are:

- Malaria
- Relapsing fever
- Sleeping sickness
- Schistosomiasis
- Typhus
- Yellow fever
- Dengue
- Leptospirosis.

VHFs are summed up in Table 7.4.

Table 7.4 Vector-borne VHFs and their clinical profiles

Disease	Infecting agent	Incubation period (days)	Diagnosis	Reservoir	Communicability	Immunisation
Dengue	Flavivirus: type 1, 2, 3, 4	3–14 days	Specific ab in serum – 5 days	Aedes aegypti mosquito	No person-to-person Human infectious 5 days Mosquito 8–12 days after feed	Vaccine for 9–16-yr-old children living in endemic areas
Ebola/Marburg	Filoviridae	2–21 days	Ab present in serum and body fluids	Unknown, possibly primates and fruit bats	Person-to-person via blood High risk during later stages of disease Semen infectious	Vaccine for Zaire strain available
Lassa fever	Arenavirus	6–21 days	Abs in serum, body fluids	Mastomys multimammate mouse	Person-to-person spread via secretions and urine up to 6 weeks	Under trial in Guinea
Crimean Congo haemorrhagic fever	Nairovirus	1–12 days	Virus isolated from blood	Ticks, farm animals as hosts	HAI – blood contact	Under development
Yellow fever	Flavivirus	3–6 days	Virus isolated from blood	Aedes aegypti in urban areas	Mosquito bite	Vaccine gives 10 years' immunity Mass immunisation

7.2.5.1.2 Public health measures for vector-borne diseases

When considering public health interventions it is always wise to include community education in the programme so that there is support and ownership of the prevention practices. As an example, a programme to eliminate or reduce yellow fever will include the following:

- Educate the public and promote behaviours to remove, destroy or manage vector and mosquito larval habitats, which for *Aedes aegypti* are usually artificial water-holding containers close to or inside human habitations. For example, old tyres, flowerpots, discarded containers for food or water storage.
- Remove contact with rodent and other animal vectors and improve reporting methods for pest control.
- Survey the community to determine the extent of the vector spread and organise treatment with appropriate larvicides.
- Ensure personal protection against day-biting mosquitoes or other vectors through repellents, screening and protective clothing.

7.2.5.1.3 Transmission of vector-borne viruses

There is no direct person-to-person transmission, but this may happen accidentally (see above). Patients usually haemorrhage into their internal organs and blood may be present in respiratory secretions, excretions and wound sites. Humans are usually infectious in the acute phase; however, the virus may be present in semen for several months after recovery. Ebola virus is known to survive in fresh dead bodies and therefore burial rituals must be carefully controlled. Insect vectors can become infected from biting humans who are in the acute phase of the illness. The vector remains infected for its life and this can prolong the transmission of infection.

7.2.5.2 IPC precautions for cases of VHF nursed at home

While it is essential that the authorities be notified immediately and the patient removed to a place where proper healthcare support can be delivered, there should be some IPC instruction to the household and/or caregiver before the patient is transferred to a secure treatment facility. Equally, there are some countries that will not admit VHF cases to a main hospital and will expect them to be cared for at home or in the community. Either way, IPC personnel and **caregivers must avoid direct contact with blood and body fluids of infected patients**. The hierarchy of control will require administrative controls including a surveillance and reporting system to a central command, engineering controls providing ventilation and good spacing in the clinical areas. Last, but not least, wearing appropriate PPE, in this case **contact plus droplet precautions**. This will require covering the body and all exposed areas, protecting the mucous membranes such as the eyes, nose and mouth, and a visor to protect the face from splashes.

Great care must be taken while donning and doffing the PPE. It should be done deliberately, carefully in a designated area. Spraying with chlorine is not recommended. A patient suffering from VHF is highly contagious during the acute phase and terminal phase; in Ebola dead bodies are particularly infectious because of a high viral load. There is a high risk to all coming into contact with even minute amounts of blood and body fluids. She or he may be unconscious, vomiting or bleeding from all orifices.

Before a person is transferred to the hospital, the family or caregiver may need to give some care and support and should consider the following IPC precautions in the interim:

- Move the patient into a separate single room (if possible), or isolate in a separate space, immediately and keep the door closed until the medical team arrives.
- Keep the room well ventilated but not cold.
- If there has to be any contact with or help given to the patient, make sure that the person dealing with him or her is aware of what to do and how to do it with appropriate protection.
- Hands should be washed thoroughly after each contact with the patient or his or her belongings (environment).
- The patient should be transferred to a medical facility as soon as possible for the best possible care.

To contain the cluster of cases or outbreak, one of the public health measures is to clean and spray the house with an insecticide. Make sure that **humans are not exposed to any of these dangerous chemicals**.

7.2.5.2.1 Caregiver

The caregiver dealing with any patient with a known blood-borne viral infection must carry out the following recommendations:

- Everyone should avoid all direct contact with the patient's secretions, blood and body fluids.
- The caregiver should be given means to look after the patient safely with adequate protection.
- Make sure the caregiver understands the clinical situation clearly and the risks involved.
- PPE should be made available as soon as possible. Gloves, face masks and plastic aprons should be provided and closed shoes worn.

In the absence of appropriate PPE for contact precautions the following may be used for emergencies but **are not recommended for routine use**:

- Wear a plastic sheet (or bin liner with a hole in it for the head) to cover the front and clothes and tie around the waist.

- If there are no gloves, use plastic bags to protect hands during contact.
- Several layers of cloth may be used to protect the nose and mouth (in the absence of a mask). Wind a scarf around your head, leaving only your eyes exposed.
- Wear glasses or goggles to protect the eyes – sunglasses will suffice.

To remove
- Turn bag covering the hand inside out on itself and discard into another plastic bag.
- Remove the plastic bag covering the body away from self and roll inside out.
- Wash hands with soap and water. Dry hands thoroughly. Use ABHR if available.
- Remove face cover and sunglasses carefully.

7.2.5.2.2 Healthcare workers

Healthcare workers who go to visit the patient or manage the patient in the community should take the following precautions:
- The healthcare worker should wear full PPE before entering the patient's room or having any contact with the patient in the home. These include:
  - Gloves, surgical masks (for splashes), visor, waterproof gown/apron (or coveralls) and closed footwear (boots)
- Wound care: If dressings are necessary, these should be done very carefully and contaminated dressings discarded into a plastic bag, which can be discarded later as highly infectious waste.
- Taking blood samples: If the patient is in the community and blood samples are required for laboratory tests prior to the medical team arriving, the healthcare worker must wear well-fitting latex gloves and use a safe closed system (such as a vacuum tube) to take blood and make sure the hands are thoroughly cleaned after the gloves are removed.
- The PPE is removed once the healthcare worker has finished attending to the patient and is discarded immediately. The healthcare worker must wash her or his hands thoroughly or use ABHR before doing anything else. This can be a difficult task.

7.2.5.2.3 Patient-care item

These should be dedicated to that person's use only (razors, toothbrushes) and should be washed very carefully by holding them under the surface of the water to avoid splashing.

7.2.5.2.4 Toilet and bathroom facilities

Most of the patients cared for at home will be bed-bound and will require care while prostrated or semi-conscious. The caregiver should always wear protective equipment when dealing with the patient's needs or providing care.

- If the patient has diarrhoea, use old clothes as nappies that can be changed and discarded immediately when soiled. Bed-bound patients require bedpans and these should be handled with great care. The caregiver should:
  - — Wear adequate protective equipment when giving the patient the bedpan.
  - — Once the patient has completed its use, the bedpan should be removed and covered with a plastic bag to reduce spillage.
  - — The contents should be discarded in toilet. In the absence of a toilet, a 1 m pit should be dug far away from dwellings. Dispose of the contents of the bedpan there and cover with a layer of soil.
  - — The bedpan should be washed carefully and thoroughly while wearing PPE, to remove all organic matter, and dried. Some recommend the use of bleach at this stage.

7.2.5.2.5 Washing and cleaning the patient

This should be performed with full protective equipment, using a separate water bowl and disposable cloth. The cloth can then be thrown away (discarded) into the bag for infectious waste.

7.2.5.2.6 Crockery and cutlery

Although there is little risk of transmission by the oro-faecal route, the cleaning of the patient's crockery and cutlery should be done carefully. The person cleaning the crockery should make sure that his or her skin is intact if gloves are not available. It is advisable to keep the patient's feeding utensils separate so that these can be thoroughly cleaned with hot water and detergent and then dried thoroughly. The water tumblers should be for the exclusive use of the patient.

7.2.5.2.7 Bedclothes, linen and patient's clothes

Washing the clothes and bed linen from an infectious patient presents particular challenges in a home with poor resources. The washing will invariably be done manually. Since the patient's linen may be contaminated with blood and body fluids, particular care should be taken during washing to avoid splashes. The person washing the linen should:

- Wear PPE (as described above) when washing clothes or bed linen.
- Soak items in very hot water with bleach for 10 minutes. Remove and wash using hot water and detergent and dry.
- Do not wash the patient's clothing or articles in communal areas like rivers or lakes.

7.2.5.2.8 Waste

The handling of waste in the home requires particular care since it is very infectious. The designated caregiver should be taught to keep a separate plastic bag or closed container for discarding all soiled and contaminated items such as nappies. Ideally, the waste should be incinerated with minimal handling. However, since this is not always possible, empty the contents into a pit approximately 1 m deep and cover to prevent access by animals.

7.2.5.2.9 The environment

The room of a patient has an effect on his or her morale so it should be clean, airy and free of clutter. It must also be free from vectors such as ticks and mosquitoes and, if possible, the room should be sprayed with an insecticide, but ONLY when the patient is out of the room. Spraying with chlorine is not recommended.

7.2.5.2.10 Social contact

Only designated caregivers should be allowed contact until the patient is transferred to a healthcare facility. Visitors, especially children, should not be allowed to come into the patient's room but can communicate through a window or open space at a distance of at least 2 m. Visitors should be instructed not to touch the patient or sit on the patient's bed. The visit should be brief.

7.2.5.3 Rituals after death

In some communities there are prolonged burial rituals where the body is touched by all the funeral attendees. Sometimes the body is bathed before being buried. **Physical contact with the corpse is not recommended.** Appropriate PPE should be worn when touching the corpse. The body is placed in double bags, which are sealed prior to burial. These are traumatic times for the family and they should be allowed to participate safely as part of the burial so that they can say their farewell to their loved ones.

There is clear evidence that dead bodies of those who succumbed to EVD had high viral counts present in their body secretions. For this reason, the corpse should not be allowed to be handled by untrained persons or the family. Postmortems are not recommended. When carrying out the last rites the family may be present and participate by helping to dig the grave, recite prayers and conduct rituals that do not involve touching the body, observe the burial and help to put the soil on top of the coffin.

7.2.5.4 Care of viral haemorrhagic fever patients in hospital

Care of patients such as these in hospitals has been covered in transmission-based precautions, but the salient features of these precautions that safeguard patients and healthcare workers are summarised here. Contact and droplet precautions must be applied.

- The hospital should be informed in advance that a suspected case of VHF is expected. The clinical condition of the patient will dictate the type of care and whether or not the patient requires respiratory support. The patient may be unconscious, incontinent or bleeding.

7.2.5.4.1 Precautions for healthcare workers in hospital

The patient must be isolated in a single room immediately upon arrival at the hospital, directly from the ambulance (see section 5.7.1 Isolation facilities). All healthcare workers entering the patient's room should apply **contact and droplet precautions** at all times when in contact with the patient. The following course of action must be carried out methodically:

- Change out of street clothes and shoes.
- Wear full PPE before any contact with the patient:
  - Gloves, surgical masks (for splashes), visor, waterproof gown/apron and covered footwear (boots).
  - Overshoes are not recommended as you might trip or slip.
- Plan the management of this case and document this plan in the form of a checklist. The plan includes:
  - Setting up a separate IPC trolley dedicated to the patient with all the necessary items needed for care.
  - Placement of the patient: (a) single room with en suite facilities; (b) negative pressure ventilation especially for Lassa and Ebola; (c) door closed at all times; (d) clear signage on the door.
  - There should be a record of all staff who carry out invasive procedures on the patient in case of accidental injury.

7.2.5.4.2 Additional IPC measures

- **Safe disposal of sharps.** In the isolation facility there should be a new sharps box dedicated to this particular patient placed within arm's reach of the bed so that once the sharp has been used, it is disposed of immediately. The sharps container should be sealed and clearly labelled when three-quarters full.
- **Urinary catheter** should be inserted very carefully, avoiding contact with the urine, especially if containing blood. The urinary bag should be connected and a closed system of drainage maintained. Staff emptying the urinary bag must wear full contact PPE. The urine should be emptied into a jug with a lid which can be disposed of immediately in an automatic washer-disinfector on the ward.
- **Intubation for mechanical ventilation** of such a patient should be carried out only by experienced staff wearing full personal protection to avoid splash contamination. A closed endotracheal suctioning system only should be used and single-use disposable endotracheal suction catheters are preferred.

- **Respiratory ventilator circuit** should either be disposable (preferable) or heat-disinfected at 80 °C for 3 minutes through an automated washer-disinfector.
- **Wound care** should be done carefully and without interruption, preferably by an experienced healthcare worker. It would require preplanning to make sure that all items needed for the dressing are present on the dressing trolley before hand (see section 4.6.6.1 Procedure for dressing a wound). Closed suction drainage should be applied if there is fluid in the wound. Dressings should be discarded directly as infectious waste.
- **Patient care articles** should be dedicated single-patient use only for the duration of the patient's stay.
- **Linen** should clearly be marked as infectious. It should be transported and washed separately from the regular load if it is sent to the laundry. The laundry should use an automated system for washing such linen.

7.2.5.5 Non-vector-borne exposure to blood-borne viruses

Blood-borne transmission more commonly occurs in the absence of insect vectors when infected blood is injected into a human. The route of transmission is inoculation and therefore the same IPC principles apply. Some of these viruses also spread via sexual contact, but it is their association with contaminated needles, sharps or medical equipment that is of relevance to IPC. All used sharps are potentially infectious and direct contact with them should be avoided.

In an order of rank of the commonly found blood-borne viruses in most communities, hepatitis B is highly infectious, hepatitis C less so and HIV is the least infectious. In fact, HIV requires a substantial amount of blood or body fluid to transmit disease. A particular challenge with HIV is that the care of patients is complicated by the opportunistic infections acquired because of suppressed immunity. Of these, pulmonary tuberculosis is of major concern and up to 38% of HIV-infected cases are co-infected with tuberculosis. Other diseases such as cryptosporidial diarrhoea, esophageal candidiasis or Kaposi's sarcoma are not infectious.

7.2.5.6 Diseases transmitted via blood (non-vector)

Communicable diseases (Table 7.5) transmitted via blood are listed below. The first three are of IPC importance:
- **Hepatitis B**
- **Hepatitis C**
- **HIV**
- VHFs (healthcare associated – see above)
- Malaria (during acute phase of illness)
- Syphilis

Table 7.5 Blood-borne viruses transmitted between humans by means other than insect vectors, their distribution and clinical profile

Disease	Infecting agent	Incubation period	Diagnosis	Reservoir	Communicability	Immunisation
Acquired immune deficiency syndrome (AIDS)	Retrovirus: HIV-1 and HIV-2	1–3 months; HIV to AIDS up to 15 years	HIV ab in serum; low CD4 counts	Humans	Exposure to high viral loads; presence of other STI	None at present; vaccines trials under way
Hepatitis B (HBV) (also delta)	Hepadnavirus	45–180 days	Specific antibodies and antigen in blood	Humans	All HbsAg positive persons via blood and body fluids	Widely available; very effective
Hepatitis C (HCV)	Enveloped RNA-virus; Flaviviridae	2 weeks – 6 months	Anti-HCV in blood	Humans	1 week before onset of symptoms Liver enzymes raised	None at present

7.2.5.6.1 Public health measures to prevent transmission of blood-borne viruses (non-vector)

The general public need to be aware of how the transmission of blood-borne pathogens occurs and the ways of avoiding infection. The following list outlines the safe behaviour that minimises the risk of blood-borne virus transmission. The first item is education of the public since it is only through being informed and convinced that people will practise safe behaviour.

- Education of the public regarding the modes of transmission. This covers the danger of contact with blood and body fluids.
- Safe sex by using condoms.
- Not sharing needles and syringes among intravenous drug users. Needle exchange programmes are available in most developed countries, where intravenous drug users can bring their used syringes and needles to a central drop-off point and these are exchanged for sterile ones while the used ones are returned and safely disposed.
- Screening of blood and blood products for blood-borne viruses.
- Preventing perinatal mother-to-infant transmission by providing anti-retroviral cover during late pregnancy and labour.
- Preventing nosocomial exposure to contaminated sharps and inadequately disinfected or sterilised equipment. Some blood-borne viruses are stable in the environment and these can be transmitted by indirect inoculation via inanimate objects.
- Use of disposable single-use needles and syringes in healthcare.
- Transmission to patients from HBsAg-positive healthcare workers has rarely been documented except from surgeons.

7.2.5.6.2 IPC precautions for non-vector blood-borne virus transmission

There is very little risk to the general population or healthcare worker from such patients unless there is a means of inoculating either accidentally or deliberately. The IPC precautions instituted here are **standard precautions** and should be applied to all risk procedures whether these are undertaken in a healthcare or home setting. However, if there is massive bleeding then **contact precautions** should be instituted.

The principles are:
- Avoid contact with all blood and body fluids.
- Avoid contaminated needles. Infection can be transmitted from person to person via needles and syringes; thus intravenous drug users are particularly at risk.
- Careful handling and disposal of sharps.

7.2.5.6.2.1 Applying IPC principles to non-vector transmission in the community

A summary of how these principles are applied in practice is given below.

7.2.5.6.2.2 The patient

Patients who are infected with hepatitis B or C and HIV may be nursed at home safely unless there is a specific reason for them to be admitted to hospital. For example, an HIV-infected patient may require hospitalisation for a serious opportunistic infection such as cryptococcal meningitis or tuberculosis pneumonia. In the home, if the risk increases, contact precautions can be applied. Most patients with blood-borne viruses manage to look after themselves. There is no need for separate facilities.

7.2.5.6.2.3 Caregiver

The caregiver, if one is needed, should be aware of what he or she can help the patient with and how best to do so. The following IPC principles apply:

- Some type of hand cover should be worn only when dealing with blood or body fluids from an infected patient. Gloves are best, but if these are not available an intact plastic bag may be used to handle items contaminated with blood and body fluids.
- Wash hands immediately after contact.
- The caregiver's hands should have intact skin.
- No special precautions are needed (if the skin is intact) when caring for the patient such as bathing, helping him or her out of bed, or feeding the patient.

7.2.5.6.2.4 Healthcare worker

Healthcare workers need to be aware that the average household will have no equipment at all. They should ensure that they carry with them:

- a supply of non-sterile gloves
- a small sharps container to carry the needles and syringes back to the clinic if injections are administered
- a small bottle of hand ABHR for personal use. Hand hygiene is of the essence.

7.2.5.6.2.5 Toilet and bathroom facilities

There are no restrictions on communal-use ablution facilities or toilets. The toilet should be clean and dry. If the patient has diarrhoea and is bedridden, hand covering should be worn to remove the bedpan and clean the patient. Hands should be washed thoroughly afterwards. The patient can be bathed without the use of protective equipment provided the patient's skin is intact.

7.2.5.6.2.6 Waste

Generally the waste from hepatitis and HIV patients needs no particular treatment except that care should be taken when disposing of contaminated sharps. It should be noted that sanitary towels and nappies can be discarded in domestic waste.

7.2.5.6.2.7 Patient-use articles

Shaving equipment, toothbrushes and other personal use items should be for the patient's use alone. Such equipment should not be shared.

7.2.5.6.2.8 Precautions for other items

No special precautions need to be taken with the following items:
- crockery and cutlery
- bed linen and clothes.

7.2.5.6.2.9 Social contact

Socialising with friends and family should be encouraged to boost the patient's morale. Visitors, including children, are allowed and, provided there is no opportunistic infection present, can freely touch, cuddle or hug the patient.

Sexual contact is only acceptable with the use of condoms.

7.2.6 Transmission of infectious agents via the respiratory route

Unlike hospitals, where transmission-based precautions for droplet and aerosol (airborne) infections are differentiated, in the domestic environment, precautions for all transmissions of pathogens via the respiratory route can be covered by applying similar IPC principles. Current thinking is that the respiratory cloud expels a large number of particles of varying sizes and depending upon the atmospheric conditions, these may travel near or far (see section 4.2.3.6.4). Generally, respiratory infections via infectious nuclei spread rapidly, particularly in poorly ventilated areas and affect a large population quickly, such as the H1N1 influenza and SARS-CoV-2 pandemics. These pandemics could end just as quickly and, depending on the season, are soon over. However, with COVID-19 there are waves of increased infection caused by various mutants, and a combination of influenza and COVID-19 could be disastrous. The challenges are to differentiate seasonal respiratory diseases from epidemic strains. The influenza and SARS-CoV-2 viruses mutate rapidly, resulting in major morbidity, particularly among those who have not been vaccinated.

Alerts are raised by the WHO and all member countries are informed of the level of infected cases across the globe. Public health authorities should be prepared for outbreaks of respiratory diseases of global significance and prevention strategies should be in place. Respiratory infections that spread by smaller airborne nuclie, such as TB, are more insidious in their transmission and affect the community for a long time, spreading slowly through it.

Table 7.6 Transmission via the respiratory route

Disease	Infecting agent	Incubation period	Diagnosis	Reservoir	Communicability	Immunisation
Influenza	Type A, B and C with many serotypes	1–3 days	Detection of virus in secretions, antibodies in blood	Humans; birds, primates, mammals	3–6 days (adults); 7 days (children)	Partial efficacy as virus mutates frequently
SARS-CoV-2	Coronavirus	3–10 days	Antibodies in serum – PCR	Birds, fowls	Probably 21 days	Vaccines widely available
Meningococcal meningitis	Neisseria meningitidis	2–10 days	CSF and blood culture positive	Humans	Up to 24 hours post-antimicrobial therapy	A and C effective for mass gatherings
Tuberculosis (pulmonary)	Mycobacterium tuberculosis	2–4 weeks; could be shorter or longer	Smear-positive sputum (or clinical suspicion of disease)	Humans and primates	As long as untreated; up to 2 weeks after appropriate therapy	BCG widely used for susceptible population
Measles	Morbillivirus	10 days	Usually clinical; antibodies in serum	Humans	1 days before prodrome to 4 days after rash	Effective vaccination

7.2.6.1 *Diseases transmitted via the respiratory route (examples)*

7.2.6.1.1 Airborne transmission (smaller infectious nuclie)

- Measles
- Tuberculosis
- Chickenpox
- SARS-CoV-2 and influenza during an outbreak

7.2.6.1.2 Droplet transmission (larger infectious nuclie)

- Meningitis
- Pertussis
- SARS-CoV-2
- Influenza (all types)

7.2.6.2 *Public health measures*

Public health control measures are based on levels of alert issued by the WHO and should be put into place urgently to prevent spread of respiratory pathogens within the local community. With increasing global travel, it is inevitable that pandemics like H1N1 influenza and COVID-19 rapidly arrive on the shores of most countries within days. It was clear that the world, and the WHO, was not prepared for the COVID-19 pandemic. Many lessons were learnt during the steep learning curve on dealing with this virus. An important message was that during a pandemic, viruses that are usually controlled with administrative, engineering (ventilation, bed spacing) and PPE (face covers) measures required deeper investigation into the routes of transmission. New evidence suggests that respiratory pathogen transmission should be considered as part of a whole, the infective cloud, which carries varying sizes of infectious particles.

How this affects IPC practices is uncertain, given that the current transmission-based precautions have stood us in good stead to date. There were clear indications that SARS-CoV-2 had to be treated like an airborne pathogen during the height of the pandemic and beyond.

The public health services usually increase the level of awareness to prepare the community for the pending outbreak or epidemic. These include:

- Media alert and awareness campaigns. The campaigns include the distribution of information via pamphlets, television and newspapers on how to prevent transmission.
- Early alerts and reporting of suspected pandemic infectious strains that occur within households or are identified at airports and other entry points for those travelling into the country.
- Public health measures widely broadcast, including basic hygiene measures such as cough etiquette, hand hygiene and appropriate disposal of waste.
- Extensive research and development into means of containing the pathogens.
- Rapid publication of relevant evidence to allow for informed decision-making.

The other public health concern currently is **tuberculosis**. Recently emerging multidrug-resistant TB has concentrated the minds of public health and IPC teams to increase awareness and, where possible, contain its spread. The transmission of TB is most common in a closed environment such as overcrowded institutions, prisons and homes. It is beyond the scope of this chapter to discuss TB in detail beyond section 7.2.6.3.2.2 below. Readers are referred to the literature on the most recent advances in TB management.[11]

7.2.6.3 IPC precautions for the respiratory route of transmission

7.2.6.3.1 IPC precautions for management of droplet-precaution respiratory diseases

For details see section 4.2.3 Transmission-based precautions.
- Isolation of suspected or confirmed cases and the application of **droplet precautions** (see (see section 4.2.3.6.4).
- Particular attention should be paid to interventions such as the use of nebulisers, chest physiotherapy, bronchoscopy or gastroscopy and other interventions that may disrupt the respiratory tract or place the healthcare worker in close proximity to the patient and to potentially infected secretions.
- PPE is discarded as infectious waste.

7.2.6.3.2 IPC principles applied at home

The general principles are as follows for those transmitted by droplet infection (see above):
- Separate the patient from other members of the household and visitors if possible.
- Open windows to increase ventilation.
- Prevent the spread from respiratory secretions by interrupting dispersal.
- Practice good hand hygiene.
- Ensure a clean and airy environment.

7.2.6.3.2.1 IPC practices for managing respiratory infections at home

7.2.6.3.2.1.1 The patient. The principles governing the care of the patient centre on minimising the spread of infection through coughing and sneezing:
- Place the patient in a single room, near a window, if possible, with the door closed.
- Provide tissues or a hanky to be used to cover the mouth and nose when sneezing or coughing (putting one's head under the blanket is also acceptable).

---

[11]   First National Tuberculosis Survey, South Africa, 2018.

- Discard tissues into a plastic bag placed near the bed – do not drop on the floor. Clean hands immediately after using tissue or hanky – ABHR or wipe works well if there are no handwashing facilities in the patient's room.
- If the patient has to leave the room, she or he may do so to go into the open air and should be reminded of complying with the cough etiquette.
- Windows may be opened in the summer; in the winter heating should be provided with the window slightly open if possible.
- Provide some entertainment (TV or radio) so that the patient remains in the room.

7.2.6.3.2.1.2 *Caregivers (household and healthcare workers).* Caregivers need to take precautions to avoid airborne transmission. They should:

- Cover nose and mouth during close contact when attending to the patient.
    - surgical mask is recommended for healthcare workers, or
    - cloth mask tied back to cover mouth and nose.
- Wash hands immediately and dry or use ABHR after each contact.

When cleaning the patient's environment they must be aware that droplet spread can contaminate surfaces, bedclothes and the carer's clothes. They should:

- clean all surfaces daily and keep them dry
- not sit on the patient's bed.

There is no need for the patient to have a face cover if he or she goes into the open air, but he or she should maintain cough etiquette and cover the nose and mouth during coughing. This is because the risk of transmission is less than in a confined space. Maintain a distance of at least 2 m between the patient and others if socialising.

7.2.6.3.2.1.3 *Toilet and washing facilities.* Some of the poorer communities may have communal toilets located outside the house.

7.2.6.3.2.1.4 *Crockery and cutlery.* Wash the crockery and cutlery in very hot water and air-dry. There is no indication to separate these utensils from those of the rest of the household. The patient's water glass should be dedicated for her or his use only (respiratory secretions).

7.2.6.3.2.1.5 *Waste.* Used tissues and other similar waste can be discarded with the ordinary domestic waste.

7.2.6.3.2.1.6 *Social contact.* Most people do not feel like socialising when they are very sick, but patients should be prevented from socialising, even when recovering, until the symptoms have cleared. If patients insists on socialising, ask them to set up a place in the open air and wear a mask where they can socialise without risk to others.

7.2.6.3.2.1.7 *Visitors*. Visitors need to be carefully instructed so that they do not come into close contact with the patient – maintain a distance of at least 2 m.

- Do not allow visitors except caregivers during the infectious phase of the disease. Visits may be allowed during convalescence, but should not sit on the patient's bed.
- Children should not be allowed to climb on the bed or come in close contact with the patient.
- Visitors should be discouraged from providing health support for the patient (unless they are trained). This should be left to the designated caregiver.

7.2.6.3.2.1.8 *Aftercare*. Once the patient has recovered, the bed linen and window covering should be changed and washed. The room should be cleaned and aired thoroughly before use.

7.2.6.3.2.2 Additional precautions for cases of tuberculosis at home

In addition to the precautions mentioned above, cases of tuberculosis require additional precautions. The caregiver and healthcare worker should wear a surgical mask when tending to the patient during the first week of starting therapy because the patient is still considered infectious. If the patient leaves the room, he or she should also be given a surgical mask to use for the first week after starting therapy.

If the patient is known to have multidrug-resistant TB, it is recommended that a surgical face mask should be worn whenever he or she leaves the room for as long as the patient remains infectious (smear results remain positive). Healthcare workers are advised to wear well-fitted respirators, while caregivers can be supplied with well fitting surgical masks. There should be minimum contact with friends and relatives, but the patient should be allowed to go into the open to sit and should wear a surgical mask.

The patient should sleep on his or her own with the windows open to improve ventilation.

If the patient is still coughing, a supply of tissues should be available to cough into, which are discarded into a plastic bag. This bag can be placed in the municipal waste and sent for landfill.

All surfaces in the room must be clean and kept dust-free to reduce environmental contamination.

7.2.6.3.2.3 *IPC principles for managing a patient with respiratory communicable disease in the hospital*

The management of patients with a suspected or confirmed respiratory disease in hospital was differentiated by the size of respiratory secretion particle into droplet or airborne transmission precautions (see (see section 4.2.3.6.2). One school of thought is that all respiratory infections should be considered airborne, thus identifying the route, or vehicle, of transmission. Either way, current IPC transmission-based precautions will remain the same for now until the matter is resolved.

The foremost task of the clinical management team is to identify all suspect and probable cases of the outbreak strain of respiratory infection such as TB, influenza or SARS-CoV-2 using the WHO case definitions. Probable cases should then be rapidly diverted by triage to a separate area and given a face mask.

During outbreaks of rapidly spreading respiratory disease such as SARS or influenza, contact tracing is required to determine the extent of the problem.

Any person (a contact) who cared for, lived with, or had direct contact with the respiratory secretions, body fluids and/or excretion (e.g. faeces) of a suspected or probable case of SARS or influenza is asked to report to a health facility if he or she develops symptoms. Usually there is such a large population affected that active contact tracing is not necessary.

7.2.6.3.3 Additional precautions for TB cases in hospitals

Ideally the patient should be isolated in a single room with negative-pressure ventilation and en suite facilities when admitted to a hospital. If this is not possible, the patient should be placed at the far end of the ward next to an open window.

For multidrug-resistant TB it is essential that a single room be found where the patient will remain until he or she either is ready for discharge or has become sputum-smear negative.

During the first week or two (infectious period) everyone coming into close proximity of the patient should wear a surgical mask and observe airborne precautions. If the patient has multidrug-resistant TB, healthcare workers should be offered well-fitting respirators. Visitors should be restricted.

It is advisable to discharge the patient as soon as he or she is well enough to leave the hospital and arrangements should be made to have medication, including injections, given to the patient in the community by a healthcare worker, as prescribed.

7.2.7 Prions

Prions are to date the smallest infectious particles identified as transmissible pathogenic agents and are unrelated to viruses, bacteria, fungi or protozoa infections. They are made up of nucleic acids alone. Prions are an abnormal conformation (PrPSc) of a normal cellular protein, known as the prion protein (PrP).

Prions cause a variety of neurodegenerative diseases in mammals and animals that include scrapie in goats and sheep, bovine spongiform encephalitis (BSE) in cattle and Creutzfeldt–Jakob disease (CJD) in humans. What happens is that when a prion from one species enters another species it replicates and changes enough as to be distinguishable from its original conformation. It accumulates in the brain and nervous tissue, which causes neuronal dysfunction. Prions cause disease that can manifest in infectious, inherited or sporadic illnesses.

The duration of illness is usually years and there is slow degeneration of nervous tissue in all the species it infects.

7.2.7.1 Transmission

Transmission to humans can occur in the following ways:
- **The food chain.** Prions cross species when offal and brain tissue of one animal, sheep with scrapie for instance, is mixed with feeds for cattle. The cattle then develop bovine spongiform encephalitis (BSE) and when consumed by humans these prions infect the human neural system and the brain resulting in vCJD.
- **Contaminated medical devices** that have been used in neurosurgical procedures and processed normally via routinely available sterile service systems.
- **Contaminated medical products**, such as human growth hormone (HGH), that were derived from cadavers of undiagnosed cases of vCJD.

There has been no person-to-person transmission reported except in Papua New Guinea, where ritual eating of a dead family member's brain and organs passed on the disease. There is also no evidence that prions can spread via blood or blood products despite concerns to the contrary.

7.2.7.2 Decontamination of medical devices and other products

Prions are very difficult to remove or kill, possibly because of the lack of cellular components, which are usually the targets of decontamination and disinfection. Robust systems should be put into place to ensure thorough cleaning, decontamination and sterilisation of all items. The difficulties are:
- Since the particles are tiny, they pass through most filter systems that will retain bacteria and viruses.
- They also have a tendency to aggregate and cannot be solubilised by detergents, except under denaturing conditions where infectivity is lost.
- Prions are not affected by nuclease enzymes, metals ion chelators, acids with pH ranges between 3 and 7, formalin, boiling or proteases. In fact, there is very little that inactivates prions.
- Two steam sterilisation cycles at 134 °C with a prolonged exposure time are recommended by some reports. More recently hydrogen peroxide chemical sterilisation has been reported to be effective.

7.2.7.3 IPC precautions

Carry out a risk assessment regarding processing the medical devices. Should these be discarded? Should these be processed? Whatever the decision, it should be made by the clinical team, IPC and SSD. The main risk lies with cutting procedures involving exposure to neural tissue such as neurosurgery or post-mortems.

7.2.7.3.1 Transmission-based precautions

There is no direct person-to-person transmission, but contact with infected neurological tissue poses a risk and therefore **contact precautions** are advised. There is no transmission via the airborne or droplet routes.

7.2.7.3.2 Cutting procedures (post-mortem or surgery)

- The case should be identified prior to starting the post-mortem.
- The area should be cleared and this case done last.
- The surfaces should be covered with disposable sheets that can be incinerated afterwards.
- Proper PPE should be made available:
  - It is strongly recommended that **cut-resistant gloves** be worn under surgical gloves – maximum protection is required to reduce exposure.
  - **Respirators and face shields** are advised because of the bony fragments when cutting into the skull.
  - Waterproof body cover should be worn.
- It is recommended that all PPE is single use and is incinerated after discarding into infectious waste.

If accidental contamination of the healthcare worker's skin occurs, 1 N sodium hydroxide should be applied to the area for five minutes and then washed thoroughly with large quantities of water. **Surface contamination** can be cleaned with repeatedly wetting with 2 N sodium hydroxide for one hour.

7.2.7.3.3 Safety cabinets

All neuro tissue should be processed (fixed or cut) in a Class 2 safety cabinet fitted with HEPA filters. These filters should be changed frequently and sterilised before being incinerated. The internal surfaces of the safety cabinet should be decontaminated with 1 N sodium hydroxide followed by 1 N hydrochloric acid and rinsed with water.

7.2.7.3.4 Recommendation for medical device decontamination for vCJD

There are differences of opinion between various countries. In the UK[12] all medical devices are single-use only and sent for incineration after the procedure, in the

---

[12] www.nice.org.uk/guidance/ipg666.

belief that steam, no matter how long it is applied for, cannot denature prions. The USA policies favour two cycles of sterilisation pre- and post-decontamination processing.

The effective decontamination of instruments used in neurosurgery should be considered for the presence of vCJD since there have been several cases of vCJD reported from South Africa over several years.

- The instrument trays should be clearly labelled if neurodegenerative disease is suspected, wrapped separately with minimal contact and sent to SSD. The processing of such items is a skilled and prolonged business and cannot be rushed.
- Infectivity of prions can be diminished by prolonged digestion with proteases or boiling in sodium dodecyl sulphate. It has been shown that autoclaving at 134 °C for 4.5 hours was able to sterilise a rodent's brain with high titres of prions.
- Of the disinfectants, denaturing organic solvents such as phenol (1 : 1), chaotropic agents such as guanidine isocyanate or hydrochloride (>4 mol/l) or alkali such as sodium hydroxide for 24 hours can dramatically reduce the infectivity of prions.

Procedure for decontamination (USA)[13]:
- The SSD should be informed that a tray of instruments either from the surgical suite or the mortuary is arriving so that they can prepare.
- All instruments are opened and placed in a large stainless steel container and soaked for one hour in 2 N sodium hydroxide or two hours in 1 N sodium hydroxide, or placed in a steriliser at 134 °C for
  − one hour in a gravity displacement steriliser
  − one 18-minute cycle at 30 psi or six 3-minute cycles at 30 psi in a porous load steam steriliser
- Instruments can then be carefully removed from the steriliser and cleaned.

The person cleaning the instruments should be properly garbed.

The instruments are cleaned very carefully by hand by an experienced person or in an automated washer-disinfector.

The items are then packed and processed for the second time through a steriliser. Anecdotally, to date approximately 25 cases of CJD have been reported from South Africa which is in keeping with 3 to 4 cases in a million of the population.[14]

13   Centers for Disease Control and Prevention CDC (2020). Prion Diseases. Available from https://www.cdc. gov/prions/index.html [accessed 5.2.2021]
14   Toovey S, Britz M & Hewlett R. 2006. *South African Medical Journal* 96(7): 592–93.

7.3 Occupational health

There is a close working relationship between occupational health (OH) and IPC teams. The latter ensures that the work environment is safe for patients and staff to perform optimally, while OH treats and manages the welfare of staff. The health and safety officer is responsible for evaluating the workplace and applying risk assessment and evaluating the work conditions according to the level of risk. These three, OH, IPC and quality improvement, form part of the quality assurance programme.

7.3.1 Legislation governing occupational health

Occupational health is regulated by several pieces of legislature, but the main one is the Occupational Health and Safety Act of 1993 (South Africa)[15] and, as in other countries such as the UK and the US, covers all aspects of safety in the workplace. It is beyond the scope of this book to detail the OH regulations, but it suffices to say that IPC works to prevent the biohazard aspects of the Act.

7.3.2 OHS Act

The Occupational Health and Safety Act 85 of 1993 and the Compensation for Occupational Injuries and Diseases Act 130 of 1993 are administered in South Africa by the Department of Labour. The OHS Act lays out what must be done to make the workplace healthy and safe for employees with the aims of creating a safe and satisfactory working environment and a healthy, active and productive worker. It has a system of inspection to make sure that the workplace conforms with safety regulations and to advise employers on how to improve working conditions.

7.3.3 Liability of employer

The employer is liable for payment of wages/salary for the first three months from the date of occupational injury and has to register the injury with the Department of Labour and complete a resumption of work report.

7.3.4 Compensation

In South Africa medical costs, transportation costs (evacuation/ongoing treatment) and funeral costs are covered by the employer and these include compensation for permanent disability and payment of wages/salary at 75% of the level of pay, but not payments for temporary disablement that lasts less than four days.

---

15   Department of Labour. South Africa. 1993. Occupational Health and Safety Act 85 of 1993.

7.3.5 Functions of occupational health

The OH department carries out medical evaluations on all staff in the facility. This includes a pre-employment questionnaire to make sure the member of staff is appointed to the correct post following the pre-placement questionnaire. Some OH departments carry out random and periodic surveys on health and all OH departments must carry out an exit interview if a member of staff leaves. There are also several other evaluations which they perform such as fitness to return to work, fitness to wear PPE, vaccination history and completion of vaccination schedules, biological monitoring of high-risk areas such as the TB wards and, very rarely, they offer some primary medical care to staff such as helping them with the Directly Observed Treatment, short-course (DOTS) programme.

OH works closely with IPC teams to evaluate risks of transmission of viable hazardous biological agents from a primary source (usually a patient or a laboratory) and the IPC team is represented on the occupational health and safety committee.

7.3.6 Staff protection

The OH department, especially in larger healthcare facilities, offers outpatients services and health evaluation. Of interest to IPC is the immune status of the patient and the availability of post-exposure prophylaxis following accidental exposure to blood-borne viruses.

7.3.6.1 Environment in the workplace

The other important aspect is that the environment in which staff work should be safe. When working in a busy healthcare facility, especially where there is a high risk of acquiring respiratory infections such as TB, adequate ventilation should be provided (see section 5.3.6.1 Ventilation). Staff should have areas for relaxation and taking breaks which are open, airy and well ventilated (transmission in enclosed and poorly ventilated tea rooms during the COVID-19 pandemic was well recognised).

7.3.6.2 Immune status of the healthcare worker

The immune status of the healthcare worker is private, but it does become relevant when there is a shortage of staff and the person is required to work in a highly infectious environment. For this reason it is essential that the following information is available at the OH department about all members of staff:

- **Immunisation** against hepatitis B should be recorded when any person starts work in a healthcare facility. See Table 7.7.
- **Post-exposure prophylaxis (PEP).** Healthcare workers exposed to HIV-infected sources should be administered PEP preferably within four hours but

not later than 48 hours. The member of staff who has been exposed should report to a designated station to have blood taken for HIV antibody levels. A sample of blood from the source is necessary, which is tested for HIV and hepatitis B and C. The healthcare worker can be started on the following regime (current treatment regime) while awaiting results:
— AZT 200 mg; 8-hourly × 28 days
— 3TC 150 mg: 12-hourly × 28 days.

If the source blood is uninfected, the PEP can be stopped. If it is found to be positive, then the regime may be modified to three drugs, depending on the findings.

Table 7.7 Immunisation schedule for hepatitis B: Immunisation for healthcare workers

Hepatitis B immunisation	HBV Status of source and treatment		
HWC	HBsAg +	HbsAg–	Unknown
Unvaccinated or documented non-response to previous vaccination. HBsAb < 10 IU/ml	Vaccinate 3 doses + HBIG × 1	Vaccinate 3 doses	Vaccinate 3 doses + HBIG × 1
Vaccinated HBsAb < 50 IU/ml	Booster + HBIG × 1	Booster	Booster + HBIG × 1
Vaccinated HBsAb > 50 IU/ml	No action	No action	No action

7.3.6.3 Work restriction for HIV- or hepatitis B-infected healthcare worker

There is one more area in which IPC should advise. HIV-infected healthcare workers should not be exposed to unnecessary risks and therefore, with consultation, should be placed where they are of little risk to themselves or the patients and public. The recommendations are that in the absence of exposure-prone invasive procedures there are generally no work restrictions. However, the following precautions are necessary:
- Healthcare workers infected with hepatitis B or HIV should not perform exposure-prone procedures unless cleared by an expert review panel, including their own physician, infectious disease specialist and health professional with expertise in the procedures performed.
- HBsAg status to be regularly monitored.
- Possible career counselling and job retraining, if indicated.
- Possibly moved to an administration job (management) with promotion.

7.3.7 Occupationally acquired HIV

Circular Instruction No 183 from the Compensation Commissioner for Occupationally Acquired HIV (South Africa) deals with HIV infection arisen out of and in the course of employment. The investigation into these claims is rigorous because of the level of compensation should it be proven to be occupationally acquired.

There should be:
- Evidence of occupational exposure to an HIV-infected source and proof of a reported work-related incident/accident involving a potentially HIV-infected source.
- Serological confirmation of absence of HIV antibodies within 72 hours of the incident.
- Confirmation (as far as reasonably practicable) that the source was HIV-infected.
- Proven seroconversion at six and/or 12 weeks or six months after the date of the incident.

Impairment has to be assessed and proved beyond doubt. Assessment of impairment is determined after maximal medical improvement (as decided by the treating medical practitioner).

HIV infection plus Clinical Stage IV AIDS will be granted 100% impairment compensation.

HIV infection plus failure of response to improvement on antiretroviral treatment will be granted 100% impairment compensation.

Benefits

Occupational disease where the employer is responsible will be supported with benefits based on:
- Eligibility for benefits lapse if no seroconversion after six months from date of incident.
- Temporary total or partial disablement will be paid for maximum 24 months.
- Confirmed occupationally acquired HIV infection is granted 15% permanent disablement.
- Confirmed occupationally acquired HIV infection plus advanced AIDS and/or a poor response to ARVs will be granted 100% permanent disablement.

Note: Medical costs will cover diagnosing HIV infection, appropriate anti-retroviral therapy plus all necessary treatment.

Providing PEP once liability is accepted. The initial report of occupational exposure to blood- or body fluids-borne pathogens should be submitted within seven days of the incident and should include the employer's report of an accident, notice of claim and the first, progress and final medical reports.

8 Gathering and applying information in IPC

Annick Lenglet & Briette du Toit Ludick

Learning outcomes

What you should know after reading this chapter:
- Best method of surveillance to be applied for maximum effect
- The use of accurate information to form evidence-based policies
- How to set up and carry out an audit
- Appropriate study design for types of research studies
- Applying basic statistics to information collected

Introduction

As referred to earlier, 'the application of evidence-based knowledge and a regular revision of policies supported by a trained IPC team have significantly improved healthcare delivery and reduced infection rates in hospitals'. The chapters that followed have illustrated how an IPC team carries out this key function and its involvement in all aspects that influence infection rates. This chapter explains how data is collected, how it is used and what evidence it can provide to the IPC and clinical teams, including reducing or preventing transmission of pathogens and reducing AMR.

8.1 Surveillance

Carrying out surveillance is part of the IPC team's function. The key objective is to detect and contain pathogens that cause infectious diseases or healthcare-associated infection (HAI) and, if not curtailed, will result in clusters or common-source outbreaks. Surveillance defines some of the core activities of an IPC team and sets priorities for the IPC committee. Rapid intervention to prevent further spread is required in collaboration with the clinical teams and occupational health.

The information gathered through surveillance is applied to quality improvement by formulating new or revising current policies. It influences education and training of healthcare workers. Surveillance has shown to effectively reduce HAI, thereby reducing cost of infection, over a period of time.

There is no defined benchmark for overall HAI rates in a healthcare facility (as it may differ depending on the local situation), but global publications suggest an overall range between 7 and 10% with approximately 5 times higher rates in low-income countries.[1] It is noteworthy, however, that an estimated 30% of these infections are preventable. Surveillance systems are now well established in most well-resourced countries, which monitor quality of care, level of infection and the impact of IPC programmes. In 2013 the additional cost to the healthcare bill in the USA was $9.8 bn, made up of five major HAIs, with SSI contributing the most to the overall cost (33.7% of total).[2]

8.1.1 What is surveillance?

Surveillance (of HAI) is defined as 'the systematic collection, collation, analysis, and interpretation of data on the frequency of disease'. The World Health Assembly (2005) further recommends 'dissemination of this information to those who need to know in order for action to be taken'. It is essential to the planning, implementation and evaluation of health practices and the timely dissemination of the data for public health action (prevention and control).[3] A key step to mitigate AMR is to prevent HAIs from occurring.

> **There is no point to surveillance if the data is not used for action!**

8.1.2 Why do surveillance?

There are several reasons for carrying out surveillance, but most commonly it is to evaluate whether a programme, for example an IPC programme, is effective in a particular clinical area. Surveillance is an essential part of risk management and quality improvement, where data collection informs further developments and modifications to the programme towards improvement.

8.1.2.1 Using data for improving quality of care[4]

Quality functions in three domains – structure, process and outcome.[5] Structure relates to the settings in which care is provided, process is the activities of the caregiver and outcome is the change in health status of the patient.

---

[1]   WHO. 2011. Report on the endemic burden of healthcare-associated infection worldwide. Geneva: World Health Organization. http://apps.who.int/iris/bitstream/ 10665/80135/1/9789241501507_eng.pdf.

[2]   Zimlichman E, Henderson D, Tamir O, et al. 2013. Health Care-Associated Infections A Meta-analysis of Costs and Financial Impact on the US Health Care System. *JAMA Intern Med* 173(22): 2039–2046.

[3]   South African National Department of Health. 2021. Practical Manual for the Implementation of the National IPC Strategic Framework. October 2021.

[4]   Agency for Healthcare Research and Quality (AHRQ). Types of Quality Healthcare Measures. https://www. ahrq.gov/talkingquality/measures/types.html.

[5]   Donabedian A. 1998. The quality of care. How can it be assessed? *JAMA* 260(12): 1743–8.

Indicators are a group of measurements that identify various aspects of quality improvement in healthcare – these are structural, process and outcome indicators. IPC concentrates mainly on process and outcome indicators, but occasionally evaluates structural indicators (see section 8.4 Key audit indicators).

8.1.3 Structure of surveillance

A multi-centre monitoring system must satisfy three requirements:
- It must have a **very clear purpose**.
- It must use **standard definitions**, data fields and protocols (including those of cohorts or groups to be monitored and periods of data collection).
- It must **identify an aggregating institution** in order to standardise definitions and protocols, receive the data, assess it for quality and standardise the approach to risk. This involves adjusting the benchmarks, and interpreting and disseminating the data.

Purpose: why is surveillance being carried out? Is it to establish a baseline of HAI in the health facilities? To assess compliance to existing IPC policies? To identify areas which require development? Or compare one establishment to another nationally or internationally? For each of these situations the data gathering tool will vary and some might be quite different. The person carrying out surveillance needs to be able to do it efficiently and accurately, gathering as much information as possible in the shortest time. Therefore, it is important to keep the tools tight, precise and short, which gives maximum information using a few parameters.

> **DO NOT collect information for the sake of it. There must be a purpose!**

Clear definitions should be agreed upon and applied consistently each time surveillance information is gathered. There are a number of national surveillance systems, but the one that is most frequently used and adapted is the definitions by the US National Healthcare Safety Network (NHSN). An example of superficial surgical site infection (SSI) as defined by CDC is shown below – the definition is clear and unambiguous.

Superficial incisional site infection – SSI[6]
- occurs within 30 days after the operation
- involves only the skin or subcutaneous tissue, and

---

[6]   A wound is not considered a superficial site infection if (a) a stitch abscess is present, (b) the infection is at an episiotomy or circumcision site or a burn wound, or (c) the SSI extends into the fascia or muscle. NHSN. 2022. Procedure-associate Module. SSI Events. https://www.cdc.gov/nhsn/pdfs/pscmanual/pcsmanual_current.pdf.

- at least one of the following:
  - purulent drainage (culture documentation not required)
  - organisms isolated from fluid/tissue of superficial incision
  - at least one sign of inflammation (e.g. pain or tenderness, induration, erythema, local warmth of the wound)
  - wound is deliberately opened by the surgeon
  - surgeon or attending physician declares the wound infected.

Most national surveillance systems are voluntary, confidential and healthcare-facility-based. These influence IPC efforts nationally and sometimes internationally.

Benchmarks for infection rates are established through standardised case definitions, data collection methods, computerised data entry and analysis. Analysis of surveillance data helps reveal changes in patterns of incidence, distribution, antibiotic resistance, sites of infection, outcomes and risk factors for infection. Most systems focus on surveillance but not for overall infection control.

One of the outcomes of surveillance is the ability of trained IPC practitioners to collect data accurately.

8.1.4 The role of surveillance

Surveillance is designed to:
- establish a baseline of infection rates before planning and implementation of interventions
- monitor patterns of infectious disease (including their causes), enabling preventive and control measures to be put in place
- prevent outbreaks or detect them early in order to initiate timely action
- identify groups of patients at risk of disease
- provide information for planning of infection control services and allocation of resources
- identify interventions which have been successful and those which have not
- detect patients with notifiable medical conditions for reporting to the national Department of Health
- identify the effectiveness of a control measure or the impact thereof to change practice and behaviour.

8.1.5 The plan

Surveillance requires great thought and meticulous planning. For example, the national surveillance programme on blood stream infection rates in South Africa required planning, training and execution to ensure the data collected is accurate.

Before starting surveillance for the first time, set up a group where each member has clearly defined roles. Identify when, where, what and how. Remember to keep it simple so that any trained person can carry out surveillance easily once s/he is used to it.

Before starting, the committee (management, clinical teams, IPC) should meet to discuss the following:

- Who will **carry out surveillance** and collect the data?
- Who will **check the data and verify the information**?
- **Clear definitions** must be provided and discussed that are not open to interpretation.
- **The period of time** over which surveillance is carried out must be defined. Ideally, this should be a minimum of six months for total (continuous) or targeted surveillance in order to get a meaningful dataset that will take into account variations in admission rates, the weather, holidays and so on. Point prevalence surveys must have a clearly structured time frame including frequency of data collection, such as a particular month or week, during a year.
- There must be a clearly defined **denominator** in order to calculate rates of infection.
- The **sample size** must be adequate to give realistic results.
- **Data entry** must be accurate with minimum transcription errors – computerised systems reduce such errors.
- **Standardised data collection tools should be available,** e.g. standardised form, spreadsheet or electronic application.
- **Channelling the information** means defining the communication and feedback reporting structures for further action.
- Assign tasks and responsibilities to the various members of the group.

Use the information effectively to improve quality of care!

There are universally accepted definitions for HAI which should be used to make comparisons and to ensure reliability. When comparing data between clinical areas or hospitals, the same definitions should be applied in exactly the same way each time, preferably by trained IPC practitioners. This system is usually applied when several health facilities in a large structure are carrying out surveillance.

Standardised definitions are available from the Centers of Disease Control (CDC), National Healthcare Safety Network (NHSN), European CDC (ECDC) or from the Hospital Infection Society (UK) and others which are freely available online. It should be mentioned that definitions continuously evolve or change depending on information from new data.

8.1.5.1 Methods of surveillance

Methods of surveillance vary in detail but all involve careful scrutiny and evaluation of a health-related problem. Global surveillance for diseases of interest are recorded by the WHO such as HIV, TB, and now COVID-19-related infections and deaths. This is an ongoing compilation of data sent in by countries worldwide. In this way a surveillance of the changing patterns and trends of the pandemic is made.

As previously mentioned, good surveillance starts with a plan with clear definitions and precise parameters to be measured. The plan must indicate the working of the method of surveillance because it should define how often these measurements are to be made and how they are recorded and stored.

8.1.5.1.1 Types of surveillance

The type of surveillance will be dictated by the number of IPC staff available to collect the information and the resources and skills to interpret the data once collected. Surveillance can be **continuous** (total or targeted) or **periodic** (also known as **point prevalence**) over a period of time. The type of surveillance will depend upon the reason for carrying out surveillance.

8.1.5.1.1.1 *Continuous total surveillance*

If a group of hospitals want to find out the overall rate of HAI over a period of time (usually 6 months), all HAI infections will be recorded by incidence, causative pathogens and outcome of infection such as morbidity or mortality. This will give a clear idea of which areas may be targeted specifically in the future.

The outcome of such surveillance will be to establish alert sites (which are the commonest sites of infection), alert organisms (the commonest pathogens) and their antimicrobial sensitivity patterns (multidrug-resistant organisms, MDROs).

Continuous total surveillance is very expensive and time-consuming, particularly for resource limited settings. Ideally, it should be followed by targeted surveillance once the parameters of interest have been established through continuous surveillance.

8.1.5.1.1.2 *Continuous alert organism surveillance*

'Alert organisms' are pathogens such as bacteria or viruses that are of interest to the IPC team and are specifically noted on laboratory reports as requiring immediate intervention. Some examples are MRSA, multiple antibiotic-resistant gram-negative bacilli, or *Mycobacterium tuberculosis* isolated from a hospital.

This involves daily review of the laboratory results for the presence of significant pathogens as an indicator of the status of infection in the hospital. Usually, the laboratory will ring the IPC team when an alert organism or a new specific pathogen has been isolated. These specific organisms have been identified by type as being problematic. Alert organisms might be only prevalent on particular wards such as the intensive care unit or neonatal unit or these could be widespread throughout the hospital.

Recently, ESKAPE (*E faecium, S aureus, K pneumoniae, A baumannii, P aeruginosa* and *Enterobacter spp*) and CPE (carbapenemase-producing Enterobacteriaceae, *C difficile* and *Candida* species) pathogens have been put on the list and these are reported regularly to international bodies such as the WHO.

8.1.5.1.1.3 *Continuous alert condition surveillance*

The same broad approach applies, but this type of surveillance is focused on those groups of patients most likely to acquire an infection or who are particularly vulnerable should they acquire an infection. This method requires close liaison between the infection control team and ward staff and relies on ward staff being able to identify those patients who should be monitored and recognise an infection from the patient's condition. Here, link nurses are particularly useful who act as eyes and ears of the IPC team.

An example is the intensive therapy units (ITUs) where bloodstream infections, intravenous therapy infections or SSIs are recorded. Another example is diarrhoeal disease or tuberculosis occurring in a particular ward.

8.1.5.2 *Targeted surveillance (point prevalence)*

Such surveys are undertaken periodically at one point in time, at each interval rather than continuously. This type involves surveillance of patients according to certain characteristics. These are patients who make up a particular case mix, are from a specific ward or unit or share the same site of infection. It could be applied to a single unit or nationally, if accurately designed. It can reflect changing patterns of HAI within an institution or geographical area. Prevalence surveys, if performed at regular intervals, can accomplish the same outcomes as continuous surveillance. Some African countries have adopted the Global Point Prevalence Survey (GPPS), which is run three times per year. For more information, go to the website.[7] The European Union also has a PPS system in place.

8.1.5.3 *Selective laboratory-based ward liaison surveillance*

Here, laboratory and ward staff review selected surveillance data. This method can reveal an increase in the incidence of infection in a healthcare setting before it becomes a problem, but a reasonably functioning laboratory is required to support IPC.

Where resources are short both in funds and staff, a simple surveillance method can be set up in the particular ward or unit that requires the most attention. For example, targeting the ITU for only bloodstream infections will give accurate information leading to intervention strategies.

8.1.6 Where there are no laboratory services

It is very difficult to report an HAI without laboratory back-up. However, if there is no laboratory service available, a well-trained IPC practitioner and clinical team can attempt to quantify certain infections by carrying out regular clinical ward

---

[7]   https://www.global-pps.com/.

rounds and a clinical assessment of the patients. For example, if there are clear signs of a SSI, or a device-related infection, the IPC practitioner can document this as a probable or suspected HAI. Mortality rates, particularly post-operative deaths, length of stay in hospital and prescribing empiric antibiotics to patients might be used as indicators to document an HAI.

While it is acknowledged that this data is not robust and probably will not be considered worthy of quality improvement or change, a cluster of cases that suddenly emerge or a new type of device-related infection not seen previously might alert management to provide some assistance to investigate further.

When the data is presented at the next meeting, an increase or decrease in particular types of infection can be discussed and commented upon. Needless to say, this is not an ideal set-up for good surveillance.

8.1.7 Levels of surveillance

Surveillance can be conducted at different levels, depending on the information required and who requires it.

8.1.7.1 Individual or unit level

Surveillance at this level will provide information about a specific problem in a specific unit, e.g. the rate of bloodstream infections in the ICU or the central-line-associated infection rate (CLABSI in the neonatal ICU (NICU)).

8.1.7.2 Healthcare facility

The surveillance at healthcare facility level is dictated by the number of available staff, the predominant disease patterns, both community and hospital-acquired, and local expertise. Usually the information collected is more than that required for national purposes. For example, overall HAI rates for the facility and/or alert organisms and alert conditions on specific units.

Specialised or tertiary referral hospitals may want to conduct surveillance pertinent to their group of units or diseases.

8.1.7.3 Provincial

Disease patterns may differ from one province to another and surveillance will reflect this. Provincial authorities will carry out their own investigations and surveillance for outbreaks of cholera or diarrohea in their specific provinces. This information is relayed to the national Department of Health.

8.1.7.4 National

Most countries have a set of data which is collected for the World Health Organization (WHO) or for national use and usually the data is for communicable (notifiable) diseases. Without a clear plan, this data can be inaccurate. Information passes through several tiers and can become distorted (see section 7.1.2.2 on notifiable diseases). The National Health Laboratory Services (South Africa) provides epidemiological data and periodic feedback. For example, COVID-19 cases across all facilities in the province can be provided by the NHLS, but some facilities might want case load in specific areas.

8.1.7.5 Global

Surveillance of diseases that are of global concern, e.g. tuberculosis data per 100 000 population in each country, are published annually and provide comparisons between countries. Other communicable diseases such as polio, measles and influenza are reported to the WHO. COVID-19 cases globally are reported and regular feedback is published on the WHO and other websites.

8.1.8 Who carries out surveillance?

It is usually the IPC team that carries out surveillance as part of the routine, but in some hospitals there are surveillance teams who do it as a full-time job. The plan should clearly identify the team with the following:
- Personnel who have had extensive training in
  - surveillance definitions
  - data collection
  - data analysis (basic)
  - methodology
  - understanding the information.
- Ability to interpret the results
- Readiness to co-operate as a team
- There must be support from
  - management
  - clinical staff
  - IPC personnel.

8.2   Data collection systems

Depending on the number of staff in the IPC team or unit, collecting information for surveillance is time-consuming and should be structured in a manageable data collection system, including frequency of data collection depending on the type of surveillance used.

When setting up a data collection system for the healthcare facility, make sure that only the necessary information is gathered and that what is necessary is agreed by the surveillance team, such as:
- Name, age, sex of patient, hospital number or unique identifying number.
- Date of admission and date of discharge.

- Clinical diagnosis and date of onset of infection.
- Antibiotic therapy started on and dates.
- Interventions such as surgical operations.
- Device insertions: intravenous lines, CVP lines, surgery, mechanical ventilation and urinary catheterisation, with dates of insertion and removal.

Before starting surveillance, get an outside evaluator to go over the data set to give unbiased advice. Do not collect data for the sake of it. It is best to get a minimum data set and apply it for maximum effect.

8.2.1 Storing the data

An electronic device, within certain limits, presents an ideal safe system for storing data efficiently and safely. For economic reasons, paper is still used as a method of collecting and storing raw data in LMICs.

> **Store data in an easily accessible system so that the information is easily accessible to inform decision-makers.**

8.2.2 Paper forms

The information can be collected on standardised paper data collection forms which can be captured on a computerised database. The forms should be stored for at least five years in case the information has to be revisited. The disadvantages of this system are (a) transcription errors, (b) no checks when entering data (the information could be incomplete or incorrect), (c) takes up storage space and it is labour intensive and (d) makes it difficult to find information retrospectively.

8.2.3 Computerised systems

Computerised systems are more efficient and reliable and there are several inexpensive (sometimes free) packages available online (WHO website).

Data from different sources can be collated electronically, for example patient admission information, laboratory results, IPC protocols implemented and so on. Each patient can be followed up individually. At the end of a period the information can be collated into a comprehensive report which allows rapid generation of reports with graphs and tables.

Small handheld computers (tablet) can be used to collect data directly during ward rounds, which is downloaded directly onto the main database. This reduces duplication and the risk of transcription errors. The information is entered by the person who is collecting the data, reducing discrepancies and saving time. This system also has the advantage of being fed directly into electronic statistical packages for analysis and generating reports.

It is essential that access to the data is limited (patient confidentiality) and password-protected so that only a few people can access it. Ideally, a named person should be responsible for managing the database and printing of reports, and work closely with the IPC team. Data analysis can be done quickly, accurately and efficiently.

All data has to be treated as confidential and stored safely with a daily backup system (cloud or server) in case the system crashes.

8.2.4 Data analysis and interpretation

The information should be analysed by a knowledgeable statistician or epidemiologist to ensure the data is accurate. Details of data analysis are discussed later in this chapter.

8.2.4.1 Using the information

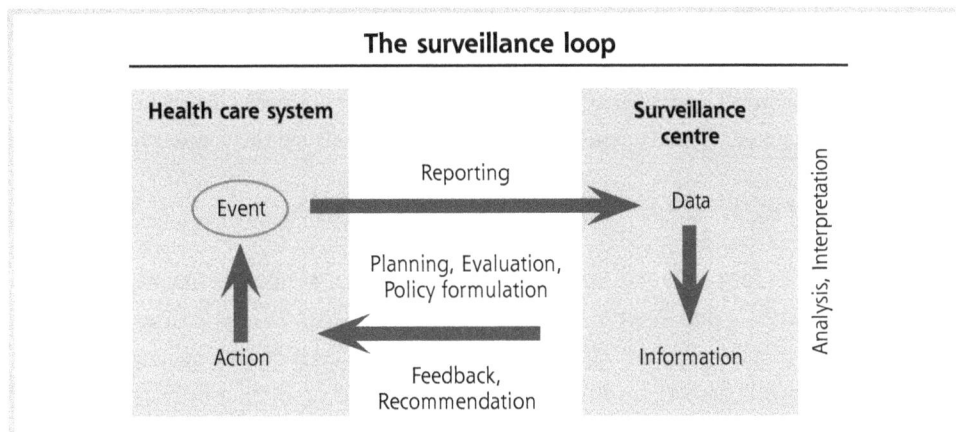

Figure 8.1 Data capturing and feedback surveillance loop for improving IPC[8]

Once data has been collected for the specified period, it should be analysed and presented to the IPC committee, clinical units and management to effect improvement in patient care. The IPC practitioner should learn to understand and interpret the information and its application to clinical practice – for this, education is essential. The data is used to develop policies and IPC structural support.

8.2.4.2 Healthcare-associated infections

One of the roles of IPC practitioners in healthcare is to detect and prevent HAIs. For this, surveillance is necessary, not only for establishing a baseline of infection rates but also to monitor the effectiveness of implemented IPC measures. Some

---

[8] Adapted from a lecture by G Kuzmanovska, National Public Health Institute, Macedonia.

basic concepts are mentioned here, but will be developed further later in the chapter (see section 8.6 Descriptive and analytical epidemiology).

8.2.4.2.1 Terms used in HAI calculations

Rate is an expression of the *frequency* with which an event (e.g. an infection) occurs in a defined population over a given time period. Rate always includes time as a part of its expression.

A constant expresses the result into a uniform quantity so comparisons between rates can be made. For example, SSI (operations) or peripheral line infection (number of peripheral lines inserted) over a period of time, let's say one month, is expressed as percentages (per 100 cases), CAUTI is expressed as number of urinary tract infections per 1 000 catheter-days and and hand hygiene compliance as a percentage of hand hygiene opportunities.

Three important things to remember when calculating a rate:

- The numerator and denominator must reflect the same population – cases that are in the numerator must also be counted in the denominator.
- All cases in the denominator are eligible to be considered for the numerator.
- Counts in the numerator and denominator must cover the same time period.

These rates can be used as indicators of monitoring HAIs.[9]

Rates can further be divided into incidence and prevalence.

An **incidence** rate is used to measure the frequency of occurrence of **new cases** of infection within a defined population during a specified time frame.

Prevalence is the number of **total (old and new)** cases of a disease or infection in a specific population at a particular point in time or over a specific period.[10] Standardised methods should be used to calculate HAI rates and should be expressed as either as a percentage or a rate. For example:

A numerator could include the following

- Number of infections
- Number of patients infected
- Number of device-associated infections

A denominator could include the following:

- Number of patients admitted in a unit or hospital
- Number of days in hospital
- Number of device days
- Number of operations

9   South African National Department of Health. Practical Manual for the Implementation of the National IPC Strategic Framework. October 2021.

10   https://s4be.cochrane.org/blog/2020/11/06/prevalence-vs-incidence-what-is-the-difference.

EXAMPLE: How to calculate a CLABSI rate:

CLABSI rates are calculated by dividing the total number of CLABSI cases by the total number of central line days. This number is multiplied by 1 000 to get a rate per 1 000 central line days.

Numerator: $\dfrac{\text{Number of CLABSI infections} \times 1\,000}{}$

Denominator: Total number of central line days

= rate of CLABSI cased per 1 000 central line days

Central line days are counted from the day of insertion of the device (day one) until the date of removal. Every day that the device is *in situ* needs to be counted to identify the total number of device days.

8.2.4.2.2 Presentation of HAI data

Surveillance data should be reported to facility management teams, clinical staff and the IPC committee. Data should be presented in a way that it makes sense to the end user, therefore graphs and tables are useful.

8.3 Audit in IPC

Audit is an important quality assurance tool using monitoring and evaluation of good clinical practice and is a means of establishing **compliance to written policies** (should be evidence-based). If there is no evaluation and measurement of the outcome of practice, certain practices may not be detected until a crisis occurs. Usually, surveillance precedes auditing.

8.3.1 What is audit?

Audit is a 'measurement of performance taken over a limited period of time to ascertain whether **pre-determined standards** are being met'. And is also 'a quality improvement process that seeks to improve patient care against explicit criteria and the implementation of change'.

By definition, an audit cannot be carried out unless policies or standards are in place. The principle of auditing is to check actual practice against a standard, report back and offer interventions which will improve the quality of care, and then re-audit after implementation. Therefore audit follows surveillance, policies, implementation of policies and setting standards. Only when these are completed is performance measured – not before.

> Audit measures against standards of good practice laid out in clearly written evidence-based policies.

8.3.2 Setting up an audit – what should be in place

Before an audit can be undertaken, the following should be in place:

- Standards or clear guidelines against which the audit will be conducted
- Access to all areas of clinical practice which are being audited
- All areas informed of when the audit will take place – no surprise element
- Available written copies of documents for inspection if required
- Willing participation of management
- A structure to report back to which can take action (to improve performance)
- A programme for re-auditing after an effective intervention has taken place
- Accountability for improving practice
- Resources to carry out audits – budget and trained personnel.

8.3.2.1 Elements of an audit

- There should be no element of surprise – inform the clinical area of an audit taking place and preferably when it will happen.
- The staff should have **knowledge** regarding a task which is established by an interview questionnaire.
- There should be **appropriate resources provided** by management for the personnel to complete a task, which is established by observation.
- **Impartial** observation of clinical practice demonstrates how the combination of the knowledge and facilities are used to provide a high standard of patient care.
- **Nothing is taken for granted.** If, on the day of the audit, one or more elements are missing, the answers will be negative irrespective of what is stated about other times outside the audit.
- A **report or feedback** mechanism which will influence improvement change.
- **Non-judgmental feedback.** Make helpful and positive recommendations.

> **Do not comment on practice or offer advice while conducting an audit – only observe and record.**

8.3.2.2 The audit tool

The audit tool is how performance is assessed. Usually this is a series of questions the auditors ask and check upon through inspection to evaluate the quality of healthcare. The findings are scored against a maximum attainable level and thus identify areas that require attention. The following points should guide the choice of an audit tool:

- When using an audit tool try to choose or develop one which has been validated in a particular location or environment.

- Applying universally accepted audit tools from different healthcare structures is acceptable as long as the standards are similar, for example Hand Hygiene Self-assessment Framework tool.[11]
- The tool should be structured as **statements not questions** (if possible) such as 'is there alcohol-based hand rub present at each bed?' Yes or No
- Occasionally certain questions are necessary, for example when assessing IPC knowledge; if a statement rather than a 'yes' or 'no' response is made by the interviewee, it should be recorded and analysed separately and put in as an appendix or addition to the report – it should be anonymous.
- The audit tool should be comprehensive but not too long, otherwise those carrying out the audit will find it difficult to complete within a given time. Ask only the most pertinent questions; inevitably some issues will not be covered. If these do not affect good clinical practice, they are irrelevant.
- There should be no room for ambiguity. The answers are simply 'yes' or 'no'. This is not as easy as it sounds because interpretations may differ.

The same audit tool cannot be applied to every section of the healthcare facility and individual tools should be developed with the same principles but reflecting the difference in practice. A particular problem of applying audit tools developed in other countries or hospitals is that the questions may not be applicable; however, these can be adapted.

- Some parts of the audit tool may not apply if a particular unit does not exist. For example, there is no point in asking a clinical nurse about steriliser validation in the sterile services department (SSD).
- Make sure the audit tool is piloted in several areas before implementation.
- Finally, the audit tools in each country or province are best developed by experts in the field who have been involved in developing guidelines, standards and key indicators.
- The tool should be developed in collaboration with quality improvement and clinical teams.

> Audit tools have to be adapted to individual facilities and local standards and guidelines, e.g. the WHO audit tools are well researched, but should be adapted to local settings.

Audit tools are designed to monitor key indicators in healthcare practice as discussed below.

---

[11] https://cdn.who.int/media/docs/default-source/integrated-health-services-(ihs)/clean-hands-2015/hhsa_framework_october_2010-3.pdf?sfvrsn=98cbf596_3&ua=1.

8.4   Key audit indicators in IPC

Key indicators are helpful tools as part of quality of care and reflect either outcome (performance) or processes, and monitoring of administrative operational function. From an IPC perspective, risk indicators are more helpful since these are proactive and identify adverse events and vulnerabilities before problems arise.

8.4.1 Types of indicators

There are different key indicators that measure different aspects of IPC practices, as shown below:

8.4.4.1   **Structure indicators** measure *physical equipment and facilities, qualification levels of staff* and administrative programmes, and usually identify how closely national and/or local organisational rules are being followed. They have also been called *compliance indicators* and are usually evidenced by internal policies and guidelines that reflect **compliance with statutory requirements**.

         For example
- Number of qualified surgeons undertaking a specified procedure who are accredited in accordance with a national standard.
- Number of nurses working in the operating theatre qualified according to the national standard.
- The ventilation in the operating theatre.
- The sterilisation of medical devices and appropriate storage.

         Structure indicators are often readily formulated and easily measured. However, it is not always a simple matter to establish a clear relationship towards achieving desired health outcomes.

8.4.1.2   **Process indicators** measure **provision of healthcare** available to the population. These indicate how members of an organisation *follow internal rules and guidelines (attending training and applying them).* In turn, these evidence-based guidelines typically reflect *good clinical practice and recommendations (best practice guidelines).*

         Observational audits of specifically stated organisational requirements (such as hand hygiene activities following patient contact) are examples of process indicators. Detailed records of the number of people who have access to, or attend, internal training courses on guideline implementation are also recognised tools to assess a process indicator.

Examples of process indicators are:

1. Attendance at infection control educational activities
2. Compliance with internal policies and guidelines for infection control
3. Observational audit of hand hygiene
4. Measuring of compliance to environmental cleaning processes
5. Compliance to the correct PPE for specific transmission-based precautions

Process indicators are usually more sensitive to differences in quality and are easier to evaluate and interpret – these may be used for public reporting to reflect quality.

8.4.1.3 *Outcome indicators* link a risk indicator to the progress or clinical outcome of patients and are considered the *gold standard of care*. These reflect the impact of health interventions on the outcome of the patient such as recovery from a clinical procedure, restoration of functionality and survival rates.[12]

HAI rates are outcome indicators.

Examples of outcome indicators

1. Alert Organisms/Alert Conditions
   - Healthcare-associated *Cl difficile* diarrhoea
   - Carbapenemase Producing Enterobacterales (CPE)
   - Penicillin-resistant *S pneumoniae*
   - *Acinetobacter baumannii* rates of infection in the intensive care unit
2. Healthcare-associated infection rates
3. Procedure-related infections, e.g. surgical site infections
4. Device-associated infections
   - Ventilator-associated pneumonia
   - Catheter-associated urinary tract infections
   - Central-line-associated bloodstream infections
   - Peripheral-line-associated bloodstream infections

12 Lorini C, Porchia BR, Pieralli F & Bonaccorsi G. 2018. Process, structural, and outcome quality indicators of nutritional care in nursing homes: a systematic review. *BMC Health Services Research* 18: 43. doi 10.1186/s12913-018-2828-0.

While outcome indicators reflect the ideal standard of care, some factors may be beyond the provider's control. For example, if there is no functioning operating theatre, or the sterilisation methods for medical devices is inadequate, or if there is an acute shortage of medical supplies or staff, this will have a profound impact on the outcome of surgical site infection.

In order to calculate a more accurate rate of outcome, risk adjustment methods might be necessary.

Outcome indicators are usually reported with process indicators.

8.4.1.4   *Surrogate indicators* attempt to relate actions to effects. As the name suggests, these represent 'proxy' markers of activity or outcome. Their relationship to the activity measured needs to be very clear and explicitly defined at the outset, and possible confounders identified.

Examples of surrogate indicators

1.   Hand hygiene – the volume of ABHR used per month
2.   Use of of disinfectants
3.   Use or commencement of antimicrobials
4.   Length of hospital stay

Each hospital or healthcare facility can develop its own indicators and audit against the defined key indicators. It is a useful way of starting an audit programme in low-resource settings.

8.4.2 The areas to be audited

It is best to inform the staff of the health facility area where the audit will take place during a given time interval; specific dates are not necessary.

It is preferable that the auditor does not carry out an audit in his or her own department because there may be a bias. For example, if asked whether an IPC policy manual exists, the interviewee may say 'no', but the auditor knows there is one at another location and prompts a 'yes' answer.

Audits are to improve performance, never to be punitive.

8.4.3 Conducting the audit

During the audit, the auditor should try not to disrupt busy clinical practice within the area being visited. As well as any curtailment of essential work being undesirable, the auditor should be auditing a functioning environment.

If possible, send in a list of documents to be viewed in advance so that those in charge can get the necessary information, such as number of beds, type of ward, number of staff and so on.

Talk to the healthcare workers at their convenience. They know there is an audit in progress and should have made arrangements to be interviewed. It also builds trust and confidence. Make sure that the interviews remain anonymous.

The auditor should not be too visible. Staff might decide to alter practice or not perform tasks while the audit is being conducted and this may give a false outcome or, as often happens, no outcome at all.

8.4.4 The audit report

The audit results should be laid out in a clear, comprehensive manner. This is best achieved using a scoring formula as shown below.

$$\frac{\text{Total number of 'yes' replies} \times 100}{\text{Total number of 'yes' plus 'no'}} = \%$$

- The outcome can be reported as a percentage.
- The sample size should be adequate to make an informed decision.
- Categories can be allocated. An example is shown below:
  — Minimum compliance: 75% or less
  — Partial compliance: 76–84%
  — Compliance: 85% or more

Additionally, those practices considered more important for good IPC practices can be graded, such as hand hygiene versus wearing headgear when carrying out a wound dressing.

8.4.5 Feedback

The report should be given to the quality assurance and management teams with an expectation to introduce improvement measures in areas identified as requiring more support, such as education, provision for carrying out transmission-based precautions or for a water supply.

A re-audit date should be set once the improvements have been carried out.

8.5 Outbreak investigation and management

Outbreaks may arise in healthcare facilities (HAI) or the community (community associated infection – CAI), but could spread to the healthcare facility or vice versa by community members seeking healthcare. IPC teams are usually responsible for investigating and containing HAI, while public health manages CAI; however, there may be an overlap between the two, depending on the expertise required to contain the outbreak.

Investigation and containment of outbreaks is a team effort made up of the clinical teams involved or communicable disease doctors, IPC team, management of the institutions involved, microbiologists, media spokespersons and others who are co-opted as required. If transport is needed for patients or staff, emergency services should be kept informed, as should the pharmacists and procurement departments.

All potential outbreaks should be reported to the provincial and national communicable diseases authorities and reference laboratories.

8.5.1 Definitions of high occurrence of a disease

There are several definitions available, but the following are appropriate:

1. **Outbreak:** An outbreak of communicable disease/infection can be defined as the incidence of disease above that normally expected. Usually this means that there are two or more linked cases of the same illness/symptoms. In some instances, only one case may be sufficient to fulfil the definition, e.g. Ebola.

2. **Endemic:** The usual level of a disease within a geographic area. These sporadic infections represent most preventable HAI, e.g. Ebola, Lassa fever.

3. **Epidemic:** The level of disease is above what is normally experienced. It can also be defined as a sudden violent occurrence of disease, e.g. severe acute respiratory syndrome (SARS), Ebola in West Africa.

4. **Pandemic:** An epidemic that spreads to several countries, usually affecting many people, e.g. H1N1 influenza, COVID-19.

8.5.2 Alert (warning) system

Often, HAI outbreaks are picked up during surveillance; this could be from laboratory or clinical reports. The clinical team might notice an increase in a particular type of infection and inform the IPC team. Global systems are set up to recognise emerging diseases across the world, such as H1N1 influenza, Ebola in West Africa or SARS-CoV-2 in China (2019). There are several websites that offer these services and it is worthwhile subscribing to them as they are free (ProMED, WHO). There are also national communicable disease control units that send out information regularly.

8.5.3 Types of outbreak

The pattern and source of an outbreak indicate its type. There are two main types: the **common source** outbreak, when all victims acquire the disease from the same source such as cholera from contaminated water or a group of people becoming ill after attending a gathering. There can be a **continuing source** outbreaks when victims acquire the disease over multiple incubation periods such as SARS-CoV-2.

The patterns are summarised below:
- Common source
  - From a single person
  - Single vehicle such as contaminated water
  - May be continuous (one peak) or intermittent (several peaks).
- Continuing source – large populations affected
  - Person-to-person transmission
  - Occurs over a longer period of time
  - Secondary or tertiary cases occur.

8.5.4 Occurrence

The occurrence is recognised by reporting of an unusual disease that has not been previously recorded or via an alert being issued by the WHO or the national department of health.

When investigating an outbreak, attention should be focused on specific groups of patients especially in healthcare facilities and other locations, for example Crimean-Congo haemorrhagic fever (CCHF) originated on cattle farms. Treatment modalities, contaminated products or devices and the effect on healthcare providers and healthcare practice should be taken into account.

The **aim** of the outbreak investigation is to identify contributing factors to control the current outbreak and prevent further outbreaks. Clusters of infections are investigated in a systematic and meticulous way, recording contributing factors such as source(s), pathogen(s), host(s), mode of transmission and other elements. Ending the outbreak involves modifying one or more of these factors. The methodology is discussed below under section 8.5.6.1.

8.5.5 Healthcare facility outbreaks

The IPC team as part of the larger outbreak team will investigate any unusual occurrence of infection identified by the laboratory or clinical reports as part of the ongoing targeted or continuous surveillance.

8.5.5.1   A **single case** (new admission or already admitted) with an 'alert organism' or 'alert clinical condition' will be visited and the clinical details noted. While present on the ward:
- The IPC team should:
  - provide on-the-spot training and advice to the clinical team
  - check hand hygiene and other IPC practices
  - reinforce necessary transmission-based precautions, including isolation.
  - ensure there is an adequate supply of appropriate PPE

    — compile a written procedure or policy to manage the clinical occurrence
    — ensure infrastructure is well supplied, such as ventilation, water supply, sanitation and isolation facilities
    — provide moral support.
- The clinical team should be informed and management of the case discussed, including the possibility of an outbreak.

Patients should be informed, especially if transmission-based precautions are being implemented. The infection control measures should be explained to the patients and efforts made to ensure they are comfortable with the process.

The IPC team should closely monitor the clinical areas for at least three incubation periods or six weeks after the last case has occurred.

8.5.5.2 **If two or more cases** are epidemiologically related, an outbreak is suspected.

The IPC team's response should be quick and prevention measures put into place as soon as possible to prevent further spread.

The IPC team should:
- Visit and talk to the ward staff in great detail.
- Make sure there are adequate facilities to contain the infection.
- If not, arrange transfer to an isolation room or another ward or hospital.
- If the patient is transferred, advise the receiving ward.
- Take a detailed history from the patient including:
    — contact with other people who may be infected
    — travel abroad
    — admissions to other hospitals
    — medication
    — co-infection
    — previous similar episodes.
- Check on and reinforce hand hygiene practices.
- Ensure transmission-based precautions are in place.
- Read through policy and update if required.
- Set up an outbreak record chart.

Following these initial procedures:
- The clinical team should follow up any further suspicious cases.
- Management should be informed.
- An outbreak response team should be set up.

8.5.6 Investigation of outbreaks

8.5.6.1 Epidemiological steps during an outbreak

The epidemiological steps of a community-based outbreak investigation are outlined in Table 8.1. The next section on steps mainly focus on HAI outbreak investigation.

Table 8.1 Epidemiologic steps of an outbreak investigation[13]

1. Prepare for field work
2. Establish the existence of an outbreak
3. Verify the diagnosis
4. Construct a working case definition
5. Find cases systematically and record information
6. Perform descriptive epidemiology
7. Develop hypotheses
8. Evaluate hypotheses epidemiologically
9. As necessary, reconsider, refine and re-evaluate hypotheses
10. Compare and reconcile with laboratory and/or environmental studies
11. Implement control and prevention measures
12. Initiate or maintain surveillance
13. Communicate findings

Step 1: Prepare for the investigation. Clearance from the facility management is required. The department of microbiology and virology should be advised to prepare for specimens taken from the investigation and to save specimens and isolates until the outbreak has ended; the samples will be required for genotyping further epidemiological investigation. If laboratory facilities do not exist on site, reference laboratories should be alerted and asked for assistance.

The IPC team should meet internally to discuss strategy. The physician responsible for IPC liaises with the medical staff, especially the head of department, and notifies them of the impending investigation. The IPC practitioner will liaise with nurse managers and ward staff to inform them of the investigation and report back on progress. The IPC team should have at least one, if not more, daily meeting(s) to discuss progress. The outbreak team should meet once a week or more frequently to discuss current and future management.

Step 2: Confirm existence of an outbreak. Develop a case definition (CD) and use it to estimate the magnitude of the problem. With new diseases such as SARS-CoV-2 the CD may need to be revised as information is gathered. It is important

---

[13]   https://www.cdc.gov/csels/dsepd/ss1978/lesson6/section2.html.

to compare incidence rates within the healthcare facility to detect any real or perceived increase in the number of cases. A literature search should be conducted to get an idea of what to expect and to learn from the experience of others.

At this point management should be alerted to a potential outbreak. The laboratory is advised to hold all samples from the outbreak.

Step 3: Establish or verify diagnosis and identify agent if possible. The CD may need to be refined as investigation proceeds with identifying agent and diagnosis confirmed. This will be based on the clinical picture, laboratory results and procedures undertaken during the outbreak to establish links.

The clinical character of the nature of disease and signs and symptoms obtained by reviewing patient charts may suggest further changes to the CD. Appropriate samples should be taken for laboratory testing and analysis.

Step 4: Search for additional cases. Cases within the geographical area or hospital setting should be documented on a ***line list*** and samples should be taken from suspected cases for screening. Use a Gantt chart (Figure 8.2) to document relationships between the patients admitted or related to the index case.

Encourage immediate reporting from wards and laboratories so that the follow-up of suspected cases is swift. Collect the information on specific data collection forms that have detailed questions relating to the CD. A data abstraction form is used to enter critical aspects from the existing information.

Step 5: Characterise cases of disease, persons, place and time. Establish who is at particular risk and who should be included in future studies. An epidemic curve is established using date of onset, the exact period of the outbreak, including the period of exposure, and the common source or propagated source of the outbreak.

Next, look for clusters of an at-risk population. The cases involved should be characterised by age, gender, location and common factors that fit the CD. Any exposure to the index case or infected cases, large or small, should be documented.

In the case of healthcare facilities, therapeutic interventions such as surgery, antibiotics, insertion of intravenous lines, urinary catheters or mechanical ventilation should be documented. Calculate attack rates (see below).

Step 6: Formulate a tentative hypothesis. Record, tabulate and review collected data and literature searched. Develop a hypothesis based on these findings that would explain the majority of the cases. There may be some cases that cannot be explained and this could be due to different risk factors, a different disease or a different source or mode of transmission. In other words, there may be two outbreaks going on simultaneously for whatever reason and both should be documented.

Step 7. Test the hypothesis. Many investigations do not reach this stage because the situations resolve themselves. Similarly it might be a pseudo-outbreak from contaminated sampling containers or equipment.

To test the hypothesis there should be an adequate number of personnel, information on the extent and severity of the problem and the available resources.

Alternatively, carry out retrospective case-control studies or cohort studies. The analysis from case investigations and sources of transmission may demonstrate significant differences of incidence and exposure in contrasted populations.

Step 8: Plan additional systematic studies. These studies will help to refine the hypothesis and carry out additional studies. In the interpretation of the results it is vital to obtain a meaningful association between risk factors and disease. This depends on many factors, many of which are eliminated with careful initial planning and adhering to the plan.

Step 9: Take immediate control measures if indicated. Increase containment or prevention measures such as reinforcing IPC measures, removing specific suspected products and assessing breaks in IPC practice. The impact of this should be documented. Many clusters of infections resolve themselves once IPC measures are reinforced. The IPC team must visit the clinical area and reassure the staff in a 'no blame' discussion. This is vital for good cooperation and gathering information. Surveillance is initiated and continued until the outbreak is over.

Step 10: Communicate frequently with stakeholders
There should be a daily meeting of the outbreak committee to keep everyone informed. Keep the clinical areas informed. It is best to visit the ward/area daily and offer support and advice.

8.5.6.2 IPC steps during an outbreak

Step 1: Collection of specimens
- Screening of other patients and staff should be carried out during the outbreak and some after the outbreak has abated.
- Environmental screening is not recommended routinely unless there is an indication that it will shed light on the outbreak. Samples of products or items used may be taken if the route of transmission suggests such a spread.
- Co-ordinate with laboratory. The initial requests are for ordinary cultures, but molecular studies can be carried out on selected isolates to prove similarity.

Step 2: Implement and evaluate IPC measures. Check on current practices during the outbreak and follow up daily with visits to ensure continuity and provide moral support.

Step 3: Initiate surveillance. Surveillance helps to evaluate the specific recommendations to stop the outbreak. It also helps the evaluation of interventions and whether further transmission has occurred or not.

Step 4: Review current policies and revise policies that are ineffective or are outdated. Use most recently published evidence-based information to support the update.

Step 5: Talk to the staff on several occasions, especially during the outbreak. Frequent visits to the clinical area are very important. The IPC team should provide the reassurance needed for the staff. They should identify training needs and help to change attitudes. It must be a no blame and safe environment so that the staff can confide in the IPC practitioner.

Step 6: Feedback should be given regularly to the clinical team, ward staff and management.
- Communicate findings – what isolates have been detected, which practices contribute to infection:
  - verbally at an emergency meeting of IPCC
  - through written reports.
- Circulate to everyone who needs to know.
- Get definite commitment with timelines of implementation.

Table 8.2 The various methods to carry out quantitative studies

Objective	Common design
Prevalence	Cross-sectional
Incidence	Cohort
Cause	Cohort, cross-sectional, case-control
Prognosis	Cohort
Treatment effect	Randomised Controlled trial (double blind)

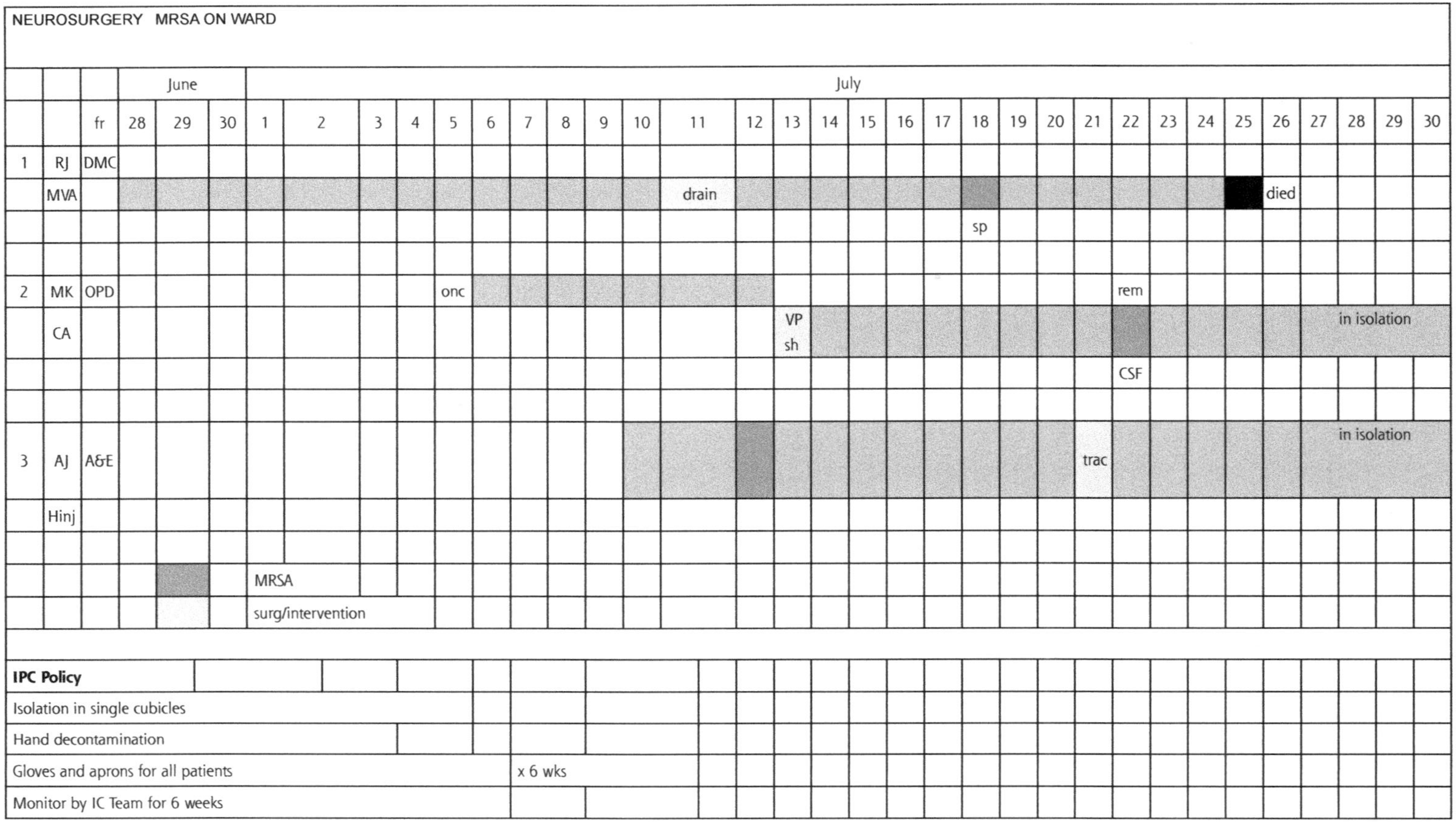

NEUROSURGERY MRSA ON WARD

			June			July																										
		fr	28	29	30	1	2	3	4	5	6	7	8	9	10	11	12	13	14	15	16	17	18	19	20	21	22	23	24	25	26	27	28	29	30
1	RJ	DMC																																		
	MVA															drain								sp							died					
2	MK	OPD								onc																		rem					in isolation			
	CA																	VP sh										CSF								
3	AJ	A&E																									trac							in isolation			
	Hinj																																			
		MRSA	surg/intervention

IPC Policy

Isolation in single cubicles		
Hand decontamination		
Gloves and aprons for all patients	x 6 wks	
Monitor by IC Team for 6 weeks		

Figure 8.2 A Gantt chart showing a cluster of MRSA cases on a neurosurgical unit. The first identified case was not the index case – Case 3 was the first MRSA isolated on the ward but went unnoticed.

8.6 Descriptive and analytical epidemiology

Epidemiology is defined as the study of the distribution (frequency, pattern) and determinants of health-related events (not just disease) in specified populations – and the use of this study to control diseases. Epidemiological indicators are useful in healthcare settings, therefore, to summarise and explain situations and contexts by defining 'time', 'place' and 'person'.

8.6.1   *Time* describes **when** something occurred (i.e. onset of symptoms), or the duration of an event (i.e. length of stay of a patient).

8.6.2   *Place* describes **where** the event happened (i.e. in the inpatient ward) or can indicate the geographic spread of an occurrence (i.e. patients come from all districts).

8.6.3   *Person* allows us to describe **who** the event affected and what their characteristic include (i.e. only patients receiving surgical intervention or patients over 70 years of age had a higher risk of dying).

We use epidemiological indicators to express different aspects of time, place and person. These indicators either express a measure of frequency (count, proportion, ratio, incidence and prevalence), association (risk ratio, odds ratio, risk difference) and impact (attributable risk, population attributable fraction) (Table 8.3). We will only address frequency and association in this chapter.

8.6.4   *Frequency indicators* are used for descriptive epidemiology (description of time, place and person). Analytical epidemiology will use association and impact indicators to quantify the risk of disease for different population groups and the potential impact of disease on those groups.

Table 8.3   Common epidemiological indicators used to express 'time', 'place' and 'person'

Frequency	Association	Impact
Count	Risk ratio	Attributable risk
Proportion	Odds ratio	Population attributable fraction
Ratio	Risk difference	
Incidence		
Prevalence		

8.6.5 Descriptive vs analytical epidemiology

Non-experimental epidemiological study design can be divided into descriptive and analytical studies (Figure 8.3). Experimental studies would include in vitro laboratory studies, clinical trials and field trials. We will not be covering experimental study designs in this chapter.

The main difference between descriptive and analytical epidemiological study designs is that descriptive epidemiology does not use a comparative group, whereas analytical studies (cohort, case-control and cross-sectional studies) all include comparison groups, which are also reflected in the indicators that are calculated in these studies.

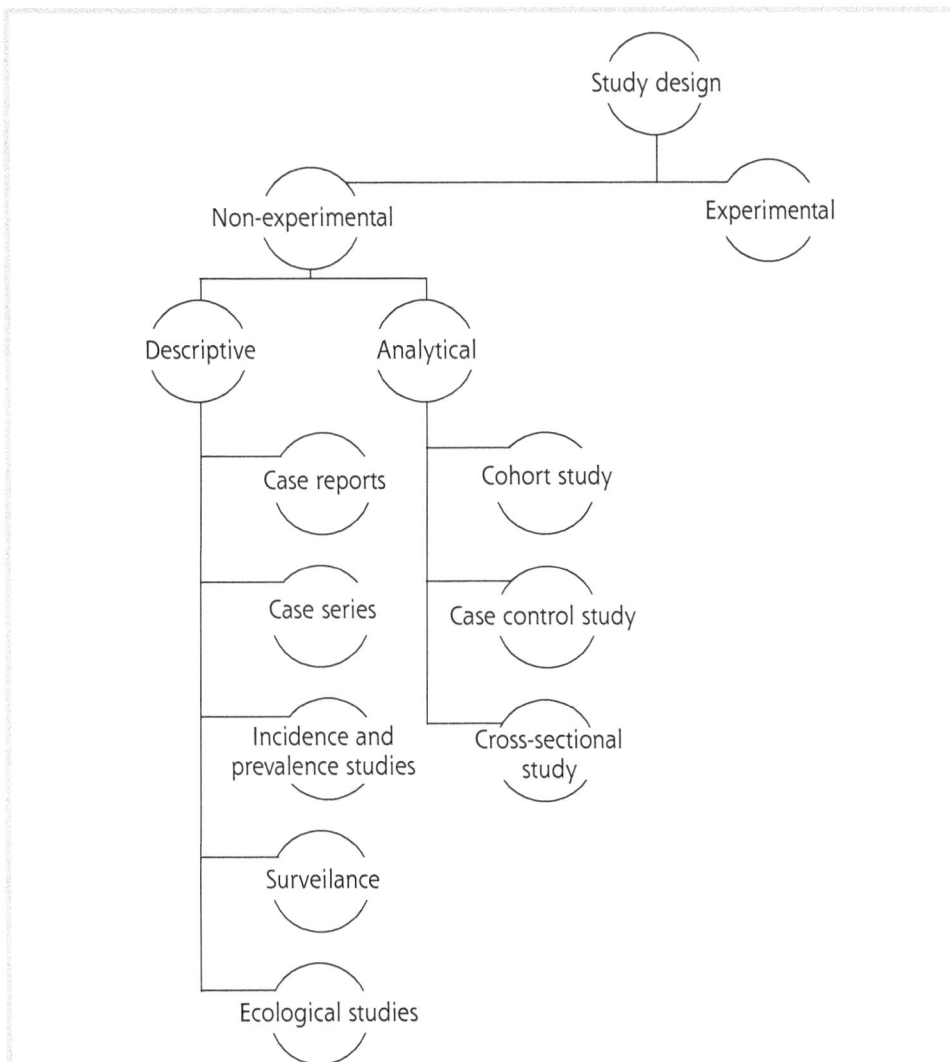

Figure 8.3 Non-experimental study designs used in epidemiology (courtesy Annick Lenglet)

8.6.5.1 Frequency indicators in descriptive studies

The following indicators are used in descriptive studies:

8.6.5.1.1 Count

A *count* is expressed an absolute number of cases, for example: 'we have 3 cases of surgical site infections'. On its own a count is not very informative as there is no denominator, no time period expressed and we have no comparison group.

> **The count alone does not represent a risk of disease.**

8.6.5.1.2 Ratio

A ratio is the division of two numbers where the top of the division (numerator) and the bottom of the division (denominator) are not of the same entity.

> **A ratio therefore compares quantities that are of a different nature.**

In healthcare, we often use ratios to describe medical programming or evaluate quality of care.

> **Box 1:**
>
> An example of a ratio: 5 nurses are the numerator and 25 patients are the denominator. In this case the ratio of nurses to patients is 5 divided by 25 = 1 nurse for each 5 patients or 0.2. Other common ratios used in healthcare include physician to patient ratio, male to female ratio etc.
>
> Nurse to patient ratio $\quad \dfrac{5 \text{ nurses}}{25 \text{ patients}}$

8.6.5.1.3 Proportion

A proportion is a division of two numbers with a numerator and denominator.

> **In contrast to the ratio, in a proportion, the numerator is always included in the denominator as the quantities are of the same nature.**

A proportion can be expressed as a number between 0 and 1 or multiplied by 100 and expressed as a percentage.

Box 2:

Proportion of children under 5 years of age admitted to hospital this month

$$\frac{35 \text{ admission in children} < 5 \text{ this month}}{69 \text{ total admissions this month}} = 0.51 = 51\%$$

Box 3:

Proportional morbidity of late onset neonatal sepsis among all admitted neonates

$$\frac{12 \text{ cases of late onset neonatal sepsis}}{15 \text{ cases of neonatal sepsis}} = 0.8 = 80\%$$

8.6.5.1.4 Incidence

The incidence (rate) is a measure of the speed of occurrence of an event over time. It takes the time period into consideration and therefore *is an expression of risk of disease*. Incidence is a useful indicator if you want to compare the speeds of disease development between different geographical areas or different groups of the population.

The incidence is a division of the number of *new cases* of a specific disease divided by the total person-time at risk in that given population.

Box 4:

Calculating incidence of HAIs in a specific hospital ward

$$\frac{\text{New cases}}{\text{Total person-time at risk}}$$

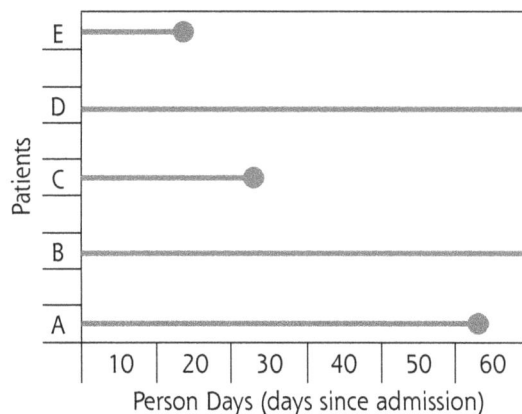

In the above example, there are 5 patients admitted to this ward. Patients E, C and A all develop HAIs (indicated by the dots at the end of their lines). Patient E develops the HAI around 18 days into admission, Patient C 23 days after admission and Patient A 54 days after admission. Both patients D and B are at risk of developing an HAI for the duration of their admission (60 days), but never develop an HAI.

To calculate the incidence rate for HAIs in this example we first need to calculate the denominator, which is the 'person-time at risk'. In this case both patients B and D spent 60 days at risk for an HAI, patient A spent 54 days at risk and then developed an HAI, patient C spent 23 days at risk and then developed an HAI and patient E spent 18 days at risk before developing the HAI. The numerator includes the total number of new cases of HAIs in this patient population, which is 3.

$$\frac{\text{Number of new cases of HAI} = 3}{\text{Person time at risk} = 60 + 60 + 54 + 23 + 18 = 215 \text{ days}}$$

$$= \frac{3}{215} = 0.0139 \times 1000 = \textbf{13.9 HAIs per 1000 person days}$$

8.6.5.1.5 Prevalence

Prevalence is a proportion of the total number of cases in a population at that *moment in time* (numerator) divided by the total population at risk at that moment in time (denominator).

It therefore expresses the proportion of people in a population at a given time with the disease. It is different to the incidence for two reasons: (1) it considers **all** cases of diseases present (not only new cases of disease) and (2) it does not include a measure of time in the denominator.

$$\frac{\text{Number of existing cases in a given population at a specific time}}{\text{Population at a specific time (average value)}}$$

Box 5:

Calculating the prevalence of colonisation with extended-spectrum beta-lactamase-producing gram-negative bacteria in mothers admitted in an obstetric emergency hospital (point prevalence survey).

In this cases all women admitted to this hospital will have a rectal swab screen; thus the denominator is total number of women screened. The numerators will be all those women who were identified as being colonised with ESBL-producing gram-negative bacteria.

$$\frac{\text{Number colonized women with ESBL-GNB}}{\text{Total women screened for colonisation}}$$

$$= \frac{3}{20} = 15\%$$

8.6.6 Frequency indicators in analytical epidemiology

The three main indicators used in analytical epidemiology are the rate ratio (RR, also known as risk ratio), the risk difference and the odds ratio.

The type of indicator one uses will depend on the study design used for data collection.

Cohort studies will generally calculate RR and risk difference. Case-control studies will generally calculate odds ratios. All indicators are calculated based on the '2 x 2 table' (see Figure 8.4).

	Diseased/Cases	Not diseased/Controls	Row totals
Exposed	a	b	a + b
Not exposed	c	d	c + d
Column totals	a + c	b + d	a + b + c + d

Figure 8.4 2 x 2 table for analytical studies

8.6.6.1 Rate ratio

The RR is the ratio between the risk of developing disease after being exposed to a specific exposure compared to the risk of developing the disease when not exposed.

The result is the division between the attack rate of disease in the exposed group divided by the attack rate in the unexposed group.

$$\frac{\text{Risk of disease in exposed group}}{\text{Risk of disease in the unexposed group}} = \frac{\text{Attack rate exposed group}}{\text{Attack rate unexposed group}}$$

In healthcare epidemiology you would usually compare the risk of developing an HAI between different patient groups (cohort) in the hospital depending on gender, age group, disease upon admission, medical intervention, invasive device insertion etc.

Box 6:

A cohort study has been conducted in an intensive care unit in a secondary-level hospital. One hundred patients were followed up from admission. All patients who received central venous catheters (CVC) were recorded, as were all patients who developed confirmed bloodstream infections (BSI). The RR of developing a confirmed BSI after having a CVC inserted was calculated (see also Figure 8.4).

- Patients with CVC who developed BSI = 20
- Patients with CVC who did not develop BSI = 18
- Patients without CVC who developed BSI = 3
- Patients without CVC who did not develop BSI = 59

	Bloodstream infection	No bloodstream infection	Row totals
CVC	a = 20	b = 18	a + b = 38
No CVC	c = 3	d = 59	c + d = 62
Column totals	a + c = 23	b + d = 77	a + b + c + d = 100

Attack rate exposed group $= a/a + b$

Attack rate unexposed group $= c/c + d$

Rate ratio $= (a/a + b)/ (c/c + d)$

Risk ratio $= ((20/38))/((3/62)) = 10.9$

The risk of developing a bloodstream infection is 10.9 times higher in patients with a CVC compared to patients who did not receive a CVC.

8.6.6.2 Risk difference

The risk difference would be the excess risk supposed in the exposed group compared to an unexposed group (and not the ratio of these two numbers). By itself the risk difference is not very informative and usually is shown with the risk ratio and individual attack rates for different exposures.

Risk difference = risk of disease in exposed group − Risk of disease in the unexposed group

Risk difference = attack rate exposed group − attack rate unexposed group

> **Box 7:**
>
> Using the same example of Box 6, risk difference between the patients who received CVC and those who did not develop bloodstream infections would be:
>
> Risk difference = attack rate CVC recipients – attack rate non-CVC patients
>
> $$= (20/38) - (3/62) = 0,53\text{-}0,05 = 0,48$$

8.6.6.3 Odds ratio

> **The odds ratio (OR) is the main indicator that is calculated for case-control studies.**

It is another measure of association that quantifies the relationship between an exposure with two categories and an health outcome. The OR calculates the odds of exposure in cases (or those with the disease in question) divided by the odds of exposure control group.

Taking into consideration the 2 × 2 table from Figure 8.4, this translates to:

OR = odds that a case was exposed / odds that a control was exposed
    = (a/b) / (c/d) = (a*d) / (b*c)

In situations where the prevalence is low the OR will approximate the RR for that specific exposure. This is why case-control studies (which sometimes are easier to implement than cohort studies) are sometimes used to identify the exposures of risk.

> **Box 8:**
>
> In a case-control study that investigates the risk for SSIs after having received elective resection of colon and the rectum. The study team identifies that, with an operative time more than three hours, the OR = 2.6.
>
> This means that patients who had an operative time of more than three hours had a 2.6 higher risk of developing a SSI compared to patients whose operative time was shorter.[14]

8.6.6.4 Interpreting risk ratios and odds ratios

The interpretation of RRs and ORs is similar:
- RR or OR of **1.0** indicates identical risk among the two groups.

---

[14] Tang R, Chen HH, Wang YL, Changchien CR, Chen JS, Hsu KC, Chiang JM & Wang JY. 2001. Risk factors for surgical site infection after elective resection of the colon and rectum: a single-center prospective study of 2 809 consecutive patients. *Ann Surg* 234(2): 181–9. doi: 10.1097/00000658-200108000-00007.

- RR or OR of **greater than 1.0** indicates an increased risk for the group in the numerator.
- RR or OR of **less than 1.0** indicates a decreased risk for the numerator.

It is important to also take into consideration the 95% confidence interval (95% CI) around the RR and OR as this is a measure of the precision around these estimates (see section below).

8.6.7 Describing time, place and persons in descriptive and analytical epidemiological studies

Using the above-described epidemiological indicators, any public health problem can be described in terms of time, place and person.

8.6.7.1 Time

To illustrate the concept of time when describing a public health problem, the two most commonly used tools are epidemic curves (for outbreaks) and graphs (for surveillance data), both based on timelines of events.

8.6.7.1.1 Epidemic curve

An epidemic curve is used to describe the start, end and duration of cases during an outbreak setting. They are also used to show the peak of outbreaks as well as outliers in the outbreak (atypical cases). In general, the time of onset since exposure is shown on the x-axis and the number of cases reported are shown on the y-axis (Figure 8.5).

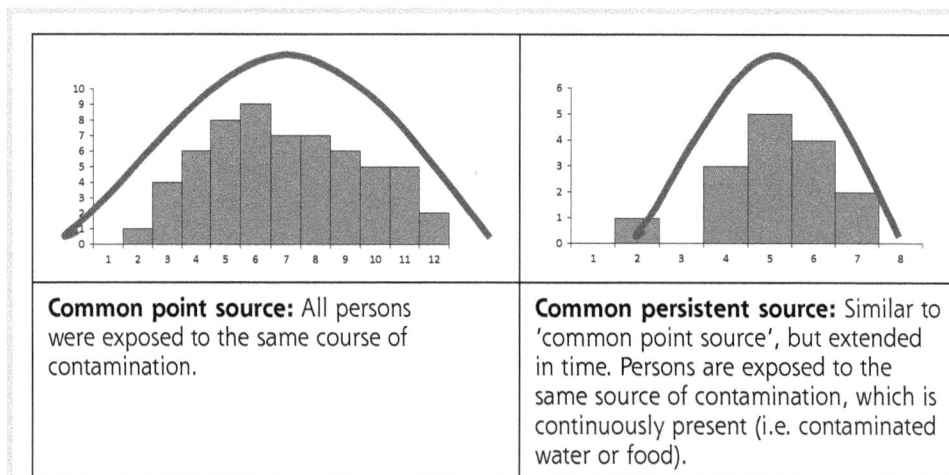

Common point source: All persons were exposed to the same course of contamination.	**Common persistent source:** Similar to 'common point source', but extended in time. Persons are exposed to the same source of contamination, which is continuously present (i.e. contaminated water or food).

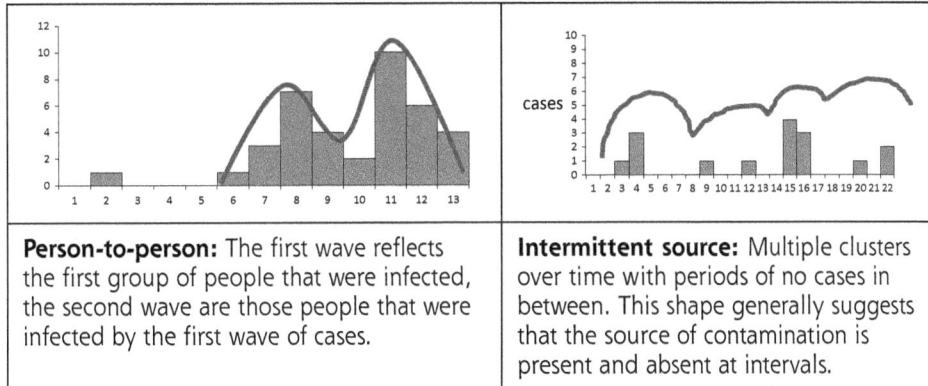

| Person-to-person: The first wave reflects the first group of people that were infected, the second wave are those people that were infected by the first wave of cases. | Intermittent source: Multiple clusters over time with periods of no cases in between. This shape generally suggests that the source of contamination is present and absent at intervals. |

Figure 8.5 Epidemic curve shapes and their transmission dynamics

The shape of an epidemic curve also give a good hint at the possible transmission dynamics at play in that outbreak (Figure 8.5).

8.6.7.1.2 Time series of surveillance data[15]

The time series is applied to the surveillance of reportable infectious diseases and is used for modelling and forecasting the progress of an epidemic over time on expected numbers of reported cases. Forecasts can be modified based on interventions or changes in the trends of the epidemic.[16] The longer the time span (months rather than days), the better. The longer the outbreak or infection surveillance lasts, the easier it is to forecast using mathematical modelling.

15   Hategeka C, Ruton H, Karamouzian M et al. 2020. Use of interrupted time series methods in the evaluation of health system quality improvement interventions: a methodological systematic review. *BMJ Global Health* 5: e003567. doi:10.1136/ bmjgh-2020-003567.
16   *Bulletin of the World Health Organization*. 1998. 76 (4): 327–33.

8.6.7.1.3 Timelines of events

Time series are also known as 'before and after studies'. A baseline data is collected for a fixed period of time, then a well-planned intervention is put in place and evaluated over another period of time, followed by a post-intervention data set. The pre- and post-intervention data sets are compared and reflect the impact of the intervention.

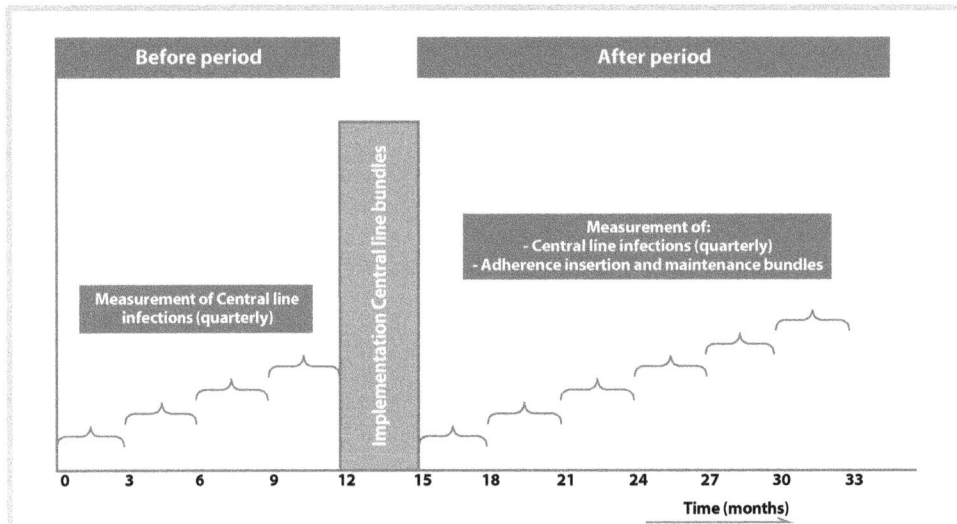

Figure 8.6 Time-interrupted series study of CVC in neonates[17]

A study to improve CVC infections in a neonatal unit was undertaken to study the impact of education and adherence to CVC bundles. The rates of CVC-BSI were measured before and after the intervention, which was the CVC bundles (Figure 8.6).

8.6.7.2 Place

The 'place' usually refers to an administrative location (country, province, district, city) when comparing data between different areas. In hospital settings this might refer to the ward patients were hospitalised in, which beds they were in etc.

17   Helder O, Kornelisse R, van der Starre C, Tibboel D, Looman C, Wijnen R, Poley M & Ista E. 2013. *BMC Health Services Research* 13: 417. http://www.biomedcentral.com/1472-6963/13/417.

8.6.7.2.1 Spot map

A spot map, also known as a geo-map, plots cases by location on a map and helps to visualise where these cases have occurred in a community or area. As an example, confirmed COVID-19 cases in Johannesburg and Cape Town South Africa in April 2020 are plotted using spot or geo-mapping. This highlights clusters and hotspots, which can be managed and contained more effectively.

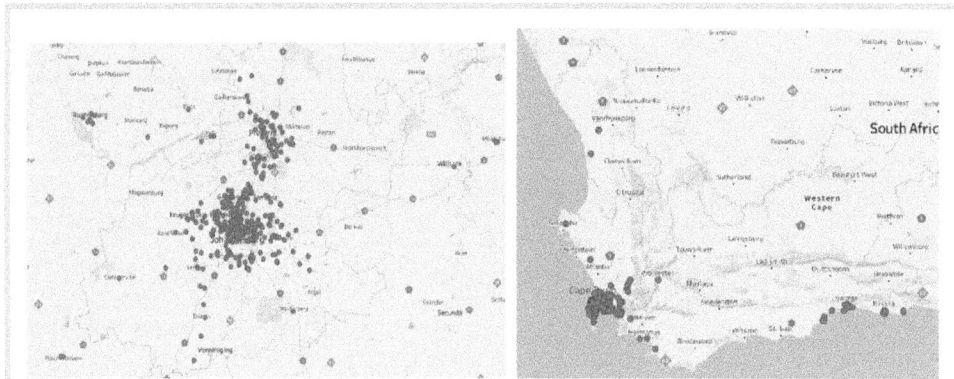

Figure 8.7 COVID-19 case distribution in Johannesburg (left) and Cape Town (right) mapped early in the pandemic. The hotspots or case clusters are easily visualised.[18]

8.6.7.3 Time and space plot (TICL)

A time and space plot, also known as a Gantt chart (see Figure 8.2 under section 8.5.6.2), is used in healthcare facilities to plot several very useful pieces of information, particularly when investigating an outbreak and trying to identify the index case or source. A chart can be established for a single ward or larger clinical unit. Data on the overlap between patient admission dates, interventions such as surgery, devices, isolates identified from the specimens sent for culture and antibiotic and other aspects of clinical management can be documented. Figure 8.8 shows an example of a multi-resistant *S pneumoniae* in a healthcare facility and the impact of good IPC measures.[19]

---

[18] National Department of Health presentation to Parliamentary health portfolio committee, 10 April 2020.

[19] Bastiaens GJH, Cremers AJH, Coolen JPM, Nillesen MT, Boeree MJ, Hopman J & Wertheim HFL. 2018. Nosocomial outbreak of multi-resistant *Streptococcus pneumoniae* serotype 15A in a centre for chronic pulmonary diseases. *Antimicrob Resist Infect Control* 27(7): 158. doi: 10.1186/s13756-018-0457-3.

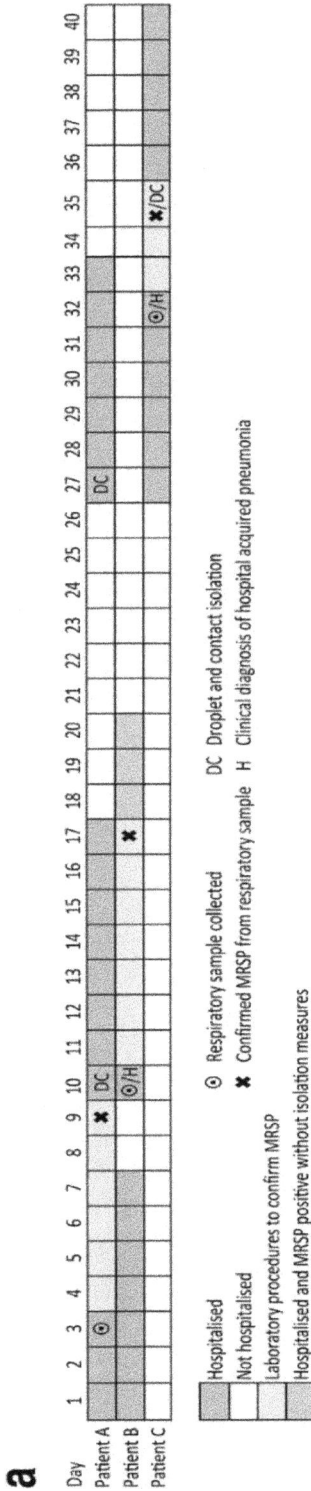

Figure 8.8 Spread of a multidrug resistant *S pneumoniae* in a health facility

8.6.8 Person

Personal characteristics of identified cases

The personal characteristics make up the case definition (CD) as discussed in the outbreak section. This essential data distinguishes a person with disease from one who is not infected, but is not always clear-cut, particularly at the start of an outbreak or epidemic, since all the facts are not known. However, as the outbreak or spread progresses these characteristics can be honed to become more precise. A narrow CD is helpful to the clinicians when dealing with a large group of exposed persons and eliminating those that do not fit the CD profile.

For example:
There is an outbreak of food poisoning that occurred at a wedding. The CD will include persons who attending the wedding, ate certain foods, met many other people and used the bathroom which had handwashing facilities. Once the pathogen, *S typhimurium*, is identified, certain foodstuffs can be eliminated. The line list will help to establish the individual characteristics of cases.

Attack rates between different groups
Following the example above, the attack rates (RR) between different groups can be established using a 2 × 2 table and exposure to each type of food and the personal characteristics of the different groups present at the wedding.

8.7   Important concepts in statistics

8.7.1 Sampling and describing samples

In epidemiological studies it would be unusual that the entire population of interest would be studied as this generally is not feasible in the situation. For this reason, most studies choose a subset of the population of interest called a **sample**. The sample should be representative of the population of interest for the different characteristics that that population might represent, such as age, disease of interest, gender etc.

Most populations will be normally distributed (Figure 8.9) for all main characteristics of interest. Samples drawn from populations therefore should also achieve normal distribution across the same characteristics.

We use indicators such as mode, median, interquartile-range, mean and standard deviation to describe these characteristics as they will identify if the sample is not normally distributed (skewed) in some way.

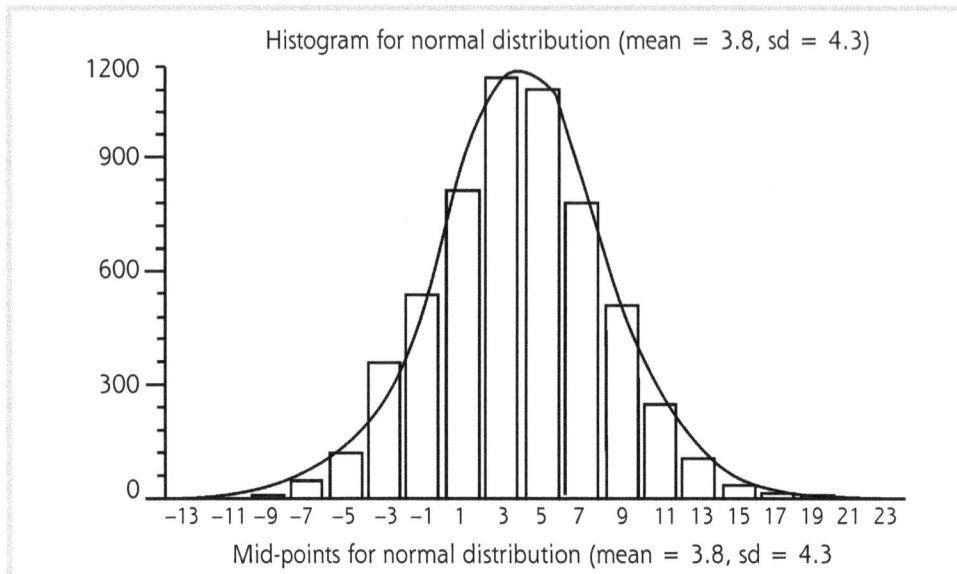

Figure 8.9 Normal distribution in a population for a characteristic of interest

The **mode** is the value that is most commonly used for an outcome of interest.

The **median** is the number that lies in the middle of all the values across that sample (i.e. at 50% of the sample).

The **interquartile range** (IQR) will identify the values that lie at 25% and 75% of all the values.

The median and IQR are always reported together.

The **mean** is the average value of all the values in the sample.

Standard deviation (SD) indicates the difference between a group of values and their mean, taking all the data into account. The larger the standard deviation, the more the values differ from the mean and are therefore widely spread out. It is used to identify the spread in a population. The mean and the SD are usually reported together.

Standard error (SE), which is another term for SD of a sampling distribution rather than just a sample, is used in hypothesis testing and the calculation of confidence levels.

Box 9:

Calculating indicators to describe the sample of patients who developed a urinary tract infection with a catheter in situ. Thirty-two patients had a catheter inserted and for the follow-up period 13 patients developed urinary tract infection (prevalence = 13/32 = 0,4 = 40%). When describing the time between the catheter insertion and the onset of the urinary tract infection, the following data is available for the 13 patients who developed the urinary tract infection.

Patient Number	Days when urinary sample became positive
1	3
2	4
3	4
4	4
5	5
6	6
7	6
8	8
9	8
10	8
11	8
12	9
13	18

- What is the mean number of days for the UTI to develop?

  Mean = (total number of days of all UTI patients)/total UTI patients

  = (3+4+4+4+5+6+6+8+8+8+8+9+18)/13 = 85/13 = 6,5

- What is the median of days for the UTI to develop? You see in the table that there is one patient who develops the UTI 18 days after the catheter was inserted, in which case showing the median might be more useful.

  Median = centre-most value (50%) in the whole list of values = 7th observation in the list = 6 days

  Mode = most common value = 3 patients with 8 days = 8 days

  IQR 25% = the value at 25% of all values = 4 days

  IQR 75% = the value at 75% of all values = 8 days

8.7.2 95% confidence interval

95% confidence intervals (95% CI) are statistical calculations of different estimates for prevalence, incidence, proportions, RRs and ORs. They are used to estimate how precise the estimates for these indicators are compared to the reference population from where the sample was drawn. The most simplistic way to think about 95% CI is to think that if you ran the same study 100 times, 95 times the estimates you calculated would fall within that range.

A wide 95% CI generally indicates: (1) the estimate is not very precise; (2) there was a high variability in the data for that indicator in your sample; (3) the sample size you drew for your study was probably too small for the outcome indicator you calculated.

When interpreting 95% CI for RR or OR, if the range includes 1, this risk factor or exposure is not statistically significantly associated with the outcome of interest. For this reason, 95% CIs are often more informative than p-values alone.

Boxes 10 and 11 have some examples on how to interpret 95% CIs.

Box 10:

You asked two different study teams to conduct a COVID vaccination coverage survey among healthcare workers in your hospital. Team 1 estimates a 90% coverage for COVID vaccination with a 95% CI = 86–93%. Team 2 also estimated a 90% coverage with a 95% CI = 7–295%. Which of the two teams' estimates would you find more reliable?

Answer: Both teams estimated a 90% coverage for vaccination among the healthcare workers in your hospital. However, Team 1 has a CI95% that is 7% wide, whereas Team 2 has a CI95% that is 13% wide. This suggests that Team 1's estimate is more precise and likely because they had a more appropriate study design and sample size for the coverage survey.

Box 11:

You have conducted a case-control study to explore risk factors associated with SSIs following elective resection of the colon and the rectum. Two exposures you looked at included duration of operative time and the number of blood units received. Your results are shown below. Considering these results, how do you interpret the 95% CI associated with the risk factors for SSIs after elective resection of the colon and rectum?
- Operative time more than three hours: OR = 2.6; CI95% = 1.4–4.8
- 1–3 blood units received: OR = 1.5; CI95% = 0.8–2.9

Answer: The ORs for both risk factors are above 1 and therefore would be considered to carry a higher risk of developing an SSI in patients that had an operative time of longer than three hours or patients that received 1–3 units of blood. However, when you look at the 95% CI for these two risk factors, you see that the risk factor for blood units received includes 1. For this reason, it is not a statistically significant risk factor. In contrast, the 95% CI for the risk factor related to operative time remains greater than 1 and therefore is a statistically significant risk factor for the development of an SSI in these patients.

8.7.3 P-values

Probability is a mathematical technique of predicting outcomes. It predicts how likely it is for a specific event to occur. It is measured on a scale from 0 to 1.0. Probability (the p-value) is usually expressed in a decimal format (50% becomes 0.5), it is never more than 1.0 and it cannot be negative.

The p-value is a number that expresses the probability that equal (or more extreme than) results can be observed by chance alone. In general, a p-value <0.05 is considered to show that what you observe is statistically significantly different to what would be observed by chance alone (in more critical studies this value might be set to <0.01).

> **Note: The presence of significance does not prove biological, clinical or public health relevance of an effect.**

Also, a lack of significance is **not** necessarily a lack of an effect: 'Absence of evidence is not evidence of absence *(of effect)*'.

P-values should be interpreted with caution, especially when rejecting the null hypothesis. Two types of errors can occur:
- Type 1 error: rejecting the true null hypothesis and accepting a false alternative
- Type 2 error: not rejecting a false null hypothesis

It is wise to report both p-values and confidence levels since the latter is considered a better way of testing a hypothesis – if the confidence level does not include the hypothetical mean, it indicates significance.

8.7.4 Chi square

x^2 (Chi square) statistics are used to compare whether observed counts in your sample for different categorical variables would be expected under the assumption of no association. In this way you can use the x^2 to test the hypothesis of no association between two or more groups, populations or criteria.

A small value for the x^2 (observed counts and expected counts are similar) supports the assumption that there is no association between the groups you are comparing.

A large value of the x^2 statistic (observed counts and expected counts would differ) would support an assumption that the groups you are comparing are associated or different.

Using a x^2 statistic table, for each value of x^2 you calculate you can identify an associate p-value that indicates the probability of obtaining a statistic of this magnitude or larger when there is no association.

8.8   Defining the research question and study objectives

Any proposal for a study needs to start with a well-defined research question (or research questions). The way that the research question is formulated will influence how you formulate the objectives for your study, the study design you choose and how you will interpret the data you collect. After you have formulated the research question you will formulate study objectives that will indicate how you will try and answer that research question.

Research objectives will generally have an overarching objective (primary study objective or study aim), but then will have other more detailed objectives that can also be addressed over the course of the study (secondary objectives).

Box 12:

Example on how to formulate research questions and objectives

Your research question is to understand the prevalence of healthcare-acquired infections among pediatric patients in your hospitals. Your main study objective would be: to determine the prevalence of HAI among pediatric patients admitted to hospital between xxx date and xxx date. Your secondary objectives then might include:
- to describe pediatric patients with HAI in clinical and epidemiological terms
- to microbiologically isolate bloodstream, urine and pus pathogens from patients with HAI and determine the antibiotic resistance profile of these bacteria
- to determine risk factors associated with the development of HAI in pediatric patients.

8.8.1 Choosing the right study design

Deciding the study design to answer your research question and address your study objectives is the next crucial step for determining the methodology and the resources required. You can choose quantitative study designs, which include non-experimental studies and experimental studies (clinical trials etc). You can also choose qualitative study designs, which are targeted more to understanding behavioural and perception aspects of certain research questions. You can also choose to combine quantitative and qualitative methods to have a mixed-methods study design. It is important to include the right expertise in your study team in order to help decide the proper study design and to help you further with methodology, implementation, data analysis and interpretation.

A few common research study designs for quantitative and qualitative studies are listed below.

8.8.1.1 Common quantitative study designs

The information during quantitative studies is collected in a precise manner and the researcher (or investigator) simply observes. There is no intervention carried out by the observer. The enquiry is into phenomena and their relationships – cause and effect. The data set is precise, usually numeric and recorded without subjective bias if possible. Examples of study designs are cross-sectional, cohort or case-control studies and are applicable to epidemiology and IPC. The process of measurement is central to quantitative research because it provides the fundamental connection between empirical observation and mathematical expression of quantitative relationships.

Case study

A case study is an in-depth analysis of a single case that can lead to further research, but is of little value in itself unless it is:

- describing an extremely complicated case (unlikely to get a number of very similar cases that one can 'pool' data from)
- as an illustration that a theory may be correct
- extending experience relating to a specific case
- challenging existing theory.

Case series

Case series are a group of cases affected by the same outcome of interest or disease. There is no time frame or controls. Its main advantage lies in collecting information about a particular disease, which may later be used to stimulate further research. It is not expected to stand up to research rigour unless it is exceptionally well defined, analysed and presented.

8.8.1.1.1 Cohort studies

The incidence and natural history of a condition are best defined by cohort studies. These may be prospective or retrospective and sometimes as a comparison of two cohorts.

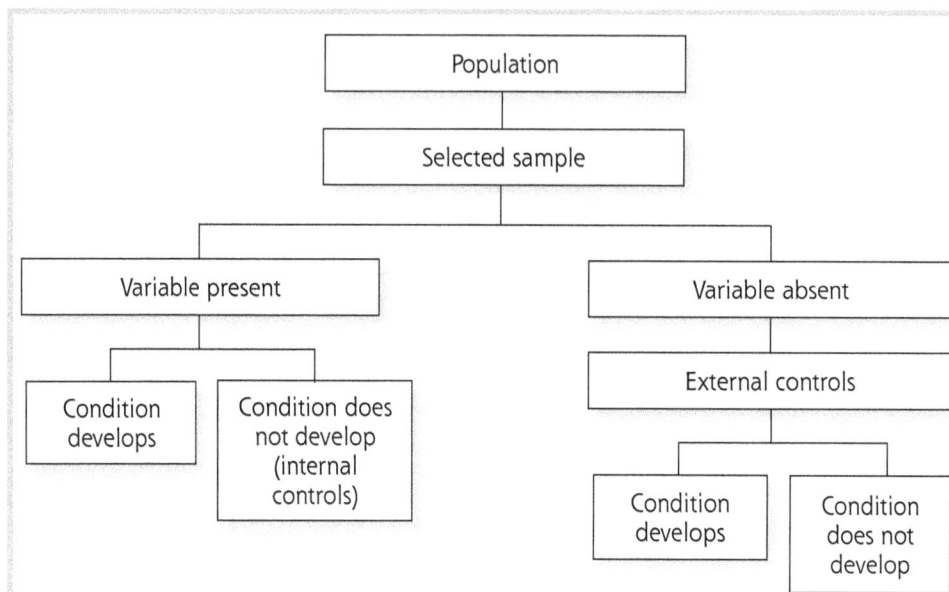

Figure 8.10 A plan for a cohort study design

8.8.1.1.2 Prospective cohort studies

These are when a group of people do not have an outcome of interest (disease) at the beginning of the study, for example a urinary catheter-associated infection. The research will measure a variety of variables (demography, method of catheterisation, type of urinary catheter etc) and the group is followed up over a period of time to see whether they develop a urinary infection. In a single cohort study those who do not develop the outcome of interest (i.e. a urinary infection) are used as internal controls. When two groups are compared, one group is given an intervention, such as antibiotics, while the other is not, the latter acting as external controls.

Advantages
- Cohorts are applicable when randomised controlled trials may be unethical; research on risk factors can effectively use cohort studies.
- As such studies measure potential causes before the outcome has occurred, the studies can demonstrate that these 'causes' preceded the outcome and avoid debate regarding cause and effect.
- Cohort studies can simultaneously look at other outcome variables from the data collected. In contrast, case-control studies only assess one outcome variable (the one they entered the study with).
- Cohorts allow calculations of the effect of each variable on the probability of developing the outcome of interest (relative risk).

Disadvantages
- A prospective cohort study is inefficient when a certain outcome is rare; the efficiency of a prospective cohort study increases as the incidence of a particular outcome increases.
- A loss of some subjects to follow up. This can significantly effect the outcome especially since the numerator decreases – the rarer the condition the more significant the effect.

8.8.1.1.3 Retrospective studies

In retrospective studies, the data has already been collected for other purposes. The methodology is the same, but the study is performed after the event and the cohort is 'followed up' afterwards. The time to complete the study is only as long as it takes to collate and analyse the data.

Advantages
- These are cheaper since the data has already been collected.
- There is a lack of bias because the current outcome of interest was the original reason for collecting the data.

Disadvantages
- The data set may not be complete for the purposes of studying the current outcome because the database was not set up for it originally – some variables may be missing.
- Recall (sampling) bias – subjects with the outcome of interest are more likely to exaggerate or minimise what they now consider risk factors.
- When two cohorts are compared, one will be exposed and the other will not; the major disadvantage is the inability to control for all other factors that might differ between the two groups – confounding variable.
- Confounding variables are independently associated with both the variable of interest and the outcome of interest The only way to eliminate all possibility of a confounding variable is by carrying out a prospective randomised controlled study so that each type of exposure is assigned by chance and the confounding variable will be present in both groups.
- Bias can occur in any study and reflects the potential that the sample is not representative of the population it was drawn from. For example, taking a sample from the employed to reflect the population at large will be inaccurate.

8.8.1.1.4 Designing a cohort study
- If the data already exists, it is easy to set up a retrospective study. If not, then a prospective study has to be designed.
- Definition of sample group. Each subject must have the potential to develop the outcome of interest.

- Descriptive. The sample must be representative of the general population if the study is primarily looking at the incidence or natural history of the condition.
- Analytical. If the aim is to analyse the relationship between predictor variables and the outcomes, then the sample should contain as many subjects as possible who are likely to develop the outcome of interest.
- Each variable should be accurately measured. Some may be fixed, such as height, and a single measurement is sufficient; some may vary (weight), when several measurements are needed.
- It reduces the risk of missing confounding variable – all relevant variables should be measured to make the study results robust.
- All subjects entered in the study should be followed up until the end of the study.

8.8.1.2 Cross-sectional study

Cross-sectional studies are primarily used to determine prevalence – the number of cases in a population at a given point in time – as a snapshot. It cannot provide an incidence rate. Each measurement is made at one point in time and could be repeated the same time each year for several years. A good example is the antenatal HIV and syphilis survey conducted each October in South Africa. These studies also infer causation. At one point in time the subjects are assessed to determine whether they were exposed to a relevant agent and have the outcome of interest (some subjects will not have either). This distinguishes this type of study from other observational studies (cohort and case-controlled) where reference to either exposure and/or outcome is made.

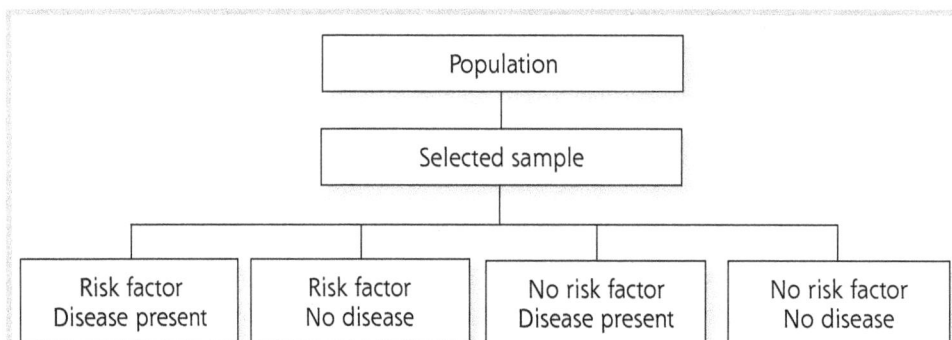

Figure 8.11 Layout for a cross-sectional study

Advantages
- Subjects have not been deliberately exposed or treated and have little or no ethical difficulties.
- Study is relatively cheap; data is collected once from one group and multiple outcomes can be studied.

- Relatively quick to do.
- Best way to establish prevalence and useful associations – good for HAI infections.
- Easy way to study multiple outcomes.

Disadvantage
- Does not differentiate cause and effect from simple association.
- Rare conditions cannot be studied using cross-sectional studies; it is best to study a sample that already has the disease (a case series).

To ensure a good response rate from a representative sample a random selection from a group should be invited to complete a questionnaire. It does not, however, take into account non-responders.

Another method is to carry out a census, but this is not applicable to medical research.

8.8.1.2.1 Designing a cross-sectional study

Such a study can be done using questionnaires or interviews. Questionnaires are cheaper to do and can reach a wide sample size, but have a low response rate. Interviews are expensive, but the response rate is high and the sample size can be smaller. A low response rate does not give a representative sample; volunteers are unlikely to be representative of a general population.

Formulate a research question and select a sample. Then decide what variables of the study group are relevant to the research questions. A method of contacting the subjects should be devised, such as phone calls or house visits. The data is collected and analysed.

For example, the natural history of HIV has been studied using cohort studies, and efficacy of treatments via case-controlled studies and randomised clinical trials.

8.8.1.3 Case-controlled studies

Case-controlled (CC) studies are usually retrospective – those with the outcome of interest are matched with a control group that does not. Retrospectively, the cause and effect is determined. **When the outcome is rare, case-controlled studies are best**. The aim is to identify predictors of an outcome.

These types of studies are more cost-effective, since there are a higher percentage of cases per study. CC studies determine the relative importance of a predictor variable in relation to the presence or absence of the disease. CC studies are retrospective and therefore cannot be used to determine relative risk (unlike a prospective cohort study), but they can be used to determine odds ratios, which in turn usually approximate to relative risk.

8.8.1.3.1 Designing a case-control study

Formulate a hypothesis and what will be measured and how. Specify the characteristics of the study group and construct a valid control group. Then compare the 'exposure' in the two groups to each variable.

Advantages

- Simple to organise.
- Can compare two groups retrospectively.
- In uncommon conditions, CC studies generate a lot of information from relatively few subjects.
- CC studies are the only feasible option when there is a long latent period between exposure (variable) and disease (outcome of interest).
- Comparatively few subjects are required so more resources are available to study each – the number of variables available for study are more.
- CC studies are useful for generating a hypothesis that can be tested using other types of study.

Disadvantages

- The flexibility of variables studied comes at the expense of the restricted outcomes studied, such as the presence or absence of disease.
- There are problems with confounding variables and bias (see above).

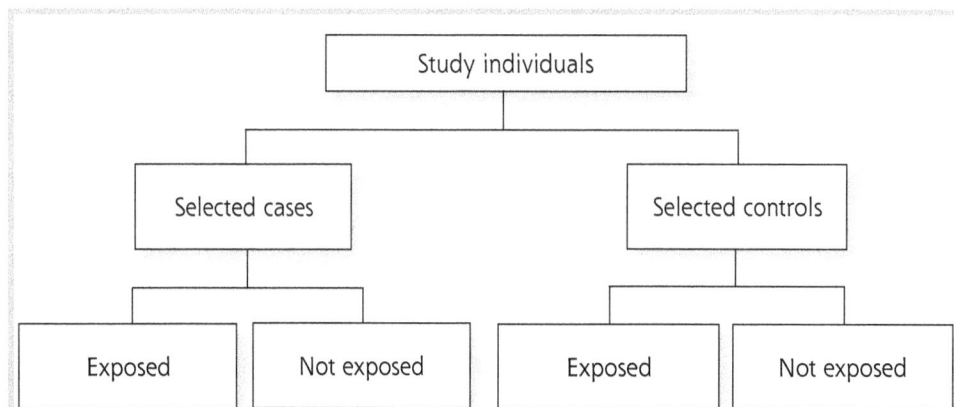

Figure 8.12 Plan for a case-control study

8.8.1.4 Overcoming sample bias

Ideally, the CC studied should be a random sample of all the patients with the disease; this is sometimes difficult if the diagnosis has not been made or there has been misdiagnosis or misinterpretation of the signs and symptoms.

1. Selection of controls is a more difficult problem. Control should represent the same population as the cases.

2. Convenience sample: Sampled in the same way as the cases. While convenient, it will reduce the external validity of the test.

3. Matching: The controls may be matched or unmatched random samples from the unaffected population. 'Overmatching' can cause a true difference to be underestimated.

4. Using two or more control groups: If the study demonstrates a significant difference between patients with disease and those without, even when the latter is sampled in several different ways, the conclusion is more robust.

5. A population-based sample of both cases and controls. One can take a random sample of all patients with a specific disease from a specific register. The control group can be constructed by matching a randomly selection from the population with the study group.

8.8.1.5 Overcoming observation and recall bias

Use of data recorded for other purposes before the outcome occurred can reduce observational bias, but is limited by the type of data collected.

Alternatively, blinding cannot be used where either subject or investigator knows if they are a case or control, nor are they aware of the study hypothesis. In practice, this is very difficult when dealing with clinical conditions and only partial blinding is possible.

8.8.2 Common qualitative study designs

Qualitative research is a field of inquiry that crosscuts disciplines and subject-matters. Qualitative researchers aim to gather an in-depth understanding of human behaviour and the reasons that govern such behaviour. The discipline investigates the why and how of decision-making, not just what, where, when. Hence, smaller but focused samples are more often needed. This method is useful to establish compliance with policies and regulations since it can answer certain important questions more efficiently and effectively than quantitative approaches. It assists to understand important questions about relevance, unintended effects and impact of (IPC) programmes. This is because establishing content validity – do measures measure what a researcher thinks they measure? – is seen as one of the strengths of qualitative research. Qualitative studies structured as a questionnaire, interviews or focus group reveal certain other factors – allergies, distance from patients too far, do not have time etc. The subjects can express their opinions on what the actual practice is and/or should be. Qualitative data is usually difficult to graph or display in mathematical terms.

8.8.2.1 *Observations*

Often, in healthcare settings, to better understand how and why certain things happen (hand hygiene adherence, clinical decision making etc) it is valuable to observe natural interactions with teams of people and just record those observations. Data collection can be done using recording sheets or checklists, observation guides (listing interactions, processes, behaviours to be observed) and field notes. Increasingly the use of digital tools (cameras, mobile data collection tools) is making this type of a methodological approach easier.

Observations can be done 'overtly', where the group under observation is aware they are being observed, or 'covertly', where the observations are done without the group's knowledge (through 'secret shopper' or camera-based observations).

Advantages
- The researchers are exposed first-hand to the natural environment where an activity is happening.
- Observations sometimes work better with people or groups that have limited time or willingness to answer questions.

Disadvantages
- Insights are susceptible to the researcher's bias.
- Observations can be time-consuming (and expensive).
- Any observation where the subjects are observed might make them behave differently, or 'better', because they know they are being observed. This is known as the Hawthorn Effect.

8.8.2.2 *Key informant interviews*

Key informant interviews are interviews conducted between the research team and someone who is considered to have an 'expert' or in-depth understanding pertaining to the research question. The interview is usually conducted in a semi-structured manner (some questions are fixed, but there is space to collect open-ended answers as well as ask additional clarifying probing questions). The interviews generally last between 60 to 90 minutes and are ideally conducted face to face.

Key informant interviews are useful for complex or sensitive topics, or when very detailed information is needed that cannot be collected in any other way. Key informant interviews are useful when trying to explain results obtained in quantitative studies as part of mixed methods design.

Advantages
- Yield in-depth understanding and new insights.
- Can capture both knowledge and emotional reactions to topics.
- Give the researcher the opportunity to clarify aspects or probe for more detailed responses.

Disadvantages
- Costly and time-consuming.
- Interviewers need to be highly trained.
- Collect a lot of information, which needs to be transcribed, coded and analysed.
- The information is only explorative and is not necessarily representative for what the study population thinks or feels.

8.8.2.3 Focus group discussions

In a focus group discussion (FGD) a researcher will speak to a group of people with similar characteristics (i.e. women of reproductive age, nurses, doctors, patients etc) and discuss their perceptions, opinions, beliefs and attitudes towards an idea, concept or topic. The same topic will be discussed with different groups in order to obtain diverse and more in-depth information. A FGD will not last longer than 90 minutes and should not contain more than 12 people (minimum 6 participants).

Advantages
- FGDs are more effective in obtaining information on perceptions, attitudes and experiences than a survey.
- They provide ways to collect very detailed data about a topic.
- Researchers are able to ask clarification questions.

Disadvantages
- The data collected in an FGD will be reflective of the participants in that group, is not generalisable to the rest of the population and might be very context-specific.
- FGD facilitators must remain neutral and not influence the direction of the conversation as well as ensure that no single participant dominates the discussion.

8.8.3 Study protocol and implementation

Designing a comprehensive study protocol is critical in research. It provides the 'recipe' book for all the questions, issues, resource needs and constraints that the study team has identified and the solutions and way forward in order to be able to carry out the research.

The research protocol should reflect as a minimum the sections listed below:
- A title which reflects the study purpose.
- Background and context in which the research is based.
- Purpose/research question: the aim of the study should be clearly stated.
- Methods:
  - Overall study design

- Study population or sample:
  - accurately reflect the population it has been drawn from
  - source of the sample should be stated
  - the sampling method should be described
  - the sample size should be justified
  - entry and exclusion criteria should be justified
  - the number of patients lost to follow up and an explanation given
- The control group (if relevant)
  - should be easily identifiable
  - the source of the controls should be explained – from the same population as the controls or not
  - are the controls matched or randomised to minimise bias and confounding
- Data to be collected and how
  - data collection tools or questionnaires
  - laboratory procedures
  - data protection and ownership
  - quality of measurements and outcome
  - validity – are the measurements regarded as valid by other investigators?
  - reproducibility – can the results be repeated or are these a 'once-off'?
  - blinded – are the investigators or subjects aware of their allocations?
  - quality control – are the methodologies rigorously adhered to?
  - completeness
  - did all the patients comply with the study?
  - how many failed to complete the study?
  - deaths?
  - missing data – how much is unavailable and why?
- Data analysis plan
  - for quantitative data this should include dummy tables and proposed statistical tests to be used.
  - for qualitative data this should include the proposed framework and coding approach to analysing the data collected.
- Limitations and bias
  - extraneous treatments – other investigations may have affected some of the subjects.
  - confounding variables – other factors that might influence the results.
  - appropriate analysis – have the right statistical tools been used to analyse the data?
  - internally valid. The conclusions can be drawn from the results produced by appropriate methodology.

    ○ externally valid. The value of the study to other populations – the generalisability of results.
- Ethical considerations
- Risks and benefits from the research proposed
- Dissemination plan following the research

Using established guidance for research protocol development is always a good idea. One place to start would be the 'Bridging research integrity and global health epidemiology (BRIDGE) statement and guidelines.'[20]

---

[20]   https://pubmed.ncbi.nlm.nih.gov/33115859/; https://pubmed.ncbi.nlm.nih.gov/33115860/.

Glossary

Aerosol. A suspension of extremely small liquid or solid particles in the air.

Air change occurs when a volume of air equivalent to the volume of the room has been supplied to or removed from that room (whichever airflow is the greater). The rate of air change is usually given in terms of air changes per hour (ACH) and is derived from the volume of a room and the ventilation rate.

Alcohol-based (hand) rub. An alcohol-containing preparation (liquid, gel or foam) designed for application to the hands to reduce the growth of micro-organisms.

Alert organisms. Organisms of IPC importance such as multi-resistant gram-negative bacilli and methicillin-resistant *Staphylococcus aureus* (MRSA). Positive microbiology reports of their presence may result in a case review, a search for other carriers or infected patients.

Antimicrobial (medicated) soap. Soap (detergent) containing an antiseptic agent at a concentration which is sufficient to reduce or inhibit the growth of micro-organisms.

Antiseptics. Substances that discourage the growth micro-organisms. They are safe to use on the skin (living tissue). The two commonly used antiseptics are chlorhexidine gluconate either 2% or 4% w/v, or povidone iodine which has replaced tincture of iodine for safety reasons.

Antiseptic handrubbing (or handrubbing). Applying an antiseptic handrub to reduce or inhibit the growth of micro-organisms without the need for an exogenous source of water and requiring no rinsing or drying with towels or other devices.

Antiseptic handwashing. Washing hands with water and soap or other detergents containing an antiseptic agent.

Aseptic. The absence of micro-organisms.

Audit. Measurement of performance taken over a limited period of time to ascertain whether pre-determined standards are being met.

Bacteria. Single-celled micro-organisms which can exist either as independent (free-living) organisms or as parasites (dependent upon another organism for life).

Binders. Chemicals which bind and remove calcium and manganese and reduce scaling.

Biofilm or **glycocalyx**. Protective covering produced by some bacteria. It is made of similar material to a capsule (see below) and serves the same purpose – to escape phagocytosis. Biofilm is formed over most inert materials, especially plastic, allowing the bacteria to survive and thrive, inside it.

Capsule. A protective covering produced by some bacteria, notably *Streptococcus pneumoniae* which protects them from an external hostile environment and phagocyctosis. In some bacteria the capsule enhances virulence or invasiveness.

Cascading system. An IPC system characterised by its spreading outward, such as the transfer of information from a government initiative through hospitals, bigger clinics to the smallest clinic.

Cell wall. Rigid structure which allows selective absorption and excretion of various substances. In gram-negative bacilli there are inlets or channels called porins which allow selective passage in and out of the cell and can be modified, if required, to restrict noxious substances from entering the cytoplasm.

Chemical waste. Waste from pharmacy, laboratories, engineering workshops and all other areas where chemicals are used.

Clinical waste. Any waste which consists wholly or partly of human blood or animal tissues, blood or other bodily fluids, excretions, drugs or other pharmaceutical products, swabs or dressings and syringes, needles or other sharp instruments.

Communicable disease. Transmission of an **infectious agent** or its toxic product from an infected person, animal, or reservoir to a **susceptible host** (a disease that can be communicated from one person to another).

Detergents (surfactants). Compounds that possess a cleaning action. They are composed of a hydrophilic and a lipophilic part and can be divided into four groups: anionic, cationic, amphoteric and non-ionic.

Disinfectants. Antimicrobial agents that are applied to non-living objects to destroy micro-organisms. They are used on inanimate objects and surfaces because these have adverse effects on living tissue.

Droplet precautions. Precautions taken to prevent and control the spread of infections from organisms spread by droplet transmission.

Droplet transmission. When oral or nasal secretions of an infected patient enter the eyes, nose or mouth of another person. The secretions are most commonly passed through coughing and sneezing.

Dryness value. A measure of the amount of water droplets in a steam supply for sterilisers.

Duty of Care. The professional standards and the responsibility of each healthcare worker to a patient.

Employee. Someone who is hired and paid to work by a person or organisation.

Employer. A person or organisation(including the State) who pays someone to work for them.

Flagellum. Long helical filaments which support motility and allow the bacterium to change its environment.

Hand hygiene. A general term referring to any action of hand cleansing.

Lysis. The dissolution or destruction of cells, such as blood cells or bacteria, as by the action of a specific lysin that disrupts the cell membrane. It can thus be the gradual subsiding of an acute infection.

Notifiable disease. Any disease that is required by law to be reported to government authorities.

Occupational disease. A disease caused by the work someone does or the workplace such as needlestick injury or asbestosis among asbestos miners.

Occupational injury. An injury that is the result of the work that someone does.

Oro-faecal. Transmitted from faeces to the mouth.

Outbreak. An occurrence of disease greater than would otherwise be expected in a particular time and place. It may be a small and localised group or impact upon thousands of people across an entire continent.

Parametric release. Declaring a product as sterile. This requires the pre-validation of all processes such as loading patterns and load configuration followed by verification that all parameters and variables are within pre-set defined limits.

Personal protective equipment (PPE). Equipment used to protect the user from transmission of infection. For example, use of gloves (and plastic aprons) when dealing with blood and body fluids including intravenous access.

Pili and fimbriae are external fine hair like rigid structures (not involved in motion), which allow the bacterium to attach itself to external surfaces – either to a host (common pili) or other bacteria (sex pili); the latter is to transfer genetic information.

Prions. Infectious agents which only have nucleic acid and are highly resistant to routine disinfection and sterilisation. They are the cause of Creutzfeldt-Jakob disease (vCJD).

Porins. Inlets or channels which allow selective passage in and out of the cell and can be modified, if required, to restrict noxious substances from entering the cytoplasm.

Procedures. Clearly structured acts according to standard operating procedures (SOPs).

Soil. Faeces and other excretions. Artificial soil is used to test the cleaning of instruments.

Standard precautions. Routine precautions that reduce the risk of transmission of micro-organisms from both recognised and unrecognised sources of infection in healthcare settings.

Sterilise. To make free from bacteria and other organisms including spores.

Validation. Documented procedure of obtaining, recording and interpreting the results required to establish that a process will consistently yield products complying with predetermined conditions.

Virus. Ultramicroscopic infectious agent that requires the host's systems to survive; therefore viruses infect every life form from bacteria, fungi, plants, to animals and humans. Viruses are classified into DNA or RNA viruses depending on the type of nucleic acid they are made of. They are further classified as single or double stranded.

Waterless antiseptic agent. An antiseptic agent that does not require the use of exogenous water. After application, the individual rubs the hands together until the agent has dried. The term includes different types of handrubs (liquid formulations, gels, foams).

Index

A

ACH *see* air, changes
acute flaccid paralysis 410
acute respiratory infection *see also* SARS-CoV-2
    cleaning 356, 443, 444
    home-based care 442-445
    linen & laundry 220, 434, 444
    PPE 355, 442, 443, 444
    treatment centre 355-356, 445
    ventilation 303, 355, 356, 442, 443
acute rheumatic fever 410
admission
    data regarding 79, 461, 462, 474, 483-486,
        491
    policy 335, 337, 342, 353
aerosols 214, 300, 320, 329, 394
    linen & laundry 223, 368, 371, 373
    mortuary 345
    PPE 230-233, 235
    short- and long-range 214, 300
    transmission route 66, 67, 86, 186, 194,
        217, 439
air *see also* ventilation
    air conditioners 120, 312, 322, 324
    air delivery systems for OTs 322-324
    air flow direction in OT 320, 328
    air handling unit 303
    air sampling OT 327-328
    air-handling unit (AHU) 120, 221, 303, 312,
        323, 329
    changes 305-306, 322
    direction in SSD 120
    HEPA filters 304, 323-324, 332, 447
    medical-grade quality 119, 318
airborne precautions 222-224
    airborne transmission 214, 217, 221-224
    cleaning 222-223, 443, 444
    hand hygiene 222
    kitchen 223
    linen & laundry 223
    medical devices 223
    patient placement 222
    PPE 222

    ventilation 303
    visitors 222, 224
alcohol-based handrub (ABHR) 197, 202, 205-209,
    225, 227
    number of dispensers 313
alert organism 22, 74-75, 458, 469
allergies 209-210, 229-230, 505
    ABHR 209
    drug 242
    latex 202, 225, 227, 229-230, 255
anthrax 410
antibiotics *see also* antimicrobial, antibacterial
    agents
    overuse 406
    prophylactic 264, 281, 282
antimicrobia 84-85
    broth microdilution 85
    disc sensitivity testing 85
    e-test 85
    VITEK 83, 85
antimicrobial resistance (AMR) 86, 88, 89, 90,
    91-94, 95, 96, 200
    AMR transmission in low resource settings
        100
    antimicrobial stewardship (AMS) 97-106
    in animal health 97-100
antimicrobials
    anti-microbial-coated urinary catheter 256
    anti-tuberculosis drugs 95
    antibacterial agents 86, 87-91
    antifungal drugs 95-96
    antimicrobial agents 86-96, 264, 281, 282
    antiviral drugs 96
    resistance 86, 88, 89, 90, 91-94, 95, 96, 200
    stewardship (AMS) 97-106
    tests *see* antimicrobia
    urinary antiseptics 95
antiseptic 207, 208, 251, 252, 263, 279, 287,
    290-292
aprons *see also* personal protective equipment
    (PPE) 235-236
    cleaning and decontamination 122, 127,
        132, 181, 392, 403

HCW 121, 213, 214, 216, 225, 330, 377, 355, 366, 423, 430, 431, 434
    kitchen 342
    linen & laundry 370, 371, 375
    mortuary 346
    waste 381
audit *see also* monitoring and evaluation (M&E) 465-471
    definition 465, 510
    areas to be audited 470
    audit report 471
    conducting the 470-471
    elements 466
    hand hygiene monitoring and audit tools 10
    key audit indicators 467-470
    re-audit 471
    requirements 466
    tools 466-467
automatic washer-disinfectors (AWD) 111, 130, 133, 135-137, 165, 261, 434
    endoscopes, for 179-180

B
bacillus *see* bacteria
bacteria 48-56
    anatomy 51-53
    classification 49-50
    growth cycle 55-56
    haemolysis 51
    morphology and growth characteristics 50-51
    protection and survival 53-55
    respiration 51
    staining characteristics 50
baths 329, 330, 399, 423
bed
    bed frame 396, 399
    cleaning 396, 399, 423, 432
    curtain 216, 220, 223, 313, 368, 375, 395, 400
    number of to calculate SSD size 116
    occupancy 14, 313
    positioning and spacing 271, 287, 313, 334
    ratio 19
bedpan 315
    cleaning 223, 315, 330, 332, 399, 423, 432
    PPE 227, 423, 432, 438
    sample taking 80
benchmarking 2, 11-12
    HAI 2, 454, 456

best practices *see also* bundles of care 8, 226, 468
biomarker 83
bladder infection *see* urinary tract infection
blood
    blood-borne virus transmission 425-439
    drawing or taking *see* phlebotomy
    spillages, cleaning of 396, 437
body fluids 66, 415, 445
    hand hygiene 198-199, 205, 392
    laundry 368, 375
    mortuary 345, 346
    PPE 226, 235, 236, 337, 438, 452
    specific diseases 429, 437, 438, 445
    standard precautions 212, 213
    surfaces 394, 396
    waste 381, 382
boiling steriliser 137, 350
bone marrow transplant unit 331-333
    cleaning 332
    design and layout 332
    food preparation 332-333
    microbiological screening 333
    pharmaceutical products 333
    staff and visitors 333
    transmission, risk of and prevention 331, 332
Bowie-Dick (BD) test 111, 158
brucellosis 53, 410
bundles of care 237, 287-289
    definition 237, 287
    CA-UTI (bladder bundle) 260
    CVP line 253
    difference to checklist 288-289
    how are they produced 288
    peripheral IV cannulation (PIVC) 249
    surgical site infections (SSI) 282
    use in practice 288
    VAP 287
burial 352, 420, 429, 433
burns unit 236, 328-331, 399
    cleaning 331
    design, layout and location 296, 320, 329
    risk of transmission 328-329

C
catering *see* kitchen
catheters
    CVP *see* central venous pressure (CVP) catheters
    suprapubic 264

urinary catheter 254-265, 434
ceilings 120, 166, 294, 311
central line-associated bloodstream infection
    (CLABSI) 190, 253, 460, 465
central venous pressure (CVP) catheters 81, 226,
    242, 249-253, 461, 486
    bundle of care 253
    CLABSI 190, 253, 460, 465
    hyperalimentation (TPN) lines 226, 250, 253
    line insertion 251-252
    line insertion and infection sites 250
    maintaining CVP lines 252
    pathophysiology 250
    selecting an CVP 251
chemical
    cleaning agents 130-131
    disinfection 168-172
    indicators for decontamination 109, 134,
       146, 149, 158-159, 160, 161
    purification of water 419
    sterilisation 148, 160-164
chlamydia 56
chlorhexidine 207, 208, 251, 252, 263, 279,
    287, 290, 291
cholera 45, 410, 416, 417, 418, 420, 421, 422,
    460, 472
cleaning 389-398
    acute respiratory infection 356, 443, 444
    airborne precautions 222-223, 443, 444
    blood spillages 396, 427
    bone marrow transplant unit 332
    burns unit 331
    chemicals used 130-131
    contact precautions 216
    daily 216, 219, 326, 332, 394
    damp dusting 326, 331, 335, 393-394, 399,
       401-402
    dialysis unit 339
    droplet precautions 219-220, 442, 443, 444
    dry dusting not recommended 389, 393
    endoscopes 178
    equipment 396-397
    frequency 216, 219, 326, 332, 393, 394
    good cleaning practice 132
    isolation rooms 395
    kitchen 365-366
    manual cleaning 181, 393
    medical devices 128-137
    methods 131-136, 393-394

monitoring 390-391
mops 331, 345, 394, 396, 401, 402
neonatal unit 10, 345
patient care articles 112, 216, 220, 223,
    330-331, 343-344, 398-405, 431
patient rooms 394-395
pest control *see* pest control
policies and protocols 10, 389, 390, 391
risk assessment 398
Sinner's Circle 130
sweeping not recommended 389, 393, 401
terminal cleaning 43, 216, 220, 223, 389,
    395-396
toilets 332, 394, 396, 404, 423, 425
transmission-based precautions 216, 219-220,
    222-223, 392, 395
validation 132, 136
weekly 326
communicable diseases
    definition 407, 511
    acute respiratory infections 439-446
    common oro-faecal diseases 426
    Communicable Diseases Control Manual 420
    control of 407-408
    control of social movement 410, 411
    factors affecting 410-412
    food-borne diseases 419-421, 446
    home-based care 422-425, 429-433, 437-439,
       442-445
    non-vector blood-borne virus 435-439
    notifiable 408-410, 412
    oro-faecal route of transmission 63-65,
       415-425
community-associated infection (CAI) *see also*
    public health 105, 471
community-based *see also* home-based care
    clinics 137, 347-350
    IPC programmes 23
    training for community-based care 44
cost
    HAI 24-26
    IPC programme 23, 26-28
coughing
    cough room 224, 349
    etiquette 212, 441, 442, 443
    patient screening 84, 192, 342, 348, 349
    reflex 68, 69, 285
    staff with cough 327, 333

tissues and masks for patients 223, 442, 444
transmission route 64, 194, 217-219, 300, 415
whooping cough 410
coveralls *see* personal protective equipment (PPE)
covid *see* SARS-CoV-2
COVID-19 pandemic
case distribution map 491
face covers 230-232
IPC recommendations 3
ventilation 293, 295, 300, 450
CPE pathogens 458, 469
Creutzfeldt-Jakob disease (CJD) 168, 180, 445-448
Crimean-Congo haemorrhagic fever (CCHF) 428, 473
cultural considerations 29, 31-32, 34, 357, 412
curtains *see* bed; window
cystitis *see* urinary tract infection

D

data *see also* epidemiology; statistics
analysis and interpretation 463-465
collection systems 461-465
computerised systems 462-463
data capturing and feedback surveillance loop 463
effective use of 10-11
storing 462-463
day hospital *see* community-based, clinics
day room 313, 317
debridement *see* wounds
decontamination *see* sterilisation; sterilisation and sterile service department (SSD)
dengue 58, 413, 417, 427, 428
dental clinics 350-352
decontamination of equipment 119, 127, 133, 149, 153, 351-352
dental work station 351
layout and ventilation 351
PPE 352
staff 121, 352
transmission 350-351
designing a new healthcare facility 293-308
building design 296-299
burns unit 329
choosing a site 295
cleaning (housekeeping) unit 345
climatic considerations 296

clinical handwash basin 313-314
engineering unit 344
furnishing of clinical areas 311-312
infrastructure requirements 299-307
IPC aspects to be considered 293-294
laundry and linen areas 345
pharmacy 345
population and disease profile 295
specialised areas of care 318-345
temperature control 312
UVGI 306-307
ventilation *see ventilation*
ward layout 297-299, 312-317
waste storage 345
workflow and healthcare delivery 308-310
dialysis unit 164, 336-339
admission policy 337
cleaning 339
cost 25
dialysis process 338
disinfection and hand hygiene 173, 337, 338
layout 336
monitoring dialysis fluids 339
PPE 235, 337
transmission, risk of and prevention 336, 337
waste management 338
water quality 318, 339
diarrhoeal disease 7, 63, 65, 68, 79, 215
patients with 335, 342, 382, 415-425, 431, 438
staff with 333, 366, 367, 375
diphtheria 410
diphtheroids 50, 72
dirty utility (sluice) area 315, 384
disease profile 7, 295
disinfection 165-173
appropriate use 17, 19, 39, 74, 99
categories of disinfectants 168
chemical 168-172
choice of disinfectant 167-168
choosing a method 165-166
disinfectant is not a sterilant 167
disinfectants spectrum 169-172
efficacious against 54, 57, 168-172
intensive therapy units (ITUs) 335
kitchen & patient cutlery and crockery 365, 400, 424
level of disinfection required 168-173
not efficacious against 58, 93, 168-172

overuse of 32, 73, 86, 99, 167, 326, 393
pasteurisation 160, 338
policy 18, 167-168
should not be used at point of use before
    cleaning 127
thermal 166, 174, 315
DNA (deoxyribonuclease)
    definition 52
    bacteria 49, 52
    inhibition of DNA replication antibacterial
        agents 90-91
    prokaryotic v eukaryotic cells 49
    viruses 48
doors 319, 322, 362, 370, 422, 430, 434
    clinical areas 311-312
    door handles 312, 331, 395
drapes 251, 279-280, 360
dust 294, 389
    damp dusting 326, 331, 335, 393-394, 399,
        401-402
    dry dusting and sweeping 389, 393, 401
    filters 303, 312, 324, 330
    packaging and storage to prevent 140, 141,
        143, 146, 316, 373, 393
    UVGI 306
dysentery 63, 64, 416, 421, 422

E
E(scherichia) coli 50, 54, 72, 76, 254, 255, 308
Ebola 352-354, 408, 410, 413, 425-439
    home-based care 429-433
    jump between host species 57, 59
    PPE 235-236, 352, 354, 429-431, 434
    transmission 58, 352
    treatment facility 352-354
education in IPC *see* training
endemic, definition 472
endoscopes 112, 133, 173-182
    decontamination 173-175, 178-180
    heat sensitive 165, 166, 173, 174
    Medical Device Regulations 175
    sources of infection 174
    storage 180-181
    traceability 180
    types and components 175-178
engineer
    engineering controls 210-211
    engineering unit 344
    maintenance of OT 326-327
    role of 18

    SSD 116, 117, 128
    training 42
environmental cleaning *see also* cleaning 389-398
    checklist 10
environmental health officers 36, 43, 366-367
epidemic, definition 472
epidemiological studies
    case-controlled studies (CC) 503-504
    cohort studies 499-502
    common qualitative study designs 505-507
    common quantitative study designs 499-503
    cross-sectional studies 502-503
    defining the research question and study
        objective 498
    focus group discussions 507
    key informant interview 506
    observations 506
    overcoming observation and recall bias 505
    overcoming sample bias 504-505
    retrospective studies 501, 503-504
    study design 481, 498-507
    study protocol and implementation 507-509
epidemiology
    descriptive and analytical 480-493
    descriptive studies 481-485
    frequency indicator 480, 482-488
    person indicator 480, 493
    place indicator 480, 490-491
    study designs *see also* epidemiological
        studies 481, 498-507
    time and space plot (TICL) or Gantt chart
        476, 479, 491-492
    time indicator 480, 488-490, 491
ESKAPE pathogens 74, 458
ethylene oxide (ETO) 141, 142-144, 148, 161-162
eukaryotes 48-49
evacuated tube system (ETS) *see* injections
evaluation *see* monitoring and evaluation (M&E)
excretions 212, 215, 368, 379, 423, 429, 445

F
face covers *see* personal protective equipment
    (PPE)
face shield *see* personal protective equipment
    (PPE), face covers
fingernails *see* nails (and nail beds)
flash steriliser *see* immediate-use steam
    sterilisers (IUSS)
floors *see also* cleaning, mops 120, 311, 401
fluid bag *see* intravenous (IV) systems

food poisoning 358, 361-362, 367, 410, 419-421, 446
food preparation *see* kitchen
formaldehyde 142, 144, 148, 163, 380
fungi 60-62
    antimicrobial resistance and disinfection required 168
    morphology 60
    reproduction 61
    types of fungal infection 61-62

G
Gantt chart *see* time and space plot (TICL) or Gantt chart
glossary 510-513
gloves 121, 124, 137, 194, 198-199, 213, 216, 225-230
    cleaning 131, 181, 392
    double gloving 226, 279
    how to wear properly 228
    indications for 226-228
    overuse 32, 122
    specifications 225
    types of 225-228
    urinary catheterisation 258-259
goggles *see* personal protective equipment (PPE), eye protection
gowning area 118, 121-123, 126
gowns *see* personal protective equipment (PPE)
gravity sterilisers 141, 143, 448
guidelines 8, 12-14, 467-468
    AMS guidelines 97, 102-104
    for precautions *see* precautions
    International Health Facility Guidelines 357-358

H
hand hygiene 14, 196-210, 214, 216, 225, 313-315, 349, 406
    ABHR *see* alcohol-based handrub (ABHR)
    airborne precautions 222
    antiseptics used in *see also* antiseptic 207, 208, 290-292
    barriers to effective 197, 209
    body fluids 198-199, 205, 392
    bone marrow transplant unit 332
    burns unit 330
    cleaning 392
    clinical handwash basin 313-314, 332
    compliance 206-207, 208
    contact precautions 216

contextually appropriate 33
damage to hands and skin *see also* skin, damaged 210
dialysis unit 337
droplet precautions 219
Ebola 354
effects of inadequate 198
fingernails 197, 209
fingernails and nail beds 197, 209
general ward 313-314
handwashing 202-205
handwash facilities, placement of 122, 204-205
intensive therapy units (ITUs) 334
kitchen 203
monitoring and audit tools 10
neonatal unit 340
oro-faecal route of transmission 422-423
principles of 198-202
reasons for poor adherence 208, 209
SSD wash (dirty) area gowning-up 121, 122
strategies for improving 208-209
transmission via hands 197, 201
WHO 5 Moments for Hand Hygiene 198-199
handwash basins 313-314, 332, 405
    kitchen 362
Hazard Analysis and Critical Control Point (HACCP) 361
head cover *see* personal protective equipment (PPE)
Health and Safety at Work Act 4
health, definition 413
healthcare-associated infections (HAI)
    benchmarking 2, 454, 456
    calculations 464-465
    cost of 24-26
    reporting without lab services 459-460
    surveillance 13, 18, 39, 101, 188, 453-461, 463-465
healthcare area 200
healthcare facilities
    access to facility 310
    AMS programme 104-106
    designing a new *see* designing a new healthcare facility
    differences in 7
    healthcare clinic 346-347
    hospital administrator 17
    IPC committee 16-19, 191
    laundry cycle 368, 369

nurse-in-charge 17, 18, 331, 395
outbreaks 352-356, 473-474
renovations 294
signage 309
surveillance *see also* surveillance 460
healthcare workers (HCW) *see also* nurses; staff
apron use *see* aprons
compliance, improve 30-32, 209-209
cough, with 327, 333
diarrhoeal disease, with 333, 366, 367, 375
education and training 12, 13, 22, 26, 36, 38, 39, 41-44
hand hygiene *see* hand hygiene
hepatitis B, with 437, 451
HIV, with 352, 451-452
immune status 193, 450-451
injuries sustained by *see also* occupational health 30-32, 208-209
movement (workflow) of 310
MRSA carrier 186
patients, non-vector blood borne disease, with 438
patients, respiratory disease, with 443, 444, 445
patients, VHFS, with 431, 434
patients, visiting at home 423, 438, 443, 444, 445
perceptions 30-32, 208-209
personal protective equipment (PPE) *see* personal protective equipment (PPE)
precautions *see* precautions
responsibility and accountability 2, 16, 184
trust with community and patients 32, 412, 414
hepatitis A 410
transmission 58, 416, 420, 421-422
waste from patients 438
hepatitis B 435-439
antimicrobial resistance and disinfection required 168, 173
isolation of HBsAg-positive dialysis patients 336, 337
transmission 58, 174, 336, 337, 437
vaccination 327, 436, 451
work restrictions for infected HCW 437, 451
hepatitis C 336, 337, 435, 436
HIV 435-439
antimicrobial resistance and disinfection required 57, 168, 173
home-based care 406, 438

occupationally acquired 452
post-exposure prophylaxis (PEP) 26, 337, 352, 450-451, 452
staff with 352, 451-452
test 337, 350, 451
transmission 58, 238, 336, 337, 415, 435
home-based care 23, 44-45, 272, 406, 414, 422
blood-borne virus patients 406, 438
communicable diseases 406, 422-425, 429-433, 437-439, 442-445
designated caregiver 414-415
education and training 44-45, 406, 407
hand hygiene *see* communicable diseases *above*; hand hygiene
linen & laundry 424, 425, 432
non-vector blood-borne virus patients 437-439
oro-faecal infected patients 422-425
respiratory communicable disease 442-445
VHFs 406, 429-433
hospital administrator 17-18
hospital-acquired pneumonia (HAP) *see* ventilator-associated pneumonia (VAP)
housekeeping 18, 345, 383-384, 396
humidity
burns unit 330, 331
humidifiers 303, 344, 401
NNU 343, 344
OT 324-325
SSD 120
ward environment 398
hydrogen peroxide 142, 162-163, 271, 446
hyperalimentation (TPN) lines 226, 250, 253

I
immediate-use steam sterilisers (IUSS) 126, 152-153
immune status *see* staff
immune system 68-71
acquired immunity 70-71
cellular immunity 69-70, 71
physical barriers 69
immunisation *see* vaccination
immunocompromised patients 255, 283, 294, 421
bacteriostatic antibiotics 87
isolation 224, 235
mycoses 61, 62, 68
PPE 230, 235
impetigo 415, 417

incidence 464, 483-484, 499-502
incubator
    infant 340, 343, 344, 401
    lab 85
indicators (audit and M&E) *see* monitoring and
    evaluation (M&E)
indicators (decontamination)
    biological 111, 158, 161
    chemical 109, 134, 146, 149, 158-159, 160,
        161
    classification of 158-159
    physical 111, 149, 152, 161
indicators (epidemiological) *see* epidemiology
indigenous knowledge 32, 411-412
infection prevention and control (IPC)
    definition 1, 3
    activities of national specialist bodies 5
    committee 15, 16-19, 23, 184, 191
    core elements of infection control practice
        188
    education *see* training
    frameworks 4, 8
    goal 1, 5-6
    information and policy hierarchy 4
    IPC doctor 19-20
    risk management control hierarchy 210-211,
        408
    team *see* IPC programmes
infection prevention and control professional
    definition 41, 47
    (IPCP) 20-23
    duties 22-23
    number of 23
    qualification and training 21-22, 40-41
    role of 21
infusion *see* intravenous (IV) systems
injections 238-242
    bolus injections 239, 246
    disposals of sharps 253-254
    injection devices advantages and
        disadvantages 240-242
    intensive therapy units (ITUs) 334
    recommended needle gauges 240
    routes of injection, methods and fluid load
        238-239
    safety-engineered devices (SEDs) 240,
        242-242
inspection, assembly and packaging (IAP)
    117, 118, 120, 122-124, 129, 138-147, 164
    accessories 146

assembly 138-139
choice of materials 182
inspection 138
packaging 139-144
sealing, indicators and labelling 145-147
SSD IAP area 123-124
SSD IAP gowning-up area 122-123
types of packaging with their advantages
    and disadvantages 142-144
validation 146
wrapping 144-145
intensive care unit *see* intensive therapy units
    (ITUs)
intensive therapy units (ITUs) 4, 23, 76,
    333-336, 459
    admission policy 335
    cost 25, 26, 27
    disinfection and decontamination 335
    IV catheterisation 242, 251, 486
    location and layout 334
    neonatal 340-341, 460
    policy 336
    recommended policies 335, 336
    representative from 17, 18-19
    surveillance 22, 458
    training 36, 335
    transmission, risk of and prevention 334-335
    VAP 284
    ventilation 335
International Health Regulations (2005) 3,
    408-409
International Postgraduate Diploma in
    Infection Control (IPDIC) *see also* training,
    courses 45
intravenous (IV) systems 242-249
    areas where contamination can occur
        243-245
    bundles of care 249, 253
    central venous pressure (CVP) catheters
        81, 226, 242, 249-253, 461, 486
    components of IV access 245-247
    fluid or infusion bags 228, 243-244, 247, 253
    hyperalimentation (TPN) lines 226, 250, 253
    multi-dose vials (MDVs) 247, 336, 337, 338
    peripheral IV access 29, 239, 242, 243, 245,
        247-249, 464, 469
    porthacaths 239, 247
IPC programmes
    aim 12

community-based 23, 44-46, 347-350
cost of 23-28
dependence on local conditions 6-7
health facility 16-23
national programme and committee 15
outcome 12
role of 6
starting a 12-23
structure 12-14
team 19-23
isolation
    cleaning of isolation rooms 395
    duration of 217, 221, 224
    facilities 318-319, 336, 341, 427, 434
    patient placement 442
    protective (source) isolation 224, 233, 336, 337
    SARS-CoV-2 213, 303, 355
    VHFs at home 420, 430

J
jewellery 113, 197, 209

K
kangaroo care *see* neonatal unit (NNU)
key indicators
    audit and M&E *see* monitoring and evaluation (M&E)
    decontamination *see* indicators (decontamination)
    epidemiological *see* epidemiology
kitchen 357-367
    airborne precautions 223
    and food preparation 332-333, 357-367, 424
    bone marrow transplant unit 332-333
    building design 297, 310, 345, 354
    cleaning 365-366
    cloths 401
    contact precautions 217, 424
    cutlery and crockery 364-365, 400, 424
    designated preparation areas 362-364
    droplet precautions 220
    food delivery to wards 364
    food-borne diseases *see* food poisoning
    handwashing 203
    Hazard Analysis and Critical Control Point (HACCP) 361
    inspection 366-367
    layout and workflow 358-359
    milk kitchen 342

pest control *see also* pest control 362, 381, 419, 420, 422
raw produce 360-361, 362-363, 419
staff, training 42, 43, 366
waste 359, 366, 381
Klebsiella pneumoniae 50, 55, 74, 76, 84, 254

L
laboratory *see* microbiological laboratory
labour ward, representative from 17, 18-19
laminar flow cabinet 253, 332, 333
language considerations 7, 29, 31, 33, 34, 412
Lassa fever 428, 434, 472
latex *see* allergies
laundry *see* linen & laundry
layout
    acute respiratory infection treatment centre 355
    administration (offices) non-clinical areas 310
    bone marrow transplant unit 332
    burns unit 329
    community-based clinic 348-350
    dental clinic 351
    dialysis unit 336
    Ebola treatment facility 353-354
    furnishing of clinical areas 311-312
    general ward 312-317
    healthcare facility 310-312
    intensive therapy units (ITUs) 334
    kitchen 358-359
    mortuary 346
    neonatal unit 296, 340
    patient waiting or day rooms 317
    play area 317
    staff area 317
    treatment room 316
    types of wards 297-299
    utility areas, clean and dirty 315-316
    visitors' toilets 317
    waste holding room (disposal room) 316
leadership
    effective 43, 106, 107, 184, 190-191, 390
    traditional 32, 411-412, 414
legislation 3-4, 378, 449
light
    clinical area 311
    dental work station 351
    examination lamps 401
    SSD 121, 123

UV light for neonates 340
UVGI 168, 306-307
linen & laundry 212, 217, 220, 223, 367-376, 401
    acute respiratory infection 220, 434, 444
    airborne precautions 223, 368, 371, 373
    body fluids 368, 371, 375, 435
    clean laundry, returning 374
    contact precautions 216, 422, 425, 434
    droplet precautions 220, 434, 444
    effectiveness factors 375-376
    heat-sensitive clothing 372
    home-based care 424, 425, 432
    infectious linen 368, 371, 435
    infested linen 368, 370
    laundry collection 368, 370-371
    laundry cycle for healthcare facilities 368, 369
    linen bags 217, 220, 223, 315, 316, 368
    manual and automated washing 371-373
    methods of processing different types of dirty linen 373
    OT 368, 370
    ozone 373-374
    policy 367, 374
    PPE for manual washing 371
    safe handling of 369
    sluicing on ward not recommended 370
    staff 375
    storage of clean linen 374-375
    storage of used linen 370
    temperature of washing cycle 372
    trolley 374
    types of dirty linen 367-368, 373
literacy 32, 45, 110

M
malaria 63, 64, 410, 417, 427, 435
MALDI-TOF MS 82-83
masks see personal protective equipment (PPE)
matron see nurses, nurse-in-charge
mattresses 330, 402
MDRO see multidrug resistant and virulent pathogens
measles 221, 303, 410, 440, 461
medical devices
    airborne precautions 223
    assembly see inspection, assembly and packaging (IAP)
    classification based on level of risk 112

    cleaning 128-137
    contact precautions 217, 447
    decontamination see sterile service department (SSD)
    droplet precautions 220
    inspection see inspection, assembly and packaging (IAP)
    operating theatre 325
    packaging see inspection, assembly and packaging (IAP)
    process of decontamination cycle 113
    reprocessing of medical devices 126-163
    single-use see single-use items
    Spaulding classification 111-112
meningitis 53, 82, 84, 218, 410, 438, 441
micro-organisms 48-66, 445-448
    classification 48
    CPE pathogens 458, 469
    ESKAPE pathogens 74, 458
    multidrug resistant and virulent see multidrug resistant and virulent pathogens
    relationship between pathogen and host 66-68
    transmission 67
microbiological laboratory 77-81, 350
    antimicrobial tests see also antimicrobia 84-85
    challenges 78
    clinical teams, relationship with 77-78
    food samples 362
    organisms that cannot be cultured 81
    request form 79
    results, interpreting 83-84
    sample processing 82-83
    sample registration 82
    sample taking 77, 78, 224, 261-262
    sampling site and transportation 80-81
    specimen container 79
    staff safety 86
    waste 381
microbiology, introduction to 47-107
microbiome 71-74
    microbes 71
    normal flora 71-72
milk and dairy
    milk kitchen 342
    neonatal unit prep area 342-343
    pasteurisation 420
monitoring and evaluation (M&E) see also audit 8-10, 14, 16, 33

cleaning 390-391
  hand hygiene audit tools 10
  key indicators 8-9, 11, 467, 468-470
monkeypox 409, 415
mops *see* cleaning
mortuaries 345-346
  body fluids 345, 346
  Ebola 353, 354
  prions 447
mosquitoes 58, 64, 65, 397, 429, 433
movement (workflow) of
  equipment and supplies 310
  patients 308
  staff (HCW) 310
MRSA *see Staph(ylococcus) aureus*
mucous membrane 69, 415
  irritants to 132, 169
  PPE 121, 131, 230, 232, 427, 429
  precautions applicable 211, 218, 427, 429
multi-dose vials (MDVs) 247, 336, 337, 338
multidrug resistant and virulent pathogens
  74-77, 86-88, 95, 406
multimodal strategy (MMS) 14, 43, 195-196
mycoplasma 50, 56
mycoses *see* fungi, types of fungal infection

N
nails (and nail beds)
  brushes 402
  flora and infections 61, 62, 72
  hand hygiene 197, 209
National IPC Strategic Framework (2020) 4, 8,
  42-43
National Nosocomial Infection Surveillance
  (NNIS) system 278
nebulisers 402, 442
necrotic tissue and debris 63, 268-270, 272,
  273-274, 276, 280
needles and syringes
  disposals of *see* sharps
  injection devices advantages and
    disadvantages 240-242
  re-use of 112, 212, 239, 242, 437
  recommended needle gauges 240
neonatal
  blindness 64
  ophthalmitis 56
  sepsis 483
  tetanus 409
neonatal unit (NNU) 23, 339-345

circumcision site 275
cleaning and checklist 10, 345
isolation 340, 341
kangaroo care 296, 341-342
layout and placement 296, 340
milk preparation area 342-343
needle and cannula gauge 240, 245
neonatal intensive care 340-341, 460
parents, screening of 342
representative from 17
surveillance 458
temperature and ventilation 312, 341
training 36, 339
transmission 75, 340
VAP 283, 285, 343
notifiable diseases and notification systems
  409-410, 412
nurses *see also* healthcare workers (HWC)
  link nurses 21, 22, 40, 42, 459
  nurse-in-charge 17, 18, 331, 395

O
occupational health 4, 449-452
  compensation 449
  functions of 450
  immune status of HCW 193, 450-451
  liability of employer 449
  Occupational Health Act 4, 449
  occupationally acquired HIV 452
  representative 17, 18
  staff protection 450-451
Office of Health Standards Compliance 4, 10
  Norms and Standards of the South African
    Office of Healthcare Standards tools 10
operating theatre (OT) 319-328
  aseptic zones 321-322
  clean zone 321
  dirty linen 368, 370
  equipment 325
  layout example 320
  maintenance 326
  outer zone 321
  staff health 327
  storage areas 325
  ventilation and air delivery 320, 322-324
  waste management 325
oro-faecal route of transmission 63-65, 415-425
  common oro-faecal diseases 426
  diseases transmitted by 421-422
  food preparation 419-420, 424

food-borne diseases 419-421
  PPE 423
  precautions against 420, 422-425
  water-related diseases 416-419
outbreak 5, 11, 19, 22, 58, 75, 407-409
  definition 472, 512
  alert (warning) system 472
  cost 26
  epidemic curve 488
  epidemiological steps 475-477
  Gantt chart *see also* epidemiological studies
    476, 479, 491-492
  healthcare facility 352-356, 473-474
  investigation and management *see* outbreak
    investigation and management
  IPC steps 477-478
  occurrence 473
  outbreak response teams 408
  patient facilities during 352-356
  policies 474, 478
  PPE 219, 235-236, 474
  public awareness 412, 427, 441
  training 28, 32, 34, 45
  types 472-473
outbreak investigation and management 471-479
  definitions of high occurrence of a disease 472
overshoes *see* personal protective equipment
  (PPE)
ozone *see also* linen & laundry 148, 163, 371,
  372, 373-374

P
packaging *see* inspection, assembly and
  packaging (IAP)
pandemic *see also* outbreak 413, 439
  definition 472
  COVID-19 *see* COVID-19 pandemic
  knowledge transfer in and for event of 34,
    35, 407
  public health measures 441
  UVGI 307
parasites 62-65
  classification 63-64
  symptoms and diagnosis 63-64
  transmission 63-64
pasteurisation 160, 338, 342, 343, 418, 420
pathogens *see* micro-organisms
patient
  care equipment 112, 216, 220, 223, 330-331,
    398-405, 431, 434, 439

crockery and cutlery 365, 400, 424, 432, 443
neonatal care equipment 343-344, 401
placement 213, 215, 219, 222, 422, 442
positioning (tissue load management) 271,
  274
toilet 297-298, 313, 318, 331, 354, 394, 438
zone 200-203, 225, 313
peripheral IV cannulation (PIVC) 247-249
  bundle of care 249
  correct technique 248-249
  pathophysiology 248
personal protective equipment (PPE) 225-237,
  335
  acute respiratory infection 355, 443, 444
  airborne precautions 222
  appropriate use of PPE 110, 114, 210-211
  aprons *see* aprons
  availability of 115
  blood-borne viruses 438
  body fluids 226, 235, 236, 337, 438, 452
  bone marrow transplant unit 332
  burns unit 330
  cleaning 392
  contact precautions 216, 447
  coveralls 236, 352, 431
  dental clinic 352
  disposal of 381, 382
  droplet precautions 219
  Ebola *see* VHFs *below*
  eye protection 121, 132, 181, 231, 232,
    236-237, 346, 431, 447
  face covers 121, 127, 132, 230-233, 236-237,
    352, 355, 371, 429, 434, 447
  gowns 117, 236, 251, 279, 321, 327, 330,
    352
  head cover 122, 237
  indications for face covering 235
  mortuary 346
  operating theatre 279
  outbreak 235-236, 474
  overshoes 121, 237, 434
  overuse 26, 32, 211
  prions 447
  respirators *see* respirators
  SARS-CoV-2 219, 235, 236, 355
  SSD wash (dirty) area gowning-up 121, 122
  VHFs 235-236, 352, 354, 429-431, 434
pest control 362, 378, 397, 420, 429
  food preparation 362, 381, 419, 420, 422

infested linen 368, 370
  officer 366, 370
pharmaceutical
  PPE in product manufacture 237
  products in bone marrow transplant unit
    332, 333
  waste 379, 380, 382
pharmacist 17, 18, 42, 104-106, 472
phlebotomy 226-227, 238, 240-242, 247, 349,
  431
piggybacking 246
planned preventive maintenance (PPM) 116, 128
policies *see also* bundles of care
  admission 335, 337, 342, 353
  audit, monitor and revise 12, 15, 109-110,
    115, 194, 453, 465, 505
  cascading system of information and IPC
    policies 4
  cleaning 10, 389, 390, 391
  development 5, 6, 11, 16-19, 22-23, 194, 463
  disinfection 18, 167-168
  ITU 336
  linen & laundry 367, 374
  outbreak 474, 478
  training and 31-32, 36, 192
  waste 378
polio
  antimicrobial resistance and disinfection
    required 168
  non-enveloped virus 57
  reportable to WHO 461
  transmission 58
  vaccination 375
population 413
  for calculations *see* epidemiology; statistics
  size and disease profile 295
  variation of 7
portacath *see* intravenous (IV) systems
porters 36, 42, 43, 383
post-exposure prophylaxis (PEP) 26, 337, 352,
  450-451, 452
povidone iodine 207, 263, 271, 279, 290
pre-vacuum sterilisers 141, 153-154, 155, 156
precautions
  airborne transmission 214, 217, 221-224
  contact transmission 214-217, 427, 434,
    437, 447

droplet transmission 214, 217-221, 427, 434
  respiratory 217-224, 442-446
  standard 33, 103, 188, 211-213, 214, 375,
    437
  transmission-based 213-224
prevalence 464, 484-485, 502-503
prions 48, 168, 445-448
  decontamination of medical devices 446,
    447-448
  transmission 446
professional bodies 4-5
prokaryotes 48-49
Proteus spp 254, 263
public awareness 412, 427, 441
public health 406-413
  meaning 413
  measures for food-borne diseases 419-420
  measures for respiratory-transmitted
    diseases 441-442
  measures for vector-borne diseases 429
  measures for blood-borne viruses (non-
    vector) 437
  Public Health Act 4
  public health emergency of international
    concern (PHEIC) 409

Q
quality *see also* monitoring and evaluation (M&E)
  cycle 1
  improvement 1, 7-12
  of care, improve and evaluate 8, 11, 100,
    454-455, 654, 482
  quality assurance (QA) 8, 109-110, 175,
    357, 449
  quality manager 115
  steam 150, 153, 154, 155, 159, 163
  water 119, 130, 173, 180, 308, 318, 339,
    375, 416
quantitative studies *see also* epidemiological
  studies
  common study designs 499-503
  various methods to carry out 478
quarantine *see also* isolation 124, 379
  VHF area 427

R
rabies 400, 410
ratios
  odds ration (OR) 487-488, 496
  rate ratio (RR) 485-486, 487, 488, 493, 496
recycling 355, 376-377, 386

air 323-324
things not to 79, 242, 402
waste 376-377, 386, 388
respirators 214, 219, 220, 221-222, 233-234, 355, 447
resuscitaires 344
rickettsia 56
risk
definition 183, 185
analysis 188-191
assessment 184, 185-188
core elements of infection control practice 188
difference 486-487
hazard v risk 184
management ch 4
minimising or reducing 186, 191-193
risk management control hierarchy 210-211, 408
risk-prone (clinical) procedures in healthcare 237-265
risk-reducing precautions 210-224
risk-reducing strategies 193-224
transmission routes and levels of risk 194
waste flow diagram 380

S

safety cabinets 86, 307, 447
safety-engineered devices (SEDs) 240, 242-242
salmonella
antimicrobial resistance 75
laboratory 51, 79, 81, 84
transmission 76, 173, 361, 421
sanitisation *see* water, Water sanitation and Hygiene (WASH)
SARS-CoV-2
continuous source outbreak 472
enveloped (lipid) virus 173
identify and warn 445, 472
isolation 213, 303, 355
jump between host species 57, 59
PPE 219, 235, 236, 355
transmission 58, 198, 218, 221, 292, 301, 439, 441
schistosomiasis 417, 427
secretions 199, 235, 368, 403, 428
contact precautions 215, 222, 235
respiratory 223, 284-287, 429, 442-445
standard precautions 211
VHFs 428-430, 433

sexual contact 56, 58, 63, 415, 425, 435, 437, 439
sharps
disposal of in box or container 194, 212, 239, 253-254, 325, 336, 380-381, 384, 385, 434, 438
end disposal 387
injuries 339, 352, 375, 378
placement of sharps box 194, 253, 335, 338
PPE 227
training in handling 194, 339, 375
transmission via 194, 337, 435, 437
shellfish 420, 424
single-use items 79, 108, 128, 199, 219, 225, 259, 314, 399, 403, 434
gloves 199
needles and syringes 112, 212, 239, 242, 437
skin 69, 197
damaged 62, 67, 89, 112, 196, 197, 210, 212
flora 66, 72
fungal infections 61, 62
intact 69, 112, 194
lesions and blisters 56, 64, 65, 327
structure and inflammatory response when breached 266
transmission via *see also* hand hygiene 58, 64, 65
soap 122, 130, 198, 202-205, 308, 314, 403, 422
South African AMR Implementation Plan 103
spirochetes 50, 51, 56
sputum 64, 78, 80, 82, 86, 218, 224, 285, 349, 445
pot 86, 224, 349, 403
staff 14, 27
awareness and training for cleaning 390, 391-392
bone marrow transplant unit 333
burns unit 331
changing rooms 121
cough, with 327, 333
dental clinics 121, 352
dialysis unit 337
diarrhoeal disease, with 333, 366, 367, 375
hepatitis B, with 451
HIV, with 352, 451-452
kitchen 42, 43, 358, 366
linen & laundry 375
movement of in OT 310
occupational health protection 450-451
OT 310, 327

SSD 113-117, 121
toilet 121, 308, 358, 359
Staph(ylococcus) aureus 275, 284, 421
  methicillin-resistant (MRSA) 26, 75-76, 88,
    186, 198, 215, 290, 291, 299, 458
statistics
  95% confidence interval 488, 495-496
  chi square 497
  important concepts in 493-497
  p-values 496, 497
  sampling and describing samples 493-495
steam 119, 126, 149-160, 163
sterile service department (SSD) 112-127
  cleaning of medical devices 128-137, 280
  cooling area (sterile store) 125
  dispatch area 126
  IAP area 123
  IAP gowning-up area 122-123
  infrastructure requirements 119-127
  ITU clinical equipment 335
  layout and workflow 112-113, 117-118,
    121-126, 345
  manager 17, 114, 115, 181
  patient care articles 112, 216, 220, 223,
    330-331, 343-344, 398-405
  prions 446, 447-448
  role 113
  routinely used items 399-405
  size 116-117
  staff 113-117, 121
  sterilisation area 124
  wash (dirty) area gowning-up area 121
  wash room (decontamination area) 121-122
sterilisation 147-165
  Bowie-Dick (BD) test 158
  chemical 148, 160-164
  decontamination process showing the flow
    of work and SOPs 129
  dental clinic 119, 127, 133, 149, 153, 351-352
  difference to disinfection 167
  dry heat 148-149
  gas sterilisation process 161
  indicators *see* indicators (decontamination)
  labelling 163
  outside SSD 126-127
  quality assurance (QA) 109-110
  standards and regulations 110
  steam 149-160
  traceability 164-165

tracking 164
types of 147-163
validation 110-111, 137, 143, 161
stratification
  social 7
  surgical 276
Streptococcus
  group A 51, 54, 72, 83, 417
  pneumoniae 51, 54, 72, 75, 284, 469, 491
surgery
  length of 278, 279
  representative from 17, 18-19
surgical patient classification (ASA) and risk
  (NNIS) 278
surgical site infections (SSI) 108, 274-283, 496
  definition 455
  antibiotic prophylaxis 281
  bundle of care 282
  classification of wounds and risk of infection
    276-278
  contamination of wounds from various
    sources 319
  cost of 454
  enhancement of host defences 282-283
  healing by primary or secondary intention
    274-275
  management of 282-283
  National Nosocomial Infection Surveillance
    (NNIS) system 278
  occurrence 275
  post-operative care 281
  prevention of 278-282
  risk determinants 276
  surgical site meaning 274
  surveillance 455-456
surgical trays 117, 123, 126, 139
surveillance 453-461
  definition 454
  continuous 458-459
  data capturing and feedback loop 463
  HAI 13, 18, 39, 101, 188, 453-461, 463-
    465
  ITU 22, 458
  National Nosocomial Infection Surveillance
    (NNIS) system 278
  NNU 458
  levels 460-461
  outbreaks 478
  periodic or point prevalence 458, 459

planning 456-457
purpose 455
reasons for carrying out 454-455
role of 456
selective laboratory-based ward liaison 459
structure 455
types 458-459
who carries out 461
sutures 275, 276, 280, 282
suture material 280
sweat 212, 342
syphilis 56, 410, 415, 435, 502
temperature
burns unit 330
control 312
dry heat 148
food storage 358, 360, 361, 362
keeping patient warm during surgery 282
linen washing cycle 372
neonatal unit 312, 341
SSD 120
steam steriliser 156, 157
thermal disinfection 166, 315
water for cleaning 130
water for hand hygiene 198
tetanus
neonatal 410
vaccination against 114, 375
thermometers 112, 216, 220, 223, 398, 403, 404
time and space plot (TICL) or Gantt chart 476, 479, 491-492
toilets 314, 344, 423
blood-borne viruses 438
cleaning 332, 394, 396, 400, 404, 423, 425
communal 410, 423, 443
home-based care 431-432
location 297-298, 313
number of 297, 308, 313
oro-faecal transmission precautions 420, 423, 425
patient 297-298, 313, 318, 331, 354, 394, 432, 438
staff 121, 308, 358, 359
toilet seat 332, 400, 404
transmission 55, 215, 410
visitors 308, 317
waiting area 348
trachoma 56, 410, 417

traditional healers 32, 411-412
traditional leaders 32, 411-412, 414
training 8, 13, 28-44
adult learning 30-31
budget 31, 33
burns unit staff 331
cleaning 389-390
community-based structures 44-46, 407
difference between education and training 29-30
home-based care 44-45, 406, 407
HCWs 12, 13, 22, 26, 36, 38, 39, 41-44
in-service (on the job) 36-37, 114
influences on learning 31-34
intensive therapy units (ITUs) 334
kitchen staff 42, 43, 366
language 29, 31, 33, 34
linen and laundry 375
mentorship 31, 36
neonatal unit 36, 339
outbreak 28, 32, 45
policies 31-32, 36, 192
porters 36, 42, 43
practical 37
risk reduction 192
SSD 114, 116
teaching methods 34-36
Train the Trainer (TTT)v39-40, 42
training courses 38, 41-44, 45-46
VHFs 427
transmission
blood-borne virus 425-439
bone marrow transplant unit 331, 332
burns unit 328-329
community-based clinic 347
dental clinic 350-351
dialysis unit 336, 337
Ebola 58, 352
food-borne diseases 65, 419-421
HIV 58, 238, 336, 337, 415, 435
intensive therapy units (ITUs) 334-335
mortuary 345
oro-faecal route 63-65, 415-425
prions 446
routes of for communicable diseases 63-65, 415-448
routes of transmission in OT 320
SARS-CoV-2 58, 198, 218, 221, 292, 301, 439, 441

sexual contact 56, 58, 63, 415, 425, 435, 437, 439
toilet 55, 215, 410
transmission routes and levels of risk 194
transmission-based precautions *see* transmission-based precautions
vectors, by 63-65, 425, 427-428
transmission-based precautions 213-224, 414, 427, 447
    cleaning 216, 219-220, 222-223, 392, 395
    isolation facilities 318-319, 368, 395
    training 33, 39, 43, 45
transport
    food delivery to wards 364
    patient 217, 220, 223-224, 310, 378
    waste 385
trolley
    decontamination area 120, 122, 123, 124
    dressing or procedure 202, 251, 282-283, 313, 316, 319, 334, 337, 400
    food 359, 363, 364
    linen 374
    patient transport 310, 378
    waste 385
tuberculosis 7, 26, 254, 342, 406, 410, 413, 442-446, 461
    anti-tuberculosis drugs 90, 95
    applying risk management 192-193
    cough room 349
    dust 389
    extra precautions 444, 445
    extra-pulmonary 221
    face covering 235, 443, 444, 445
    home-based care 406, 442-444
    MDR and XDR 222, 224, 442, 445
    Mycobacterium tuberculosis 55, 70, 80, 82
    pulmonary 192, 221, 222, 224, 435
    sampling site 80
    UVGI 168, 306, 307
    ventilation 221, 292, 300, 302, 317, 347, 450
    waiting room 317, 347
typhoid 410, 416, 417, 421, 422
typhus 427
ulcers, chronic and pressure 266-274, 286
    assessment of 268-269, 271
    cause 267-268
    infection 266, 272
    management of 269-270, 271

ultrasonicators 133-134, 352
ultraviolet germicidal irradiation (UVGI) 168, 306-307
urinal *see* bedpan
urinary tract infection 254-265
    CA-UTI bundle of care 260
    catheter-associated urinary tract infection (CA-UTI) 254-255
    pathophysiology 254
    prophylactic antibiotics 264
    urinary catheter 255-265
    urine sampling 261-262
utility area 296
    clean 316
    dirty 315
vaccination 114, 337, 408, 412, 420, 426, 436
    immunisation schedule for hepatitis B 451
vagina 72, 226, 227
    urinal catheterisation 260
    vaginal speculum 112, 350
    vaginal swab 63, 80
validation
    definition 110, 512
    cleaning 132, 136
    endoscope decontamination 180
    external indicators (decontamination) 111, 139, 141, 146
    inspection, assembly and packaging (IAP) 146
    sterilisation 110-111, 137, 143, 161
vectors
    diseases transmitted by 425, 427-428
    organisms and transmission 63-65
ventilation
    acute respiratory infection 303, 355, 356, 442, 443
    air changes 305-306
    burns unit 329-30
    community-based clinic 348
    considerations when designing a new healthcare facility 295, 296-297, 300-305
    COVID-19 pandemic 293, 295, 300, 450
    dental clinic 351
    Ebola 353
    HEPA filters 304, 323-324, 332, 447
    intensive therapy units (ITUs) 335
    mechanical 303-305, 318, 435
    natural 301-302
    neonatal unit 341

neutral ('balanced') 302
operating theatre 320, 322-324
types of 300-301
ultra-clean ventilation 323-324
ventilator-associated pneumonia (VAP) 283-287
diagnosis 285
pathophysiology 284-285
prevalence 284
reducing risk for 285-287
risk factors 285
VAP bundle of care 287
ventilators 331, 335, 343, 404-405, 434-435
viral haemorrhagic fevers (VHFs) 58, 308, 410, 413, 425-439
Ebola *see* Ebola
healthcare facility care 433-435
home-based care 429-433
viruses 48, 57-60
classification 57-58
DNA or RNA 48, 57
enveloped 57-60, 173, 205
mutation 57, 59
non-enveloped or unenveloped 57, 58, 205, 418
replication 59-60
structure 57
transmission 58-59
visitors
acute respiratory infections 220-221, 443-444
airborne precautions 222, 224
blood-borne virus patients 439
bone marrow transplant unit 333
burns unit 331
contact precautions 217, 425-426
droplet precautions 220-221, 443-444
oro-faecal transmission precaution 217, 425-426
social movement 410, 411, 433
toilets 308, 317
VHFs 433
visor *see* personal protective equipment (PPE), face covers
waiting area 235, 308, 317, 341, 346, 347, 348, 351, 355
wall-mounted
air conditioners 120, 324
dispensers 202, 314, 403

walls 120, 311, 321, 326, 394, 395
wards
bay ward 299
dormitory (Florence Nightingale) ward 297-298
food delivery to 364
frequency of dirty linen collection 370
racetrack ward 298-299
waste 376-388
'5 Rs' 376
blood-borne viruses 438
cleaners, training of 36, 42, 43
Ebola 353, 354
end disposal 385-388
incineration 386-387
infectious 379-381, 386, 424, 433
kitchen 359, 366, 381
non-infectious 380-382, 384, 385-386, 443
pharmaceutical 379, 380, 382
policy 378
recycling 376-377, 386, 388
risk waste flow diagram 380
sharps *see* sharps, disposal of in box or container
source segregation 382-383
storage, collection and transportation 384-385, 394
types of 378, 379-382
waste containers 383-384
waste management hierarchyv376
waste management team 378-379
waste stream generation and disposal 377
water
AWD *see* automatic washer-disinfectors (AWD)
bath water 399
guidelines when building a new healthcare facility 295
handwashing 202-205
handwash basin 313-314
kitchen 359, 366, 381
quality 119, 130, 308, 318, 339
temperature and products 198
training 43
Water and Sanitation for Health Facility Improvement Tool (WASH FIT) 10, 307
water containers 417, 418, 429
Water sanitation and Hygiene (WASH) 43, 307-308

water treatment 418-419

water-associated diseases 416-419, 427, 429

WHO

  core components (2016) 4, 9, 10, 12, 38

  5 Moments for Hand Hygiene 198-199

  antimicrobial stewardship 97-106

  classification of waste 379-382

  Decontamination Manual (2016) 114, 142, 159

  Domestic water supply 416

  Ebola Facility design and layout (2015) 354

  Guidelines for core component of an IPC programme (2016) 12-14

  Guidelines on decontamination and reprocessing of medical devices for health-care facilities (2016) 109

  Guidelines on drawing blood best practices in phlebotomy (2010) 238 n28

  Guidelines on safe injections 238

  Guidelines on sanitation and health (2018) 308

  hand hygiene monitoring and audit tools 10

  International Health Regulations (2005) 3, 408-409

  multimodal strategy (MMS) 195, 207

  national infection prevention and control assessment tool 2 (IPCAT2) 10

  recommended needle gauges 240

  technique on handwashing 203

  ventilation, natural 301-302

  waste management hierarchy 376

  water, sanitation and hygiene (WASH) standards 43, 307-308

whooping cough 410

window 301, 312, 433

  closed 120, 303, 331, 335

  curtain 201, 375, 395, 400, 444

  open 222, 296, 297, 302, 318, 348, 349, 442, 443

wounds 266-274

  clean, contaminated and dirty 277-278

  contamination of from various sources 319

  debridement 273-274

  determinants for healing 276

  dressings 269-270, 272, 282, 431, 434

  pathophysiology 266-267

  pressure ulcers 266-274

  skin structure and inflammatory response when breached 266

  surgical wounds *see* surgical site infections (SSI)

  types of and management 272

yellow fever 58, 413, 417, 427, 428, 429